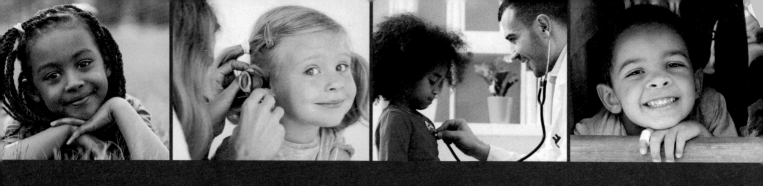

Pediatric Nursing Care

A Concept-Based Approach

Luanne Linnard-Palmer, EdD, MSN, RN, CPN

Professor

Department of Nursing

Dominican University of California

San Rafael, California

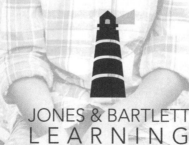

JONES & BARTLETT LEARNING

World Headquarters
Jones & Bartlett Learning
5 Wall Street
Burlington, MA 01803
978-443-5000
info@jblearning.com
www.jblearning.com

Jones & Bartlett Learning books and products are available through most bookstores and online booksellers. To contact Jones & Bartlett Learning directly, call 800-832-0034, fax 978-443-8000, or visit our website, www.jblearning.com.

Substantial discounts on bulk quantities of Jones & Bartlett Learning publications are available to corporations, professional associations, and other qualified organizations. For details and specific discount information, contact the special sales department at Jones & Bartlett Learning via the above contact information or send an email to specialsales@jblearning.com.

37547-3

Production Credits

VP, Executive Publisher: David D. Cella
Executive Editor: Amanda Martin
Editorial Assistant: Christina Freitas
Developmental Editors: Nancy Hoffman, Elizabeth Hamblin
Production Manager: Carolyn Rogers Pershouse
Senior Marketing Manager: Jennifer Scherzay
Product Fulfillment Manager: Wendy Kilborn
Composition: S4Carlisle Publishing Services
Cover and Text Design: Scott Moden

Rights & Media Specialist: Wes DeShano
Media Development Editor: Troy Liston
Cover and Title Page Images: top left © Samuel Borges Photography/Shutterstock; top middle left © luckyraccoon/Shutterstock; top middle right © didesign021/Shutterstock; top right © Rob Hainer/Shutterstock; bottom © Rawpixel.com/Shutterstock
Printing and Binding: LSC Communications
Cover Printing: LSC Communications

Library of Congress Cataloging-in-Publication Data
Names: Linnard-Palmer, Luanne, author.
Title: Pediatric nursing care : a concept-based approach/Luanne Linnard-Palmer.
Description: Burlington, MA : Jones & Bartlett Learning, [2019] | Includes bibliographical references and index.
Identifiers: LCCN 2017013154 | ISBN 9781284081428 (pbk.)
Subjects: | MESH: Pediatric Nursing
Classification: LCC RJ245 | NLM WY 159 | DDC 618.92/00231--dc23
LC record available at https://lccn.loc.gov/2017013154

6048

Printed in the United States of America
21 20 19 18 17   10 9 8 7 6 5 4 3 2 1

Contents

Preface

Caring for children and their families is a complex and emotional endeavor. Many struggles and barriers in accessing comprehensive health care for children continue to plague families across the United States. Current data from the U.S. Census Bureau (2016) reveal that as many as 19.7% of American children younger than age 18 are living at the poverty level and 5% to 7% of American families have inadequate health care for their children (Kaiser Family Foundation, 2017). Other challenges faced by many families include food insecurity, homelessness, unsafe neighborhoods, unemployment, and single-parent households. These stressors, as well as concerns about the promotion of health and security of safety for children, add to the complexity of providing holistic care. Nurses must be confident and well prepared to assist a family, no matter what the family's constellation, economic status, or level of health. Pediatric nursing is challenging, rewarding, and increasingly more complex in the current times.

The foundation for excellence in clinical care of children and their families starts with knowledge of growth and development according to the expected milestones and clinical presentation for each stage. Knowledge of the significant anatomic, physiologic, developmental and cognitive differences between children and adults will provide the new pediatric nurse with information on which to base the child's assessments and care. Children are not "little adults." The pediatric nurse must use both unique theoretical and skills-based foundations to make safe decisions about these vulnerable patients.

This text presents material for the new pediatric nurse, whether that nurse is new to the profession or is transitioning from adult care to pediatric care. It provides vital information about the various settings in which the pediatric nurse can encounter children—inpatient acute care, pediatric intensive care, school nursing, outpatient nursing, and so on. As most children do not experience a hospitalization during their developmental period, it is important for a pediatric nurse to be well prepared to conduct assessments, implement the nursing process, work as an interdisciplinary team member, and provide care to both the child and the family regardless of the setting. The book stresses the importance of using family-centered care as a foundation for respect, no matter what the family is facing or experiencing in their lives. Empowering and enabling parents or caregivers to provide care for their child are two important concepts of family-centered care.

This text has been written by a very experienced pediatric nurse. The author is both a professor of pediatric/family healthcare nursing and an actively practicing pediatric nurse in the greater San Francisco Bay Area. She works in the inpatient pediatrics unit at California Pacific Medical Center with children who have a wide variety of acute, surgical, and traumatic injuries. She also works per diem for Lucille Packard Stanford Hospital at a pediatric hematology oncology clinic in San Francisco; her role there is as a clinical coordinator providing children with outpatient chemotherapy, education, and supportive care during cancer treatment.

Many pediatric and family healthcare textbooks are currently available. What is unique about this text is that it provides a concept-based perspective as well as a great deal of information on pathologies and diagnoses unique to children. Its many features provide the latest information on family education, research, safety, and pharmacology. The author has used a variety of national standards of practice as well as position papers by national pediatric organizations to inform the content provided. Chapters unique to this text include those focusing on symptoms assessment and management for children, working and communicating in interdisciplinary teams, caring for children across healthcare settings, cultural care models, essential safety models. and pediatric-specific skills. Each chapter has been written to provide the essential components of pediatric nursing theory as well as the corresponding skills. The carefully selected appendices also enhance the text by providing specifics on pediatric calculations, nutrition, safe and effective handoffs, growth charts, prevention of errors, and tips for maintaining professional boundaries, among other resources.

The author hopes that the reader finds this text to be a helpful guide and a reference for attaining deeper understanding of the unique aspects of pediatric nursing.

References

Kaiser Family Foundation. (2017). Health insurance coverage of children. Timeframe: 2013–2015. Retrieved from kff.org/other/state-indicator/children-0-18

U.S. Census Bureau. (2016). Income and poverty in the United States: 2015. Retrieved from https://www.census.gov/library/publications/2016/demo/p60-256.html

Acknowledgments

I would like to express my sincere appreciation for the highly professional editorial, production, and rights & media teams at Jones & Bartlett Learning: Amanda Martin, Christina Freitas, Nancy Hoffman, Elizabeth Hamblin, Carolyn Pershouse, Wes DeShano, and Troy Liston, thank you so much for your expert guidance.

I would like to also express my deepest appreciation to my family for being patient with me as I spend so much time writing. Evan, my generous husband, I thank you with all my heart. My children, Logan and Christina, thank you for your support and words of encouragement. To my incredible mother, thank you so much for providing our family with the best role model of a strong work ethic that one could possibly imagine. You are our inspiration, and the unbelievable devotion you express to our entire family is much appreciated. Loren, my kind, thoughtful, and funny brother, blessings to you in heaven. When we lost you last year, I wasn't sure I could continue on. Your words of encouragement before you became an angel kept me going. I miss you. I love you.

Reviewers

Christine M. Berté, EdD(c), APRN-BC, CPN
Professor of Nursing
Western Connecticut State University
Danbury, Connecticut

Nathania Bush, DNP, PHCNS-BC
Associate Professor of Nursing
Morehead State University
Morehead, Kentucky

Stephanie Evans Butkus, PhD, APRN,
    CPNP-PC, CLC
Assistant Professor of Nursing
Texas Christian University
Aledo, Texas

Vicki L. Caldwell, MSN, RN
Instructor of Nursing
Millikin University
Decatur, Illinois

Jeffrey K. Carmack, DNP, RN, CHSE
Assistant Professor of Nursing
University of Arkansas, Little Rock
Little Rock, Arkansas

Rhonda Conner-Warren, PhD, RN,
    CPNP-PC, BC
Assistant Professor of Health Practice
Michigan State University College of Nursing
East Lansing, Michigan

Linda Del Vecchio-Gilbert, DNP, CPNP-PC,
    ACHPN, CPON
Associate Professor, New England Institute of
    Technology
Associate Professor of Practice and Coordinator
    of the Core Clinical Curriculum, Simmons
    College of Nursing and Health Sciences
Pediatric Nurse Practitioner Consultant,
    Notre Dame Pediatric Palliative Program

Susan B. Dickey, PhD, RN
Associate Professor of Nursing
Temple University, College of Public Health,
    Department of Nursing
Philadelphia, Pennsylvania

Kimberly Dimino, MSN, CCRN
Professor of Nursing
William Paterson University
Wayne, New Jersey

Karen Dublin, MEd, BSN, RN
Professor of Nursing
Tyler Junior College
Tyler, Texas

Michele Faxel, EdD, MS, RN
Assistant Professor of Nursing
Samuel Merritt University
Oakland, California

Heather Janiszewski Goodin, PhD, RN,
    AHN-BC, CPN
Professor of Nursing and Chair of Post-Licensure
    Nursing Program
Capital University
Columbus, Ohio

Faith Irving, MSN, ARNP-BC

Joann Kapa, MSNed, FNP-BC, CPN
Professor
Oakland University
Rochester, Michigan

Christina Kiger, MSN, RN-CPN
Assistant Professor
Marian University Leighton School of Nursing
Indianapolis, Indiana

Sherry Knoppers, PhD, RN
Professor of Nursing
Grand Rapids Community College
Grand Rapids, Michigan

Jill M. Krell, DNP, RN
Assistant Professor of Nursing
Concordia University Wisconsin
Mequon, Wisconsin

Cynthia Glawe Mailloux, PhD, RN, CNE
Professor and Chairperson
Misericordia University
Dallas, Pennsylvania

Kathleen Motacki, MSN, RN, BC
Clinical Professor of Nursing
Saint Peter's University School of Nursing
Jersey City, New Jersey

Patricia O'Connor, MSN, RN, CNE
Assistant Professor of Nursing
Saint Francis Medical Center College of Nursing
Peoria, Illinois

Catherine Pankonien, MSN, RNC-NIC
Assistant Professor of Nursing
Midwestern State University
Wichita Falls, Texas

Mechelle Perea-Ryan, MS, FNP-BC, RN-BC, PHN
Associate Professor of Nursing
California State University, Stanislaus,
    School of Nursing
Turlock, California

Rhonda Phillips, MSN, CNS, RN
Assistant Professor of Nursing
City Colleges of Chicago
Chicago, Illinois

Michele Polfuss, PhD, RN, APNP-AC/PC
Assistant Professor, University of Wisconsin
Nurse Researcher, Children's Hospital of Wisconsin
Milwaukee, Wisconsin

Rebecca Presswood, MS, RN
Professor, Associate Degree Nursing Program
Blinn College
Bryan, Texas

Linda S. Rodebaugh, EdD, MSN, RN, CNE
Associate Professor
University of Indianapolis, School of Nursing
Indianapolis, Indiana

Margaret Rudd-Arieta, DNP
Full-Time Lecturer
University of Massachusetts–Dartmouth,
    School of Nursing
North Dartmouth, Massachusetts

Andrea Seay, MS, RN, PPCNP-BC
Professor of Nursing
Lone Star College Cy-Fair
Woodlands, Texas

Theresa Turick-Gibson, MA, PNP-BC, RN-BC
Professor, Department of Nursing
Hartwick College
Oneonta, New York

Linda Kaye Walters, PhD, MSN, RN, CNE
Professor and Program Director
Indiana State University School of Nursing
Terre Haute, Indiana

Irish Patrick Williams, PhD, RN, MSN,
    CRRN, CFN
Hinds Community College
Raymond, Mississippi

Overview of Pediatric Nursing Care

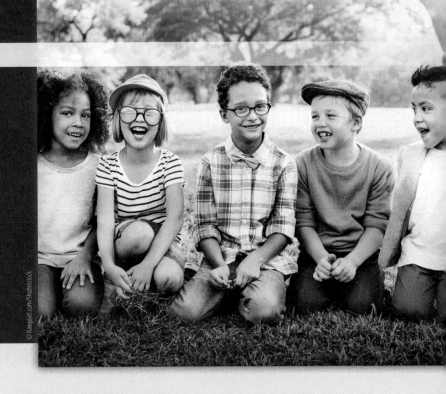

© Rawpixel.com/Shutterstock

CHAPTER 1

Introduction to Children's Health Care

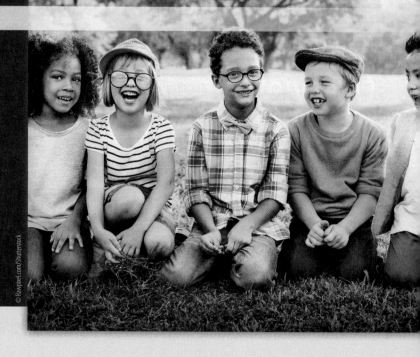

© Rawpixel.com/Shutterstock

LEARNING OBJECTIVES

1. Analyze how contemporary issues in children's health may be encountered in pediatric nursing practice.
2. Identify and apply the components of "Bright Futures" created by the American Academy of Pediatrics.
3. Identify how the concept of "new morbidity" for children in urban rural and suburban environments may affect nursing practice.
4. Analyze models of critical thinking that can be applied to the complexities of pediatric nursing.
5. Analyze the care needs of families of diverse constellations (teen parents, single parents, parenting by grandparents, extended families, blended families and culturally diverse families).
6. Apply the philosophy of family-centered care to common pediatric staff–family encounters.

KEY TERMS

Anticipatory guidance
Binuclear family
Clinical judgment
Concept-based learning
Critical thinking
Empowerment
Enabling
Extended family
Family-centered care
Family strengths
New morbidity

Introduction: Contemporary Issues in Children's Health

Providing comprehensive well-child and health restoration nursing care for children across the developmental period is a complex endeavor. Children are part of families, and families are unique in their composition, strengths, and needs. Children progress from total dependence on caregivers as babies to independence as young adults. This time period—from birth to young adulthood—is dynamic and can be challenging. Pediatric nurses must be prepared to provide support, education, and meticulous care to children from diverse cultural, racial, and ethnic backgrounds, and from diverse family structures. Some families are able to provide for their children's basic needs such as health care, whereas others experience stressors that adversely influence their children's health and well-being (**Figure 1-1**). Contemporary times have brought both economic and health challenges that can greatly influence a pediatric nurse's experiences in caring for children and their families.

In today's world, any given child may experience many socioeconomic factors that influence his or her health. Current research shows that large numbers of families in the United States and elsewhere are experiencing unemployment, frequent moves, food insecurity, and lack of consistent health care and insurance. Hunger—a basic human experience—has been documented as a national problem with adverse health and cognitive consequences, affecting physical, academic, and social functioning during childhood (Coleman-Jensen, Rabbitt, Gregory, & Singh, 2015a, 2015b; Kushel, Gupta, Gee, & Haas, 2006; Melchior et al., 2012; Weinreb et al., 2002) and contributing to long-term mental health issues from adolescence into adulthood (McIntyre, Williams,

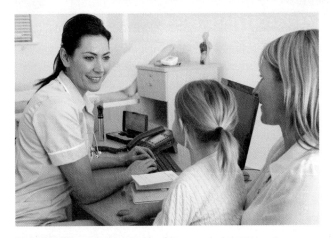

Figure 1-2

© Monkey Business Images/Shutterstock

Lavorato, & Patten, 2013). A comprehensive plan for a child's health should include early assessments and screenings, immunizations, disease prevention, acute care for illness and injuries, and, if needed, chronic care for lifelong conditions that first present in childhood. The term **anticipatory guidance** is used to denote the process of preparing parents, guardians, or caregivers for what to expect as the child grows, develops, and matures (**Figure 1-2**).

FAMILY EDUCATION

Definitions of Anticipatory Guidance

Anticipatory guidance is a phrase used to define information provided to parents so they can expect, plan for, and cope with actual or potential problems associated with normal growth and development of a child before those problems arise. As a child progresses from infancy to adolescence, particular points along the developmental path require preparation. Anticipatory guidance gives the healthcare team the opportunity to teach parents or caregivers about what to expect. For instance, teaching about the increasing mobility of infants, which progresses from rolling over to crawling to walking, will help parents plan for a safe environment and prevent falls or other accidents. Teaching parents about toddlers' needs for constant supervision and their inherent clumsiness can help parents plan to prevent accidents and injuries.

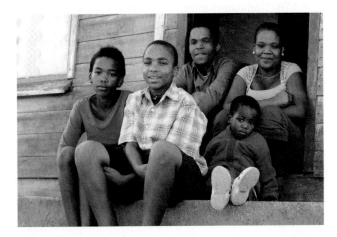

Figure 1-1

© Nolte Lourens/Shutterstock

Pediatric nurses must be committed to viewing their patients and families in a holistic and comprehensive light. The key to understanding the complexity of providing pediatric nursing care is to understand the important role that childhood plays in a developing person. Child health

With globalization and immigration, pediatric healthcare teams must be aware of international child health concerns. One major concern that arises on an international scale is poverty. Currently, approximately 20% of U.S. families are living in poverty. On a global scale, poverty affects approximately 50% of the world's pediatric population. There are currently 2.2 billion children in the world, 1 billion of whom live in poverty (Shah, 2013).

Research shows that "persistent poverty" has more detrimental effects on a child's socioemotional functioning, IQ, and school achievement than "transient poverty." Poor children experience less home-based cognitive stimulation, lower teacher expectations, inconsistent parenting, and poorer academic-readiness skills—all factors that can slow their development (Kursmark & Weitzman, 2009).

is one of the most influential factors in adult health and well-being, so it should be focused on the prevention of illness, injury, and development of chronic conditions. High priority must be given to performing comprehensive assessments, promoting good health, fostering family life, and creating support systems and safe home/school/neighborhood environments to help children grow, play, learn, and become healthy and productive adults.

Frameworks of Pediatric Health

The care of children is oriented toward the child's developmental stage, rather than chronological age. Nevertheless, for classification purposes, childhood is divided into seven developmental stages corresponding with average age groupings (**Figure 1-3**):

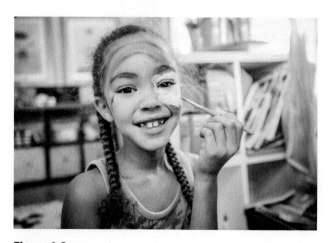

Figure 1-3

©Inti St Clair/Blend Images LLC/Getty

- Preterm infant: Born prior to 36 weeks' gestation
- Neonate: First 28–30 days of life
- Infant: One month to end of the first year
- Toddler: One year old through second year of life
- Preschooler: Third birthday through fifth year of life
- School-age child: Sixth birthday through 12th year of life
- Adolescence: 13th birthday up to 18th birthday

New Morbidity

The term **new morbidity** was coined in the 1980s by pediatrician Robert Haggerty to denote concerns that are brought about by current environmental and social issues that decrease quality of life, as distinguished from issues of the past centuries such as infectious disease (Haggerty, 1995). Attention difficulties, adolescent mood and anxiety disorders, suicide, homicide, access to firearms, school bullying and violence, and the effects of media on obesity, sexual activity, and violence are all considered contemporary issues that create concerns about health and injury and, therefore, are titled new morbidities. Contemporary scholars and practitioners have since added to Haggerty's list and incorporated evidence-based best practices to address these issues, leading to a revised set of "New Morbidities 2.0" (Giardino & Sanborn, 2013). Nurses, as part of their roles in caring for children, are in a good position to assess for morbidity concerns and provide direction, support, referrals, and counseling. Four general categories of concerns related to these new morbidities have been identified (Lucey, 2001):

- Physical and environmental factors affecting behavior and risk taking, such as access to drugs and illegal substances, cigarettes, and alcohol
- Variations of behavior and emotional development: helping parents adapt to the unexpected and learn uniqueness of each child's development
- Child behaviors affecting physical risk, such as smoking, drug use, and medical adherence
- Severe behavioral deviations and their management needs

Healthy People 2020

Healthy People 2020 is a federal initiative that promotes a set of national goals and objectives for improving the health of all people living in the United States over a 10-year period. The current series includes 1,200 objectives that are divided into 42 health-related topic areas, several of which pertain to the health and well-being of children (**Table 1-1**). The objectives reflect health indicators that encourage prioritization of key health issues and actions to be taken toward achieving maximal health for the population.

TABLE 1-1   *Healthy People 2020:* Children's Health Concerns and Goals

Goals for Maternal, Infant, and Child Health

Improve the health and well-being of women, infants, children, and families.

› Determines the health of the next generation and helps to predict public health challenges for families in the future (morbidity, mortality, poverty, and ethnic disparities).

› Risks of maternal and infant mortality and morbidity, as well as pregnancy-related complications, can be reduced by increasing access to care and identifying early any health conditions of infants related to disease, disability, or death.

› The health, nutrition, and behaviors of mothers highly influence the physical and cognitive development of infants. Breastfeeding has been widely acknowledged as beneficial for growth, health, development, and immunity (**Figure 1-4**). Promoting breastfeeding is a primary goal.

› Some objectives include:
  - Reduce the rate of fetal and infant deaths
  - Reduce cesarean births among low-risk women
  - Reduce the number of infants with low birth weight and very low birth weight
  - Reduce preterm births
  - Increase abstinence from alcohol, cigarettes, and illicit drugs among pregnant women
  - Increase the proportion of infants who are breastfed

Goals for Early and Middle Childhood

Improve the health and well-being of the early (birth to year 8) and middle (ages 6 to 12) childhood developmental periods.

› The period of early and middle childhood provides the social, emotional, physical, and cognitive foundation for lifelong health and well-being.

› Goals include research and interventions in reducing obesity, increasing physical activity, and preventing injury and violence.

› The three top developmental milestones of this period include motor skills, language development, and emotional regulation and attachment. These milestones can become significantly delayed when children experience negative risk factors and environmental stressors.

› Early and middle childhood also set the stage for the following accomplishments:
  - Eating habits
  - Self-discipline
  - School success
  - Health literacy
  - Conflict negotiation
  - Ability to make decisions during risky situations

› Children in early and middle childhood are at particular risk for:
  - Asthma
  - Obesity
  - Dental caries
  - Child maltreatment
  - Developmental and behavioral disorders
  - Unintentional injuries

(continues)

Goals for Adolescent Health

Improve the health and well-being of the adolescent developmental period (ages 10 to 19).

› Behavioral patterns during this developmental period influence not only current health state, but also risk for chronic illness and diseases during later adulthood.

› During this developmental transition period, teens are sensitive to contextual influences (surroundings) such as family, peers, environment, school, and neighborhood.

› Teens are negotiating puberty, increasing independence, and exploring many aspects of their lives.

› Adolescents who perceive that they have good communication and are bonded with an adult are less likely to engage in risky behaviors.

› Parents who provide supervision and are involved with their adolescent's activities promote a safe environment in which to explore opportunities.

› Adolescents who live in distressed neighborhoods with high poverty rates are at increased risk for poor physical and mental health, delinquency, and risky sexual behavior.

› Health disparities are related to outcomes among ethnic and racial groups, in that those persons who live in poverty or who are African American, Hispanic, or American Indian have greater obesity, higher rates of teen pregnancy, more tooth decay, and poorer educational achievement.

› Adolescent public health and social problems include, but are not limited to, the following conditions:

- Smoking
- Homelessness
- Homicide
- Suicide
- Motor vehicle crashes, including those caused by drinking and driving
- Substance use and abuse
- Sexually transmitted infections (STIs)
- Unplanned pregnancies

Data from Office of Disease Prevention and Health Promotion. (2014). Maternal, infant, and child health. Retrieved from https://www.healthypeople.gov/2020/; Office of Disease Prevention and Health Promotion. (2014). Early and middle childhood. Retrieved from https://www.healthypeople.gov/2020/; Office of Disease Prevention and Health Promotion. (2014). Adolescent health. Retrieved from https://www.healthypeople.gov/2020/

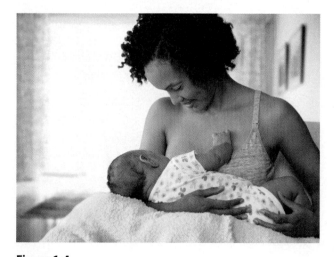

Figure 1-4

© KidStock/Blend Images/Getty

Nurses, as the largest workforce in health care, can be highly influential in developing and evaluating programs that address the identified healthcare concerns over each 10-year span of time covered by the *Healthy People* initiative. Top priorities for pediatric nurses include education and interventions for children before birth through young adulthood.

Bright Futures

The American Academy of Pediatrics has developed a national health promotion and disease prevention program addressing the healthcare needs of children, known as Bright Futures (https://brightfutures.aap.org/Pages/default.aspx). This program provides direction in the context of both family and community. It includes tools, principles, and guidelines intended to strengthen the ties and interactions between local, regional, and state programs. The Bright Futures tool and resource kit provides a variety of assessment forms and screening tools to identify high-risk behaviors, all of which can be used during child/family healthcare encounters. Pediatric nurses can benefit from reviewing the Bright Futures visit forms that offer guidance on assessments, health screenings, and interviews of families with children in infancy, early childhood, middle childhood, and adolescence. Components of the tool kit, which can enhance the quality and thoroughness of a healthcare visit, include educational handouts, screening/assessment tools, ideas for preventive care, and instructions on how to develop linkages between families and community resources.

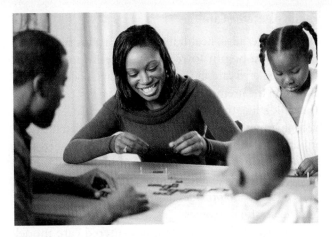

Figure 1-5

© FatCamera/E+/Getty

Caring for Families

The definition of a family can be a complex one. Many potential constellations exist, including nuclear, group, extended, blended, adoptive, foster, single-parent, same-sex parents, and untraditional such as a reconstituted or communal. Given today's high rates of marital separation and divorce, growing up in a **binuclear family**, in which a child's living time is divided between two or more households, is not uncommon. The most important consideration when assessing the structure of a child's family is highlighted by a commonly used phrase: A family is who they say they are.

Family Strengths

Every family is unique. As a family grows, interacts, and has experiences, the formation of **family strengths** provides a foundation for growth. These assets provide an optimal support system for individuals within the family as well as for the family as a whole (**Figure 1-5**). According to Sittner, Hudson, and Defrain (2007), family strengths include the following characteristics:

- Affection and appreciation
- Commitment
- Ability to cope with stress and crisis
- Positive communication
- Time spent together as a unit
- Spiritual well-being

Nurses can be instrumental in assisting families who are experiencing a crisis. A child with a new diagnosis of chronic illness, acute illness, or injury can be supported by assisting family members to develop or demonstrate components of the family strengths model. Identifying and supporting existing family strengths components, and helping the family to implement those strengths, will help the family identify and achieve goals for their child (Feeley & Gottlieb, 2000).

Family-Centered Care

In recent decades, health institutions across the United States have begun to recognize the importance of family-centered care and adopt the principles of this model. Based on the premise that the family is a key constant in the child's life, the **family-centered care** model suggests recognizing that all family members are affected by the injury, illness, hospitalization, or healthcare need that the child is experiencing. Providing support based on encouragement, enhancement of strengths, competence, and collaboration provides the foundation for interactions and successful outcomes.

The principles of the family-centered care model promote a partnership approach in which the family and healthcare team work together to identify the best way to provide care for the child (Kuo et al., 2012). Issues are prioritized based on the family's identified critical issues, and the team provides support based on what the family identifies as most important. For example, if the child has a chronic illness and the family cares for the child, the family will know the details of what the child needs and how to best respond to these needs. Family-centered care provides a structure to support the strengths of the family through a families-as-partners approach, while providing for the child's medical and nursing needs.

Although different variations of a family-centered care approach exist, they all rely on five main principles (Kuo et al., 2012):

- Information sharing
- Respecting and honoring differences
- Partnership and collaboration
- Negotiation
- Care in context of family and community

These principles are exemplified by two key ideas: enabling and empowerment. **Enabling** a family and child means that the professional healthcare team provides opportunities for the family to gain and show mastery of the care required by the child. Learning required skills such as suctioning, catheterizing, changing dressings, providing enteric nutrition, and organizing needed supplies are examples. The pediatric team should provide the time, supplies, support, and education that build the family's sense of enabling. **Empowerment** suggests that the family feels competent to provide care for their child as a result of the support, education, and trust built through interacting with the team. For example, one healthcare institution successfully incorporated family-centered care into its pediatric unit through an emphasis on hope, engaged care, and love, with the family's skills and interactions being supported and strengthened; this model allowed for the development of a collaborative partnership between care providers and family members (Frost, Green, Gance-Cleveland, Kersten, & Irby, 2010). Family-centered care can be implemented regardless of the clinical setting or environment.

Siblings and **extended family** members should be invited to interact and provide care for the child (**Figure 1-6**). The family should be supported with respect to its constellation, ability, presence (many care providers have to continue to work and may be absent for periods of time), economic status, and family functioning, without care providers making judgments based on these aspects. Child Life specialists should be involved with the assessment of the family's needs and available to assist with medical play, education, and guidance for all family members. Reaching out beyond the clinical settings is also important to family-centered care, with schools, primary providers and community resources being identified and engaged as necessary.

In a family-centered care model, the nursing staff will recognize that a child-friendly environment is a crucial component of pediatric care. Play areas, brightly colored walls and decorations, and avenues for distraction and developmental growth are all essential.

BEST PRACTICES

Pediatric healthcare team members should adhere to the following guidelines when delivering family-centered care:

- The family is the constant in the child's life.
- The family is one unit and should be treated as such.
- The family caring for a child with a chronic illness knows what the child needs and should be encouraged to demonstrate the best-care practices with which they are familiar.
- The family should be assisted to develop or continue to grow in both empowerment (competence and confidence) and enabling (provision of sound care).
- The family should be provided with education and educational materials; information sharing is a priority.
- The family and providers are collegial care team members and should be treated with dignity, respect, and collaboration.
- The family should be encouraged to take on decision-making roles.
- The family should be provided support to live with normalcy and should be given information about outside resources, community support networks, and education.
- Siblings and extended family members should be included in care and planning.

Data from American Hospital Association. (2015). Resources: Strategies for leadership: Patient and family-centered care. Retrieved from http://www.aha.org/advocacy-issues/quality/strategies-patientcentered.shtml; Institute for Family-Centered Care. (2015). Patient- and family-centered care. Retrieved from http://www.ipfcc.org; Institute for Healthcare Improvement. (2016). Person- and family-centered care. Retrieved from http://www.ihi.org/topics/pfcc/pages /default.aspx

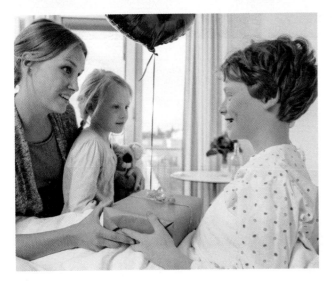

Figure 1-6

© Westend61/Getty

Concept-Based Care in Pediatrics

Historically, the education of nurses has been based on highly structured theory courses that use memorization, linear thinking, and theoretical application. More recently, concept-based nursing has gained great respect and interest as an alternative to traditional nursing education and learning. **Concept-based learning** uses a dynamic approach to the ever-growing body of scientific nursing knowledge; it focuses on key concepts that can be applied to various situations and settings. The understanding of interrelated concepts helps with the mental organization of large amounts of information, and in turns makes learning logical. An example of concept-based learning is presented in **Table 1-2**.

Critical Thinking in Pediatrics

The complexity of pediatric nursing is such that the application of a mode of thinking clearly and efficiently to complex child/family clinical presentations helps to solve problems. **Critical thinking**, in general, is a problem-solving means of thinking through a complex situation and drawing conclusions that will best help a child and their family. Critical thinking in pediatric nursing is used to separate what is known from what is unknown while helping a team of concerned healthcare providers devise a plan to assist a child in need. According to Papathanasiou et al. (2014), critical thinking is a method of problem solving that combines creativity with a specific set of cognitive skills—specifically, critical analysis (e.g., the Socratic method), inference, and concluding justification—to assess and evaluate information. By using a critical thinking mode of problem solving, pediatric nurses can identify problems early and devise systems and interventions to assist a child in need. **Table 1-3** summarizes the components of the Papathanasiou et al. critical thinking model.

Sometimes critical thinking is considered a program outcome. In Staib's (2003) interactive model of critical thinking, the basic structures of thought are what create sound thinking and effective problem solving. Staid describes eight essential components of thinking that are needed in the development of a program with distinct outcomes:

- Raise questions.
- Generate a purpose.
- Use information.
- Utilize concepts.
- Make inferences.
- Make assumptions.
- Generate implications.
- Embody a point of view.

TABLE 1-2 Concept Versus Traditional Learning		
Example of Content	**Traditional Learning**	**Concept-Based Learning**
Issues with respiratory system	Disease-based content such as asthma, cystic fibrosis, bronchiolitis, and epiglottitis, and their associated symptoms, treatments, and nursing care	Ventilation
		Oxygenation
		Perfusion
		Safety
		Infection control
		Comfort
Skin diseases	Disease-based content such as rashes, contact dermatitis, poison ivy, pressure ulcers, and acne, and their associated symptoms, treatments, and nursing care.	Skin integrity
		Infection control
		Comfort
		Symptom management

TABLE 1-3	Components of Papathanasiou et al. Model of Critical Thinking

Recognize Assumptions

› Separate fact from opinion; use a Socratic question-and-answer method to distinguish knowledge from assumptions.

› Do not assume information is true; notice, question, reveal, and identify gaps or unfounded logic.

› When listening, do not assume information is reliable; look for real evidence.

› Seek common ground with patient in basic assumptions about values.

Critical Thinking Enhancement Behaviors

› Seek to maintain impartiality, integrity, and independence of thought.

› Maintain awareness of limitations of knowledge and personal prejudices.

› Use perseverance and spiritual courage in seeking solutions.

Problem Solving

› Approach issues using empirical methods, the research process, and the scientific method.

› The value of intuition is greater with longer nursing experience.

› In making decisions, prioritize patients' multiple needs.

› Use worded, rational, and systematic approach to problem solving.

Stages of Decision Making

› Recognition of objective or purpose

› Definition of criteria

› Exploration and consideration of alternative solutions

› Design, implementation, and evaluation of solution

Data from Papathanasiou, I. V., Kleisiaris, C. F., Fradelos, E. C., Kakou, K., & Kourkouta, L. (2014). Critical thinking: The development of an essential skill for nursing students. *Acta Informatica Medica, 22*(4), 283–286.

QUALITY AND SAFETY

Critical Thinking for Safety

Critical thinking can be applied to safety in pediatric nursing. For example, if a pediatric nurse is caring for a child with complicated family dynamics, a diagnosis of severe cerebral palsy and failure to thrive, and possible evidence of abuse and neglect, using components of critical thinking can help to formulate a plan for safety.

- *Recognize assumptions.* Children with severe cerebral palsy may be considered vulnerable to child abuse because they are dependent, often nonverbal, sometimes technology dependent, skills demanding, and seen as "different." Care providers may not be able to provide for their complex needs. The failure to thrive may be assumed to be based on neglect, the most common form of child maltreatment.

- *Evaluate arguments.* Does evidence exist that the child is at risk for poor care? Does evidence exist that the child has been neglected? Do the complications of the family dynamics place the child at risk for neglect? Are the basic care needs of this child being met at home?

- *Draw conclusions.* The child's safety is paramount. The physical and emotional needs of the child must be met. Supportive resources such as nutrition, warmth, rest, appropriate clothes, medicine and medical care, play and distraction, and safe supervision must be secured. If the family cannot provide for the child with severe cerebral palsy and complex medical needs, then reporting the evidence of child abuse/neglect is warranted.

Clinical Judgment

Clinical judgment is a term that is sometimes considered interchangeable with "problem solving," "decision making," and "critical thinking." It comprises the analysis, interpretation, and drawing of conclusions about a patient's condition, including the patient's holistic needs, concerns, health problems, and areas of needed action or intervention (Tanner, 2006). Pediatric nurses must use sound clinical judgment to provide high-level holistic care. Nurses' clinical judgment is influenced by their experience, expertise, relationships with patients and families, and working as a team member. According to Tanner (2006), five conclusions can be drawn about the use and application of clinical judgment:

- Clinical judgments are more strongly influenced by what nurses bring to the situation than by the data (objective) collected concerning the situation.
- Clinical judgments about patients are highly influenced by the situational context and the culture of the nursing environment.
- Knowledge of both the patient and the patient's typical pattern of responses, complemented by engagement with the patient and family, have the greatest influence on sound clinical judgment.
- Improved clinical reasoning and the development of clinical knowledge follow from reflection upon one's practice.
- Nurses make clinical judgments based on a variety of single or combined reasoning patterns.

Professional Pediatric Nursing Care

Pediatric nurses care for both the child and the family. Nurses who care for children with complex health conditions understand the need for professional care based on concepts, theory, and skills specific to children while applying a knowledge base that focuses on the promotion of normal growth and development.

Many professional organizations provide education, best practices information, and collegial support for pediatric nurses. The Society of Pediatric Nurses (SPN) is an internationally focused, U.S.-based organization that provides a multitude of opportunities for mentoring, education, research, and scholarly development. SPN publishes *Journal of Pediatric Nursing*, which provides state-of-the-science research and best practices information on caring for children and families. Other professional nursing organizations have focus groups or specialty practice subgroups that provide support for pediatric nurses.

Because most hospitalized patients are adults, pediatric nurses are fewer in number and often practice in isolation, such as in pediatric clinics or pediatric units, contributing to the need for collaboration among the profession as a whole. It is imperative that these nurses become aware of national initiatives, research endeavors, and best practices projects to move the profession of pediatric nursing forward. **Table 1-4** lists selected organizations that support the profession of pediatric nursing.

TABLE 1-4 Selected Professional Organizations That Support Pediatric Nursing
Society of Pediatric Nurses (www.pedsnurses.org)
Sigma Theta Tau International Nursing Honor Society (www.nursingsociety.org)
Association for Vascular Access (www.avainfo.org)
Association of Pediatric Hematology/Oncology Nurses (www.aphon.org)
American Academy of Pediatrics (www.aap.org)
Pediatric Nursing Certification Board (www.pncb.org)
Transcultural Nursing Society (www.tcns.org)
National League for Nursing (www.nln.org)
Emergency Nurses Association (www.ena.org)
Association of Camp Nurses (www.acn.org)
American Nurses Association (www.nursingworld.org)
National Association of Pediatric Nurse Practitioners (www.napnap.org)

Case Study

Zack, a 3-month-old infant, has been admitted to the pediatric unit from the emergency department (ED). Zack has a history of poor feeding, weight loss, irritability, low-grade fevers, and intermittent periods of shortness of breath and tachypnea. The family brought Zack to the emergency department after he vomited four times in one day and became listless. The ED staff evaluated Zack and found him to be anemic, with an abdominal mass and organic failure to thrive. The on-call pediatric oncologist was called and immediately admitted Zack into the ward with a diagnosis of neuroblastoma. The family was stunned, very emotional, and frightened. The team immediately began to prepare Zack for placement of a central line and evaluation for cancer treatment.

Case Study Questions

1. How can the staff use the principles of family-centered care to provide support for Zack and his family?
2. Which team members should be involved with the delivery of family-centered care?
3. What does the family need during the first 24 to 48 hours after admission to the pediatric ward?

As the Case Evolves. . .

Zack has been admitted and evaluated by a pediatric oncologist. His parents, a working-class East African immigrant couple in their early 20s, are meeting with an oncology nurse-practitioner to discuss the next steps in their son's care. It quickly becomes apparent that although both speak English fluently, the parents are having difficulty understanding what is wrong with Zack and how treatment usually progresses in neuroblastoma. The father, who is self-employed running the family's restaurant, asks if delaying treatment until he can save up extra money is an option.

4. Which of the following aspects of the family's background is likely to have the greatest impact on their son's care?
   A. Cultural background
   B. Ethnic background
   C. Language fluency
   D. Socioeconomic background

After explaining to Zack's parents why his treatment cannot be delayed, the father—who until now has done all the talking—states that he cannot authorize treatment until he has conferred with Zack's grandmother. He excuses himself to make a phone call. Left alone with Zack's mother, the nurse asks if she has any questions about her son's condition and treatment, stating, "I know these treatment decisions are difficult, so anything I can tell you to help you, I'm happy to explain." The mother replies that any decisions about Zack's care will come from her husband's mother, the family matriarch.

5. According to family theory in pediatric nursing, which of the following statements would be considered correct?
   A. A family represents its cultural and/or ethnic group.
   B. A family is considered extended if multiple generations reside in the home.
   C. A family has a distinct decision maker who is easy to identify.
   D. A family is whoever they state they are.
6. Which of the following key principles are most important in implementing a family-centered care plan for Zack, given the complexities of his family situation?
   A. Empowerment and enabling
   B. Respect and independence
   C. Support and collaboration
   D. Supervision and teaching

Chapter Summary

- Contemporary issues in children's health include a variety of concerns. Issues surrounding poverty, nutrition, education, family support, and medical adherence all influence a pediatric nurse's care foci.
- A variety of frameworks can be used to examine pediatric health care. The *Healthy People 2020* initiative sets goals for the health of all Americans, while the American Academy of Pediatrics has developed Bright Futures, a national health promotion and disease prevention program that addresses the healthcare needs of children in the context of family and community.
- The term "new morbidity" is used to denote concerns associated with current environmental and social issues. Attention difficulties, adolescent mood and anxiety disorders, suicide, homicide, access to firearms, school bullying and violence, and the effects of media on obesity, sexual activity, and violence are all considered contemporary issues that create concerns about health and injury.

- Tools, principles, and guidelines have been developed to strengthen the ties and interactions among local, regional, and state programs. For example, the Bright Futures tool kit provides a variety of assessment forms and screening tools to identify high-risk behaviors, all of which can be used during child/family healthcare encounters.

- Based on the premise that the family is the constant in the child's life, the family-centered care model suggests that all family members are affected by the injury, illness, hospitalization, or healthcare need that the child is experiencing. Providing support based on encouragement, enhancement of strengths, competence, and collaboration establishes a solid foundation for positive interactions and successful outcomes.

- Two ideas underlying the principles of the family-centered care model—empowerment and enabling—promote an approach in which the family and healthcare team work together to identify the best way to provide care for the child.

- Critical thinking can be applied to the complexities of pediatric nursing. In pediatric nursing, it is used to separate what is known from what is unknown while helping a team of concerned healthcare providers devise a plan to assist a child in need. Papathanasiou et al.'s model of critical thinking includes recognizing assumptions, enhancing critical thinking behaviors, taking a reasoned approach to problem solving, and following a four-stage decision-making process.

- Many professional organizations provide education, best practices information, and collegial support for pediatric nurses.

Bibliography

American Hospital Association. (2015). Resources: Strategies for leadership: Patient and family-centered care. Retrieved from http://www.aha.org/advocacy-issues/quality/strategies-patientcentered.shtml

Centers for Disease Control and Prevention. (2010, June 4). Youth risk behavior surveillance—United States, 2009. *Morbidity and Mortality Weekly Report, 59*(SS-5), 8. Retrieved from http://www.cdc.gov/mmwr/pdf/ss/ss5905.pdf

Coleman-Jensen, A., Rabbitt, M. P., Gregory, C., & Singh, A. (2015a). *Household food security in the United States in 2014.* U.S. Department of Agriculture, Economic Research Service, September 2015. Retrieved from https://www.ers.usda.gov/webdocs/publications/err215/err-215.pdf

Coleman-Jensen, A., Rabbitt, M. P., Gregory, C., & Singh, A. (2015b). *Report summary: Household food security in the United States in 2014.* U.S. Department of Agriculture, Economic Research Service, September 2014. Retrieved from https://www.ers.usda.gov/webdocs/publications/err194/53740_err194

Feeley, N., & Gottlieb, L. (2000). Nursing approaches for working with family strengths and resources. *Journal of Family Nursing, 6,* 9–24.

Frost, M., Green, A., Gance-Cleveland, B., Kersten, R., & Irby, C. (2010). Improving family-centered care through research. *Journal of Pediatric Nursing, 25,* 144–147.

Giardino, A. P., & Sanborn, R. D. (2013). New morbidities 2.0. *Journal of Applied Research on Children: Informing Policy for Children at Risk, 4*(1), 2.

Haggerty, R. J. (1995, October). Child health 2000: New pediatrics in the changing environment of children's needs in the 21st century. *Pediatrics, 96*(4), 804–812.

Institute for Family-Centered Care. (2015). Patient- and family-centered care. Retrieved from http://www.ipfcc.org

Institute for Healthcare Improvement. (2016). Person- and family-centered care. Retrieved from http://www.ihi.org/topics/pfcc/pages/default.aspx

Kuo, D. Z., Houtrow, A. J., Arango, P., Kuhlthau, K. A., Simmons, J. M., & Neff, J. M. (2012). Family-centered care: Current applications and future directions in pediatric health care. *Maternal and Child Health Journal, 16*(2), 297–305.

Kursmark, M., & Weitzman, M. (2009, May). Recent findings concerning childhood food insecurity. *Current Opinion in Clinical Nutrition and Metabolic Care, 12*(3), 310–316.

Kushel, M. B., Gupta, R., Gee, L., & Haas, J. S. (2006). Housing instability and food insecurity as barriers to health care among low-income Americans. *Journal of General Internal Medicine, 21*(1), 71–77.

Lucey, J. (2001). The new morbidity revisited: A renewed commitment to the psychosocial aspects of pediatric care. *Pediatrics, 108*(5), 1227–1230.

McIntyre, L., Williams, J. V. A., Lavorato, D. H., & Patten, S. (2013). Depression and suicide ideation in late adolescence and early adulthood are an outcome of child hunger. *Journal of Affective Disorders, 150*(1), 123–129.

Melchior, M., Chastang, J.-F., Falissard, B., Galéra, C., Tremblay, R. E., Côté, S. M., & Boivin, M. (2012). Food insecurity and children's mental health: A prospective birth cohort. *PLOS One, 7*(12), e52615.

Papathanasiou, I. V., Kleisiaris, C. F., Fradelos, E. C., Kakou, K., & Kourkouta, L. (2014, August). Critical thinking: The development of an essential skill for nursing students. *Acta Informatica Medica, 22*(4), 283–286.

Shah, A. (2013). Poverty facts and stats. Retrieved from http://www.globalissues.org/article/26/poverty

Sittner, B., Hudson, D. B., & Defrain, J. (2007). Using the concept of family strengths to enhance nursing care. *American Journal of Maternal/Child Nursing, 32*(6), 353–357.

Staib, S. (2003). Teaching and measuring critical thinking. *Journal of Nursing Education, 42*(11), 498–508.

Tanner, C. (2006). Thinking like a nurse: A research-based model of clinical judgment in nursing. *Journal of Nursing Education, 45*(6), 204–211.

Weinreb, L., Wehler, C., Perloff, J., Scott, R., Hosmer, D., Sagor, L. & Gundersen, C. (2002). Hunger: Its impact on children's health and mental health. *Pediatrics, 110*(4), 41.

CHAPTER 2

Care Across Clinical Settings

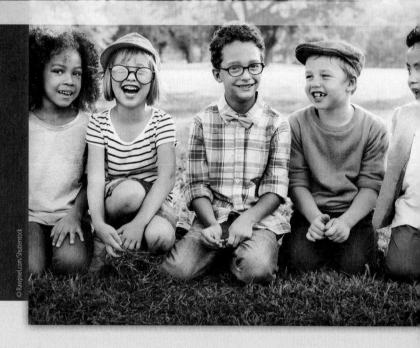

© Rawpixel.com/Shutterstock

LEARNING OBJECTIVES

1. Distinguish how goals and expectations of pediatric nursing care in outpatient and community settings differ from those in acute care environments, including emergency departments, intensive care, and hospice care.
2. Analyze how the context of varying care settings affects the way pediatric nurses execute the competencies required by the Society of Pediatric Nurses.
3. Use knowledge of child development to ensure effective, age-appropriate interactions with patients and caregivers.
4. Describe in detail different methods for providing anticipatory guidance and education appropriate to each care setting.
5. Apply key techniques of effective communication during interactions with healthcare team members, including SBAR, CUS, I-PASS, morning huddles, and STAT reporting.
6. Provide adequate measures to ensure the safety of patients in both outpatient and acute care clinical settings.

KEY TERMS

Acute care pediatric nursing
Anticipatory guidance
Camp nursing
Competencies
CUS protocol
Hospice nursing
I-PASS
Morning huddle
Neonatal intensive care unit (NICU)
Palliative care
Pediatric intensive care unit (PICU)
SBAR protocol
School nursing
Well-child visits

Introduction

Health care for children is provided across many diverse settings. The hospital setting that may be widely viewed as a major focus of pediatric nursing care is, in reality, the site of only a small subset of caregiving. Hospital-based nursing for children may be associated with many pediatric-specific skills and competencies, but nurses work in many other settings to provide both health promotion and health restoration to children. Moreover, few children experience hospitalization, and even fewer have chronic conditions, congenital conditions, or acute illnesses that require multiple hospitalizations. In short, the majority of care provided to children across the age 0–18 years developmental period occurs in clinical settings outside the traditional hospital environment. Consequently, pediatric nurses need an awareness of how the context of care influences the goals and expectations of caregiving (**Figure 2-1**).

Wellness and Health Maintenance

In the vast majority of circumstances, pediatric nursing care consists of routine care to maintain health, teach parents and patients about wellness-promoting choices, and support normal development. The setting in which such care is delivered, particularly in early childhood, is typically the primary care setting. During early childhood, children need multiple visits to their healthcare providers for assessment of their physical, mental, and emotional development; immunization; and education of parents on meeting children's health and social needs. Children require at least six **well-child visits** during their first year of life, and three to five more during their second year. These visits should include a recent health history, complete physical examination, plotting of measurements on a standardized growth chart, immunizations as indicated, and a discussion of wellness topics and anticipatory guidance. During the span from approximately age 3 through adolescence, a child should have annual well-child checkups for health screening and education. Most anticipatory guidance is provided to parents or guardians in a clinic setting during these wellness visits. **Table 2-1** provides information on suggested well-child visits across the developmental period.

Another common setting in which children's healthcare services are provided is primary and secondary school clinics, where nurses provide short-term care for children who become ill or injured during the school day, or management of symptoms or problems associated with chronic illness. Recreational settings such as camps, athletic programs, and before- or after-school programs may also include nursing care as part of the service.

Basic Competencies in Pediatric Nursing

Regardless of the setting in which a pediatric nurse practices, basic care **competencies** (i.e., the skills and knowledge needed to provide care appropriately and effectively) are expected. Pediatric nursing utilizes skills and knowledge that differ from those employed in adult nursing care. Children differ from adults in terms of their physiology and emotional development, and pediatric subpopulations have unique developmental needs. Pediatric nurses must be able to adapt their skills to care for children who range from neonate through adolescence (**Figure 2-2**).

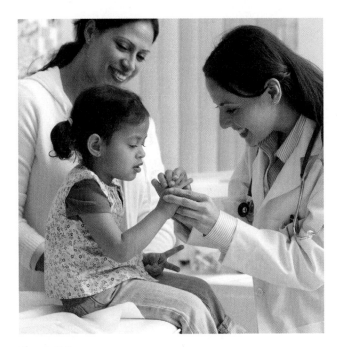

Figure 2-1

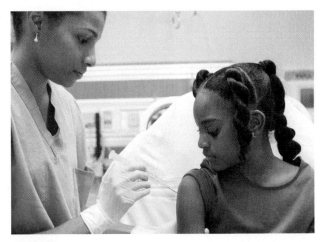

Figure 2-2

TABLE 2-1 Suggested Well-Child Visits Across Childhood (2016 American Academy of Pediatrics Recommendations)

Age at Visit	Content of Visit	Rationale
All visits	Family health assessment Immunization adherence Social and mental health Vision/hearing	› Assess family health at every visit › Check immunization adherence at each visit following the initiation of immunization protocols › Assess social/mental health at every visit from 2 years of age on, or earlier if developmental indicators suggest a need for it › Perform objective assessment of vision/hearing at each visit; subjective measurement can begin at 4 years
3 days after birth up to 1 week	Physical assessment Health risk assessment	› Visual check of infant's skin, neurological status, primitive reflexes, vital signs › Ensure breastfeeding success/nutritional needs being met › Assess for hyperbilirubinemia › Assess bonding, stressors, and support
1 month, 2 months, 4 months, 6 months, 9 months, 12 months, 15 months, 18 months	Physical assessment Health risk assessment Anticipatory guidance	› Assess for health risks, growth, and development › Perform immunizations according to schedule › Check lead levels if indicated › Perform complete blood count (CBC) if anemia is suspected › Assess for neglect or child abuse
1 year	Dental assessment Speech assessment	› Dental assessment and referral should start at 1 year › Speech assessment begins at 1 year and continues at all subsequent visits
2–10 years		› Check immunization adherence › Assess for health risks › Assess for growth and development
≥ 11 years, annually to 21 years of age	Influenza immunization and other required immunizations such as meningococcal and tetanus vaccination Reproductive/sexual assessments and education, treatment, and care Breast self-exam and testicular cancer self-exam teaching Assessment of high-risk behaviors, substance abuse, depression and other mental health-related concerns	› Continue ongoing assessments for health risks, growth, and development

Data from American Academy of Pediatrics. (2016). 2016 recommendations for preventative pediatric health care. *Pediatrics, 137*(1), 25–27.

Understanding Physical and Anatomical Distinctions

One of the most important competencies for a pediatric nurse practicing in any clinical setting is knowing how the differences between children and adults affect nursing practice. There are several major differences between children and adults in terms of anatomy, physiology, growth, and development (see **Unique for Kids: Thirteen Differences Between Children and Adults**). Knowledge of these differences is essential to ensure the delivery of safe, holistic pediatric nursing care. Other pediatric nursing competencies include knowing how to apply anticipatory guidance, respond to pediatric emergencies, participate in teamwork, and engage in play. These competencies are described in detail in **Best Practices: Pediatric Nursing Competencies**.

UNIQUE FOR KIDS

Thirteen Differences Between Children and Adults

1. A child's airway is anatomically smaller and narrower than an adult's airway. The pediatric airway has a triangular shape, which renders children more susceptible to airway obstruction and compromise. A child's tongue is also disproportionally larger, further increasing the risk of airway obstruction.
2. Infants are obligate nose breathers for the first 8–12 weeks of life. Thus, it is important to suction to ensure patency when the infant is congested.
3. Infants have larger occipital cranial bones compared to adults. Place young infants (younger than approximately 1 year) experiencing pulmonary illnesses in a sniffing position so as to not occlude their airway.
4. Young infants have poorly developed intercostal muscles. Nurses should assess for respiratory distress and retractions. When these muscles become fatigued, an infant may experience respiratory compromise and distress or respiratory failure and require resuscitation efforts. Report and act on all presentations of intercostal retractions.
5. Children have less pulmonary tidal volume compared to adults, and may need oxygen when experiencing early respiratory distress due to pulmonary obstruction, inflammation, or secretions.
6. Children have an overall larger ratio of body surface to mass compared to adults. As a consequence, infants can experience heat loss readily. They should always be dressed warmly, and young infants should wear hats to prevent heat loss when exposed to environmental elements.
7. Children have less total circulating blood compared to adults. Any bleeding, especially occult (hidden) bleeds, should be identified. Repeated phlebotomy can cause a decrease in the young child's hemoglobin and hematocrit; only laboratory microcontainers should be used.
8. Children will compensate for dehydration, trauma with blood loss, and other insults to the cardiovascular system for a period of time, but then their blood pressure will drop rapidly. By comparison, adults demonstrate a longer period of cardiovascular demise. Children compensate first, and then their overall clinical picture deteriorates rapidly.
9. Children younger than 5 years have higher glucose needs than adults and minimal storage of glycogen in the liver, and should be offered frequent feedings or snacks to maintain their blood sugar levels. Infants have variability in gastric motility, gastric emptying, and gastric contents.
10. Children have higher metabolic rates and, in general, need more calories per kilogram of weight than adults do. Always calculate a child's kilocalorie needs per weight.
11. Children pose challenges in pain management, especially in terms of assessment. Use age/development-appropriate subjective and objective pain scales in conjunction with physiologic measurements of pain (e.g., vital signs, oxygen saturation) to thoroughly assess pain in children, and treat pain appropriately.
12. Young children are at risk for dehydration. It is important to use the pediatric fluid maintenance calculation to determine minimal daily fluid needs. Electrolyte blood values differ in the various age groups; narrow fluctuations in values can reflect dehydration and electrolyte imbalances. Frequently, fluid boluses are required to reverse moderate to severe dehydration.
13. An infant's skin is very thin and can easily absorb topical medications, creams, and ointments. It is important to use only those medications ordered and to apply a thin layer.

BEST PRACTICES

Pediatric Nursing Competencies

Pediatric nurses must be able to demonstrate the following competencies:

1. Gather essential and accurate information about the child and family throughout each developmental stage (prematurity, newborn, early infancy, late infancy, toddler, preschooler, early school age, later school age, and adolescence).
2. Perform a physical assessment of a child throughout the developmental stages, including assessment of respiratory, neurosensory, cardiovascular, metabolic, gastrointestinal, genitourinary, immunologic, and musculoskeletal status. Keep in mind the anatomic

(continues)

and physiological differences between children and adults while performing these assessments.

3. Perform developmentally appropriate emotional, cognitive, and social assessment throughout the developmental stages.
4. Assess a child's age/development-specific needs for nutrition, fluid maintenance, vital signs, laboratory evaluations, and immunizations.
5. Assess a child's developmental milestones, including play needs and abilities.
6. Accurately assess a child's pain using subjective and objective pain scales appropriate to the child's development as well as physiological measurements.
7. Assess and address the learning, emotional, social and spiritual needs of the family.
8. Assess and respect a family's cultural and ethnic background and needs and desires.
9. Assess, collaborate to assess, and report actual or suspected child abuse.
10. Address the needs of a family whose members are dealing with loss, grieving, trauma, and acute, chronic, or terminal illness.
11. Advocate for a family within all areas of health care and in all settings where care is provided, applying the principle of assent, and using developmentally appropriate communication techniques with all members of the family.

12. Apply family-centered care principles.
13. Assess and provide for a family's educational needs, including anticipatory guidance to prevent injuries, illness, or trauma.
14. Refer families in need to community resources at the local, regional, state, and national level (e.g., the American Cancer Society or Leukemia and Lymphoma Foundation).
15. Demonstrate pediatric nursing skills such as suctioning, maintaining an open airway, administering pediatric cardiopulmonary resuscitation, catheterizing, administering medications safely, maintaining infection control practices, performing phlebotomy with peripheral sticks and heel sticks, performing accurate measures of intake and output (e.g., weighing diapers), providing comfort holds or restraints during procedures, and inserting and maintaining intravenous lines.
16. Assess for concerns about safety in all settings (home, car, school, work) and across the various developmental periods, including discussion of appropriate discipline and the potential for self-harm or destructive behaviors during adolescence.

Data from the Society of Pediatric Nurses (www.pedsnurses.org), American Nursing Association (www.nursingworld.org), and California Organization of Associate Degree Nursing Program Directors (www.coadn.org/north/files/resource/98.pdf).

Anticipatory Guidance

Regardless of the clinical setting in which it takes, each well-child or illness visit provides an opportunity to give parents or guardians **anticipatory guidance**. Anticipatory guidance should include education, specific to the age of the patient, about the benefits of healthy lifestyles, practices that can help prevent injury (e.g., wearing helmets and other protective gear when participating in sports), and disease prevention. The child's or teen's entry into a new developmental stage offers an opportunity to provide education, support, and referrals related to opportunities for growth or areas of concern. Written educational handouts can be distributed that provide information on expected child behavior, physical development, emotional status, and other parental concerns. Various age-appropriate forms of anticipatory guidance are described in **Family Education: Anticipatory Guidance Across Settings**.

 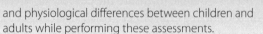

Anticipatory Guidance Across Settings

The following list includes ideas for areas of anticipatory guidance:

Infant
- Prevention of falls, aspiration, and choking
- When and how to introduce solid foods
- Play, stimulation, and sleeping needs
- Bath tub safety and drowning prevention
- Prevention of shaken baby syndrome and abusive head trauma
- "Back to sleep" to prevent sudden infant death syndrome

Toddler
- Nutrition and picky eaters
- Need for constant supervision
- Bath tub safety and drowning prevention
- Poison control numbers
- Choking hazards (e.g., food, toys, objects)

Preschooler
- Bicycle helmets
- Magical thinking
- Injury prevention

(continues)

- Socialization needs
- School readiness
- Media usage limits

School Age
- Mental health and identifying depression
- Socialization needs
- School success or problems
- Sports padding and safety equipment
- Healthful eating for overweight and obesity avoidance
- Exercise and sleep needs
- Sex education (begins at approximately age 11)
- Media usage limits
- Avoidance of smoking, drinking, and other unhealthy behaviors
- Reporting bullying

Adolescent
- Weight management
- Exercise
- Work/school balance
- Avoidance of smoking, drinking, drugs, and other unhealthy behaviors
- Sex education
- Driving safety
- Risk taking
- Reduction of media usage
- Reporting bullying
- Mental health and identifying depression
- Prevention of eating disorders

When providing anticipatory guidance, it is important to utilize strong communication skills. Some of the key points with respect to how this competency is managed are listed in **Family Education: Communicating Anticipatory Guidance**.

FAMILY EDUCATION

Communicating Anticipatory Guidance

- Use active listening techniques, talk slowly, use an interpreter as needed, and use simple nonmedical terms. Deliver handouts.
- Build trust, be kind, and be nonjudgmental.
- Recognize a "teachable moment" and jump on the opportunity.
- Use developmental assessments and observations to guide the teachable moment, including information from child development theory, expected milestones, social interactions between parent and child, and language development/skills.
- Assess for abuse, injuries, neglect, or any concerns that would prompt a "teachable moment."

Data from Schuster, M. A., Duan, N., Regalado, M., & Klein, D. J. (2000). Anticipatory guidance: What information do parents receive? What information do they want? *Archives of Pediatric and Adolescent Medicine, 154*(12), 1191–1198.

Communication Across Pediatric Clinical Settings

Communication is also a key competency for ensuring effective interactions among providers in situations where the child's care is being managed by a multidisciplinary team. Communication within the multidisciplinary pediatric healthcare team is imperative for safe and effective care of a child. Conducting a visual and physical assessment with a complete set of vital signs, head circumference (for children younger than 2 years), and weight, and then communicating areas of concern to the team rapidly and with clarity, can be lifesaving (see **Unique for Kids: Use of Anthropometric Measurements, Laboratory Testing, and Screening Across Settings**) (**Figure 2-3**). Taking the time to organize one's thinking before communicating concerns or deviations in the findings can lead to greater clarity of the information shared. Indeed, rapid communication using a thoughtful means of organization is now a practice promoted throughout healthcare institutions.

UNIQUE FOR KIDS

Use of Anthropometric Measurements, Laboratory Testing, and Screening Across Settings

- Growth charts (can be found at www.cdc.gov or www.nih.gov)
- Head circumference to monitor for increased intracranial pressure (ICP), space-occupying lesions, or failure to thrive
- Weight to monitor for failure to thrive or overweight/obesity risk
- Height to monitor for growth abnormalities and failure to thrive
- Abdominal circumference to monitor for overweight/obesity
- Ear canal check for otitis media and foreign objects
- Kilocalorie needs across the developmental periods
- Fluid maintenance calculation to implement dehydration prevention or fluid replacement
- Child maltreatment screening
- Blood pressure screening
- Laboratory testing for children
  - Lead toxicity
  - Complete blood cell count if anemia is suspected
  - Toxicology screens as needed for substance abuse if suspected
  - Vitamin deficiencies as required

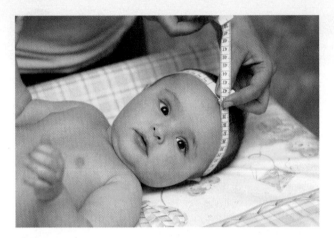

Figure 2-3

Effective Communication Within a Healthcare Team

Although the health science literature describes many communication techniques, those that have been validated may be considered most effective. Two examples of communication techniques that have been found to be effective are SBAR and CUS:

- *SBAR:* Situation, background, assessment, recommendation
- *CUS:* "I am *concerned* about. . .," "I am *uncomfortable* with. . .," "I think we have a *safety* issue. . ."

The **SBAR protocol** is a relatively simple set of steps that has been found to be effective for healthcare professionals in numerous settings (e.g., Cornell, Gervis, Yates, & Vardaman, 2014; Funk et al., 2016; Lancaster, Westphal, & Jambunathan, 2015). This protocol ensures the appropriate communication of key information and increases the efficiency of team interactions.

The **CUS protocol** is a means of encoding a level of concern by selecting key phrases that staff must be trained to recognize as indicating that a red-flag issue exists. Whereas SBAR is a formal process indicating how information is to be routinely communicated, CUS is intended as a means of communicating a need for heightened awareness or increased prioritization of the information embedded in the "trigger" words. Both protocols have been described as generally helpful in the literature; it benefits a nurse to learn and practice them in nearly every setting.

Huddles

A widely used method for intrateam communication is the **morning huddle**. This method involves setting a predetermined time each morning to discuss the day's schedule and clarify patient needs (**Figure 2-4**). Although a variety of processes may be followed for huddles, several key points make huddles effective:

- The format ensures that all interested parties are present to exchange information in a regular, organized fashion.
- Each patient's status and needs are reviewed daily.
- The huddle can be targeted toward specific areas of communication concern that need support, rather than reiterating communication that is already effective.

Handoffs

An area of specific concern with respect to communication is the handoff of patients from one provider to another, including shift-to-shift reporting within a department,

QUALITY AND SAFETY

When a child presents to a pediatric healthcare team, regardless of the clinical setting, the following clinical signs and symptoms should be reported *immediately* to the team:

- Respiratory distress, shortness of breath, increased work of breathing, and retractions
- Vital signs out of the expected value range
- Changes in perfusion such as delayed capillary refill time, decreased diastolic blood pressure, and evidence of dehydration
- Changes in level of consciousness, including lethargy
- Decreased oxygen saturation
- Significant pain
- Evidence of actual or suspected child abuse

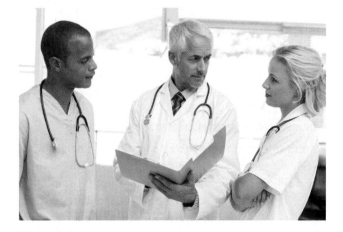

Figure 2-4

transferring a child between units or departments within a facility, and transferring a child from one facility to another. In such situations, those providers who are assuming control of the child's care need to be appropriately informed of the specific details of the child's condition in a clear, concise manner. The importance of effective communication during patient handoffs is paramount: Miscommunication or lack of communication during handoff has been identified as a precipitating factor in nearly one-third of all medical errors (Starmer et al., 2012).

Communication techniques that can be used to organize the information shared during handoffs should include three distinct phases (Riesenberg, 2012):

1. *Anticipation and preparation for the handoff* prework, including preparing the patient and the family for transitions and reviewing recent lab work, diagnostics, and outstanding orders.
2. *Actual handoff* of communication given in an organized and thoughtful way.
3. Transferring responsibility with an explicit *acknowledgment of the transfer of care*, including documenting the full name of the person receiving care of the child and family.

An example of an effective handoff mnemonic is **I-PASS** (Starmer et al., 2012), which identifies key points that *must* be reported by the transferring provider to the recipient provider to ensure adequate care:

I = Illness severity
P = Patient summary
A = Action list
S = Situation awareness and contingency planning
S = Synthesis by receiver

An especially important aspect of the I-PASS mnemonic is the last *S*—synthesis by the receiver. This stage offers an opportunity for the transferring provider to correct misunderstandings about the information provided (**Figure 2-5**).

Certification of Competency

Organizations such as the American Association of Colleges of Nursing, the American Nurses Association, and the Society for Pediatric Nurses provide lists of what are considered basic knowledge and skills competencies for practicing pediatric nurses. Keeping current in the ever-changing field of pediatrics is important to maintain awareness of contemporary issues in children's health. Most healthcare institutions require pediatric nurses to participate in mandatory annual skills competency workshops, a step that is intended to ensure that they maintain

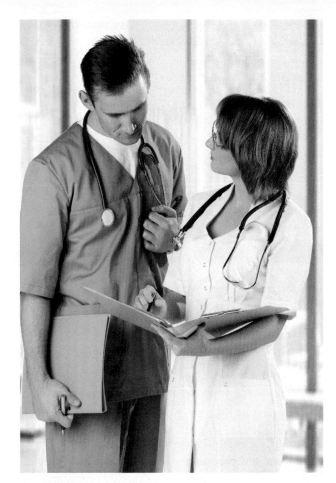

Figure 2-5

the knowledge and psychomotor skills required to be safe and competent in care.

Seeking national certification in pediatric nursing and associated specialty areas is highly beneficial for the pediatric nurse who seeks to demonstrate ongoing competency. Certification in pediatric nursing demonstrates a commitment, regardless of the clinical setting in which one practices, to a distinct body of knowledge that can be tested and recognized on a national basis. **Box 2-1** lists available pediatric nursing certifications.

Competencies According to Setting

Pediatric Nursing in Primary Care and Outpatient Settings

Most health care provided to children across childhood takes the form of wellness checks or minor illness care in outpatient settings such as clinics and physicians' offices. General care pediatrician offices provide the largest amount of care, followed by pediatric specialty clinics such as those run by pulmonologists, endocrinologists, and orthopedists.

Accordingly, clinic settings require emergency preparedness equipment and procedures; **Box 2-2** provides examples. Many children who require minor surgical procedures will receive care at outpatient (ambulatory) surgical centers. Since many of the newest technologies reduce the risk of adverse reactions, many minor surgeries can be performed in one day with explicit discharge care instructions for the parent or guardian.

Nurses working in primary care and outpatient settings need to perform appropriate physical and developmental assessments of the child as well as assess whether the child's and family's psychosocial, educational, spiritual, and emotional needs are being met. Care must be evidence based and comply with both established standards of ethical practice and Health Insurance Portability and Accountability Act (HIPAA) regulations. Sensitivity to cultural identity and advocacy for family self-determination are also important aspects of practice.

In the outpatient setting, nurses must be prepared to participate in patient care procedures and respond to unexpected changes in patient status, including initiating and participating in a code. Because complete cardiopulmonary arrests are uncommon in children, practicing pediatric emergency skills with a team approach can be lifesaving.

School Nursing

School nursing involves consultation and hands-on care for children in academic settings. The roles of the school nurse are to provide safety for all and to oversee the school district's health programs and policies, such as medication administration at school. Providing health education, health screenings, and serving as a liaison between the family, community, and school personnel are critical aspects of the school nurse's services. Given the close ties between academic performance and success and a child's health, the school nurse provides support, education, and programs to increase the health of the children within the academic setting.

According to the National Association of School Nurses (2016), there are five primary areas of specialized practice in the school nursing setting:

- Leadership in promoting health and safety, including promoting a healthy academic and community environment
- Expertise in facilitating growth and development, especially for those students with special needs
- Interventions for potential and actual healthcare problems and needs

BOX 2-2 Preparation for Emergencies: Equipment Required in All Clinical Settings

- Crash carts
- Printed algorithms to respond to various arrhythmias (code blue algorithms)
- Tanks of oxygen, regulators, and oxygen delivery systems
- Cardiopulmonary resuscitation (CPR) poster explaining this procedure for infants, children, adolescents, and adults
- Choking poster including guidelines to remove a foreign body

- Means to call 911 or another appropriate emergency response telephone number
- Emergency number for the American Association of Poison Control Centers (800-222-1222)
- Rapid Response Team's contact number
- Color-coded length-based emergency response tapes
- Defibrillator

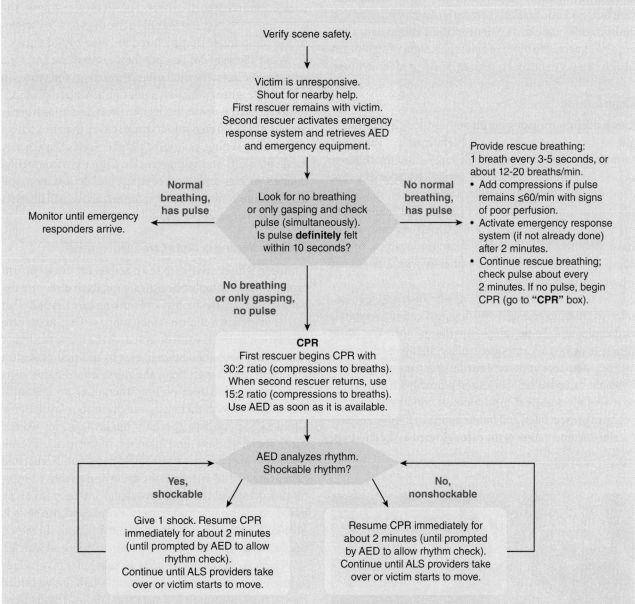

PALS Algorithm

- Clinical judgment in case management of services needed for children with individualized healthcare plans (IHPs) and clinical judgment in providing for emergencies
- Collaboration with interdisciplinary teams to build capacity for self-management, adaptation, advocacy, and learning

Nurses working in schools provide care and healthcare education, but are not expected to administer therapeutic care beyond basic first aid (barring emergencies) except as authorized by the child's parent and/or pediatrician. They are also expected to observe and report signs of significant health or safety concerns, such as abuse or malnutrition.

Camp Nursing

Camp nursing provides health support for children who attend day or overnight camps. Performed in a variety of settings, camp nursing can include care for healthy children or care for children with specific conditions. Specialty care camps include those for children with cancer, sickle cell disease, asthma, diabetes, HIV/AIDS, and many other medical conditions (**Figure 2-6**). Children's camps may have members of the medical team on location, or the camp nurse may communicate directly with a physician when concerns arise.

The camp nurse is in charge of administering medications to children and safely storing medications, supplies, and equipment. Some camps provide an infirmary, while others may have a camp nurse office. Being independent and organized are important attributes for any camp nurse. Often the camp has set policies and procedures for the nurse to assess for and treat mild medical conditions such as sunburns, insect bites, and minor injuries, all while keeping careful documentation of the care delivered to the children.

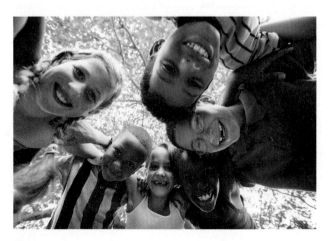

Figure 2-6

The Association of Camp Nurses (http://www.acn.org) provides guidelines on the scope of and standards for camp nursing practice. Providing campers with careful prescreening, directing camp counselors on ways to identify when nursing care is needed, using the nursing process, communicating effectively, and assessing for camp activities that may have increased injury risks are all part of the standards of practice. The camp nurse must be prepared to care for children with differing backgrounds, socioeconomic status, cultures, ethnicities, and ages. The camp nurse job may last for only a few days or a few weeks, or the camp nurse may be hired for year-round duties.

While the scope of practice for a camp nurse and for a school nurse has some similarities, the settings and venues in which these nurses work have some fundamental differences. Concerns such as drowning, hypothermia, and broken bones are more likely in an outdoor camp setting than in a school or day camp setting, calling for a higher level of emergency medicine skills and competencies. Other environmental injuries, such as sunburn, bee stings, and dehydration, will also be more common in the camp setting, as will illnesses such as urinary tract or respiratory infections.

Pediatric Nursing in Acute Care Environments

Children who receive care in an acute care environment typically have complex healthcare needs that require expanded medical treatments and nursing care beyond what can be offered in a clinic or ambulatory setting. **Acute care pediatric nursing** is team oriented, as the nurse facilitates the smooth implementation of care by multiple providers and team members. Often, the nurse coordinates visits and care provided by respiratory therapists, occupational therapists, physical therapists, nutritionists, play therapy/Child Life specialists, specialty nurses (e.g., for wound care), social workers, and members of the medical team. The acute care pediatric nurse implements family-centered care principles to ensure a satisfying and effective hospitalization for children, with providers' interactions being based on collegiality and respect. Families whose child is hospitalized may be experiencing stress and, therefore, need a team approach to reduce their anxiety and worries.

A typical assignment for an acute care nurse may include as many as four pediatric patients, although this workload may vary by institution and state regulations. The environment is demanding, fast-paced, and challenging. Children who are hospitalized in acute care settings have either an acute condition, such as appendicitis or bronchiolitis, or an acute episode of a chronic illness, such as asthma-related pneumonia. The pediatric acute care nurse provides nursing care, medical treatments, care coordination, communication with family, and frequent assessments while the child's condition remains guarded. When the child is ready to leave the hospital, extensive discharge teaching is often required for families and may help prevent readmissions for complications. After a thorough verbal explanation, the nurse should provide written discharge instructions to the family using simple terms and after securing assistance from an interpreter as needed.

Pediatric Nursing in Emergency Departments

Pediatric emergency department nursing is considered one of the most challenging areas of nursing care. Most of the patient care interactions stem from incidents involving injury or trauma; many cases present as life-threatening situations for the child. Immediate issues need to be assessed, diagnosed, and treated or triaged, even if the child presents with an illness versus an injury, accident, or trauma (**Figure 2-7**). Specialty training is required for pediatric emergency department nurses, including training in teamwork with air medical teams, ground medical teams, and other pediatric medical specialists.

Children who present to the emergency department have unique needs. They are inherently vulnerable, span ages and developmental stages from newborn through adolescence, and have to experience a fast-paced process of rapid care—diagnosis through treatment. According to Majumdar (2014), pediatric emergency room nursing requires the nurses to demonstrate the following abilities:

- Handle multifaceted cases of illness, injury, or trauma calmly while balancing the feeling of urgency related to the situation for the family
- Rapidly stabilize the child's clinical presentation
- Quickly implement diagnostic and treatment solutions
- Work within a fast-paced environment
- Administer correct nursing interventions and accurate medications, while reducing errors
- Master new skills and seek further knowledge/certification
- Be caring, patient, and supportive, and reduce stressors and anxiety for the patient and family
- Not feel heartbreak and despair when a child does not make it through a life-threatening illness, injury, or trauma

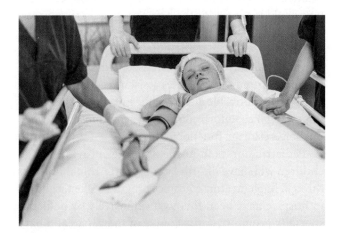

Figure 2-7
© Westend61 Premium/Shutterstock

Nursing in Pediatric Intensive Care Environments

Caring for pediatric patients in intensive care environments is a specialty practice requiring advanced training and experience (**Figure 2-8**). Because a child's clinical picture can change rapidly when the child is critically ill, nurses working in **pediatric intensive care unit (PICU)** or **neonatal intensive care unit (NICU)** environments must have the skills to rapidly assess and act on emergencies and severe conditions. Some healthcare organizations have adult intensive care unit (ICU) nurses who are cross-trained for pediatric intensive care and provide for children's needs within an adult ICU setting. Other, larger hospitals—mostly in urban environments—provide PICU beds and nurses who have specialty training and certification in caring for very ill children. An example of a specialty certification for PICU nurses is the Critical Care Registered Nurse (CCRN) certificate offered by the American Association of Critical-Care Nurses.

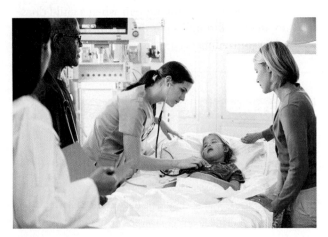

Figure 2-8

© Monkey Business Images/Shutterstock

QUALITY AND SAFETY

Preventing Injuries in Pediatric ICU Environments

Children with severe injury or illness who require a PICU stay are considered vulnerable. The following areas of concern must be addressed:

- Injury due to vulnerability of the child's health state, including severity of illness or injury
- Respiratory compromise and pulmonary tissue injury when ventilated
- Skin breakdown with prolonged bed rest
- Bloodstream infections due to placement of multiple invasive lines and central lines
- Nutritional deficiency if intubated on a ventilator or too ill to eat
- Pain and discomfort with repeated diagnostics, phlebotomy, and other procedures

- Family stressors, grief, and fear associated with PICU stay
- Adverse events due to the chaotic, complex, high-technological and fast-paced critical care environment

Safety Checklist for Pediatric Intensive Care Environment

KIDS SAFE mnemonic (Ullman, Long, Horn, Woosley, & Coulthard, 2013):

K = Kid's developmental needs, including coping, distraction, and minimizing stress

I = Infection; reducing the incidence with care bundles

D = Deep-vein thrombosis prophylaxis prevention

S = Skin integrity; preventing breakdown and pressure ulcers

S = Sedation; management of sedatives and their adverse effects

A = Analgesia to control discomfort and pain

F = Family; encourage involvement and provide family-centered care

E = Enteral needs; nutritional support, gastric ulcer prevention, enhancing immune function, and maintaining the integrity of the gut mucosa

Pediatric Nursing in Home Care Settings

Home care nurses provide assistance at home to maintain the continuum of care. Many provide care to pediatric patients who are discharged from the hospital with extensive medical needs. Parenteral nutrition, continuation of antibiotics, respiratory assessment, support, education, and follow-up can all be provided in the home setting. Infants with special needs such as phototherapy for hyperbilirubinemia, feeding tube care, tracheostomies, and mechanical ventilation can now transition from a hospital setting to home safely, with the assistance and expertise of a home health nurse. Focusing on the needs of all members of the household is a must for the home care pediatric nurse.

Pediatric Hospice Settings

The term **palliative care** is often used to describe the area of specialization that provides assistance so as to give the child the best possible quality of life by reducing suffering, improving discomfort, controlling symptoms, and, when possible, restoring functional capacity.

Pediatric nurses in hospice settings provide care to children who have life-threatening or terminal illnesses through implementing a hospice program. Often, children in hospice have been followed extensively by pediatric specialty groups over the course of their lives and have not successfully responded to medical treatment for a cure. Pediatric patients with cancer, those with cystic fibrosis, and infants with cardiac defects who do not respond to medical care and are experiencing impending death may all be cared for by a hospice team. Typically, the child has less than a 6-month life expectancy, and the care can be provided either at home or in a pediatric hospice center.

The hospice nurse provides direct care geared toward symptom management for children with life-limiting conditions. Support for the grieving family and bereavement care are offered to all of those involved with the child's care. The focus of **hospice nursing** care is on the comprehensive emotional, spiritual, psychosocial, and physical care of the terminally ill child and the family members. The hospice nurse works in close collaboration with a variety of health-care team members, including social workers, chaplains, physicians, and volunteers, to provide support and care to the child and family members.

Case Study

Stuart, a 14-year-old child with autism and moderate developmental delay, is being seen by the pediatric healthcare team in an outpatient setting for an annual check-up, influenza vaccine, diphtheria/pertussis/tetanus (DPT) booster, and ear wax removal. Stuart has a history of becoming frightened, agitated, and combative when he comes to the clinic for his appointments. Although he knows the entire staff, his behavior has become more difficult to manage as he gets older, as he has grown too large to be placed in comfort holds or blanket mummy wraps to reduce his agitation during procedures. Both parents have told the clinic schedulers that they will come in to provide assistance for the assessments and procedures. The outpatient staff performs their morning huddle and makes a plan for Stuart's visit.

Case Study Questions

1. What typically occurs during a "morning huddle" in the outpatient setting? Who attends the huddle?
2. How can the staff best prepare for Stuart's arrival in the outpatient setting? What will the parents' role be for his visit?
3. Which team members should be present for his visit?

As the Case Evolves. . .

Stuart has arrived for his appointment. Although his parents, who are divorced, had both said they would provide assistance at the appointment, Stuart's mother arrives with Stuart alone. Stuart's father called at the last minute to say he could not make it to the appointment. On cursory examination, Stuart appears restless but not overtly combative, and greets one of the staff by name.

4. Which of the following represents the best course of action to ensure that Stuart's examination can proceed safely?
   A. Perform a safety sweep of the examination room to ensure there are no hazardous items that could cause injury if Stuart becomes combative.
   B. Ensure the presence of emergency airway supplies such as suction, valve/bag/mask resuscitative equipment and oxygen as well as a crash cart and back board.
   C. Call staff together for a "huddle" to discuss how to address the change in the approach originally developed for the visit.
   D. Ask Stuart's mother to reschedule the visit for a time when both parents can be present.

Stuart is being examined by the staff at his pediatrician's office, who note Stuart has cold symptoms and a slightly elevated temperature and recommend delaying vaccination until he is well. The exam is uneventful until the attempt at ear wax removal. Upon being approached by the nurse with instruments for wax extraction, Stuart becomes agitated and uncooperative, sticking his fingers in his ears to block them. His mother states her concern that Stuart might have an ear infection, because he has said to her that his ears hurt and has had previous ear infections.

5. Which of the following should the nurse consider as the priority in caring for this client?
   A. Confirming a diagnosis of ear infection without being able to see inside the ear
   B. Adequately medicating for pain based on a child's subjective report of pain
   C. Empiric use of antibiotics to treat an infection that cannot be confirmed
   D. Educating the patient about the consequences of putting fingers or other objects in his ears

Chapter Summary

- Pediatric nursing care can occur in a variety of settings, including acute care and intensive care environments, emergency departments, outpatient clinics and observation/surgical centers, school settings, home care settings, hospice, and day and overnight camps.
- According to the Society of Pediatric Nurses, basic competencies required in pediatric nursing include a health history and physical assessment of the child during each developmental stage. Cognitive, social, nutritional, pain, and emotional assessments should also be performed.
- Effective team communication is a key nursing competency. Opportunities for communication include morning huddles and handoffs. Helpful tools include the SBAR, CUS, and I-PASS protocols.
- The application of family-centered care principles attends to the needs of the family, regardless of the clinical setting.
- Safety across clinical settings should include referral of families to needed community resources at the local, regional, state, and national levels. Safety is confirmed through active assessment of families' needs and referral to organizations that provide continuous care.
- Nurses can choose to obtain competency certification in a variety of specialties, such as diabetes education, wound care, oncology, or critical care.
- The majority of nurses work in settings outside of traditional hospital care. These venues include schools, camps, acute care and other clinics, emergency departments, home care, and hospice settings.

Bibliography

American Academy of Pediatrics (AAP). (2001, November). The role of the school nurse in providing school health services. *Pediatrics, 108*(5). Retrieved from http://pediatrics.aap publications.org/content/108/5/1231

American Academy of Pediatrics. (2016). 2016 recommendations for preventative pediatric health care. *Pediatrics, 137*(1), 25–27.

American Nursing Association. (2015). *Scope and standards of practice: Pediatric nursing* (2nd ed.). Silver Spring, MD: Nursesbooks.org.

Bond, G. R., Woodward, R. W., & Ho, M. (2011). The growing impact of pediatric pharmaceutical poisoning. *Journal of Pediatrics, 160*(2), 265–270.

Cohen, L. L., Lemanek, K., Blount, R. L., Dahlquist, L. M., Lim, C. S., Palermo, T. M., . . . Weiss, K. E. (2008). Evidence-based assessment of pediatric pain. *Journal of Pediatric Psychology, 33*(9), 939–955.

Cornell, P., Gervis, M. T., Yates, L., & Vardaman, J. M. (2014). Impact of SBAR on nurse shift reports and staff rounding. *Medsurg Nursing, 23*(5), 334–342.

Funk, E., Taicher, B., Thompson, J., Iannello, K., Morgan, B., & Hawks, S. (2016). Structured handover in the pediatric postanesthesia care unit. *Journal of Perianesthesia Nursing, 31*(1), 63–72.

Hartman, R. (2012). Minimum pediatric clinical competencies. Retrieved from http://www.coadn.org/north/files/resource/98.pdf

Institute for Healthcare Improvement. (n.d.). Use regular huddles and staff meetings to plan production and to optimize team communication. Retrieved from http://www.ihi.org/resources/Pages/Changes/UseRegularHuddlesandStaffMeetingstoPlanProductionandtoOptimizeTeamCommunication.aspx

Kling, J. (2011, September 16). Pediatric drug poisoning on the rise. *Medscape Medical News*. Retrieved from http://www.medscape.com/viewarticle/749820

Kohn, L. T., Corrigan, J. M., & Donaldson, M. S. (Eds.). (2000). To err is human: Building a safer health system. Committee on Quality of Health Care in America, Institute of Medicine. Retrieved from http://www.nap.edu/catalog/9728.html

Lancaster, R. J., Westphal, J., & Jambunathan, J. (2015). Using SBAR to promote clinical judgment in undergraduate nursing students. *Journal of Nursing Education, 54*(3 suppl), S31–S34.

Lubinensky, M., Kratzer, C. R., & Bergstol, J. (2015). Huddle up for patient safety. *American Nurse Today, 10*(2). Retrieved from http://www.americannursetoday.com/huddle-patient-safety/

Majumdar, A. (2014). Role of pediatric emergency nursing. Retrieved from http://www.multibriefs.com/briefs/exclusive/role_of_pediatric_emergency_nursing.html#.VbESpsnT31U

National Association of School Nurses. (2016). The role of the 21st century school nurse. Retrieved from https://www.nasn.org/PolicyAdvocacy/PositionPapersandReports/NASNPositionStatementsFullView/tabid/462/ArticleId/87/The-Role-of-the-21st-Century-School-Nurse-Adopted-June-2016

Riesenberg, L. (2012). Shift-to-shift handoff research: Where do we go from here? *Journal of Graduate Medical Education, 4*(1), 4–8.

Safe Kids Worldwide Media Center. (2014, March 12). Every 8 minutes a child goes to an emergency room for medicine poisoning. Retrieved from http://www.safekids.org/press-release/every-8-minutes-child-goes-emergency-room-medicine-poisoning

Safe Kids Worldwide Media Center. (2016, March). The rise of medicine in the home: Implications for today's children. Retrieved from http://www.safekids.org/research-report/rise-medicine-home-implications-todays-children-march-2016

Schuster, M. A., Duan, N., Regalado, M., & Klein, D. J. (2000). Anticipatory guidance: What information do parents receive? What information do they want? *Archives of Pediatric and Adolescent Medicine, 154*, 1191–1198.

Starmer, A. J., Spector, N., Srivastava, R., Allen, A., Landrigan, C. P., Setish, T., & I-Pass Study Group. (2012). I-PASS: A mnemonic to standardize verbal handoffs. *Pediatrics, 129*(2), 201–204.

Ullman, A., Long, D., Horn, D., Woosley, J., & Coulthard, M. (2013). The KIDS SAFE checklist for pediatric intensive care units. *American Journal of Critical Care, 22*(1), 61–69.

U.S. Department of Health and Human Services. (2015). Health information privacy. Retrieved from http://www.hhs.gov/ocr/privacy/

Von Baeyer, C. L. (2006). Children's self-reports of pain intensity: Scale selection, limitations and interpretation. *Pain Research & Management: The Journal of the Canadian Pain Society, 11*(3), 157–162.

Design credits: Magnifying Glass, Open Book, and Checkmark icons designed by Freepik from Flaticon; Clipboard designed by Vectors Market from Flaticon; ABC Blocks designed by Prosymbols from Flaticon.

Safety in Caring for Children and Families

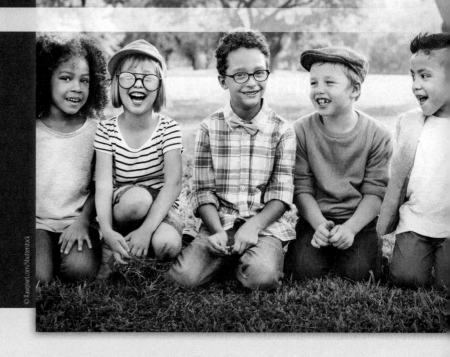

© Rawpixel.com/Shutterstock

CHAPTER 3 Essential Safety Models

Essential Safety Models

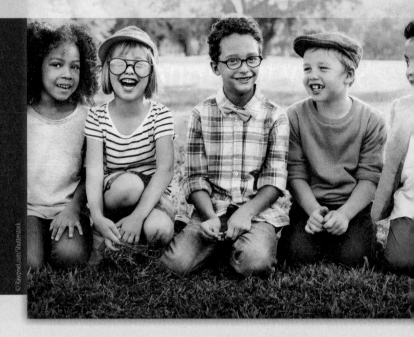

© Rawpixel.com/Shutterstock.

LEARNING OBJECTIVES

1. Apply the goals of national safety initiatives for children and their families in nursing practice.
2. Analyze how the Quality and Safety Education for Nurses (QSEN) competencies relate to direct care of children across clinical settings.
3. Incorporate safety principles into anticipatory guidance offered to parents, educators, and caregivers.
4. Analyze and apply principles of safety in the various nonclinical settings such as the home, school, daycare, and play areas.
5. Identify and apply setting-specific methods to reduce the frequency of medical and medication errors in pediatric nursing care across settings.
6. Identify and apply methods to both prevent the major types of errors in pediatric care and reduce the impact of these errors on families if they do occur.
7. Evaluate how various communication tips and concept thinking can provide a safer environment for children across clinical settings, including handoff protocols and mnemonics.

KEY TERMS

Concept-based learning
Evidence-based practice
Holistic
Informatics
Mnemonics
Quality and Safety Education for Nurses (QSEN)
Special needs

Introduction

The concept of safety within pediatrics is a key component of **holistic** (i.e., caring for the whole person, including not only his or her medical condition, but also any mental, social, and environment concerns) and comprehensive pediatric nursing care. Young children are inherently unsafe and require more than just supervision; that is, they require safe environments in which to play, grow, develop, and thrive. They require responsible adults to provide anticipated safety measures at home and in day-care, school, and playground settings, and they require an emerging sense of safety within that manifests as safe decisions as they mature. Neither infants nor young toddlers can be expected to understand what is "safe" and what is "unsafe," but by a child's third birthday, there should be a basic understanding that certain behaviors will put the child in harm's way.

Many national organizations have developed safety guidelines for children of all ages. Pediatric nurses are in the unique position of being able to discuss safety regardless of the clinical setting in which they see a patient. The Society of Pediatric Nurses, American Academy of Pediatrics, and Association of Critical Care Nurses all promote safety as a high priority. Being an excellent safety role model is one of the most important responsibilities of the pediatric nurse, so as to teach families, caregivers, teachers, and children what is and is not safe, and how to plan for safety (advice given as part of anticipatory guidance). The pediatric nurse is instrumental in demonstrating safe care for children all across the developmental period, including those with **special needs** (i.e., disabilities in medical, psychological, or mental functioning that affect a child's development), such as developmentally disabled or medically fragile children. This chapter discusses pediatric safety concerns and provides guidance on how to plan ahead for safe environments for children.

National Safety Initiatives

Every year, a staggering number of children experience significant unintentional injuries. Children are exposed to a large number of risks and hazards while they grow, learn, and explore their environments (**Figure 3-1**). Notably, their inexperience and curiosity contribute to many childhood injuries. Most injuries across childhood occur in the following general areas:

- Falls
- Burns related to heat and fire
- Motor vehicle accidents as either a pedestrian or a passenger
- Suffocation, asphyxiation, or choking

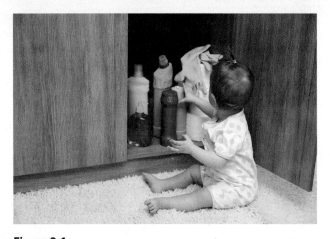

Figure 3-1

© Africa Studio/Shutterstock

- Drowning or near drowning
- Sports, recreation, and related injuries
- Poisoning

Multiple national safety initiatives have been created to provide a safety structure for those persons caring for children. Each year, approximately 9 million children seek care in U.S. emergency departments for injuries; 225,000 children require hospitalization for injuries; and 9000 children die (Centers for Disease Control and Prevention [CDC], 2015). Both governmental bodies and professional organizations have published guidelines to conceptualize and anticipate safety concerns for children.

QSEN Competencies

One of the most recently introduced national initiatives for nurses on safety across the lifespan is **Quality and Safety Education for Nurses (QSEN)**. The QSEN project was launched in 2005 to address some of the challenges encountered when trying to prepare nurses for professional practice (Cronenwett et al., 2007; Dolansky & Moore, 2013; Sherwood & Zomorodi, 2014). The project, which is funded by the Robert Wood Johnson Foundation, focuses on the knowledge, skills, and attitudes needed to consistently and continuously improve the practice of professional nursing. Multidisciplinary teams worked collaboratively to create guidelines for six competencies: patient-centered care, **evidence-based practice** (best practice based on the integration of clinical expertise, scientific evidence, and the patient's and family's perspectives), quality improvement, teamwork and collaboration, **informatics** (the application of information and computer science to health care), and safety. The founders partnered with organizations that represent current practice and proposed a set of knowledge, skills, and attitudes required for safe nursing education and practice. **Table 3-1** summarizes the main safety competencies within this initiative.

TABLE 3-1   QSEN Competencies: A Summary of Application to Pediatrics

1. **Patient-Centered Care**: Recognizes the family as a full partner in care and the source of control for the child, and provides compassionate coordinated care based on a foundation of the child's and family's needs, preferences, and cultural practices/values.

   Knowledge: Pain theory, ethics, legal implications, effective communication principles, cultural care, care for specific forms of special medical or behavioral needs.

   Skills: Assessment of pain or suffering, providing emotional support, coordinating care needs, applying effective treatments and nursing interventions, facilitating informed consent, resolving conflicts, recognizing the need for boundaries, and providing comprehensive safety.

   Attitudes: Valuing partnerships; acknowledging tension; appreciating shared decision making; respecting individual expressions of values, needs, and preferences; and recognizing the need to continuously improve one's own conflict and communications skills.

2. **Evidence-Based Practice**: The investigation, application, and integration of the best current evidence found for the improvement of clinical expertise and family preferences.

   Knowledge: Know the scientific research process, apply principles of literature searching and critiquing, secure reliable and reputable sources of information, and discriminate between best published practices and current clinical practice.

   Skills: Apply skills of data collection, research review, criticism, and protocol revision.

   Attitudes: Appreciate scientific-based practice and the importance of frequent assessment of relevant and accessible knowledge.

3. **Quality Improvement:** Consistently monitor outcomes of care and use methods of change to improve all aspects of the safety and quality of healthcare systems.

   Knowledge: Learn about outcome theory, recognize the parts of systems that can be reviewed, validate processes of outcome measurements, and learn how to approach making changes in care within systems.

   Skills: Use the outcomes of quality improvement projects, participate in such projects, identify gaps in best practice, and apply new skills to care scenarios.

   Attitudes: Appreciate the importance of quality improvement projects, value measurement skills, and be open to change.

4. **Teamwork and Collaboration:** Within nursing and interprofessional teams, the nurse functions effectively, fosters strong open communication, promotes mutual respect, and applies the principles of shared decision making to the team members and to the combination of the family and team members.

   Knowledge: Describes the scope of practice, the roles of team members, and personal strengths and limitations, and understands the impact of team function and communication on the outcome of patient safety and quality of care provided.

   Skills: Initiates a plan for self-improvement, functions within the scope of practice, integrates the skills and contributions of team members, and solicits input from members of the care team.

   Attitudes: Appreciates the importance of teamwork, values the perspectives of others, and respects team members' unique attributes.

5. **Informatics**: Communicate using information technology that assists with managing knowledge and supports decision making.

   Knowledge: Understand the importance of information and technology, describe how technology and information management improve quality and safety, and understand the time and skill needed to effectively use the tools.

   Skills: Seek information and technology skill improvements, navigate the technology using the assistance of others, and use the information generated to understand and improve patient outcomes.

   Attitudes: Appreciate the need for lifelong learning that continuously provides opportunities for improvement and change, and value the care coordination, error prevention, safety improvements, and decision making that information and technology provide.

(continues)

6. **Safety**: Maximize assessment of safety issues and minimize risk of harm to patients.

  Knowledge: Describe unsafe practices (poor communication, use of do-not-use abbreviations, and work-arounds), discuss strategies to effectively reduce reliance on memory, and describe factors that promote a culture of safety for individuals, teams, and healthcare systems.

  Skills: Use technology, practice new methods of error reduction, communicate unsafe practices, engage in root-cause analysis, and participate in designing safe systems.

  Attitudes: Value the creativity and contributions of safety measures, value the nurse's own role in error prevention, and value vigilance, monitoring, and implementation strategies.

Data from QSEN Institute. (2014). Pre-licensure KSAs. Retrieved from http://qsen.org/competencies/pre-licensure-ksas

Thinking in Concepts to Promote Safety

Applying the QSEN competencies to pediatrics provides a holistic foundation for safety, but the care of children also requires a thinking process whereby the nurse reflects on the knowledge needed to predict a child's care requirements; the skills required to provide safe, evidence-based holistic care; and the attitudes assumed by a pediatric nurse who is committed to change and improving quality and safety in all aspects of care. Given the vast amount of knowledge that a pediatric nurse must have to function with competency and safety, nurses can feel overloaded with information. The application of **concept-based learning**—a dynamic approach to the ever-growing body of scientific nursing knowledge that focuses on learning key concepts that can be applied to various situations and settings—promotes building a mental bridge between large quantities of factual knowledge and conceptual understanding. These bridges allow one to rely less on facts and more on organizing concepts that create mental links. Instead of memorizing facts and trying to retrieve them, the nurse uses concepts to quickly link and integrate information within patient scenarios to provide "the big picture." Safety as a concept is widely used to promote a cascade of thinking about identifying harm, reducing errors, and promoting safety. Thinking conceptually about safety allows the nurse to readily transfer existing knowledge to an actual clinical situation (**Figure 3-2**).

  Safety, as a concept, reflects the many needs of a person. By studying exemplars of clinical situations and thinking through the components of safety present in those scenarios, the nurse can improve his or her rapid application of integrated safety knowledge. For instance, if a nurse encounters a child with developmental delay who has a new postoperative incisional wound, cannot provide basic care for herself, and requires many treatments and medications, the nurse can use the concept of safety to think about all of the safety concerns that might arise for the child. These concerns include the

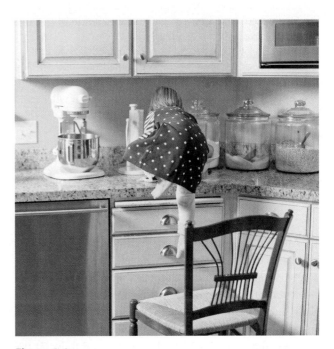

Figure 3-2
© Tetra Images/Shutterstock

following questions: What is the best way to prevent the child from touching the wound or pulling out sutures in light of her developmental delay? How can the child's caretakers best avoid medication errors or interactions in the medications used for her postsurgical therapy—and what are the potential risks of such mistakes? How can the nurse ensure that the child's pain is adequately treated in light of her special needs? How can these concerns be addressed both in the clinical setting and in the home after the child is discharged? Using safety as a concept in care should trigger a cascade of potential and actual concerns for the child. When such a conceptual lens is not used, the nurse must rely on memorization and superficial thinking and is unlikely to develop the deeper understanding that accompanies integrated thinking (Miller, 2012).

Another safety issue present in contemporary pediatric nursing is the identification of neglect. Children can suffer safety issues associated with intentional or unintentional neglect of their basic needs. According to Mennen, Kim, Sang, and Trickett (2010), child neglect is most prominent in families who are considered child welfare clients. Neglect for these high-risk families was found to be 71.0% with 95% of the cases associated with other forms of child maltreatment. Pediatric nurses must associate cases of child neglect with other forms of safety issues and assess for other forms of child abuse.

Model of Thinking: Basics of Safety During Specific Developmental Stages

Children between 1 and 4 years of age and adolescents age 15 and older have the highest rates of accidental injuries in the United States. According to the CDC (2016), boys are twice as likely as girls to die from accidents associated with unintentional injuries. The younger the child, the greater the chance the injury will be related to transportation (pedestrian, motor vehicle, or bicycles) or related to drowning or burns. Infants and toddlers are at greater risk for aspiration, choking, or poisoning deaths. Young children have newly mastered locomotion, yet have no real sense of danger versus safety—factors that put them at high risk of accidents.

Injury prevention and safety education for families based on the child's specific developmental stage is a nursing imperative. Such education should also incorporate the special needs of children with intellectual or physical disabilities. **Table 3-2** lists injury prevention topics based on developmental stage that should be discussed with families.

Identifying and Addressing Safety Issues in the Community

A child's environment can be a source of safety concerns. Industrialized areas contain hazards in the air, water, and soil. Urban households in high-traffic zones may be exposed to automobile-related hazards due to both increased risk of pedestrian accidents and poor air quality. The pediatric nurse must assess a family's concerns about the environment in which the child lives (**Figure 3-3**). Areas to assess include the following:

- *Water contamination.* Water contamination is a global concern for children. In the United States, contaminated well water is a threat monitored by the National Institute of Environmental Health (Mishamandani, 2015). Arsenic-, lead-, and mercury-contaminated water can affect a child's cognitive development and behavior. Dirty and contaminated water is considered the planet's biggest health threat to children (National Resources Defense Council, 2015).
- *Lead poisoning.* Children can be exposed to lead through water, food, air, deteriorating paint, dust, and contaminated soil. Although use of lead is now banned in both gasoline and paint products, lead poisoning remains a serious safety concern owing to lead's persistent presence in the soil, old paint, industrial emissions, and air. Health effects of lead exposure may include delays in mental and physical development, increased behavioral problems, and short attention span. Younger children are more sensitive to the damage of lead exposure as their bones grow and tissues are more susceptible.
- *Air quality.* According the U.S. Environmental Protection Agency (2017), millions of children live in areas where air quality poses potential and actual serious threats to their health with low-income families and communities of color being at high risk. Air pollution is linked to development of bronchitis and asthma, with these conditions being especially prevalent in urban areas with heavy traffic (Milligan, Matsui, & Sharma, 2016). Asbestos—a mineral fiber used in building construction materials, insulation, and fire-retardants—has detrimental health effects as well. Second-hand smoke poses serious health risks for children in both the short

TABLE 3-2 Developmental Stage–Related Injury Prevention

Young Infants

› Prevent aspiration and choking by diligently stopping the infant from reaching toys smaller than the diameter of the center of a toilet paper roll.

› Keep plastic bags away from their reach.

› Strap infants down for diaper changes; never leave an infant on a surface where the child could roll and fall.

› Do not ever drink hot liquids while holding an infant.

Older Infants

› As infants become mobile, prevent falls and injuries related to stairs and poisonings as they move and explore their environments.

› Never leave a child unattended in a high chair, shopping cart, or motor vehicle.

› Make sure older infants are provided with foods that they can eat safely. Do not give hard foods such as carrots, and chop soft foods up into very small pieces.

Toddlers

› Prevent falls, drowning, electrical burns, and heat burns by providing constant supervision while the child is awake, at play, and outside.

› Do not allow toddlers to climb on surfaces or chairs to reach desirable items.

› Use safety gates, window guards, cabinet locks, and toilet seat locks throughout their environments.

› Turn pot handles toward the back of the stove.

› Do not allow toddlers near unsupervised pets.

› Have toddlers wear helmets while learning to ride a tricycle.

› Do not leave electrical appliances plugged in and do not let electrical cords hang down.

› Teach toddlers what "hot" and "danger" mean.

Preschoolers

› Teach preschoolers about car/pedestrian safety.

› Require preschoolers to consistently wear safety devices such as helmets, padding, and straps.

› Never call medicine "candy."

› Continue to use safe barriers, safety gates, and locked cabinets.

› Teach animal safety.

› Teach and practice saying "no" to others when in an uncomfortable situation or environment.

School Age

› Teach school-age children fire safety.

› Keep matches stored in a safe area.

› Insist on seat belt safety and sports safety devices.

› Teach about car safety, stranger safety, and animal safety.

› Practice a fire escape plan and a natural disaster plan.

› Teach Internet safety.

Adolescents

› Role model safety, as teens will mimic and follow what adults do in most situations. Wear seat belts, do not participate in substance abuse, and do not smoke.

› Talk frankly with teens about sex, drugs, alcohol, and risk taking.

Special Needs

› Identify safety concerns particular to the mental, emotional, or physical impairment of a special-needs child (e.g., the need for a 504 Plan or individualized education plan [IEP] in school).

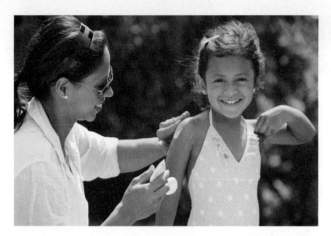

Figure 3-3
© Amble Design/Shutterstock

and long terms; notably, it is directly linked to development of ear infections, bronchitis, asthma, and sudden infant death syndrome (SIDS) (Treyster & Gitterman, 2011).

- *Sun exposure.* Most lifetime sun exposure occurs in the first 18 years of life. Children must be protected from the harmful consequences of lengthy sun exposure and sunburns, as these events are directly linked to development of skin cancer, premature aging, inflammation of the cornea and conjunctiva of the eye, accelerated cataract development, and effectiveness of the immune system (World Health Organization, 2001).

RESEARCH EVIDENCE

Well Water Contamination and Intelligence

The U.S. Environmental Protection Agency has found that children who are exposed to drinking water containing levels of arsenic greater than 5 μg/L experience a reduction of 5–6 points in most aspects of measured intelligence. Arsenic, which is naturally found in the groundwater in certain geographic areas, can have serious health consequences for children, including increasing their risks of neurodevelopmental disruption, diabetes, and cardiovascular disease (Wasserman et al., 2014).

Safety at Home

Children live in a variety of settings—rural, farm, urban, and suburban. Socioeconomic factors play a large role in determining the safety of the environment in which a child lives. Unsafe neighborhoods where crime, drug trafficking, and unemployment levels are high create greater safety concerns for children. According to the National

Center for Children in Poverty (2016), in 2014, 32% of U.S. children lived in a family at the poverty level—defined as a household with income less than $24,008 per year for a family of four. Forty-eight percent of children live in low-income families.

Clinicians should be aware of and screen for the many health and safety issues related to poverty (Chung et al., 2016). Families from lower socioeconomic backgrounds may have safety issues associated with their residence in lower-income neighborhoods, exposure to crime, and risk of substance abuse (Consumer Federation of America [CFA], 2013). Lower-income homes may lack supervision, as not all working parents can afford complete childcare coverage. Children from lower-income households also have more chronic illnesses such as asthma (Clark et al., 2015), reduced access to routine preventive health care (Center for Poverty Research, 2014), and greater risk of unintentional injuries generally as well as specifically from pedestrian, fire, burn, drowning, and fall injuries than do other children (CFA, 2013). Poverty exacerbates concerns such as food insecurity and exposure to environmental hazards such as lead paint, which may affect child development (Chung et al., 2016).

The pediatric nurse should be aware of the various resources available within the community and refer families in need to specific community organizations that can provide needed assistance. These resources may include low-cost childcare services or early childhood education programs such as Head Start, public health clinics, low-cost immunization clinics, community-based safety fairs, food banks, and community kitchens where free or low-cost meals can be secured.

RESEARCH EVIDENCE

Children who have been diagnosed with attention-deficit/hyperactivity disorder (ADHD) are at a much greater risk of injury than children without ADHD, as they are distracted quite easily and experience more motor vehicle-versus-pedestrian accidents. Research has shown that although they may follow curbside behaviors, children with ADHD are at a higher risk due to their failure to process safety factors while crossing streets and are especially prone to choosing small traffic gaps while crossing (Nikolas et al., 2016).

One major concern for families who cannot afford after-school care is "latchkey" children, referring to children who are not supervised by a responsible adult after school. The percentages of latchkey children have been reported as 2% of 8-year-olds, 4% of 9-year-olds, 6% of 10-year-olds, 11% of 11-year-olds, and 14% of 12-year-olds (Bureau of

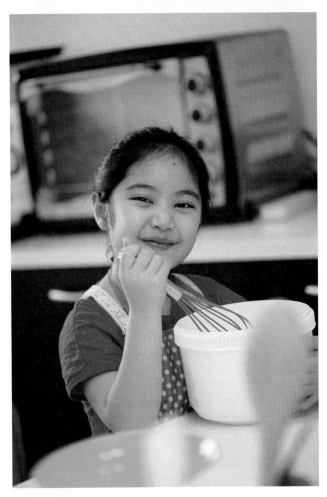

Figure 3-4

© Ronnachai Palas/Shutterstock

the Census, 1991). Approximately 10% of children age 4–12 years in 2013 spent 3 or more hours alone on each school day, and 51% of latchkey children showed poor academic performance (Lant, 2013). Latchkey children have increased safety risks, including unsafe food preparation and cooking, unsupervised computer play, unsupervised social contacts, and emotional concerns such as fear, loneliness, stress, and feelings of abandonment (**Figure 3-4**). Overall, they are twice as likely to participate in drugs and sexual activity as children who have adult after-school supervision (Lant, 2013).

One model of safety proposed for latchkey children includes the following measures to decrease their risks (Lant, 2013):

- Have consistent contact times during the unsupervised time at home.
- Have unannounced visits or come home early without notice.
- Assign chores and praise the child for completing responsibilities.
- Ask a trustworthy neighbor or friend to be a backup.
- Reinforce self-protection by locking windows and doors.
- Keep keys handy but out of sight (do not wear house keys around neck).
- Provide and support after-school activities.
- Set clear rules as to what is expected regarding friends, food preparation, screen time, and homework.
- Set controls for media, TV, and computers.

Creating a safe home environment for children is considered paramount, though the specific risks differ to some extent for boys and girls. Girls typically experience injuries within the house (burns, falls, and bodily injury), whereas boys experience injuries outside or in garage or storage areas (burns, suffocation, drowning, and bodily injury). Preparing the home environment requires understanding the physical and mental capacities of children across the developmental period. Emergency preparedness, fire safety (**Table 3-3**), and knowledge about medication safety are key areas where families need

TABLE 3-3   Prevent Burns Through Fire Safety
› Teach the family a fire escape plan and practice fire drills as a family.
› Keep the fireplace clean and safe with tight-fitting screens or doors.
› Keep fire extinguishers up-to-date and check their expiration dates annually.
› Know how to use a fire extinguisher.
› Use safe, reliable, and double-checked smoke detectors in each room.
› Store lighters, matches, candles, and cigarettes away from children.
› Store gasoline or any flammable substances away from children, heat, and sparks. Do not store them in accessible locations.
› Keep children out of the kitchen while cooking, use safety gates as needed, and cook on the back burners only.
› Do not store food in cabinets above the stove or oven.
› Keep children away from gas or charcoal grills or outdoor fireplaces or pits.
› Teach children how to "stop, drop, and roll," and practice this technique often.

anticipatory guidance, as these issues affect all children. For example, an estimated 500,000 children younger than 5 years of age accidentally ingest medications each year. Approximately 15% of these victims end up in the emergency department—one child every 8 minutes—and 70% of these patients are children age 2 years or younger. (Safe Kids Worldwide, 2012a, 2012b)

A study in the *Journal of Pediatrics* examined more than 540,000 cases of children younger than age 5 who were treated in an emergency department for medicine poisoning over a period of 8 years. Nearly 95% of single-agent poisonings were self-administered—that is, the child ingested medications kept in an unsafe location such as an open bottle, open purse, bathroom counter, kitchen counter, table, or shelf—and 55% involved prescription medications belonging to a parent or grandparent, such as oral hypoglycemic agents, opioids, and sedatives. The authors concluded that the inadequacy of safety measures intended to keep medications out of children's hands was a significant factor in these outcomes (Bond, Woodward, & Ho, 2011).

Children are at high risk for emergency hospitalizations when they have access to and ingest prescription medications in the home (Lovegrove, Mathew, Hampp, Governale, Wysowski, & Budnitz, 2014).

FAMILY EDUCATION

Home Preparation for Emergencies

- Keep a clear and easy-to-read large-print record of emergency numbers, including phone numbers for law enforcement, poison control, the local hospital, pediatricians, 911, and a local taxi service.
- Have all members of the family who are old enough take cardiopulmonary resuscitation (CPR) classes; recertify often.
- Keep emergency flashlights, matches, and candles handy but out of reach.
- Keep a well-stocked first-aid kit.
- Take the American Red Cross first-aid course; recertify often.
- Maintain an appropriate emergency supply box in case of flood, fire, earthquake, or other regional emergency. Stock this box with water, food, clothes, space blankets, candles, matches, medications and copies of prescriptions, extra eyeglasses, pet supplies, and solid shoes for all members of the family.
- Know the location of the gas, water, and electrical emergency shut-off switches.
- Teach children how to call 911.
- Have a family plan for where to meet and how to reach one another if an emergency happens.

Prevention of Poisonings at Home

- Post the poison control center's number by the phone and near poisonous materials and substances (**800-555-1212**).
- Keep medications in the original child-proof containers—never in unlabeled pill organizers or in purses, briefcases, or other storage areas where children are interested and have access.
- Do not ever call medications "candy."
- Store all chemicals, cleaning agents, and paint supplies in locked cabinets.
- Keep all plastic bags (kitchen, dry cleaning, and packaging materials) away from children.
- Keep potentially harmful materials and substances in their original packaging with clear labels, and make sure they have tight child-safety lids.
- Materials such as cleaners, vinegar, or bleaches with ammonia should never be used or stored together.
- Keep poisonous and toxic substances locked up *and* out of reach of children.
- Do not store gasoline in the garage.
- Be consistent with children about not touching anything stored, locked, or dangerous.

Medications and Substances for Poisonings

Recommendations are to call the poison control center (**800-222-1222**) for guidance.

- *Ipecac syrup* is an emetic that, when taken with a quantity of water, induces vomiting. Its long shelf life has left many households with the medication available, but it is not recommended for poisonings.
- *Charcoal* is an adsorbent used in patients with intact airways to adsorb (bind) toxic substances in the stomach. After charcoal is ingested, a nasogastric tube should be used to lavage the toxin or substance as rapidly as possible.

FAMILY EDUCATION

Motor Vehicle Restraints: Applying Safety Across Childhood

Anticipatory guidance on state car seat laws is one of the most important discussions that can take place between a pediatric nurse and the families the nurse serves. Motor vehicle accidents (MVAs) are a leading cause of injury and deaths for children between 1 year and 12 years of age. Of the 638 children younger than 12 who died from MVAs in 2013, nearly 40% were not wearing seat belts (CDC, 2013).

Numerous resources are available for explaining to parents how car restraints should be used for different age groups.

(continues)

Websites such as http://www.dmv.org and https://www.safercar.gov/parents/index.htm clarify a multitude of safety issues related to children in and around cars. In addition, numerous YouTube videos show how to install car seats correctly, and many local police or fire departments are willing to inspect car seats and assist parents with their correct installation. Nurses should keep a list of such resources available for guiding parents.

Talking to Parents About Car Safety

- Children should not be left alone in a car if the keys are in the ignition.
- Children younger than age 7 should never be left in a car without a person who is at least 12 years old.
- Drivers must be careful to "look before they lock," as heatstroke from leaving a quiet or sleeping child in a locked car with the windows up can be fatal.
- Children need to be taught about blind zones because of the risk of "frontovers" and "backovers"; discuss the blind zones of a car.

Parents must know how to properly and safely install a car seat. Double-checking that the car seat or booster seat is belted into the car, and not just the child into the car seat, can save lives.

Safety at Daycare Centers and Schools

Daycare programs, preschools, and schools should all be a safe place for children to play, learn, and thrive. Each setting, whether private or public, should have safety procedures that are written down and periodically reviewed. Nurses can be instrumental in reviewing facilities, playgrounds, procedures, sports equipment, and safety devices for safety deficiencies. Playgrounds should have shade, soft padding under climbing structures, safety fences to prevent wandering or intruders, and supervision between classes and during breaks and recesses. Policies should include safety procedures for when children are departing the facility, whether accompanied by a parent, riding on a school bus, or walking or biking home by themselves. Policies should also cover caring for an injured child and protocols for administering first aid; at least some personnel supervising children should have specific first aid and CPR training. Emergency phone numbers for fire, poison control, and 911 calls for ambulance and police should be posted in all rooms of all buildings. Policies against bullying, violence, drugs, smoking, and alcohol should be enforced.

Safety at Play

Children need guidance and supervision while at play. Nurses, in turn, should provide support and anticipatory guidance to families concerning safe play. Each developmental stage is associated with its own set of fine and gross motor milestones, and play activities can promote the achievement of those milestones. Promoting safety during play includes being aware of the potential injuries or accidents that can occur, and providing rules and structure to prevent them. The following list outlines concerns that should be anticipated during play:

- Children must consistently wear protective gear and helmets (e.g., during skateboarding, biking, snow sports, contact sports, and extreme sports).
- Supervision must be provided to prevent deviations from sports rules (e.g., young children swimming without life vests or safety floatation devices).
- Climbing structures should be free of splinters, loose screws, or nails, and should have padding or soft material underneath for protection during falls.
- Children should not be allowed to play on equipment, bikes, or other devices not made for their age or developmental level (e.g., toddlers on skateboards).

Safety in Clinical Settings

Hospitals

Hospitals are inherently unsafe places for children. Hospital environments are often fast-paced, chaotic, filled with acutely or critically ill patients, busy with a host of healthcare professionals, and populated with complicated security measures. It is the pediatric nurse's priority to provide a safe environment to hospitalized children—and doing so effectively takes concerted effort (**Figure 3-5**). Environmental sweeps for safety concerns need to be conducted on every shift, and prompt reporting of unsafe conditions,

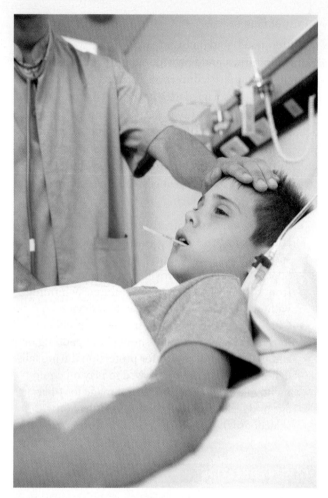

Figure 3-5

© PhotoAlto/Laurence Mouton/PhotoAlto Agency RF Collections/Getty

Rates of Medical and Medication Errors in Pediatric Care

Medical errors are responsible for more deaths among adults and children alike than motor vehicle accidents, according to Bleich's (2005) report from the Commonwealth Fund. While the majority of medication errors occur in adults—as many as 14 errors per 100 doses—children experience from approximately 2.3 to 6 adverse drug events per 100 hospital admissions (Sharek & Classen, 2006). Pediatric medication doses must be calculated using a weight-based measurement (such as milligrams per kilogram or milligrams per body surface area) and double-checked for safety. Due to the need to calculate doses individually for children, pediatric patients are up to three times more likely to experience "near-miss" errors (Kaufmann, Laschat, & Wappler, 2012; Kaushal et al., 2001).

Some pediatric institutions require that all medications administered to children be subjected to double-checking by nursing staff members against documentation and electronic/written signatures (**Figure 3-6**). Examples of medications/infusions for which pediatric registered nurses may be expected to double-check the rights of medication administration (right patient, drug, dose, time, and route) include the following therapies:

- Cardiac medications such as antihypertensives and antiarrhythmics (digoxin)
- Blood products
- Insulins and hypoglycemics
- Total parenteral nutrition and intralipids
- Chemotherapies and any medications associated with cancer treatments

broken equipment, or safety breaches is required. It is everyone's responsibility to prioritize safety for children in the hospital. Young children are particularly vulnerable to adverse effects as they explore their environment and test limits (**Table 3-4**).

Four major issues have been identified that put hospitalized children at greater safety risks (Lacey, Smith, & Cox, 2008):

- A child's fluid developmental status, as new milestones are implemented and boundaries are tested
- The dependency level inherent to children, especially the nonverbal status of young children
- An acute (rather than chronic) episode, which leads to a higher level of required care
- Poverty, racial, and ethnic disparities, which place children at greater risk for poor outcomes

Other concerns inherent to hospitalization of children include medical errors, medication errors, communication errors, falls, injuries, abductions, and poor outcomes directly linked to hospital staffing.

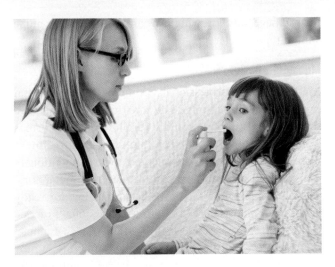

Figure 3-6

© Ermolaev Alexander/Shutterstock

- Anticoagulants
- Electrolytes
- Narcotics

Types of Errors in Pediatric Care

In general, medication errors in pediatrics can be classified into one of four categories:

- Acts of omission
- Acts of commission
- Scheduling misperceptions
- Noncompliance on the part of the family or child

Omissions are errors where a team member did not do or provide something for a child that should have been implemented. Omitting a dose of antibiotic, forgetting to open the clamp on an intravenous electrolyte replacement solution to correct a significant serum depletion, and missing a prescribed application of a topical steroidal anti-inflammatory drug are all errors of omission.

Acts of commission occur when a pediatric team member does something in error to a child that was not supposed to happen. Examples include treating a child for a condition that the child has not been diagnosed with and administering a medication to a child who does not have a standing order for this therapy.

Scheduling misperceptions involve the incorrect timing of a medication or treatment, such as administering a pain medication before it is due or administering an antibiotic to a child recently transferred from the emergency department who just received the medication in the emergency department (i.e., giving the medication too soon after the last dose). Compliance concerns may arise regarding whether the family participated in administering a medication or treatment as it was ordered, or whether the family filled a prescription that was ordered for a child.

According to McDowell, Ferner, and Ferner (2009), medication errors can be thought of as having a "pathophysiology" in that errors can be classified in one of many types: when an *action* that was intended to take place is not performed; when errors take place due to inadequate knowledge known as a *mistake*; when a well-formulated plan is not executed *(slip)* and an *erroneous act* or lapse of the plan occurs; or when *inaccurate calculation* of the required dose occurs. These authors stress that healthcare systems are complex and errors occur at various stages and steps of orders, communication, preparation, and administration.

Impact of Errors in Pediatric Care

Young children are inherently vulnerable, as they do not question or monitor their care. The impact of errors on young children exceeds the effects on adults, with such errors causing more harm and having a more significant impact on pediatric patients' safety. Children need to be protected from errors, and pediatric nurses must adhere to safety protocols to ensure that the risks of errors are reduced. The implementation of electronic order entry and computerized medication administration programs (scanning) has reduced the number of errors, but communication remains the single most important factor in errors involving pediatric patients. Reducing the impact of errors in the pediatric population requires individual dedication, team effort, and institutional commitment.

BEST PRACTICES

Reducing Miscommunications and Errors by Using Handoff Bundles

Handoff bundles have been shown to reduce medical errors in pediatric healthcare settings by reducing miscommunication. In research conducted by Starmer et al. (2014), the use of a standardized communication tool, handoff training, team handoff structure, and a verbal mnemonic reduced errors from 33.8 errors per 100 admissions to 18.3 errors per 100 admissions. Use of the SIGNOUT? mnemonic was recognized as a key factor in the improved rates, along with a "patient summary," "to-do list," and "contingency planning." The SIGNOUT? mnemonic, which was developed by Horwitz, Moin, and Green (2007), includes the following elements:

S = Sick? Do not resuscitate? Unstable?

I = Identifying data, gender, weight, age, and diagnosis

G = General course of hospitalization

N = New events of the day, including vital signs, diagnostics, lab results, and medications

O = Overall health status/clinical condition

U = Upcoming possibilities, with their plan and rationale

T = Tasks to complete, plan, rationale, and time frame

? = Any questions? Concerns?

Communication Tips

Thorough professional communication in the field of pediatrics will reduce the chance of errors. Areas where communication mishaps are prone to happen include handoffs between caregivers (also known as handovers, sign-offs, and shift reports) and handoffs between units or departments, such as between the emergency department and the nursing unit, or between the nursing unit and the radiology department. Handoffs include not only the communication of essential care information, but also the transfer of primary responsibility and authority for the child. Consistently using a formal handoff format that provides structure, critical information, and safety assurance is a best practice for minimizing errors. Conversely, insufficient handoffs may cause safety breaches and failures in safe care.

for each age, and knowing how and to whom the nurse should report a change.

Mnemonics for Safety

Many healthcare professionals promote the use of mental mnemonics to encourage safe practice. **Mnemonics** are memory tools used to rapidly recall complex information, sets of steps for skills, or components of treatment plans. Most mnemonics are intended to help practitioners either recall information or recall steps of behaviors. These tools promote safety in that they allow for ready recall of standards agreed upon in professional practice (Hagerman, Varughese, & Kurth, 2014). CAB is an example; it is used to recall the first three steps of cardiopulmonary resuscitation—compression, airway, breathing. The **Best Practices: Using Mnemonics** feature highlights this kind of memory tool for double-checking use of medications in children.

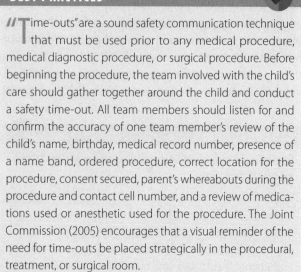

BEST PRACTICES

"Time-outs" are a sound safety communication technique that must be used prior to any medical procedure, medical diagnostic procedure, or surgical procedure. Before beginning the procedure, the team involved with the child's care should gather together around the child and conduct a safety time-out. All team members should listen for and confirm the accuracy of one team member's review of the child's name, birthday, medical record number, presence of a name band, ordered procedure, correct location for the procedure, consent secured, parent's whereabouts during the procedure and contact cell number, and a review of medications used or anesthetic used for the procedure. The Joint Commission (2005) encourages that a visual reminder of the need for time-outs be placed strategically in the procedural, treatment, or surgical room.

One of the most important aspects of promoting safety for children is rapidly identifying any change in the patient's clinical status, and then rapidly reporting the change to the proper physician for guidance or orders. Children's conditions can change very abruptly; thus, an important skill for nurses is the ability to quickly assess a child and discover a change in clinical status, and then know when and to whom to report this change. Safety in pediatric nursing is based on skills that are tailored toward children, including knowing the expected average vital signs

BEST PRACTICES

Using Mnemonics

An example of a mnemonic that assists with a child's safety is one used to remember which medications, at a minimum, should be double-checked by two licensed caregivers. (Some institutions will have additional requirements, so the nurse should always check the specific institution's policy.) The mnemonic D'BITCH'EN can be used to remind a caregiver which categories of medications should be doubled-checked with a second nurse:

D = Digoxin or any heart medication

B = Blood products of any kind, including red blood cells, platelets, plasma, intravenous immunoglobulin (IVIG), and clotting factors

I = Insulins and oral hypoglycemics

T = Total parenteral nutrition and lipids

C = Chemotherapeutics and any medication given as part of cancer treatments, including oral prednisone or intravenous steroidal anti-inflammatory drugs

H = Heparin or any anticoagulant

E = Electrolytes given to replace serum values or given as a treatment, such as magnesium for intractable asthma symptoms

N = Narcotics or any pain medication that has the potential to cause altered mental status, respiratory depression, or any other significant symptoms

Case Study

At a home-based toddler care program, a 2-year-old boy was playing in the backyard with 12 other children. Three supervising adults were engaging in play with the other toddlers. The young boy ran along the side of the home, over to some trashcans that had collected water during a recent rainstorm. The child threw a toy into one of the cans, and then scrambled up onto a bush next to the trashcan so he could climb in and retrieve the toy. The child fell into approximately 9 inches of water; he was quickly found but was unconscious.

Emergency medical personnel were called and brought to the scene. The child was resuscitated at the site and brought into the local emergency department, where his heart rate after administration of epinephrine was found to be 50 beats per minute, his respiratory rate was 8 breaths per minute, and his blood pressure was 72/30 mm Hg. The child was admitted into the pediatric intensive care unit (PICU) and quickly placed on a ventilator for respiratory support. The child's admitting diagnosis was hypoxic ischemia encephalopathy, also known as a "near-drowning."

Case Study Questions

1. State the safety breaches found within the home-based toddler care program described in the scenario.
2. What are the immediate needs of the family during the child's emergency room stay and transfer to the PICU?

As the Case Evolves...

Following the near-drowning incident in this case study, the facility's owner seeks training for employees to prevent similar incidents from happening again.

3. Which of the following represents an appropriate level of intervention to improve the safety profile of the facility?
   A. A nurse should visit the facility and perform a safety sweep of the facility yard to identify hazards.
   B. Recommend to the facility's owner that all employees be provided with training in first aid and CPR on a regular basis, at least annually.
   C. A nurse should create a binder of educational resources to give to the facility's owner so that employees can be offered safety training when they are first hired.
   D. All of these actions described should be offered to the facility as part of a comprehensive and ongoing training program.

The toddler in this case study is being cared for in the PICU. To the parents' relief, initial indications are that the child was resuscitated quickly enough to avoid severe neurologic injury. However, less than 24 hours after admission, a nurse monitoring the child notices that he has developed a low-grade fever just before she is due to go off shift.

4. Which of the following actions represents an appropriate response to ensure the child's safety in the PICU when the nurse goes off shift?
   A. Note the change and the time of observation on the child's chart and recommend administration of antibiotics.
   B. Verbally communicate that the child has developed a fever to another nurse coming in on the next shift.
   C. Formally hand off the child to the next-shift nurse using both verbal and written forms of communication, including all background information, current status, and concerns raised by the change in status.
   D. Remain for 1 hour after the shift ends to ensure that the child's status does not further deteriorate.

Chapter Summary

- Safety is a critical issue in holistic and comprehensive pediatric nursing care. Young children are inherently unsafe and require more than supervision; that is, they require safe environments in which to play, grow, develop, and thrive.
- Many national organizations have developed safety guidelines for parents of children of all ages, including the American Academy of Pediatrics and the Society of Pediatric Nursing.

- The Quality and Safety Education for Nurses (QSEN) project was created to address challenges encountered when trying to prepare nurses for professional safe practice. This program focuses on the knowledge, skills, and attitudes needed to consistently and continuously improve the practice of professional nursing while providing a foundation of safety.
- Safety as a concept is widely used to trigger a cascade of thinking about identifying harm, reducing errors, and

promoting safety. Thinking conceptually about safety allows the nurse to transfer existing knowledge about this issue to an actual clinical situation.

- Injury prevention and safety education for families across developmental stages is a nursing imperative.
- Neither infants nor young toddlers can be expected to understand what is "safe" and what is "unsafe." By a child's third birthday, however, children should have some understanding that certain behaviors will put them in harm's way.
- Children require responsible adults to provide anticipated safety measures at home, in daycare or school facilities, and on playgrounds, and they require an emerging sense of safety within that manifests as safe decisions as they mature.
- Lower household income is associated with a number of safety issues and risk factors that clinicians should understand, assess, and help families to mitigate through available resources.
- Pediatric nurses are in a unique position to offer anticipatory guidance to parents and caregivers about safety for children. Safety must be ensured in play, school, and home environments, and nurses should provide education on measures to achieve this goal.
- In pediatric clinical settings, thorough professional communication will reduce the risk of errors. Areas that are especially prone to communication mishaps include handoffs between caregivers and handoffs between units or departments.
- One of the most important aspects of promoting safety for children is the rapid identification of a change in clinical status, followed by the rapid reporting of the change to the proper physician for guidance or orders.
- Many healthcare professionals use mental mnemonics as means to encourage safe practice. Mnemonics allow recall of standards agreed upon in professional practice.

Bibliography

Bleich, S. (Commonwealth Fund). (2005). Medical errors: Five years after the IOM report. Retrieved from http://www.commonwealth fund.org/usr_doc/830_Bleich_errors.pdf

Bond, G. R., Woodward, R. W., & Ho, M. (2011). The growing impact of pediatric pharmaceutical poisoning. *Journal of Pediatrics, 160*(2), 265–270.

Bureau of the Census. (1991). Statistic brief: Who is minding the kids? Retrieved from www.census.gov/prod/2013pubs/p70-135.pdf

Center for Poverty Research, University of California, Davis. (2014). How is poverty related to access to care and preventive healthcare? Data from the Centers for Disease Control. Retrieved from http://poverty.ucdavis.edu/faq/how -poverty-related-access-care-and-preventive-healthcare

Centers for Disease Control and Prevention (CDC). (2013). Child passenger safety: Get the facts. Retrieved from http://www.cdc .gov/motorvehiclesafety/child_passenger_safety/cps-factsheet.html

Centers for Disease Control and Prevention (CDC). (2015). Injury prevention & control: Protect the ones you love: Child injuries are preventable. Retrieved from https://www.cdc.gov/safechild

Centers for Disease Control and Prevention (CDC). (2016). Protect the ones you love: Child injuries are preventable. Retrieved from https://www.cdc.gov/safechild

Chung, E. K., Siegel, B. S., Garg, A., Conroy, K., Gross, R. S., Long, D. A., . . . Fierman, A. H. (2016, April 18). Screening for social determinants of health among children and families living in poverty: A guide for clinicians. *Current Problems in Pediatric and Adolescent Health Care.* [Epub ahead of print]. pii: S1538-5442(16)00034-1. doi: 10.1016/j.cppeds.2016.02.004

Clark, N. M., Lachance, L., Benedict, M. B., Little, R., Leo, H., Awad, D. F., & Wilkin, M. K. (2015). The extent and patterns of multiple chronic conditions in low-income children. *Clinical Pediatrics (Philadelphia), 54*(4), 353–358. doi:

Consumer Federation of America (CFA). (2013). Child poverty, unintentional injuries, and foodborne illness: Are low-income children at greater risk? Retrieved from http://www.consumerfed .org/pdfs/Child-Poverty-Report.pdf

Cronenwett, L., Sherwood, G., Barnsteiner, J., Disch, J., Johnson, J., Mitchell, P., . . . Warren, J. (2007). Quality and safety education for nurses. *Nursing Outlook, 55*(3), 122–131.

Dolansky, M. A., & Moore, S. M. (2013, September 30). Quality and Safety Education for Nurses (QSEN): The key is systems thinking. *Online Journal of Issues in Nursing, 18*(3), Manuscript 1.

Hagerman, N. S., Varughese, A. M., & Kurth, C. D. (2014). Quality and safety in pediatric anesthesia: How can guidelines, checklists, and initiatives improve the outcome? *Current Opinion in Anaesthesiology, 27*(3), 323–329.

Horwitz, L., Moin, T., & Green, M. (2007). Development and implementation of an oral sign-out skills curriculum. *Journal of General Internal Medicine, 22*(10), 1470–1474.

Joint Commission, International Center for Patient Safety. (2005). Strategies to improve hand-off communication: Implementing a process to resolve questions. Retrieved from http://www.jci patientsafety.org/15274

Kaufmann, J., Laschat, M., & Wappler, F. (2012). Medication errors in pediatric emergencies: A systematic analysis. *Deutsches Ärzteblatt International, 109*(38), 609-616.

Kaushal, R., Bates, D. W., Landrigan, C., McKenna, K. J., Clapp, M. D., Federico, F., & Goldmann, D. A. (2001). Medication errors and adverse drug events in pediatric inpatients. *Journal of the American Medical Association, 285*, 2114–2120.

Lacey, S., Smith, J. B., & Cox, K. (2008). Pediatric safety and quality. In R. G. Hughes (Ed.). *Patient safety and quality: An evidence-based handbook for nurses* (Chapter 15). Rockville, MD: Agency for Healthcare Research and Quality. Retrieved from https://www .ncbi.nlm.nih.gov/books/NBK2662

Lant, K. (2013). Latchkey kid: Make home-alone time happy and healthy. Retrieved from http://www.education.com/magazine /article/latchkey-kid

Lovegrove, M. C., Mathew, J., Hampp, C., Governale, L., Wysowski, D. K., & Budnitz, D. S. (2014). Emergency hospitalizations for unsupervised prescription medication ingestions by young children. *Pediatrics, 134*(4), e1009–e1016.

McDowell, S. E., Ferner, H. S., & Ferner, R. E. (2009). The pathophysiology of medication errors: How and where they arise. *British Journal of Clinical Pharmacology, 67*(6), 605–613.

Mennen, F. E., Kim, K., Sang, J., & Trickett, P. K. (2010). Child neglect: Definition and identification of youth's experiences in official reports of maltreatment. *Child Abuse & Neglect, 34*(9), 647–658.

Miller, S. (2012). Concept-based curriculum to transform nursing education. Retrieved from http://www.mynursingcommunity .com/wp-content/uploads/2012/04/Considering-a-concept -based-curriculum.pdf

Milligan, K. L., Matsui, E., & Sharma, H. (2016). Asthma in urban children: Epidemiology, environmental risk factors, and the public health domain. *Current Allergy and Asthma Reports, 16*(4), 33.

Mishamandani, S. (2015). Summit addresses safe drinking water from private wells. *Environmental Factor.* National Institute of Environmental Health Sciences. Retrieved from https://www .niehs.nih.gov/news/newsletter/2015/12/spotlight-water

National Center for Children in Poverty. (2016). Basic facts about low-income children. Children under 18 years, 2014. Retrieved from http://www.nccp.org/publications/pub_1145.html

National Resources Defense Council. (2015). Water. Retrieved from http://www.nrdc.org/water

Nikolas, M. A., Elmore, A. L., Franzen, L., O'Neal, E., Kearney, J. K., & Plumert, J. M. (2016). Risky bicycling behavior among youth with and without attention-deficit hyperactivity disorder. *Journal of Child Psychology and Psychiatry, 57*(2), 141-148.

Quality and Safety Education for Nurses (QSEN). (2015). QSEN competencies. Retrieved from http://qsen.org/competencies /pre-licensure-ksas

Safe Kids Worldwide. (2012a). New research reveals medications are the leading cause of accidental poisoning deaths among children today. Retrieved from https://www.safekids.org/press -release/new-research-reveals-medications-are-leading-cause -accidental-poisoning-deaths-among

Safe Kids Worldwide. (2012b). Safe storage, safe dosing, safe kids: A report to the nation on safe medication. Retrieved from https:// www.safekids.org/research-report/safe-storage-safe-dosing-safe -kids-report-nation-safe-medication-march-2012

Sharek, P., & Classen, D. (2006). The incidence of adverse events and medical errors in pediatrics. *Pediatric Clinics of North America, 53*(6), 1067–1077.

Sherwood, G., & Zomorodi, M. (2014). A new mindset for quality and safety: The QSEN competencies redefining nurses' roles in practice. *Journal of Nursing Administration, 44*(10), S10–S18.

Starmer, A,. Spector, N., Srivastava, R., West, D., Rosenbluth, G., Allen, A., . . . Landrigan, C. (2014). Changes in medical errors after implementation of a handoff program. *New England Journal of Medicine, 371*(19), 1803–1812. doi: 10.1056/NEJMsa1405556

Treyster, Z., & Gitterman, B. (2011). Second-hand smoke exposure in children: Environmental factors, physiological effects, and interventions within pediatrics. *Reviews on Environmental Health, 26*(3), 187–195.

U.S. Environmental Protection Agency. (2017). Air pollution: Current and future challenges. Retrieved from https://www.epa.gov/clean -air-act-overview/air-pollution-current-and-future-challenges%20

Wasserman, G. A., Liu, X., LoIacono, N. J., Kline, J., Factor-Litvak, P., van Geen, A., . . . Graziano, J. H. (2014). A cross-sectional study of well water arsenic and child IQ in Maine schoolchildren. *Environmental Health, 13*, 23.

World Health Organization, Unit of Radiation and Environmental Health. (2001, July). Protecting children from ultraviolet radiation: Fact Sheet No. 261. Retrieved from http://www.who.int.uv /resources/fact/en/fs261protectchild.pdf

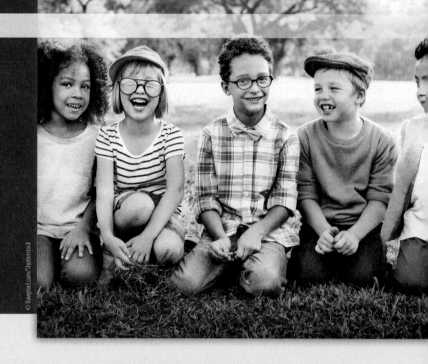

UNIT III

Models of Care

CHAPTER 4

Cultural and Religious Influences to Care

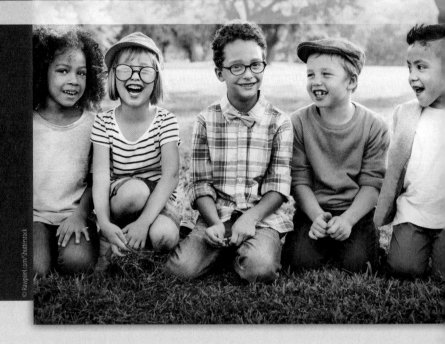

© Rawpixel.com/Shutterstock

LEARNING OBJECTIVES

1. Apply the concept of cultural care to children and their families.
2. Analyze the National Standards for Culturally and Linguistically Appropriate Services in Health Care developed by the Department of Health and Human Services Office of Minority Health as they pertain to pediatric nursing and family-centered care.
3. Discuss how culture, ethnicity, spirituality, and religious beliefs influence health and health care for children and their families.
4. Compare the merits of cultural diversity assessment tools and incorporate these tools in healthcare practice.
5. Apply cultural awareness, cultural sensitivity, cultural humility, and cultural competence across pediatric healthcare settings.
6. Examine religious influences on pediatric and family care (including treatment decisions) and identify specific religious faiths whose doctrines influence care (e.g., Christian Scientists, Jehovah's Witnesses, evangelical Christian, Orthodox Jew, Roman Catholic).
7. Analyze how disparities in healthcare outcomes relate to a family's culture, ethnicity or race, and sociopolitical or spiritual/religious beliefs.

KEY TERMS

Cultural assessment tools
Cultural awareness
Cultural beliefs
Cultural competence
Cultural diversity
Cultural humility
Cultural intelligence
Cultural sensitivity
Culture
Disparities of health outcomes
Ethnicity
Health literacy
Healthcare disparity
National Standards for Culturally and Linguistically Appropriate Services in Health Care (CLAS)
Race
Religion
Spirituality

Introduction

The United States continues to attract immigrants from all over the world. Over the years, demographic changes linked to immigration and differing birth rates have produced a culturally diverse population of patients as well as culturally diverse healthcare practitioners within the country (**Table 4-1**); this diversity can have a considerable impact on the implementation of health care and on the healthcare industry as a whole (Department of Finance, 2013; Hearnden, 2008; Laves, Reclose, & Seaway, 2008; Wilson-Stronks & Murtha, 2010). According to Leong, Wieland, and Dent (2010), their cultural backgrounds influence the behavior of both patients and providers, regardless of the healthcare setting in which they interact. Notably, differences in their cultural preferences and communication styles require individuals to listen carefully and negotiate and, through this process, to understand and overcome barriers related to their communication patterns.

Both the demographic changes and the increasing diversity of the U.S. population also compel healthcare providers to commit to improving culturally competent care. **Cultural competence** entails first developing an awareness of one's own cultural preferences and practices, and then respecting and accepting the cultural preferences and practices of others (Flowers, 2004).

Cultural preferences, factors related to their ethnic backgrounds, and religious and spiritual beliefs add richness to the interaction between a family and a healthcare provider. Both culture and ethnic diversity tend to produce exciting new perspectives on worldviews, art, music, emotional expression, beauty, family life, health practices, birth and death rituals, and expression (**Figure 4-1**). Sometimes, however, cultural and religious influences on healthcare decision making may result in ethical dilemmas and create a "storm" between families and healthcare providers (Linnard-Palmer, 2006). Such ethical dilemmas are especially likely to arise when a certain belief system leads to

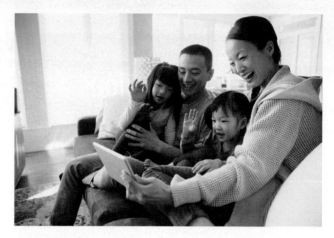

Figure 4-1

© Hero Images/Getty

a delay in treatment, refusal of treatment, or preferences to limit medical treatment for a child. A lack of understanding and non-appreciation of cultural influences in a healthcare setting can lead to negative patient outcomes, including higher risk of making medical errors, profound financial implications, and a widened healthcare disparity gap (Bagchi, Ursin, & Leonard, 2012; Laves et al., 2008). According to EthnoMed (2015), Harborview Medical Center's ethnic medicine website, "It is important to remember that simply because a person is identified as a member of a particular ethnic group or religion [it] does not necessarily mean that the person or the person's family has the set of beliefs that may be associated with the ethnicity or religion."

Pediatric nurses are in a unique position to influence healthcare outcomes through careful cultural assessments, negotiations, and culturally sensitive communication, as the amount of time they spend directly with patients and families, regardless of the setting, far exceeds that committed by other healthcare providers. Therefore, it is critical for a pediatric nurse to understand the cultural preferences and cultural communication patterns of

TABLE 4-1 Cultural Diversity
Cultural diversity is a term that refers to many groups defined on bases other than those that distinguish traditional cultural or ethnic groups:
› Sexual orientation, such as lesbian, gay, bisexual, pansexual, androsexual, skoliosexual, asexual, or questioning
› Gender identity, such as transgender, nonbinary, or fluid
› Deaf culture, representing those with hearing impairments
› Physical disabilities, such as the "wheelchair culture"
› Geriatric identity, representing the needs and perspectives of the older generation
› Adolescent identity, representing the struggles, concerns, desires, and perspectives of teens

their patients so as to influence patient care outcomes in a positive way, including by avoiding errors and by engaging in successful negotiations. A lack of awareness of a patient's and family's cultural background and failure to provide culturally competent care increase the stresses experienced in healthcare settings (Flowers, 2004; Giger, 2014).

Influences on Health Care

Culture

Culture is a set of learned behaviors or beliefs that are shared among members of a group. Families and cultural groups teach their children about cultural behaviors, preferences, and communication styles (**Figure 4-2**). Culture is influenced by customs, language, history, family structure, religion, and other environmental factors (Bird & Osland, 2006; Giger, 2014; Migliore, 2011; Self, Self, & Bell-Haynes, 2011; Soderberg & Holden, 2002; Wu, Batmunkh, & Lai, 2011). Cultures can be viewed as operating as an "iceberg," with the cultural beliefs, assumptions, and behaviors found deep beneath the surface and often not being seen by an outsider. Such hidden aspects of culture can create misunderstandings between parties, especially during communication (Chang, 2011).

Communication—the most powerful of the various cultural forces that shape interactions among patients, families, and healthcare providers—has several dimensions that influence its effectiveness. These dimensions include power distance (perceptions of inequality between individuals), short-term versus long-term orientation, individualism versus collectivism, gender roles and perception, and uncertainty avoidance (Hofstede, 2001; Hofstede, Hofstede, & Minkov, 2005; Moran, Harris, & Moran, 2010; Rudd & Lawson, 2007).

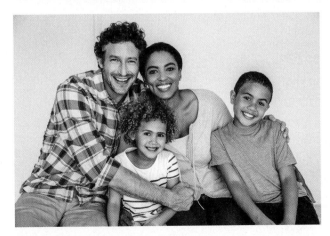

Figure 4-2

© Portra Images/Digital Vision/Getty

RESEARCH EVIDENCE

Communication and negotiations may be negatively influenced by a lack of **cultural intelligence** (CQ). The concept of cultural intelligence implies that someone with a high CQ will be able to differentiate whether a behavior is driven by an individual's cultural background or whether that behavior is characteristic of a specific person (Earley & Mosakowsko, 2004; Speedy, 2015). Some examples can clarify this concept:

- A response of "yes" during a consent interaction for a child's upcoming diagnostics exam may mean that the individual hears what is said, but does not imply that the person agrees or understands the issue. Being able to interpret this response as a culturally driven communication behavior will allow the healthcare provider to alter the teaching/consenting interaction and incorporate another means to secure understanding.
- A person may be very sensitive to both verbal and nonverbal communication techniques. These techniques, which affect one's ability to talk effectively with someone of another culture, can include the following:
  - Eye contact
  - Tone of voice
  - Space
  - Silence
  - Distance
  - Auditory volume
  - Body language, such as folding arms over chest
  - Asking personal questions
  - Touch, including needing an attendant or guardian present when conducting physical exams on areas deemed private

Ethnicity

The term **ethnicity** has a different meaning than the term "culture." Ethnicity comprises the beliefs and practices of a group whose members identify with one another based on common language, ancestry, nationality, or other factors. The group's shared beliefs and practices may include childrearing, food choices and preparation, dress, customs, and life practices such as birthing, marriage ceremonies, and death practices (**Figure 4-3; Table 4-2**). The term "culture" is used in a broader sense, whereas the term "ethnicity" denotes specific practices that are common within an ethnic group.

Religion

Religion is the practice of one's spiritual beliefs. Although religion can be separate from one's culture or ethnicity, appreciating the practice of religious faith is important in providing holistic care to patients and their families. Many religious practices are performed when a child is sick or injured. Further, religions often have very specific rituals surrounding birth and death. Individualized prayer, group prayer, visits from

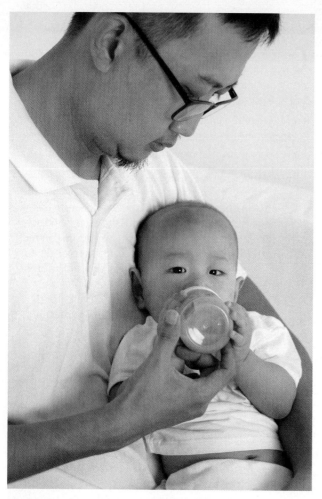

Figure 4-3
© szefei/Shutterstock

family's needs. Often, offering a visitation from a hospital chaplain can be very soothing to families who are experiencing a crisis. For others who may be agnostic or atheist, providing time for rest, silence, and contemplation may be sufficient.

Spirituality in Children

The term **spirituality** is often used interchangeably with "religion." Religion should be considered a system of beliefs, often shared by groups, that may influence a family's lifestyle, behavioral choices, attitudes toward such things as gender role identity, aspirations, conflict resolution practices, and standards for individual and group behaviors. Spirituality, by comparison, is a broader concept. A person's spirituality influences how that individual views situations and one experiences a sense of well-being and internal peace. Spirituality influences how a person connects to others, sees meaning in life, and interacts with and finds pleasure in nature.

A child's and family's religiosity may be structured around an organized religion that features a structured set of doctrines, techniques of worship, and shared beliefs. Shared beliefs may include such aspects of life as choice of relationships, healthcare choices, birth and death practices, circumcision practices, and even food, clothing, and work decisions. Spirituality is broader and more open, fluid, and influential in more personally directed aspects of an individual's life. Religion is often very structured and incorporates use of sacred texts and prayer practices, whereas spirituality is unstructured, not formalized, and very personal.

The five major religions in the world have been described as Hinduism, Christianity, Judaism, Buddhism and Islam. Within those major religions, healthcare decisions may be influenced by the belief practices, prayer activities, and doctrines held by the leaders and members. Influential aspects of religious faith on health decisions include limitations of care provisions, such as the refusal of all transfused blood

clergy or religious leaders, meditation, silence, and laying on of hands are common religious practices that the pediatric healthcare team may encounter. Religious beliefs should be supported and incorporated into care designed to meet the

TABLE 4-2 Ethnic Groups and Healthcare Treatments	
Ethnic groups known to have beliefs, doctrines, or religious influences that may affect healthcare treatments for children include the following:	
› African American	› Korean
› American Indian	› Lao
› Amhara	› Mein/Yao
› Arab	› Native Hawaiian
› Asian (South)	› Pakistani
› Cambodian	› Samoan
› Chinese	› Somali
› Ethiopian	› Soviet Jewish
› Filipino	› Ukrainian
› Hispanic	› Vietnamese

Data from EthnoMed. (2015). Cultures. Retrieved from https://ethnomed.org/culture

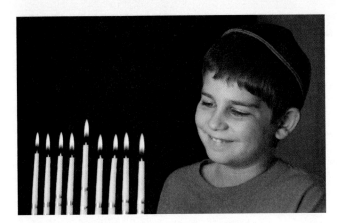

Figure 4-4

© tovfla/iStock/Getty Images Plus/Getty

products by Jehovah's Witness members, delays for prayer before care by several fundamental Christian organizations, and refusal of certain medical treatments by Christian Scientists (Linnard-Palmer, 2006). The healthcare team, after assessing the religious faith or doctrine influencing healthcare decisions, should work together to better understand the faith needs of the family, be flexible and accommodating whenever possible, and include the family's faith by ensuring the safety of their child (**Figure 4-4**).

QUALITY AND SAFETY

Jehovah's Witnesses Doctrine on Blood Transfusion

Since 1927, the Watchtower Bible and Tract Society of Pennsylvania (the legal entity of Jehovah's Witnesses) has published rules forbidding the reception of blood on the penalty of losing eternal life in the Kingdom of God. In the biblical chapters of Genesis (9:4), Acts (15:28-29) and Leviticus (17:10-12; 13-14), reference to abstaining from blood is tied to one's soul. In 1945, Jehovah's Witnesses leaders made an official denouncement of the receipt of blood transfusion (Linnard-Palmer, 2006).

Faithful parents who worship as Jehovah's Witnesses may face a situation in which they must decide whether to adhere to their faith if their child requires blood product transfusions. In cases where parents have refused consent for a lifesaving required transfusion, pediatric healthcare teams have gone through the courts to secure state guardianship for mandated transfusion therapy.

According to Jehovah's Witnesses doctrine, the following procedures are unacceptable:

- Whole blood transfusions
- Packed red blood cells transfusions
- Autologous blood transfusions if the tube from body to body is interrupted
- Plasma proteins transfusions
- Stem cell transfusions
- Epidural blood patches if the blood leaves the body and is injected back in
- Blood product donations (some flexibility allowed)

The need for religious consultation and time for prayer can be assessed by inquiring how the pediatric nurse can be of assistance in providing for a religious ceremony, prayer, or time with religious leaders. Ideally, the assessment of spirituality and spiritual needs will lead to a more open discussion of these issues. According to The Joint Commission (TJC) (2008), the healthcare provider should ask the family three important questions about their religious orientation:

- Do you have a religious preference?
- Are there any spiritual or religious preferences that are important to you and your family?
- Do you wish to contact your clergy member or religious advisor?

Other questions to ask a child and family about their spiritual background and needs are as follows:

- How do you make sense of what has happened to you?
- In what ways has your illness/injury/disorder affected your view of yourself or others or your faith?
- What is your source of support for meaning in this life experience?
- How do you decide what you could do next?
- Which kind of support do you currently have? Faith?
- What is your source of hope?

Spirituality Versus Ethnicity and Culture

Spirituality should not be confused with ethnicity or culture. Culture is considered a way in which a group of individual people interact, live, and adapt to a set of life's circumstances. It is expressed through socially transmitted behaviors, values, arts, and "human works of life." Ethnicity is more specific. For example, a group's customs such as food preparation and choices, music, dress, expressions of emotions, hierarchy of decision making, and language are all influenced by their ethnicity.

It is vitally important that a pediatric nurse working in an interdisciplinary team understand cultural, ethnic, and spiritual influences on care. Indeed, the decisions that a family makes regarding their child's health care may be based on the interwoven influences of spiritual practices, ethnic leadership, cultural values, and religious preferences (**Table 4-3**). Understanding how the nurse's own religious and cultural beliefs influence daily practices and thoughts will strengthen the nurse's understanding of and sensitivity to the influence of the same factors on a family's way of interacting with the healthcare team, deciding on treatment for their child, and making decisions about health, food, affection, childrearing and accepting or adapting to a situation such as injury, illness, or disease.

TABLE 4-3 Religious, Spiritual, and Belief Systems That Influence Children's Health Care

Religious/ Spiritual Group	Basic Beliefs	Influence to Healthcare Decisions for Children
Catholic	Sickness, illness, or injury may be God's will or based on sin (evident in last rites).	Prayer is used to ask for forgiveness and assistance in healing. For many Catholic families, the request for a visit from a priest is very important as part of the healing process of their child. Baptism is very important for their child, such that a Catholic family with a newborn who has a critical condition may request accommodation for this ceremony to take place within a healthcare institution.
Christian Science	Divine healing takes place through Jesus's healing practices. Doctrine supports that God is the only reality, and that a relationship with God can trump illness, sin, and evil by understanding spiritual practices.	Christian Science followers may not seek health care, choosing to participate in prayer over conventional medical therapies. The commitment to not naming disease, disorders, infections. or injuries may place children at risk.
Jehovah's Witness	A person's relationship with God and destiny for eternal life in God's Kingdom is dependent on religious practices.	Blood transfusions are not acceptable, even in light of impending death, due to refusal of blood and most whole blood products. Crystalloid intravenous solutions and colloids for volume expansion are acceptable, as is the use of erythropoietin.
Hindu	Religious practice of many East Indian cultures and ethnicities, including persons from Nepal. One of the oldest known religions, dating back to 500 B.C. Hinduism is the third largest religion, with more than 1 billion followers worldwide. There are as many as 330 million gods and goddesses, who are representations of the one supreme creator God, Brahma. A key belief is that everyone is divine and reincarnation is expected.	Hindus will refuse any product that is beef based. They may request time to implement spiritual practices that promote a child's healing prior to consenting to use of traditional medical diagnostics and treatments.
Fundamental Christian	This faith is based on a relationship with God and adhering to the word of the Bible. The Holy Trinity of God, Jesus, and the Holy Spirit are the foundation of faith.	Adherents may request time for "laying on of hands" or prayer groups prior to consenting to medical treatment.
Wiccan	Wicca is a pagan practice sometimes labeled "contemporary witchcraft." The principles of the practice are based on pagan rituals and theological structures, worshiping both a God and a Goddess.	Wiccans may believe in manipulative forces, witchcraft, and magic. Magic may be regarded as a law of nature. Sacred circles and spells may be used for healing, fertility, protection, and banishment of negative forces. Classical elements of air, fire, earth, and water are important. Prayers and spells are used as a form of "raising powers." Wiccan families may participate in a "Wiccaning" of their newborn infant rather than a christening.

RESEARCH EVIDENCE

Perspectives on Circumcision

The surgical procedure of circumcision (removal of the infant's foreskin) has religious undertones for many families. It might not be performed in the immediate neonatal period for various health and religious reasons. The Jewish faith advises families to wait 8 days and have the act performed by a mohel ("circumcisor") in a ceremony called a bris.

It is important for the pediatric nurse to understand that circumcision continues to be performed globally on both male and female children. Although the practice is illegal in all 50 U.S. states, a pediatric nurse may encounter a female who was circumcised in another country (e.g., Somaliland, Gambia, Sierra Leone) (Sundby, Essén, & Johansen, 2013). Female circumcision is performed for various cultural reasons and has no medical value (Tilly, 2015). The World Health Organization (WHO) considers this practice to be "female genital mutilation."

In general, there are four types of female genital mutilation:

- Clitoridectomy: removal of the clitoris.
- Excision: partial or total removal of the clitoris and the labia minora.
- Infibulation: may or may not involve removal of the clitoris. The labia majora and minora are surgically repositioned to create closure or narrowing of the vaginal opening. A small opening for urination and menstruation is kept.
- All other female genital mutilation procedures, such as piercing, scraping, and cauterizing (WHO, 2016).

Female genital mutilation has potentially devastating health and emotional consequences (Johnsdotter, 2015; WHO, 2016). Many organizations are working to put a stop to this kind of "female circumcision."

Imperative of Cultural Knowledge in Pediatric Health Care

Caring for culturally diverse children means the nurse is caring for culturally diverse families. The child is not separate from the family; rather, the child's cultural background, cultural behaviors, and cultural preferences will likely match those of the family. It is imperative that the pediatric nurse approach the child with culturally sensitive care. The nurse must ask the family how best to care for the child and how the nurse can be of assistance in providing culturally appropriate care that incorporates the family's cultural practices.

For instance, if a practicing Muslim woman is with her child in the hospital, it will be important to ask if the mother needs time and undisturbed privacy to participate in daily prayer sessions (**Figure 4-5**). If she answers affirmatively, the mother should be given time, space, and support to

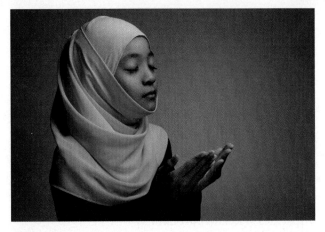

Figure 4-5
© Patrick Foto/Moment/Getty

participate in this very important cultural and religious practice. She may want the door closed during her five daily prayer sessions, and she will most likely pray on a rug while facing the direction of Mecca. She should not be disturbed, and care should be planned around her spiritual needs.

Both cultural preferences and religious doctrines can influence pediatric healthcare decisions. **Box 4-1** identifies the basic tenets of several commonly encountered cultural groups in the United States whose beliefs and cultural practices influence the provision of care to children. **Box 4-2** provides examples of religious doctrines that influence how care is provided to children and how healthcare team members are to provide care to children and families.

BOX 4-1   Components of Cultural and Ethnic Groups

Although the following practices may be applied, disregarded, or modified for individual members or groups, the following list gives examples of how culture or ethnicity may influence healthcare decisions and practices. (It is important, however, to steer clear of the "trait list approach.")

- Dietary restrictions such as a vegan diet for black Muslims and no beef for Hindus
- Restrictions on pork consumption and use of pork-based medicines by Islamic Muslims and kosher-observant Jews
- Perspective on causes of illness (supernatural = *loa*) for Haitians
- Strong relationship between theology and medicine for Native American Indians
- Conservation of energy for children healing from surgery for Arabs
- Desire for cultural healing practices such as acupuncture and herbs before application of Western medicine practices for Chinese
- Illness as a punishment by God for traditional Mexican Catholics

---

BOX 4-2 Basic Aspects of Religious Doctrines That Influence Pediatric Healthcare Decisions

- Desire for prayer in place of or prior to the participation in traditional healthcare provision
- Refusal, delay, or limitation of care based on religious doctrine or group processes
- Need for elders' or church leader's influence or say in treatment decisions
- Use of alternative healing approaches

Disparities of Health Outcomes

The term **disparities of health outcomes** is used to denote poorer clinical or health outcomes associated with particular **races** (groups identified on the basis of supposedly shared genetic or physical traits), ethnicities, and cultural groups due to, among other things, the intersection of cultural factors with acceptance of therapy. It should not be confused with the term **healthcare disparities**, which refers to differences in access to healthcare services among different groups.

Disparities of health outcomes are of great concern, as some can be rectified by providing care that takes into account the health beliefs held by various individuals and groups. Some health concerns have a genetic predisposition, such as sickle cell anemia in the African American community, thalassemia in patients of Mediterranean heritage, and Tay-Sachs disease in the Ashkenazi Jewish community. Other disparities in health outcomes relate directly to behaviors, customs, or genetics associated with cultural or ethnic groups. A higher incidence of hypertension in the African American community, sudden infant death syndrome (SIDS) in the African American and Native American communities (Pickett, Luo, & Lauderdale, 2005), and diabetes in the American Indian/Native Alaskan community, as well as differing levels of drug response or food sensitivities, are associated with lifestyle, diet, and cultural practices. Some of these cultural practices may delay screening, limit treatment options, or influence prevention. In another example of disparities in health outcomes, lesbian, gay, and transgender youth have been disproportionally affected by the human immunodeficiency virus (HIV) (American Academy of Pediatrics, 2004).

Trust is an important part of cultural connection, as some cultural groups view traditional Western medicine as being patriarchal and unfair owing to its biases, racism, and exclusionary practices. Pediatric nurses are in an important position to provide education and support to cultural groups with higher risks for certain diseases, conditions, and health states (**Figure 4-6**). Because disparities of health outcomes are harmful and lead to higher levels of morbidity and mortality, nurses should take steps to

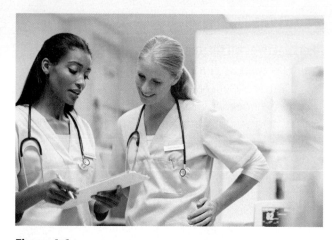

Figure 4-6
© Morsa Images/DigitalVision/Getty

BOX 4-3 Examples of Contemporary Disparities in Health Outcomes

According to *Healthy People 2020* (U.S. Department of Health and Human Services, Office of Disease Prevention and Health Promotion, 2017a), disparities in health outcomes reflect differences in overall care outcomes related to low economic or social status, race, ethnicity, culture, and environmental influences. These disparities include the differences in the following outcomes for specific groups:

- Cognitive or sensory disabilities
- Cancer
- Diabetes
- Hypertension
- Injuries and accidents leading to bodily harm
- Death rates associated with chronic and acute illnesses

---

explicitly address them. **Box 4-3** identifies some contemporary disparities in health outcomes that are predicted to persist into the future.

Health Literacy

Consistent with the relationship between culture and communication is the concept of health literacy. **Health literacy** has been defined as the ability of an individual or group to "obtain, process and understand basic health information and services needed to make appropriate health decisions" (U.S. Department of Health and Human Services [USDHHS], 2003). Recognizing that health literacy highly influences clinical outcomes, safety, informed consent, adherence, and compliance (USDHHS, 2003) can help guide a pediatric nurse to carefully assess a family's level of understanding. Even for families in which English is the first language, complex medical terms and the high levels of English-language literacy needed to understand treatment plans may mean that a family does not fully understand what is happening to their child's health and misses important information on care and treatment plans. All documents given to families should be written to reflect the language and literacy level of the responsible adult, guardian, or primary caregiver of the child (Joint Commission, 2007; Joint Commission, 2008).

Cultural Awareness Across Settings

Healthcare work settings are complex and can be very diverse environments. Indeed, many cultural and ethnic groups may interact within the same clinical setting. Not only do pediatric nurses work with and care for people with diverse cultural and ethnic backgrounds, but the staff providing the care are also influenced by their own cultural, ethnic, and religious perspectives. If the nurse is both culturally sensitive and culturally aware, the work setting can be enriched by an emerging respect for diversity and the joys of celebrating diversity through the sharing of health practices, dress, food, music, and communication styles.

It is important, however, to maintain a "patient-centered template" approach to pediatric health care (Javier, Hendriksz, Chamberlain, & Stuart, 2013). This approach encourages the healthcare provider to view each patient through a unique lens, trying to understand *this* particular patient and the influences on *this* patient's world. Practitioners are cautioned not to fall into the trap of assuming that cultural factors are always central to a case or to follow the "trait list approach" in which one assumes that certain traits apply to an entire group (Kleinman & Benson, 2006). Doing so leads to dangerous stereotyping.

Each member of the healthcare team should seek to create a positive and sensitive work environment in which diverse perspectives and care practices are respected, valued, and incorporated. The value of diversity among patients, families, groups and healthcare team members can greatly enrich the experience of pediatric healthcare practices.

It is important to be mindful of the potential for communication disconnects. If some members of the healthcare team are members of a particular ethnic group and

speak a language that is not shared by all team members, a disconnect may occur, in which some team members feel ostracized and like "outsiders." The communication of patient information, reports or handoffs, and critical findings should not occur solely in a language that is considered the collective norm (e.g., English in the United States). In other words, bilingual healthcare providers may need to repeat information in both languages—once to ensure that the patient understands the information, and a second time to ensure that all healthcare team members are likewise informed. Conscious effort should be made to be inclusive, and safety must always be the primary concern.

Cultural Assessment and Cultural Considerations

A number of **cultural assessment tools** can provide a structure for nurses to provide culturally driven care for pediatric patients and their families. A meta-analysis by Higginbottom and colleagues (2011) identified eight such tools that were informed by rigorous research perspectives; the first of these tools to be developed—Leininger's Sunrise Model (Leininger, 1997)—has been analyzed and critiqued repeatedly during the past decades. More recent models described in the analysis include the Culturally Competent Community Care (CCCC) model developed by Kim-Godwyn and colleagues (2001); the Family Cultural Heritage Assessment Tool (FAMCHAT) created by Davidson et al. (2001); and the ACCESS model (*Assessment, Communication, Cultural negotiation and Compromise, Establishing respect and rapport, Sensitivity, Safety*) developed by Narayanasamy (2002).

Sometimes, just asking the right questions at the right time to the right family member will allow for a kind and supportive conversation that increases cultural understanding. Questions can include how the nurse and healthcare team can provide the best care for the child and the family. Quality questions asked in a supportive tone can make a person feel respected and valued. **Table 4-4** lists some cultural questions that can provoke disclosure of the family's cultural background and associated preferences and needs. A nurse should be aware of each family's cultural practices and needs if the nurse is to assure trust, complete disclosure, and collaboration.

Parental Refusal of Medical Treatment

Among certain religious and cultural groups, their beliefs and doctrines may influence whether a family will consent for treatment, refuse treatment, delay seeking medical care, or limit which medical care their child receives. Treatment refusal is complicated when the child is a minor and treatments are considered essential or lifesaving. Some religious doctrines require that families refuse certain forms of medical care, or that they seek "prayer healing" prior to or instead of traditional medical care (Offit, 2015). In other instances, parents may hold sociopolitical concepts about science and medicine (e.g., anti-vaccine or anti-pharmaceutical sentiments) that conflict with the standard of care required to adequately treat the child's health issue.

In cases where the child is critically ill, refusal or delay of medical care rooted in religious practice or sociopolitical concepts can be life threatening. Most states have laws that protect the health and well-being of a child by preventing parental authority from superseding a child's safety. Most states also have laws that allow the state to take guardianship of a child for a specific time period to make sure the

TABLE 4-4	Cultural Questions for the Disclosure of Cultural Needs

› "Which ethnic group or cultural group do you identify with? Is this the same for your child?"

› "How would you and your child like to be addressed here?"

› "Who is the major decision maker in your family? Will that person be involved in your child's care and treatment plans?"

› "We very much want to honor your cultural beliefs. Is there anything you would like your care providers to know about your cultural needs?"

› "Can you share with me what you believe caused your child's illness?"

› "Are there any cultural or religious practices that we can support or provide for?"

› "Does your family need private time for prayer or any religious practice?"

› "Are there religious or cultural leaders we can call for you?"

› "Would you like to have a visit from our hospital chaplain?"

› "What do you fear most about this illness?"

› "Are there any particular cultural care provisions you give your child, such as certain foods, fluids, or medicines?"

› "Are you administering any natural remedies to your child, such as herbal medicines or supplements?"

› "Do you participate in any cultural health practices with your child, such as acupressure, acupuncture, or moxibustion?"

child receives required medical care. **Table 4-5** lists some religious and sociopolitical groups with doctrines that have been known to influence pediatric medical treatment decisions.

It is imperative that pediatric nurses understand their role in the sometimes distressing scenario of treatment refusal, delay, or limitation. All members of the healthcare team must be aware of and identify when families of diverse cultures or religious groups refuse treatment; they must know their state laws, know how to act quickly, and acknowledge that the situation is an ethical dilemma that requires communication and decision making by staff, administration, and family members. **Table 4-6** offers guidelines for staff who encounter parental refusal, delay, or limitation of health care for children. Many factors affect parental delay, limitation, or refusal of medical care for children, but cultural and religious beliefs are among the most influential, problematic, and distressing for both the healthcare team and the faithful family.

TABLE 4-5 Religious and Sociopolitical Groups That Influence Pediatric Medical Treatment Decisions

Religious doctrines	
	› Roman Catholic Church
	› Christian Science
	› Christ Miracle Healing Center
	› End Time Ministries
	› Faith Assembly of God
	› Faith Temple Church of God in Christ
	› Followers of Christ
	› Foursquare Church
	› Jehovah's Witnesses
	› Jesus Through Jon and Judy
	› The Believers' Fellowship
	› The Body
	› The "No Name" Fellowship
	› Everyday Church
Sociopolitical perspectives	› Antivaccine activists
	› Liberal anti-corporatist perspective
	› Neoconservative anti-science perspective
	› Holistic, naturopathic, or homeopathic health perspective

TABLE 4-6 Guidelines for Staff Who Encounter Parental Refusal, Delay, or Limitation of Health Care for Children

1. Maintain consistent safety for the child, and be mindful of the risk that the family may leave against medical advice (AMA).

2. Continue respectful communication with the family but be firm that the priority for all is the safety and well-being of the child.

3. Identify the family's primary decision maker and provide clarity regarding impending diagnostics, treatments, and care paths.

4. Request the name and contact information for the religious or cultural group whose doctrine is influencing the child's treatment.

5. Notify important healthcare providers, including social workers, who are involved with the child's care.

6. Coordinate a conference for the family, key healthcare professionals, and leaders in the culture or religious group, if able and appropriate.

7. Document all conversations carefully, include critical debriefing sessions.

Reproduced from Linnard-Palmer, L. (2006). *When parents say no: Religious and cultural influences on pediatric healthcare decisions.* Indianapolis, IN: Sigma Theta Tau International Publishing Co.

National Standards for Healthcare Services

The Office of Minority Health within the U.S. Department of Health and Human Services created the **National Standards for Culturally and Linguistically Appropriate Services in Health Care (CLAS)** for use as a guide for healthcare providers (USDHHS, Office of Minority Health, n.d.). This document comprises a set of mandates, guidelines, and recommendations to inform, guide, and facilitate recommended and required practices related to culturally and linguistically appropriate health services (USDHHS, Office of Minority Health, 2001). The CLAS standards provide healthcare team members with vital information on how to learn, implement, and sustain services to give the best and most respectful care to diverse communities, families, and patients. The 15 standards are divided into four main categories, including principles of the standards, governance and leadership, language and communication, and engagement. Five of the CLAS standards closely relate to the professional practice of family-centered care and pediatric nursing:

1. Provide safe, effective, equitable, respectful, and understandable care and services that take into account diversity, cultural beliefs and practices, literacy, languages, and communication requirements.
2. Recruit and support a workforce that is culturally diverse and represents many languages.
3. Participate in continued education on cultural diversity and diverse cultural healthcare practices.
4. Engage in assessment of the healthcare institution's CLAS-related policies, goals, and practices.
5. Create conflict, grievance, and resolution skills and practices that will allow a healthcare team and family to resolve issues related to diverse perspectives and needs.

In 2010, a review of implementation of these policies found that only a very small number of hospital facilities met the standards completely; indeed, more facilities met none of the standards than met all of them (Diamond, Wilson-Stronks, & Jacobs, 2010). The U.S. Department of Health and Human Services (n.d.) subsequently issued an enhanced standard that targeted these disparities. Thus,

---

BOX 4-4 Additional Resources

- Seattle's Harborview Medical Center's ethnic medicine website for cultural understanding and patient education (www.ethnomed.org)
- National Center for Cultural Competence (https://nccc.georgetown.edu)
- National Coalition for LGBT Health (www.lgbthealtheducation.org/lgbt-education/lgbt-health-resources)
- Indian Health Services (www.ihs.gov)
- *Healthy People 2020* (www.healthypeople.gov/2020/default.aspx)
- International Medical Interpreters Association (www.imiaweb.org/default.asp)
- National Center for Complementary and Alternative Medicine (http://nccam.nih.gov/health)
- Office of Minority Health (http://minorityhealth.hhs.gov)
- National Standards on Culturally and Linguistically Appropriate Services (http://minorityhealth.hhs.gov/templates/browse.aspx?lvl=2&lvlID=15)
- The Community Toolbox: Cultural Competence in a Multicultural World, Workgroup for Community Health and Development, University of Kansas (http://ctb.ku.edu/en/tablecontents/chapter_1027.aspx)
- Transcultural Nursing Society (www.tcns.org)

---

care providers may need to put in extra effort to ensure that these standards are utilized in practice. **Box 4-4** identifies additional sources of information that can help providers and institutions meet the CLAS standards.

Case Study

A 3-year-old child is being seen in the pediatric hematology oncology clinic as a follow-up after her initial induction chemotherapy phase for a new diagnosis of leukemia. The child is from a Sri Lankan immigrant family; her father has a limited command of English and the mother speaks only Tamil. The mother works two jobs to care for her three children, and the father works in another city and has a more than 90-minute commute each day. On this visit, the mother is the only parent present. Using interpreter services, the mother explains that the health condition of the child and the frequently required clinic visits are imposing stress on the family. The child is very shy and fights against having any physical exams performed. She also protests loudly when her implanted port needs to be accessed for

laboratory draws or chemotherapy infusions. The mother breaks down in tears and asks if there is a way to combine Ayurvedic medicine administered at home with fewer traditional Western medical treatments at the clinic and hospital for her daughter's condition.

Case Study Questions

1. How can the healthcare team provide culturally sensitive care to this family during this clinic visit?
2. For clarity, which questions should be asked of the mother concerning her desire to provide Ayurvedic medicine with traditional Western medical treatments?
3. For safety, how can the team provide care to the child who is fighting against physical exams and access to her implanted port?

(continues)

Case Study *(continued)*

As the Case Evolves...

Suppose that this child, instead of being 3 years old, is 14. Unlike her parents, she was born and raised in the United States and speaks fluent English as well as Tamil. Although she is able to interpret for her mother, a Tamil-speaking staff member has noticed that she sometimes does not translate all of the information, or translates it incompletely. The patient does not share her mother's wish to initiate Ayurvedic therapies and displays impatience when the nursing staff attempts to draw out her mother's wishes in the matter.

4. Which of the following actions is the top priority for staff seeking to appropriately care for the adolescent patient and her parents?
   A. A child and family psychologist should be added to the team to provide counseling for the family to limit conflict over treatment modalities.
   B. A professional interpreter unrelated to the family should be called in to ensure the parents get the appropriate information from the staff.
   C. A Child Life professional should work with the daughter to help her be more accepting of her mother's treatment perspectives.
   D. The issues faced by this family require no additional services.

Chapter Summary

- It is important that the pediatric nurse can distinguish between the terms "culture," "ethnicity," "race," and "religious beliefs" in relation to health care for children and their families. The pediatric nurse's care should be based on assessment, understanding, and application of care processes that take into account a child's and family's belief systems and cultural practices.

- Tools and guidelines are available to guide pediatric nurses' and healthcare teams' assessments of a family's cultural and religious needs. The findings can be used to determine which cultural and religious practices influence the medical and nursing treatment plans, and can inform the development of a respectful and mutual care plan that both the team and the family can understand. Specific questions should be posed early in the health encounter to clarify what is needed to provide culturally sensitive care.

- Cultural awareness, cultural sensitivity, cultural humility, and cultural competence across pediatric healthcare settings are goals of effective family-centered care. A pediatric nurse should be committed to lifelong learning about diverse cultures, ethnic groups, and religious frameworks so that the nurse can continue to practice with safety and respect.

- Religious beliefs can be highly influential in pediatric and family care, including pediatric care treatment decisions. Some religious groups desire a delay in treatment for prayer first, seek to limit treatments based on their beliefs, or refuse treatments. A pediatric nurse should be able to identify and understand those specific religious faiths whose doctrines influence care.

- The term "disparities in health outcomes" denotes poorer clinical or health outcomes associated with particular races, ethnicities, and cultural groups. Many of these disparities can be rectified by providing care that takes into account the health beliefs held by various individuals and groups. Some health outcomes disparities have a genetic predisposition, whereas others reflect behaviors associated with specific cultural or ethnic groups.

- The Office of Minority Health has developed National Standards for Culturally and Linguistically Appropriate Services in Health Care to help guide healthcare team members in providing safe, effective, respectful, and mutually satisfying care.

Bibliography

American Academy of Pediatrics, Committee on Pediatric Workforce. (2004). Ensuring culturally effective pediatric care: Implication for education and health policy. *Pediatrics, 114*(4), 1677–1685.

Bagchi, A. D., Ursin, R., & Leonard, A. (2012). Assessing cultural perspectives on healthcare quality. *Journal of Immigrant and Minority Health, 14*, 175–182.

Bird, A., & Osland, J. S. (2006). Making sense of intercultural collaboration. *International Studies of Management and Organization, 35*, 115–132.

Brotanek, J. M., Seeley, C. E., & Flores, G. (2008). The importance of cultural competency in general pediatrics. *Current Opinion in Pediatrics, 20*(6), 711–718.

Chang, L. (2011). A comparison of Taiwan and Malaysia in negotiation styles. *Journal of International Management Studies, 6*, 1–8.

Davidson, J. U., Reigier, T., & Boos, S. (2001). Assessing family cultural heritage in Kansas: Research and development of the FAMCHAT companion tool for family health assessment. *Kansas Nurse, 76*, 5–7.

Department of Finance. (2013, January 31). New population projections: California to surpass 50 million in 2049. Retrieved from http://www.tularecog.org/wp-content/uploads/2015/06/Appendix-F-Demographic-Forecast-Department-of-Finance-New-population-projections.pdf

Diamond, L. C., Wilson-Stronks, A., & Jacobs, E. A. (2010). Do hospitals measure up to the national culturally and linguistically appropriate services standards? *Medical Care, 48*(12), 1080–1087.

Earley, C. P., & Mosakowsko, E. (2004, October). Cultural intelligence. *Harvard Business Review*, 139–147.

EthnoMed. (2015). Cultures. Retrieved from https://ethnomed.org/culture

Flowers, D. (2004). Culturally competent nursing care: A challenge for the 21st century. *Critical Care Nursing, 24*(40), 48–52.

Giger, J. N. (2014). *Transcultural nursing: Assessment and intervention* (6th ed.). St. Louis, MO: Elsevier-Mosby.

Hearnden, M. (2008). Coping with differences in culture and communication in health care. *Nursing Standard, 23,* 49–57.

Higginbottom, G. M. A., Richter, M. S., Mogale, R. S., Ortiz, L., Young, S., & Mollel, O. (2011, August 3). Identification of nursing assessment models/tools validated in clinical practice for use with diverse ethno-cultural groups: An integrative review of the literature. *BMC Nursing, 10,* 16.

Hofstede, G. (2001). *Culture's consequences: Comparing values, behaviors, institutions, and organizations across nations* (2nd ed.). Thousand Oaks, CA: Sage.

Hofstede, G., Hofstede, G. J., & Minkov, M. (2005). *Cultures and organizations: Software of the mind* (3rd ed.). New York, NY: McGraw-Hill.

Javier, J. R., Hendriksz, T., Chamberlain, L. J., & Stuart, E. (2013). Cross-cultural training in pediatric residency: Every encounter is a cross-cultural encounter. *Academic Pediatrics, 13*(6), 495–498.

Johnsdotter, S. (2015, April 20). Genital cutting, female. *International Encyclopedia of Human Sexuality.* doi: 10.1002/9781118896877.wbiehs180

Joint Commission. (2007). What did the doctor say? Improving health literacy to protect patient safety. Retrieved from http://www.jointcommission.org/PublicPolicy/health_literacy.htm

Joint Commission. (2008). Promoting effective communication: Language access services in healthcare. *Joint Commission Perspectives, 28,* 8–11.

Kim-Godwin, Y. S., Clarke, P. N., & Barton, L. (2001). A model for the delivery of culturally competent community care. *Journal of Advanced Nursing, 35,* 918–925.

Kleinman, A., & Benson, P. (2006). Anthropology in the clinic: The problem of cultural competency and how to fix it. *PLoS Medicine, 3*(10), e294.

Laves, T. A., Reclose, R., & Seaway, N. (2008). The COA360: A tool for assessing the cultural competency of healthcare organizations. *Journal of Healthcare Management, 53,* 257–267.

Leininger, M. (1997). Overview of the theory of culture care with the ethnonursing research method. *Journal of Transcultural Nursing, 8,* 32–52.

Leong, K. E., Wieland, T. J., & Dent, A. W. (2010). Exploring beliefs of the four major ethnic groups in Melbourne regarding healthcare and treatment. *Australian Health Review, 34,* 458–466.

Linnard-Palmer, L. (2006). *When parents say no: Religious and cultural influences on pediatric healthcare decisions.* Indianapolis, IN: Sigma Theta Tau International.

Migliore, L. A. (2011). Relation between big five personality traits and Hofstede's cultural dimensions. *Cross Cultural Management: An International Journal, 18,* 38–54.

Moran, R. T., Harris, P. R., & Moran, S. (2010). *Managing cultural differences: Global leadership strategies for the 21st century* (8th ed.). Burlington, MA: Elsevier Butterworth Heinemann.

Narayanasamy, A. (2002). The ACCESS model: A transcultural nursing practice framework. *British Journal of Nursing, 11,* 643–650.

Offit, P. M. (2015). *Bad faith: When religious beliefs undermine modern medicine.* New York, NY: Basic Books.

Pickett, K. E., Luo, Y., & Lauderdale, D. S. (2005). Widening social inequalities in risk for sudden infant death syndrome. *American Journal of Public Health, 95*(11), 1976–1981.

Rudd, J. E., & Lawson, D. R. (2007). *Communication in global business negotiations: A geocentric approach.* Thousand Oaks, CA: Sage.

Self, R., Self, D. R., & Bell-Haynes, J. (2011). Intercultural human resource management: South Korea and the United States. *International Journal of Management and Information Systems, 15,* 41–48.

Soderberg, A., & Holden, N. (2002). Rethinking cross cultural management in a globalizing world. *International Journal of Cross Cultural Management, 2,* 103–121.

Speedy, S. (2015). Psychological influences on leadership style. In J. Daly, S. Speedy, & D. Jackson (Eds.), *Leadership and nursing: Contemporary perspectives* (2nd ed., pp. 21–36). Chatswood, Australia: Elsevier Australia.

Sundby, J., Essén, B., & Johansen, R. E. B. (2013). Female genital mutilation, cutting, or circumcision. *Obstetrics and Gynecology International, 2013,* 240421.

Tilley, D. S. (2015). Nursing care of women who have undergone genital cutting. *Nursing for Women's Health, 19,* 445–449.

U.S. Department of Health and Human Services (USDHHS), Office of Disease Prevention and Health Promotion. (n.d.). Healthy People 2010. Retrieved from https://www.healthypeople.gov/Document/HTML/Volume1/11HealthCom.htm#_Toc490471359

U.S. Department of Health and Human Services (USDHHS), Office of Disease Prevention and Health Promotion. (2003). Quick guide to health literacy: What is health literacy? Retrieved from https://health.gov/communication/literacy/quickguide/factsbasic.htm

U.S. Department of Health and Human Services (USDHHS), Office of Disease Prevention and Health Promotion. (2017a). Healthy People 2020: Disparities. Retrieved from https://www.healthypeople.gov/2020/about/foundation-health-measures/Disparities

U.S. Department of Health and Human Services (USDHHS), Office of Disease Prevention and Health Promotion. (2017b). Social determinants of health. Retrieved from http://www.healthypeople.gov/2020/topicsobjectives2020/overview.aspx?topicid=39

U.S. Department of Health and Human Services (USDHHS), Office of Minority Health. (2001). National standards for culturally and linguistically appropriate services in healthcare final report. Retrieved from http://minorityhealth.hhs.gove/assets/pdf/checked/finalreport.pdf

U.S. Department of Health and Human Services (USDHHS), Office of Minority Health. (n.d.). National Standards for Culturally and Linguistically Appropriate Services in Health Care: The case for the enhanced national standard. Retrieved from https://www.think-culturalhealth.hhs.gov/pdfs/enhancednationalclassstandards.pdf

Wilson-Stronks, A., & Murtha, S. (2010). From the perspective of CEOs: What motivates hospitals to embrace cultural competence? *Journal of Healthcare Management, 55,* 339–352.

World Health Organization (WHO). (2016, February). Female genital mutilation: Fact sheet. Retrieved from http://www.who.int/mediacentre/factsheets/fs241/en/

Wu, T.-F., Batmunkh, M.-U., & Lai, A. S. R. (2011). Cross-cultural perspectives on personality and values: A case study of Mongolian vs. Taiwanese doctors and nurses. *International Journal of Business Anthropology, 2*(1), 68–92.

CHAPTER 5

Working and Communicating with an Interdisciplinary Team

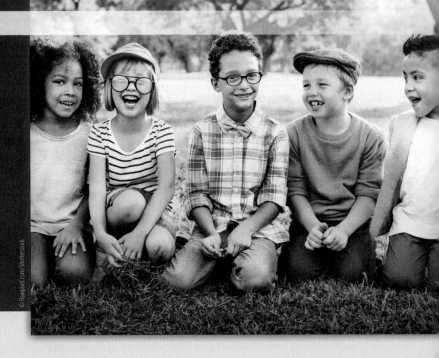

LEARNING OBJECTIVES

1. Analyze the complexities of children's care in relation to the need for effective and safe interdisciplinary communication.
2. Apply successful communication techniques that are supported by nursing, medicine, and ancillary health science literature.
3. Implement the components of SBAR in various interactions and settings.
4. Critically evaluate communication models used by pediatric healthcare teams.
5. Analyze the concept of safety during handoffs.

KEY TERMS

Child Protective Services (CPS)
Communication
CUS protocol
Empowerment
Handoffs
Interdisciplinary team
Power distance
SBAR protocol
Specialists
Therapeutic relationship

Introduction

Communication—defined as the sharing of information and meaning—is an essential part of safe pediatric health care. Communication needs to be accurate, concise, and purposeful if care is to be coordinated and safe. During every encounter, the pediatric nurse is instrumental in providing information to team members, to outside agencies and referrals, and, most importantly, to the family. Unfortunately, miscommunication remains the primary source of medical and medication errors. Nurses can be leaders in decreasing errors by providing clear communication using a structured approach.

Complexities in working with children require that team members communicate clearly, thoroughly, professionally, and often with urgency. Identifying healthcare problems in children often requires that members of an **interdisciplinary team** work closely together to provide for the needs of the child and family; such a team comprises a group of healthcare professionals from diverse fields who work in a coordinated fashion toward a common goal for the patient. In an environment characterized by high unemployment rates, insurance coverage concerns, frequent geographical moves for employment, high divorce rates, and increasing diversity in languages, cultures, and lifestyles, families can present with complicated needs requiring a team effort to meet them. Sometimes it takes immediate action to care for a child and family while they are in the healthcare arena, before they leave and the team misses the opportunity to provide continued care.

This chapter presents ideas about how strong communication skills between interdisciplinary team members can be fostered and implemented. If a child presents with an exacerbation of a chronic illness such as type 1 diabetes mellitus, severe asthma, or cystic fibrosis, the team must first identify the child's immediate healthcare needs, then identify the professional team members who have been involved with the child's care. These team members may be found across clinical settings—from providers of outpatient services to home care providers to providers during previous hospitalizations.

Prioritizing the child's needs is essential. If a child presents to the emergency department with respiratory syncytial virus (RSV)-related bronchiolitis and pneumonia, but is found to have evidence of physical child abuse or neglect, the team must provide for the child's immediate health care needs first. They must also piece together the puzzle of associated concerns and communicate with previous care providers, including social services and government agencies such as **Child Protective Services (CPS)**, which investigates cases and protects children from further abuse or maltreatment. Much more so than with adult patients, the vulnerability of a child requires all healthcare team members to work closely together, communicate assessments findings and concerns, and work collaboratively to create a comprehensive and agreed-upon plan of care.

Team Members

The provision of pediatric health care requires team members identify and communicate the needs of the child, and subsequently plan for treatment and care. When children are hospitalized with continuing medical needs, the team must work with case managers, home-care providers, community services, and the child's regular healthcare provider and office. The child might require services such as therapy, follow-up laboratory tests or diagnostic exams, and consultations with **specialists** (i.e., healthcare professionals with extensive knowledge in a particular area). The **Quality and Safety: Communicating with Team Members** box identifies team members who may potentially be involved with providing holistic and comprehensive care to children and their families (**Figure 5-1**).

for psychological evaluation, intervention, teaching, and support.

- *Community pediatricians:* Clinicians who provide historical perspectives on a child's health and communicate current health concerns and treatment plans. They may confirm immunization records and well- and ill-child encounters.
- *Developmental therapists:* Therapists who offer assessments, information, and guidance to team members and families of children with developmental issues, and locate developmental services in the community.
- *Lactation consultants/educators:* Specialists who assist a nursing mother to learn, practice, and be successful at breastfeeding, especially when a health concern arises in regard to the infant (e.g., cleft lip, cleft palate, neurologic impairment, illness, motor impairments), and who provide instructions for pumping and storing breast milk.
- *Licensed vocational nurses (LVNs)/licensed practical nurses (LPNs):* Nursing staff who assist the interdisciplinary team to provide direct nursing care to children and families while staying within their scope of practice; they communicate directly and frequently with the registered nurse assigned to supervise their care of patients.
- *Medical specialists:* Physicians with specialist credentials who work with the team to address a specific subset of medical issues (e.g., endocrinologist, cardiologist, pulmonologist).
- *Nursing assistants:* Clinicians who support the child's physical and emotional needs while assisting the nursing team in many aspects of care; they also support the family in adjusting to their child's hospitalization.
- *Occupational therapists:* Specialists who enable a child to learn and adapt to new circumstances or disruptions in lifestyle, preventing loss of function and improving psychological well-being.
- *Pediatric nutritionists:* Specialists who coordinate appropriate diets for children with a variety of healthcare needs (e.g., failure to thrive, malnutrition, weight

management, special diet needs, food alternatives in the presence of allergies) and provide education and a plan of care for the child at home.

- *Pediatric pharmacists:* Pharmacy specialists who provide accurate pharmacologic medical treatments in weight-based safe doses while children are hospitalized; prepare plans for medications needed at home; and teach or provide information to families concerning home medications.
- *Physical therapists:* Specialists who enable a child to reduce pain, improve or restore mobility, and treat physical dysfunction or injury through therapeutic exercise and restorative activity.
- *Physician assistants:* Practitioners who provide primary care in a team-based approach or in the absence of physicians.
- *Respiratory therapists:* Clinicians who support a child with airway management concerns by providing direct respiratory support skills; managing respiratory equipment such as oxygen, chest physiotherapy, pulmonary toileting, and ventilator services; and offer education on new or ongoing respiratory-related diagnoses such as asthma, bronchiolitis, or cystic fibrosis.
- *Social workers/case managers:* Social services professionals who assist the team to coordinate efforts to meet the needs of the family, including shelter, financial resources, resources, community referrals, counseling, insurance issues such as enrolling in Medicare or Medicaid, and planning for care beyond the immediate need (i.e., hospitalization).
- *Speech therapists:* Providers who evaluate a child with speech impairment or delay and develop a plan to address any physical, emotional, or neurologic issues associated with the structures of speech.
- *Spiritual care providers:* Individuals who provide religious, cultural, and spiritual support to families, especially during difficult times of crisis, loss, or emotional distress.

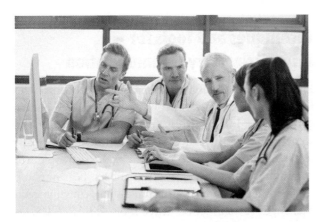

Figure 5-1

Communication Techniques

Establishing a **therapeutic relationship** is a central task for nurses working with children and families (Roberts, Fenton, & Barnard, 2015). In a therapeutic relationship, the nurse uses a style of communication that puts a person at ease, makes the individual feel reassured knowing that he or she is being taken seriously, and allows patients and families to express their concerns, questions, and emotions. Therapeutic relationships improve motivation and promote **empowerment**, the process through which a family comes to feel competent to provide care for their child (Collins, 2015). Numerous studies have found that parents' satisfaction with their child's care is correlated with their perception of the quality of communication—whether it is communication between the team and the family (Corlett & Twycross, 2006; October et al., 2016) or communication among team members (Giambra, Stiffler, & Broome, 2014; Khan et al., 2015).

A therapeutic relationship is goal oriented, has a definitive purpose, and ends with closure. The development of an effective therapeutic relationship requires 12 elements to be in place (Collins, 2015; Nursing Association of New Brunswick, 2000; Pullen & Mathias, 2010):

1. Establishing rapport with child and family
2. Showing respect to all members
3. Building trust by being honest, genuine, and authentic in all relationships; never making promises one cannot keep and never breaching privacy or Health Insurance Portability and Accountability Act (HIPAA) guidelines
4. Actively listening to the child and family while maintaining eye contact, direct attention, and solicitation of concerns, feelings, and emotions
5. Being aware of one's verbal and nonverbal communication
6. Showing empathy, understanding, and concern
7. Providing conflict management using creativity, clarification of feelings, negotiation techniques, and safety
8. Clarifying, verbally and nonverbally, the true concerns of the child and family
9. Maintaining professional boundaries; not sharing personal information (e.g., via social media)
10. Using humor when appropriate to encourage disclosure of feelings and promote relaxation
11. Being aware of feelings of inequality, shyness, resistance to disclosure, or any other boundaries that might prevent the establishment of a therapeutic relationship
12. Acknowledging when a therapeutic relationship is experiencing closure and being forthcoming in respectful goodbyes

The pediatric nurse's role in developing a therapeutic relationship is to develop trust, solicit information, support the child and family, and offer solutions and education. Because the pediatric nurse has more contact with a child and family during a hospitalization than any other team member, it is important to understand the meaning of this relationship, do the "connecting work" needed to support the family, and act as the "glue" by identifying what the family needs and how to get it. The therapeutic relationship is a positive alliance in which the nurse–patient relationship is based on trust, respect, sensitivity, helpfulness, and emotional/spiritual support (Pullen & Mathias, 2010). Regardless of the clinical setting where the nurse-family-patient

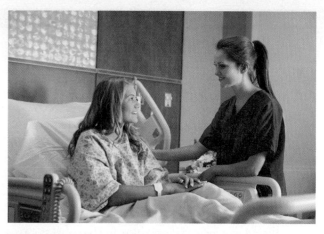

Figure 5-2
© Monkey Business Images/Shutterstock

relationship is established, the principles underlying this relationship are the same (**Figure 5-2**). The nurse, in any setting, must give his or her full attention, establish trust, provide care, and communicate all pertinent information to all team members.

BEST PRACTICES

A therapeutic relationship includes four critical components:

- *Trust:* Securing this critical component when a patient/family is in a vulnerable state.
- *Power:* Knowing there is an unequal relationship and using specialized knowledge and education to assist the child and family who may feel vulnerable.
- *Respect:* Protecting dignity, worth, culture, and all aspects of individuality.
- *Intimacy:* Providing closeness, privacy, and emotional support.

Data from Nursing Association of New Brunswick. (2000). Standards for the therapeutic nurse-client relationship. Retrieved from http://www.nanb.nb.ca/PDF/practice/Standards_for_the_therapeutic_Nurse-Client_Relationship_English.pdf

Techniques and Tools for Interdisciplinary Communication

Effective communication within a healthcare team lays the foundation for successful communication with patients and families. In high-stress environments, including the sometimes chaotic healthcare environment, it is helpful to use tools to organize one's thinking before and during communication between team members. Learning to be confident and organized during professional communication exchanges takes practice. Three tools—SBAR, CUS, and handoffs—have been shown to improve the effectiveness of interdisciplinary communication.

Structuring Communications with SBAR

The **SBAR protocol**, which was developed by the military and adopted by a network of physicians and nurses from Kaiser Permanente, is a mnemonic that represents a series of steps to organize one's thinking prior to communicating (Institute for Health Care Improvement, 2015). It provides structure when communicating with others in high-pressure or stressful situations. Using SBAR allows a nurse, or any other team member, to prepare for a conversation. Communication that follows this protocol is purposive, direct, and structured to promote an exchange of information between communicating parties such as a bedside nurse or clinic nurse and a primary care provider, while maximizing clarity and securing a plan.

SBAR includes four elements:

- **S**ituation: A concise description of the problem at hand.
- **B**ackground: A brief summary of information related to the problem at hand (i.e., what led up to the problem).
- **A**ssessment: A summary of what was found and is pertinent to the problem, such as the nurse's most recent assessment of the child.
- **R**ecommendation: A request for action in the form of a recommendation to help alleviate the problem.

Nurses can benefit from the structure of SBAR when they face a clinical problem that must be communicated. This protocol, which is considered the healthcare industry's best practice for standardized communication, promotes safety and quality by providing an efficient and well-structured format. SBAR is particularly helpful for new nurses who might feel uncertain about calling physicians to report changes in clinical status that need rapid interventions.

The CUS Protocol for Expressing Concerns

Expressing concerns can be difficult in certain circumstances—for instance, if a nurse is new to a team or setting, if there is a power differential in the relationship, or if the changes in process or status are happening rapidly. Using the **CUS protocol** allows for the expression of concerns in a respectful and professional manner. CUS stands for Concerned, Uncomfortable, and Safety (Agency for Healthcare Research and Quality, 2013, 2014):

C = "I am **concerned** about. . ."
U = "I am **uncomfortable** with. . ."
S = "I think we have a **safety** issue that needs to be addressed. . ."

Handoff Processes

An integral part of interdisciplinary and intradisciplinary communication is the passing or transfer of critical information and responsibility between healthcare providers through **handoffs**. Structured handoffs can be of enormous assistance when time is of the essence or the situation has a critical component. Although the literature includes many recommendations for specific handoff procedures and processes (see **Best Practices: Strategies for Effective Handoffs**), it is important that teams identify which set of processes is most likely to work in the context of their specific patient-care setting and given the needs of the individual patient and family. Team members should contribute to the discussion at patient intake and evaluate how the processes worked (or did not work) at discharge or, in the case of long-term patient care, at intervals throughout the care process. It may be useful to identify a nurse case manager or patient advocate to coordinate complex interactions involving multiple handoffs: Such coordination not only helps the team to avoid errors, but also increases the parents' and family members' understanding of who is on the team and what their role is in caring for the child.

Essential Formats for Handoffs

Safe and thorough handoffs also reduce errors. Nurses should share specific data about a child prior to handing the care of the child off to another healthcare professional (**Figure 5-3**). According to The Institute of Medicine (2001), "it is in inadequate handoffs that safety often fails first." Components of a safe handoff should include the following:

- Demographics, including age, developmental stage, weight, allergies, and medical diagnosis
- The child's current condition, associated previous hospitalizations and any recent or anticipated changes in the child's condition
- Up-to-date information on treatments, care needs, orders, lab values, and results of diagnostics

- Code status and level of severity (i.e., condition is currently stable, guarded or critical in nature)
- Recent medications administered or medications soon to be due (emphasis on medications administered in another department requiring re-timing, serum therapeutic levels, required patient or family education, or any consideration to medication safety)
- Any other pertinent data related to the child's condition or status

QUALITY AND SAFETY

Problems with ineffective handoffs affect the team function. Having to go back, find who gave the report, and clarify missing information takes time and creates havoc, breaches, failures, and gaps in vital information. Nurses may transfer between 40% and 70% of their patients every day (National Center for Biotechnology Information, n.d.)—rates that show how frequent and important the process is. According to Frank et al. (2005), error rates are as high as 68% in handoff sheets, including failure to include vitally important data such as accurate anthropometrics (especially accurate weights required for safe medication calculations), current allergies, and accurate information about medications.

Human Errors

- Omissions (left-out critical pieces of care information)
- Commissions (errors in information shared)
- Illegible documentation
- Lack of standardized form and lack of organization in thinking
- Lack of clarity or solicitation for clarity
- Being in a hurry

Environmental Issues

- Distractions and noise
- Interruptions
- Lack of clear space in which to work
- Poorly functioning or unavailable equipment, including computers
- Poor lighting

Patient Name: Age: Weight: Height: Known Allergies: Code Status: Developmental Stage:	IV in Place: Date of Insertion: Gauge: Location: Last Flush: Next Tubing Change:	Pertinent Medical History:
Presence of Family/ Support Systems:	Developmental Pain Scale Used: Last Pain Score: Last Pain Med Administered:	Pertinent Lab Values: Date Drawn: Reported?
Play Needs:	Other Symptoms:	Pending Labs to Draw:
Medical Diagnosis:	Pulse Oximetry:	Pertinent Diagnostic Exams:
Isolation Precautions:	Oxygen Therapy in Use:	Findings Reported?:
Diet:	Type of Oxygen Delivery Device:	Pending Diagnostics?
Activity Orders:	Wounds or Drains:	Output:
Previous Nurse:		Toileting Needs:
Body System Assessment: Respiratory: Cardiac: Neuro: Endocrine: Skin: GI: GU: MS: Sensory: Nutrition: Cognition: Emotional State:	Medications Due: 0800: 0900: 1000: 1100: 1200: 1300: 1400: 1500: PRNS Ordered:	Vital Signs: _____ _____

Figure 5-3 *Example of a handoff sheet.*

BEST PRACTICES

Strategies for Effective Handoffs

- Use only clear language that is universally known.
- Use only acceptable abbreviations, mnemonics, or shortened phrases that all team members would know.
- Limit any interruptions, but keep care safe.
- Ask clarifying questions. If you have a question, other team members will as well.

(continues)

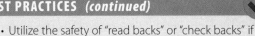
Barriers to Effective Communication

Challenges in establishing effective communication are real. The diversity and uniqueness of people, previous experiences with healthcare teams, and the environment in which communication takes place all influence whether a therapeutic relationship can be developed and fostered. In general, two types of barriers may hinder effective communication: physical barriers that need attention, and psychosocial barriers that need to be acknowledged and overcome.

Physical barriers:

- Physical space—crowding, lack of privacy, distractions (e.g., a television or computer taking attention from the speakers and listeners)
- Acoustics and ambient noise
- Qualities of the environment such as temperature, lighting, and seating

Psychosocial barriers:

- The emotional state of communicating parties (stressful healthcare environments and the child's acute state can add to distress)
- Trust within and between communicating persons
- Previous experiences with pediatric healthcare teams
- Cultural beliefs, expectations, and personal values that may influence effective communication
- Resistance to new processes and procedures or new technology

Power Distance

Power distance is a term used to capture the feelings and perceptions of inequality that exist between people and teams. It also refers to the extent to which individuals and groups accept the fact that inequality exists in society (Hofstede, 2001; Hofstede & Hofstede, 2005). As a result of power distance, communication barriers can develop between individuals who are perceived as having differing amounts of power. This imbalance, in turn, impacts the nonverbal aspects of communication (Richardson & Smith, 2007). When a perception of high power distance exists, persons deemed to have less power tend to be more polite, show more respect, and express agreement (whether they actually agree or not) in the presence of the person with the perceived higher power.

In the United States, power distance can be perceived to be very low. As such, it is common practice to address individuals by their first names irrespective of their positions in a perceived hierarchy. At the same time, differential status may be accorded to some providers due to greater specialization of practice or training than to others who are equally engaged in patient care (Zwarenstein, Rice, Gotlib-Conn, Kenaszchuk, & Reeves, 2013). In U.S. healthcare settings, which are often characterized by rich cultural diversity, healthcare providers are often seen to have higher power distance, since they have expertise that a patient does not possess. Unfortunately, the concept of power distance may also result in inequities and disparities in health care (Joint Commission, 2007, 2008).

Perceptions of power distance can be detrimental to the relationships among healthcare providers on a team as well as to the relationships between healthcare providers and family members. Errors may be introduced when higher-ranking team members (physicians or specialists) fail to communicate effectively with other team members due to power distance. In one study focused on intraprofessional communication, interactions among nursing and allied health professionals were frequent and in-depth, but few of these discussions involved physicians (Zwarenstein et al., 2013). For the most part, physician communication was limited to discussions with other physicians; when it included non-physicians, the discussion was often "one-way" in nature (Reeves et al., 2009). Such issues must be addressed if the team is to function effectively.

Greater power distance can add to errors if family members perceive that they are on an unequal footing, hold back information, do not disclose pertinent cultural practices, or simply do not wish to share their family health practices. Pediatric nurses must act as the conduit between a family and the healthcare team by whom the family feels intimidated.

Culture and Power Distance

Consider a scenario in which a Chinese immigrant father of a two-year-old girl who was recently diagnosed with leukemia expresses to the nurse—and only to the nurse—that he does not intend to sign consent forms for diagnostic exams, chemotherapy protocols, or surgical procedures such as the insertion of a central line. The father tells the nurse that he will be taking the child away from the large healthcare setting and plans to use traditional Chinese medicine to treat his child. When asked if he discussed this intention with the interdisciplinary team, the father says no, as he felt "bombarded with information," "not respected" for his culture, "not listened to," and "not allowed to speak." The father describes feeling intimidated and believes that if he shared his intent for treatment for his child, the team members would not respect him. Further care conferences held between the family and the oncology team that focus on reducing feelings of power distance ultimately may lead to the father's consenting to combine Western medicine with Chinese cultural practices to treat his daughter's leukemia.

As illustrated in this scenario, if the nurse finds that family members are demonstrating evidence of power distance or feelings of inequality, further support is needed. The pediatric nurse is in a key position to provide support; to encourage patients and families to speak up, express concerns, and give cultural guidance; and to work with team members who might be seen as intimidating by the parents, child, and extended family.

Written Communication

Current professional practice requires pediatric nurses to use a variety of written communication techniques. These techniques include electronic medical charting, sharing of electronic charting between departments and institutions, and confirmation of the accuracy of electronic checklists, notes, and entries. Computerized communication may be brief and concise—but unless the nurse takes a cautious approach, excessive brevity can lead to legal consequences. It is imperative that attention is given to learning electronic charting techniques and adhering to institutional policy and protocols concerning charting, as failure to do so has been associated with an increased rate of errors (Jylhä, Bates, & Saranto, 2016). The value of electronic communications in decreasing power distance among healthcare professionals has also been noted (Zwarenstein et al., 2013).

Case Study

The parents of twin girls, age 4 months, presented to the hospital's pediatric emergency department (ED) with both infants demonstrating weight loss, inconsolable crying, and bruises to the upper thighs. The parents both work full-time, have no respite infant care, and depend on each other to flex their demanding work schedules to attend to the twins. The father expressed concern about the girls' persistent crying and their changing eating patterns.

Upon assessment, the pediatric nurse noticed extreme crying during a diaper change. The ED staff ordered an X-ray of one of the girl's lower extremities and found a hair-line fracture on the inner aspect of the femur. Both girls underwent a complete skeletal survey, and the second twin demonstrated a healing fracture on the left fourth rib.

The mother, when interviewed in private, broke down in tears and described verbal threats, yelling, and physical abuse meted out by her husband and asked for help. Subsequently, the infants were placed on a police hold. After their acute healthcare needs were met, they were transferred under the direction of Child Protective Services to a medical foster home for care while an investigation of the potential abuse and neglect was conducted. The smooth interdisciplinary team communication efforts ensured a rapid sequence of safety and extended care.

Case Study Questions

1. Who were the members of the healthcare team who provided for the safety of the family?

(continues)

Case Study *(continued)*

2. How can interdisciplinary team members best communicate to ensure all aspects of this complicated case are addressed?
3. Which tools can be used for interdisciplinary team communication?

As the Case Evolves...

Suppose that during the process of examining the twin girls, one of the attending clinicians noted a bluish tint in the sclera of one child's eyes. She verified that this condition was present in the second child as well, and noted that both infants have loose joints and somewhat curved spines. The X-ray studies revealed the same fractures described in the original scenario, but the mother denied any conflict with the father and stated that all is well in the home. She anxiously indicated that she could not understand how her children came to have fractures as they have not yet begun crawling. One team member suggests that the infants might potentially suffer from a rare condition called osteogenesis imperfecta, in which bones are brittle and prone to low-impact fractures (Osteogenesis Imperfecta Foundation, n.d.).

4. Which of the following actions should be taken, and who should be added to the team, to appropriately care for the infants and their parents?
   A. After completing acute treatment, obtain a complete family medical and social history and request a consult with a clinical geneticist.
   B. After completing acute treatment, obtain a bone scan on both parents to determine whether they also have brittle bones and call for a consult with an osteologist.
   C. After completing acute treatment, obtain blood samples from the parents for DNA analysis and call for a consult with a hematologist.
   D. After completing acute treatment, obtain evaluations of the parents from social welfare and psychiatric professionals to determine whether a call to Child Protective Services may be warranted.

Chapter Summary

- Communication is an essential part of safe pediatric health care. Communication needs to be accurate, concise, and purposeful if care is to be coordinated and safe. During every encounter, the pediatric nurse is instrumental in providing information to team members, to outside agencies and referrals, and, most importantly, to the family.
- Complexities in working with children require that team members communicate clearly, thoroughly, professionally, and often with urgency. Identifying healthcare problems in children often requires that an interdisciplinary team work closely together to provide for the needs of the child and family.
- Use of successful communication techniques is supported by the health science literature, including SBAR, CUS, and safe handoff procedures and practice.
- Two types of barriers may hinder effective communication: physical barriers that need attention, and psychosocial barriers that need to be acknowledged and overcome.
- Power distance (the perception of inequality between people or parties) is a very real concern and poses challenges to effective communication, both within interdisciplinary teams and between team members and patients' families.
- Written communication is an important part of teamwork. Techniques include electronic medical charting, sharing of electronic charting between departments and institutions, and confirmation of the accuracy of electronic checklists, notes, and entries.

Bibliography

Agency for Healthcare Research and Quality. (2013). Team strategies and tools to enhance performance and patient safety. In Agency for Healthcare Research and Quality (AHRQ). *TeamSTEPPS pocket guide (2.0)*. Retrieved from http://www.ahrq.gov/professionals/education/curriculum-tools/teamstepps/index.html

Agency for Healthcare Research and Quality. (2014, October). *Examples of the SBAR and CUS tools: Improving patient safety in long-term care facilities: Module 2*. Rockville, MD: Author. Retrieved from http://www.ahrq.gov/professionals/systems/long-term-care/resources/facilities/ptsafety/ltcmod2ap.html

Collins, S. (2015, May 14). Good communication helps to build a therapeutic relationship. *Nursing Times*. Retrieved from https://www.nursingtimes.net/roles/nurse-educators/good-communication-helps-to-build-a-therapeutic-relationship/5003004.article

Corlett, J., & Twycross, A. (2006). Negotiation of parental roles within family-centered care: A review of the research. *Journal of Clinical Nursing, 15*(10), 1308–1316.

Curley, C., McEachern, J. E., & Speroff, T. (1998). A firm trial of interdisciplinary rounds on the inpatient medical wards: An intervention designed using continuous quality improvement. *Medical Care, 36*(8 suppl), AS4–A12.

Frank, G., Lawler, L. A., Jackson, A. A., Steinberg, T. H., & Lawless, S. T. (2005). Resident miscommunication: Accuracy of the resident sign-out sheet. *Journal of Healthcare Quality*. Retrieved from http://lists.amctec.net/email/link_redir/176/www.nahq.org/journal/online/pdf/webex0305.pdf

Giambra, B. K., Stiffler, D., & Broome, M. E. (2014). An integrative review of communication between parents and nurses of hospitalized technology-dependent children. *Worldviews on Evidence Based Nursing, 11*(6), 369–375.

Hofstede, G. (2001). *Culture's consequences: Comparing values, behaviors, institutions, and organizations across nations.* Thousand Oaks, CA: Sage.

Hofstede, G., & Hofstede, G. J. (2005). *Cultures and organizations: Software of the mind.* New York, NY: McGraw-Hill.

Institute for Health Care Improvement. (2015). SBAR Toolkit by Kaiser Permanente, Oakland California. Retrieved from http://www.ihi.org/resources/Pages/Tools/sbartoolkit.aspx

Institute of Medicine. (2001). *Crossing the quality chasm: A new health system of the 21st century.* Washington, DC: National Academy Press.

Joint Commission. (2007). What did the doctor say? Improving health literacy to protect patient safety. Retrieved from http://www.jointcommission.org/assets/1/18/improving_health_literacy.pdf

Joint Commission. (2008). Promoting effective communication: Language access services in health care. *Joint Commission Perspectives, 28*(2), 8–11.

Joint Commission, International Center for Patient Safety. (2005). Strategies to improve handoff communication: Implementing a process to resolve questions. Retrieved from http://www.jcipatientsafety.org/15274

Jylhä, V., Bates, D. W., & Saranto, K. (2016, April 14). Adverse events and near misses relating to information management in a hospital. *Health Information Management Journal.* [Epub ahead of print]. pii: 1833358316641551

Khan, A., Rogers, J. E., Melvin, P., Furtak, S. L., Faboyede, G. M., Schuster, M. A., & Landrigan, C. P. (2015). Physician and nurse nighttime communication and parents' hospital experience. *Pediatrics, 136*(5), e1249–e1258.

National Center for Biotechnology Information. (n.d.). Retrieved from https://www.ncbi.nlm.nih.gov

Nursing Association of New Brunswick. (2000). Standards for the therapeutic nurse-client relationship. Retrieved from http://www.nanb.nb.ca/PDF/practice/Standards_for_the_therapeutic_Nurse-Client_Relationship_English.pdf

October, T. W., Hinds, P. S., Wang, J., Dizon, Z. B., Cheng, Y. I., & Roter, D. L. (2016, April 7). Parent satisfaction with communication is associated with physicians patient-centered communication patterns during family conferences. *Pediatric Critical Care Medicine.* [Epub ahead of print]. doi: 10.1097/PCC.0000000000000719

O'Mahony, S., Mazur, E., Charney, P., Wang, Y. & Fine, J. (2007). Use of multidisciplinary rounds to simultaneously improve quality outcomes, enhance resident education, and shorten length of stay. *Journal of General Internal Medicine, 22*(8), 1073–1079. doi:10.1007/s11606-007-0225-1

Osteogenesis Imperfecta Foundation. (n.d.). Child abuse or osteogenesis imperfecta? Retrieved from http://www.oif.org/site/DocServer/_Child_Abuse__Child_Abuse_or_Ostegenesis_Imperfecta.pdf?docID=7189

Pullen, R., & Mathias, T. (2010). Fostering therapeutic nurse–patient relationships. *Nursing Made Incredibly Easy!, 8*(3), 4.

Reeves, S., Rice, K., Conn, L. G., Miller, K. L., Kenaszchuk, C., & Zwarenstein, M. (2009). Interprofessional interaction, negotiation and non-negotiation on general internal medicine wards. *Journal of Interprofessional Care, 23*(6), 633–645.

Richardson, R. M., & Smith, S. W. (2007). The influence of high/low-context culture and distance on choice of communication media: Students' media choice to communicate with professors in Japan and America. *International Journal of Intercultural Relations, 31,* 479–501.

Roberts, J., Fenton, G., & Barnard, M. (2015). Developing effective therapeutic relationships with children, young people and their families. *Nursing Children and Young People, 27*(4), 30–35; quiz 36.

Zwarenstein, M., Rice, K., Gotlib-Conn, L., Kenaszchuk, C., & Reeves, S. (2013). Disengaged: A qualitative study of communication and collaboration between physicians and other professions on general internal medicine wards. *BMC Health Services Research, 13,* 494.

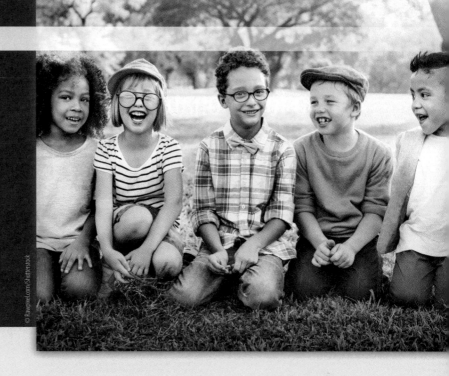

UNIT IV

Developmentally Focused Care and Developmental Milestones

CHAPTER 6

Caring for Neonates and Infants

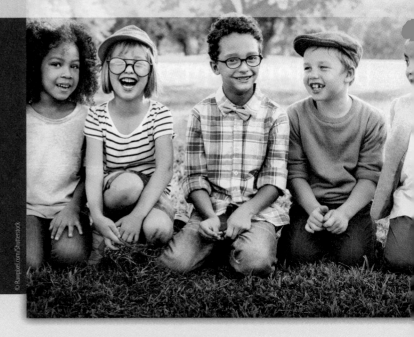

© Rawpixel.com/Shutterstock.

LEARNING OBJECTIVES

1. Apply developmentally appropriate techniques and perspectives in caring for children in the neonate and infant developmental stages.
2. Apply the classic psychosocial and developmental theories to children in the infant developmental stage.
3. Analyze patients' progress in relation to expected growth and development occurring during the neonatal and infant developmental periods.
4. Evaluate the play needs and play behaviors expected for children in the early and late infancy developmental periods.
5. Critically evaluate common health concerns during the infant developmental period.
6. Analyze safety concerns for parents caring for a rapidly growing and developing infant.
7. Apply components of anticipatory guidance for parents who have an infant.

KEY TERMS

Anthropometric measurements
Apgar scores
Asphyxiation
Aspiration
Cephalocaudal growth pattern
Colic
Deciduous teeth
Immunization schedule
Neonatal intensive care unit (NICU)
Proximal–distal growth pattern

Introduction

Pediatric nurses must have a tremendous foundation of knowledge on the principles of growth and development, as these are key pediatric concerns. When assessing their young patients, pediatric healthcare professionals focus on whether the children are achieving the expected or normal growth and development from the neonate through adolescent periods. Pediatric nurses must know what to expect regarding an infant's growth and development if they are to provide anticipatory guidance to parents and caregivers.

The infant developmental stage is marked by rapid growth in height, weight, head circumference, and body mass index, which are collectively referred to as **anthropometric measurements.** Infants typically can be expected to double their birth weight by 6 months of age and triple their birth weight by 1 year. Height typically increases by 50% from birth to 1 year of age. This tremendous growth influences the infant's motor ability. The infant learns to hold her head up within a few weeks of life and may be walking by her first birthday. Providing safety as the infant masters these motor milestones is one of the most important roles and responsibilities of caregiving during the infancy period (**Figure 6-1**).

The infant developmental stage is divided into three distinct periods: the neonatal period (birth to 28 days), the young infancy period (1 month to 6 months), and the older infancy period (6 months to 1 year). Each time frame has unique cognitive and motor milestones.

Neonates

Neonates, who must adapt to extrauterine life, experience the highest rate of infant mortality. The majority of neonates who die due to congenital anomalies, complications of birth, complications of prematurity, or a life-threatening condition, will die within the first week after birth, with one-fourth of those deaths occurring within the first 24 hours of life (Jehan et al., 2009). The stability of the transition from the uterine environment and the first few hours to days of life depends on the infant's ability to establish and maintain a healthy breathing pattern.

When caring for a neonate, the pediatric nurse should have access to the patient's birth history and Apgar scores; both provide information on the stability of the newborn's first few hours and days of life. **Apgar scores,** which assess the stability of the newborn, are performed at 1 minute and again at 5 minutes of life (**Box 6-1**; **Figure 6-2**). If the score is less than 7, assessment is repeated at 1-minute intervals until the newborn is stable (National Library of Medicine, 2015). The 1-minute score informs healthcare providers how the neonate tolerated the process of birthing. The 5-minute score indicates how the neonate is adapting to breathing and extrauterine life. The lower the score, the more interventions

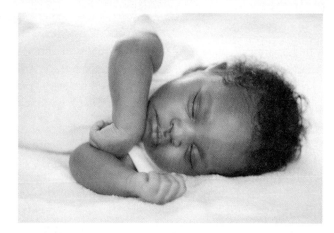

Figure 6-1 *The infant developmental stage is marked by rapid growth.*
© FatCamera/E+/Getty

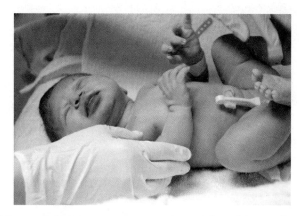

Figure 6-2 *Apgar scores assess the stability of the newborn immediately after birth.*
© Brian McEntire/Shutterstock

that will be required to support the infant's transition. Consistently low scores will mean a transfer to a **neonatal intensive care unit (NICU)**, a specialty unit for neonatal patients whose care requires advanced training and experience.

Neonates have unique presentations and unique challenges in many of their body systems:

- Neonates need inspired environmental oxygen to dilate their pulmonary vessels for ventilation, and closure of the three fetal shunts—the foreman ovale, ductus arteriosus, and ductus venosus.
- They need adequate surfactant to maintain oxygenation across the alveolar membrane.
- Neonates exhibit shallow and irregular breathing patterns and fast respiratory rates (40–60 breaths/min).
- Their rapid metabolic rates require more kilocalories (100–110 kilocalories/kilogram/day) and leave the newborn at risk for acidosis.
- Poor concentration of waste products due to immaturity of the kidneys (lower specific gravity) and fluid and electrolyte disturbances may lead to rapid dehydration and electrolyte imbalances.

BOX 6-1 Apgar Scoring

This system for scoring the stability of newborns was first developed in 1952 by anesthesiologist Dr. Virginia Apgar. The tool is implemented for all births; the newborn is scored twice, at 1 minute and 5 minutes, with repeated measures as indicated for a score of less than 7. Total scores can range from 0 to 10. For most institutions, any score of less than 7 provokes further assessment and possible immediate interventions to support the newborn's transition (tactile stimulation, nasal and oral suctioning, oxygen, chest compressions, etc.).

Classic Component	Acronym	Score of 0	Score of 1	Score of 2
Color	**A**ppearance	Blue/pale over entire body	Acrocyanosis Body pink	Body and extremities pink
Heart rate	**P**ulse	Absent	< 100	≥ 100
Reflex irritability	**G**rimace	No response to stimulation	Grimace/weak cry when stimulated	Cry or attempt to pull away when stimulated
Muscle tone	**A**ctivity	None	Some flexion	Flexed extremities that resist extension
Respiratory efforts	**R**espirations	Absent	Weak, irregular, gasping	Strong cry

Reproduced from Apgar, V. (1953). A proposal for a new method of evaluation of the newborn infant. *Current Researches in Anesthesia and Analgesia,* 32(4), 260–267. http://journals.lww.com/anesthesia-analgesia /Citation/1953/07000/A_Proposal_for_a_New_Method_of_Evaluation_of_the.6.aspx. Reprinted by permission of the Publisher, Wolters Kluwer.

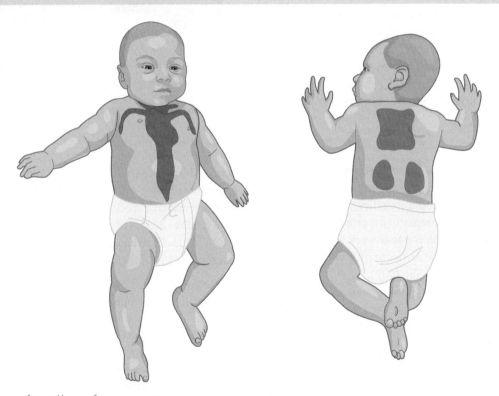

Figure 6-3 *Areas of stored brown fat on a neonate.*

- Challenges in thermoregulation include neonates' reduced stores of brown fat, a type of mitochondrial-rich fat that provides energy for thermoregulation (**Figure 6-3**).
- A neonate's immature gastrointestinal system leads to poor absorption of fats from decreased lipase production; poor storage of glycogen, which increases the risk of hypoglycemia; and increased regurgitation risk from the immature cardiac sphincter valve at the base of the esophagus.
- Neonates have a primarily cartilage-based musculoskeletal system, rather than bone tissue.

- Their primitive nervous systems rely on primitive reflexes and are not widely myelinated.
- A neonate's large occiput may contribute to airway occlusion (**Figure 6-4**).

Unexpected changes in status can affect even infants who are released in good health after birth. Health concerns arising during the neonatal period that may bring the infant into the pediatric acute care setting include fevers of unknown origin, hyperbilirubinemia, respiratory distress, and jaundice. Premature infants, low-birth-weight infants, and those with congenital anomalies are more likely to need acute care. In the acute setting, neonates may require monitoring devices and observation; for example, if a neonate experiences a brief, resolved, unexplained event (BRUE; previously described as an apparent life-threatening event [ALTE]), the neonate will be placed on an apnea monitor (**Figure 6-5**) and will likely need long-term follow-up (Rabasco et al., 2016; Tieder et al., 2016).

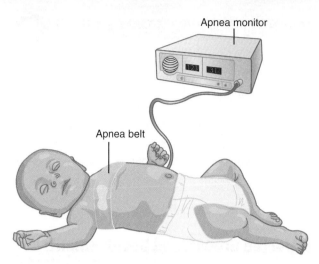

Figure 6-5 *An infant on an apnea monitor.*

Developmental Theory

In all settings in which they work, members of the pediatric healthcare team apply the theoretical concepts and constructs introduced by developmental theorists, especially the theories of Erikson, Piaget, and Freud. From birth through the various developmental stages, application of these theories allows providers to assess what is considered expected at an infant's particular stage, and provide anticipatory guidance to parents about what is coming next for the infant.

Erik Erikson's Theory of Psychosocial Development

Erikson described trust versus mistrust as the challenge for the infant during the first year of life. If the infant fails to develop a sense of trust in the environment and care providers, the infant will demonstrate signs of mistrust (frustration and anxiety). Consistently providing for an infant's basic needs, such as warmth, feedings, dry diapers, holding/cuddling, sensory exploration, and consistent caregiving, gives the infant the sense of security needed to develop trust.

Jean Piaget's Theory of Cognitive Development

Piaget describes the period of infancy up to the second birthday as the sensorimotor stage. During this stage, the infant uses his or her senses to explore the environment and objects. The infant develops more coordinated movements that allow for object manipulation and exploration. The recognition of object permanence emerges, such that the infant searches for items taken out of sight. Differentiation of self from environment is established.

Sigmund Freud's Theory of Psychosexual Development

According to Freud, infancy is the oral phase, in which the primary focus of exploration and sensation is the mouth. Infants, when developmentally able, will place all items in their mouth to explore and learn. Freud describes how sucking and biting are the primary sources of pleasure at this time.

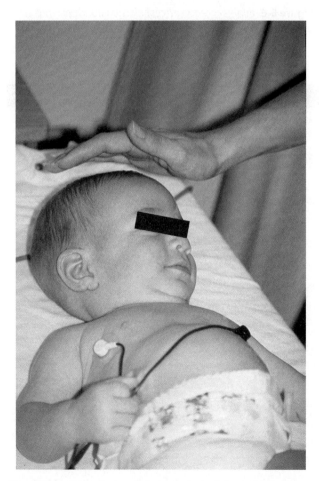

Figure 6-4 *Neonates have a large occiput relative to body size.*
Courtesy of Ron Deickmann, MD

Expected Growth and Development: Infant

The period of infancy is marked by rapid growth and development. The neonate quickly moves from complete dependency and motor movements based on primitive reflexes to rapidly developing gross and fine motor control. Infants experience a growth pattern that is described as **cephalocaudal** (from the head downward) and **proximal–distal** (from the center point outward). **Figure 6-6** illustrates this growth pattern. The pediatric nurse can expect the infant to demonstrate a series of milestones in the following order (**Table 6-1**):

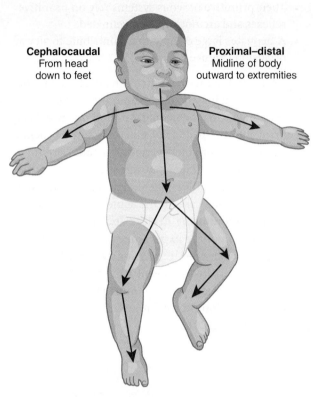

Cephalocaudal
From head down to feet

Proximal–distal
Midline of body outward to extremities

Figure 6-6 *Infants experience a cephalocaudal and proximal–distal growth pattern.*

TABLE 6-1	Infant Developmental Milestones
Height and weight	› Doubles birth weight by 6 months of age (gains, on average, 1.5 pounds per month)
	› Triples weight by 12 months of age
	› Grows on average 9–11 inches the first year, which represents a 50% increase in length (grows an average of 2.5 cm per month for first 6 months, then slows gradually)
Nutritional needs	› Premature infants need at least 110–120 kilocalories/kilogram of weight daily
	› Neonates need 100 kilocalories/kilogram of weight daily
	› Infants require 90–100 kilocalories/kilogram of weight daily up to 5 months
	› Older infants need 70–90 kilocalories/kilogram of weight daily
Sleep needs	› Newborns typically sleep 11–18 hours daily, at irregular times
	› Infants older than 4 months sleep 9–12 hours at night, with an additional 2–6 hours of nap time during the day
	› Circadian rhythm begins to develop at approximately 6 weeks of age
	› Infants younger than 6 months spend equal time in REM and NREM sleep; by approximately 6 months, the REM component is 30% of total sleep
	› Disrupted sleep can impact developmental milestones (Blumberg, Gall, & Todd, 2014; Scher & Cohen, 2015; Spruyt et al., 2008)
Sensory development	› All of the sensory organs are intact and functioning except for vision. The infant's eyes continue to be immature in visual acuity for most of the first year of life. Bringing items close (8–10 inches) to the child's visual field will help the child appreciate the item.

(continues)

TABLE 6-1	Infant Developmental Milestones *(continued)*	
	› Pain during infancy is real (**Figure 6-7**) and should be assessed on a regular basis using developmentally appropriate objective infant pain scales such as CRIES (Krechel & Bildner, 1995), NIPS (Hudson-Barr et al., 2002), or the revised FLACC (Malviya, Voepel-Lewis, Burke, Merkel, & Tait, 2006)
Eating behaviors	› Young infants are dependent on breastfeeding and bottles being held by the caregiver
	› Older infants hold their own bottle
	› Solid foods should not be introduced before 6 months of age and should start with iron-fortified baby cereals
Dentition	› First teeth erupt between 4 and 6 months
	› Teeth need twice-daily brushing; do not use fluoride toothpaste
	› Sugar should not be introduced in any foods during infancy
	› One to six **deciduous teeth** (baby teeth) should erupt during the first year of life; rarely do neonates have teeth at birth
	› Sippy cups should replace bottles and pacifiers by the first birthday
Expected vital signs	Temperature: 36.5–37.5°C
	Pulse: 100–200 beats/min for a younger infant; 80–150 beats/min for an older infant
	Oxygen saturation: 98–100%
	Blood pressure: 60–80/40–50 mm Hg
	Respiratory rate: 40–60 breaths/min for neonates; 22–30 breaths/min for infants

- One month: Cries, watches faces intently, closes hand, quiets when hears sounds and voices, grasp reflex present, fixes vision on objects 8–10 inches away.
- Two months: Lifts head up when prone; smiles socially; searches around for sounds with head and eyes; differentiates cries between hunger, discomfort, and distress; posterior fontanel closes.
- Three months: Demonstrates binocular vision, watches one hand, makes cooing and babbling sounds, shows increasing interest in the environment and surroundings.
- Four months: Rolls from back to side, holds head up while held in a vertical position, shows recognition of familiar objects and faces.
- Six months: Sits with support; grasps objects using the palm of the hand; rolls from stomach to back first, then from back to stomach.
- Seven to eight months: Begins to show stranger anxiety, sits unsupported for brief periods of time, begins using a pincer grasp to pick up small objects, scoots well.
- Eight to nine months: Shows hand dominance, pulls self up to stand, crawls well on hands and knees, knows the word "no."
- Ten months: Says recognizable sounds, typically "dada"; picks up objects and throws them.
- Twelve months: Eats with fingers, drinks from sippy cup.

UNIQUE FOR KIDS

Neurologic Assessments for Infants

Primitive reflexes are typically gone by the time the child reaches four to six months of age:

- Suck: Elicited by stroking the infant's cheek or the edge of the infant's mouth.
- Rooting: Elicited by stroking the infant's cheek on the desired side.
- Palmar: When an object is placed in either of the infant's hands, the infant will grasp the object.
- Plantar: Elicited by touching the sole of the infant's foot; the infant's toes will curl downward (**Figure 6-8**).
- Moro/startle: A slight change in equilibrium or sudden noise will cause the infant's arms and legs to extend and abduct.
- Dance or stepping: When the infant is held upright, with feet touching a surface, the infant will take tiny stepping movements with both feet.
- Fencing (tonic neck): When the infant is lying flat, if the head is turned to one side, the infant will make small arm movements that mimic a fencing stance.
- Babinski: Elicited by stroking the outer edges of the sole of the foot; the infant's toes will fan outward and upward (**Figure 6-9**).

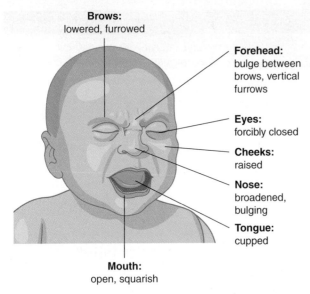

Brows:
lowered, furrowed

Forehead:
bulge between
brows, vertical
furrows

Eyes:
forcibly closed

Cheeks:
raised

Nose:
broadened,
bulging

Tongue:
cupped

Mouth:
open, squarish

Figure 6-7 *Infant in pain with classic squared mouth.*

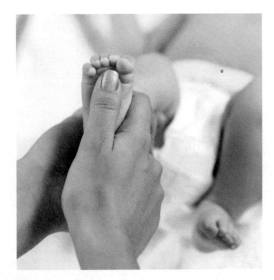

Figure 6-8 *Plantar reflex.*

© Dmytro Vietrov/Shutterstock

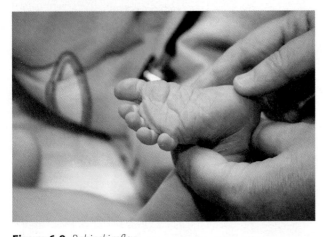

Figure 6-9 *Babinski reflex.*

© In The Light Photography/Shutterstock

FAMILY EDUCATION

Anticipatory Guidance for Family with an Older Infant: Food Introduction

Proper introduction of foods is a very important topic to discuss with parents of young infants in preparation for this 6-month milestone. Infants younger than 6 months should not be fed any food other than breastmilk or formula. The best anticipatory guidance to give on food introduction is to try one new food item every 3 to 5 days to assess for allergies. Infants' sucking reflex causes them to protrude their tongue when they first are offered foods on a spoon. Parents need to understand this is not a demonstration of the infant not liking the taste of the food.

Parents should introduce foods in the following order:

1. Iron-fortified baby cereals such as rice mixed with breastmilk or formula
2. Green vegetables first, then the sweeter yellow and orange vegetables
3. Mixtures of fruits and vegetables
4. Fruits
5. Meats at 10 months (beef, pork, chicken, and tofu)
6. Egg yolks at 10 to 11 months (no egg whites until 1 year of age)

Parents should follow these safety tips when feeding infants:

1. Do not given an infant any source of sugar.
2. Avoid common allergy-trigger foods: citrus juices, egg whites, cow's milk, and peanut butter.
3. Provide infant-safe biscuits only when the infant is able to gum and swallow well.
4. Avoid honey during infancy due to the risk of infantile botulism.

Communication

Language development begins during early infancy with cooing sounds. Infants should babble freely by seven months of age; if they do not, a hearing impairment should be ruled out. Infants move from cooing to making many unique sounds, including imitating sounds made by those people with whom they are interacting. Indeed, these sounds are the basis of learning words later (Graf Estes & Bowen, 2013). Most infants will say at least one purposive word by one year of age. The first recognizable sound is usually "dada" (a sound made by infants around the world), which can occur as young as 4 months of age. Reading, talking, and singing to the infant will help expand the child's language acquisition and cognitive development.

Providing Anticipatory Guidance to Parents: Milestones Needing Caution

- Rolling over can happen rapidly and unexpectedly; prevent serious head injuries by not placing infants on beds, tables, or surfaces where they can roll and sustain injuries.
- Avoid choking hazards. Do not allow young siblings to feed an infant; deaths have occurred from toddler and preschool siblings feeding infants, causing **aspiration** (inhalation of a substance or foreign body so that it enters the larynx or lower respiratory tract) and **asphyxiation** (choking).
- Older infants with pincer grasps will pick up all small objects they can find, including buttons, coins, watch batteries, candy, and medications. Do not leave purses, bags, backpacks, or other open containers containing hazards within their reach.
- Turn down all water heaters to 120° F to prevent burns.
- Prevent poisoning: Remove houseplants that are toxic, sweep and vacuum frequently, and have an adult lie on the floor and look for dangerous objects.
- Cover all electrical outlets to prevent electrocution.
- Do not place a crib by curtains with strings or ropes that might cause strangulation.
- Place cabinet locks on all cupboards that contain cleaning products, detergents, or any hazardous materials.
- Infants become more progressively social when exposed to others outside of the family. The infant must be given all of the childhood immunizations required during the first year of life; an **immunization schedule** will identify the recommended doses and agents for routine vaccinations (**Table 6-2**).

Play and Recreation Needs of the Infant

Infants participate in what is called solitary play (**Figure 6-10**). This does not mean the infant plays alone; rather, the infant enjoys visual and auditory stimulation and typically plays with objects presented by a partner. Older infants have short attention spans, so they benefit from the availability of a variety of objects in bright colors that make noise. Appropriate toys and activities for infants include the following:

- Crib mirrors
- Crib busy boxes
- Rattles
- Mobiles hung above the crib
- Teething toys
- Nesting toys
- Playing pat-a-cake
- Soft toys that make noise
- Reading board books to the older infant

Infant Health Conditions

Infants are especially prone to the following health conditions:

- Head injuries due to falls and motor vehicle accidents
- Anemia due to poor nutrition and lack of iron-fortified cereals (Maternal stores of iron are depleted by six months of age.)
- Sudden infant death syndrome (SIDS) (Place an infant on the back for sleeping ["back to sleep"], and do not smoke around the infant or hold infant in clothing with smoke on it.)
- Shaken baby syndrome (abusive head trauma) due to vigorous shaking of infant
- Failure to thrive, demonstrated by growth plot points below the 5th percentile on multiple occasions
- Significant diaper rashes caused by *Candida* (yeast with satellite lesions)
- Otitis media
- Lead poisoning from oral fixation
- Aspiration, choking, and asphyxiation
- Hyperbilirubinemia
- Dehydration and acid–base imbalances
- Neonatal seizures related to a metabolic disorder, birth trauma, prenatal infection, or neurologic malformation
- Sepsis due to immune system immaturity and development of an infectious process
- Exposure to maternal infections, including TORCH: **T**oxoplasmosis, **O**ther (syphilis varicella, HIV, or parvovirus B19), **R**ubella, **C**ytomegalovirus infection, **H**erpes simplex (Hockenberry & Wilson, 2013)
- Exposure to drugs in utero or fetal alcohol spectrum disorders
- Inborn errors of metabolism (phenylketonuria [PKU], congenital hypothyroidism, galactosemia, sickle cell disease, thalassemia, cystic fibrosis and congenital adrenal hyperplasia) (Cole & Lanham, 2011; Hockenberry & Wilson, 2013; Hopkins Medicine, 2015)

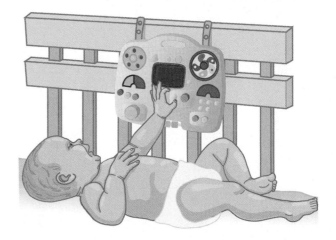

Figure 6-10 *Young infant in solitary play.*

TABLE 6-2 Childhood Immunization Schedule with Infant Recommendations

Vaccine	Birth	1 mo	2 mos	4 mos	6 mos	9 mos	12 mos	15 mos	18 mos	19–23 mos	2–3 yrs	4–6 yrs	7–10 yrs	11–12 yrs	13–15 yrs	16 yrs	17-18 yrs
Hepatitis B[1] (HepB)	1st dose	←— 2nd dose —→			←———————————————— 3rd dose ————————————————→												
Rotavirus[2] (RV) RV1 (2-dose series); RV5 (3-dose series)			1st dose	2nd dose	See footnote 2												
Diphtheria, tetanus, & acellular pertussis[3] (DTaP: <7 yrs)			1st dose	2nd dose	3rd dose		←———— 4th dose ————→					5th dose					
Haemophilus influenzae type b[4] (Hib)			1st dose	2nd dose	See footnote 4		←— 3rd or 4th dose, See footnote 4 —→										
Pneumococcal conjugate[5] (PCV13)			1st dose	2nd dose	3rd dose		←———— 4th dose ————→										
Inactivated poliovirus[6] (IPV: <18 yrs)			1st dose	2nd dose	←——————————————— 3rd dose ———————————————→							4th dose					
Influenza[7] (IIV)						←————————————— Annual vaccination (IIV) 1 or 2 doses —————————————→							Annual vaccination (IIV) 1 dose only				
Measles, mumps, rubella[8] (MMR)					See footnote 8		←—— 1st dose ——→					2nd dose					
Varicella[9] (VAR)							←—— 1st dose ——→					2nd dose					
Hepatitis A[10] (HepA)							←— 2 dose series, See footnote 10 —→										
Meningococcal[11] (Hib-MenCY ≥6 weeks; MenACWY-D ≥9 mos; MenACWY-CRM ≥2 mos)										See footnote 11				1st dose		2nd dose	
Tetanus, diphtheria, & acellular pertussis[12] (Tdap: ≥7 yrs)														Tdap			
Human papillomavirus[13] (HPV)														See footnote 13			
Meningococcal B[11]														See footnote 11			
Pneumococcal polysaccharide[5] (PPSV23)												See footnote 5					

Range of recommended ages for all children

Range of recommended ages for catch-up immunization

Range of recommended ages for certain high-risk groups

Range of recommended ages for non-high-risk groups that may receive vaccine, subject to individual clinical decision making

No recommendation

Note: These recommendations must be read with the footnotes in the original source. For those who fall behind or start late, provide catch-up vaccination at the earliest opportunity as indicated by the green bars in the table. To determine minimum intervals between doses, see the catch-up schedule in the original source. School entry and adolescent vaccine age groups are shaded in gray.

Reproduced from Centers for Disease Control and Prevention (CDC). (2017). Recommended immunization schedule for children and adolescents aged 18 years or younger, United States, 2017. Retrieved from https://www.cdc.gov/vaccines/schedules/downloads/child/0-18yrs-child-combined-schedule.pdf

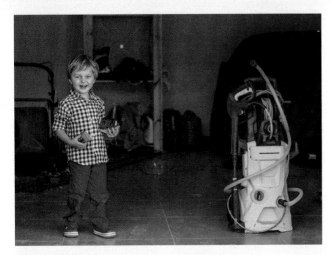

Figure 6-11 *Common areas for poisoning.*
© Ksenia Lev/Shutterstock

Poison Facts

Young children in infancy and young toddlerhood are a particular risk for poisoning due to their inquisitive nature, their tendency to mouth all objects they can reach, and being placed in circumstances where hazards exist (**Figure 6-11**). An estimated 44% of poisonings occur in children younger than 6 years old, 7% in children age 6 to 12 years, and 8% in teens (National Capital Poison Center, 2014). The following substances are most commonly implicated in infant and young-child poisonings (National Capital Poison Center, 2014):

- Cosmetics
- Cleaners
- Pain medications
- Foreign bodies
- Topical medications
- Vitamins and antihistamines
- Batteries
- Plants and mushrooms
- Office supplies, and arts and craft supplies
- Pesticides

Worldwide, acute poisoning is the fourth most common cause of unintentional deaths, after traffic injuries, fires, and drownings (World Health Organization, 2014).

Safety Concerns During Infancy

Infants are inherently dependent on others to provide all aspects of safety. As infants learn to control their movements, become mobile through crawling, and then develop the ability to stand, cruise while holding onto a surface, and walk, they become a greater safety risk with each passing month. Even their sleeping environment requires considerable thought to ensure safety: Parental co-sleeping, overly soft sleeping surfaces and bedding, "clutter" in the bed, and the possibility of overheating are all sleep-related concerns (Scheers, Woodard, & Thach, 2016; Task Force on Sudden Death Syndrome & Moon, 2011). The first major safety concern arises when an infant is able to push up on the hands and arms and roll over, but it is followed by many more. The prevention of head injuries during infancy is paramount. **Table 6-3** outlines safety concerns for the infant from birth to one year.

Treating Colic

Colic is a nonpathologic condition in which an infant cries for more than 3 hours per day for more than 3 days per week. Colic affects approximately one in six families and is the most common complaint seen by pediatricians in many parts of the world. It typically starts at 2 weeks of age and goes away without treatment by 3 to 4 months of age. Although the infant appears to be in gastric pain, infants with colic actually feed, grow, and thrive despite the long periods of crying.

The exact cause of colic is unknown, but theories of its etiology include gas, overstimulation, development of the nervous system, acid reflux, and hormones causing discomfort. There is no one, single cause of colic.

For safety, parents must be reminded to never shake their baby and that it is okay to put the baby down safely in the crib and take a break to take care of themselves during this trying time. Having a colicky baby can be frustrating and exhausting, as there is no cure for this condition. Some ideas for reducing the crying include taking the baby outside or using a safe baby swing. Keeping calm, asking others for help, finding respite, and providing safety for the infant is the best advice a pediatric nurse can give (Dobson et al., 2012; Johnson, Cocker, & Chang, 2015; mayoclinic.org, 2014).

Administering Medications to Infants

- Double-check all medications being administered in a healthcare setting (i.e., two nurses should check each medication).
- Use the most current weight to calculate doses of medications that are determined on a milligram per kilogram of weight basis.
- Do not administer medications to crying infants.
- Most medications administered to infants will have a longer clearance time; monitor for toxic effects.
- Some medications require higher doses to cross the blood–brain barrier.

(continues)

- When mixing a medication of formula, breast milk, juice, or flavored syrup (not recommended), use the smallest amount of fluid possible to ensure the entire dose will be consumed. Do not mix medications in bottles.
- Topical medications are readily absorbed into infants' skin; use them sparingly.

Topical Medications

- Place only a small amount of topical medications on infants' skin.
- Use only prescription medications or medications suggested by a primary provider, as over-the-counter medications may not be safe for young infants.
- Do not put any topical medication on open diaper rashes without the guidance of a primary care provider, as the medication will have systemic distribution within the infant's body.
- Do not allow infants to be in the sun for any period of time; do not apply sunscreen until infants are older than 6 months.

Antibiotics

- Teach parents to administer the entire prescription of oral antibiotics to an infant so that the pathogen does not return and resistant strains are not produced.

Antipyretics

- Use antipyretics with caution in infants. Fevers in young infancy should be reported.
- Indiscriminate use of acetaminophen can have serious side effects in the infant's hepatic system.
- Nonsteroidal anti-inflammatory drugs such as ibuprofen can reduce platelet aggregation.
- Do not administer more medicine than is recommended within a 24-hour period.

Teething

- Parents should not treat teething discomfort with alcohol (e.g., rubbing brandy on an infant's gums).
- A teething infant may benefit from a dose of acetaminophen.

Colic

- Colic should not be treated with over-the-counter medications such as diphenhydramine (Benadryl). Medications such as simethicone and proton pump inhibitors are ineffective, and dicyclomine (Bentyl) is contraindicated.
- For breastfed infants, use of a probiotic *Lactobacillus reuteri* (strain DSM17938) and reduction of maternal allergen intake may be effective. For formula-fed infants, switching to hydrolyzed formula may help.
- Always suggest that families talk to their physician before administering medications to children (Johnson et al., 2015).

TABLE 6-3 Safety Concerns During Infancy

Suffocation

› Infants will readily pull plastic bags over their head.

› Balloons should never be given to an infant or kept in the home environment.

› Plastic crib mattress covers must be removed.

› Crib slats must not be spaced wider than $2^5/_8$ inches.

› No pillows, toys, or stuffed animals should be placed in a crib.

› Strings and drawstrings must be removed from blankets or clothing.

› Infants should always be placed on their back to sleep to reduce risk of suffocation and SIDS.

Aspiration and Asphyxiation

› Small toys should not be given to infants. Use the cardboard toilet tissue tube check: If a toy can slip through the diameter of the tube, it is too small for young toddlers and infants. (**Figure 6-12** shows some common items that infants may choke on.)

› Toys must be labeled as safe for infants; small parts such as plastic wheels, buttons, and glued bits of plastic can be gummed or chewed off and cause aspiration.

Falls

› Infants will progress from rolling from front to back, to then rolling from back to front.

› Infants are at risk for severe head injuries from falling from surfaces or falling from highchairs, strollers when not buckled in, bouncy chairs, or other child devices where constant supervision is required.

(continues)

TABLE 6-3 Safety Concerns During Infancy *(continued)*

Burns

› Infants are at risk for burns from hot beverages consumed by the caregiver when the child is held.

› Infants who can stand are at risk for pulling over hot dishes and cups of hot liquids.

› Scalding burns can occur in the bath with water that is too hot.

› Infants can suffer sunburns. Infants younger than 6 months should not have sunscreen placed on their skin, but rather should not be exposed to the sun.

› Breast milk, formula, and baby foods should not be microwaved due to the risk of hot spots that can cause significant mouth, pharyngeal, and esophageal burns.

Drowning

› Crawling infants are at risk for moving through pet doors and subsequently drowning in pools.

› No standing water should ever be left in the presence of infants or toddlers.

› Young children do not have the arm strength to push themselves out of containers of water (trashcans, buckets) and will drown silently.

Head Injuries

› Infants must not be left alone for any period of time while being placed in an infant bouncy seat, highchair, or play-station chair.

› Infants should never be left alone on a changing station, even with straps in place.

Electrocution

› Older infants playing with objects may try to put the object (e.g., keys) into an electrical socket.

› Infants must be kept away from electrical appliances and water (especially in the bathroom near electric toothbrush docking stations, shavers, and curling irons).

› Teething infants should not be allowed around electrical cords.

› While hospitalized, infants are at risk for strangulation from wires and tubes.

Motor-Vehicle Injuries

› Infants are at risk for serious injuries if their car seats are not installed properly per state guidelines, or if the infant is not buckled in as directed.

› Infants should be rear facing, center seat in the back seat to prevent acceleration–deceleration head injuries.

› Infants should never be left unattended in a car.

Bodily Harm

› Infants will try to pull down heavy or harmful objects such as irons on ironing boards and house plants dangling down from a shelf.

› Infants should not be left alone with animals of any type.

› Sharp objects such as nails, scissors, clippers, and razors must be kept out of infants' reach.

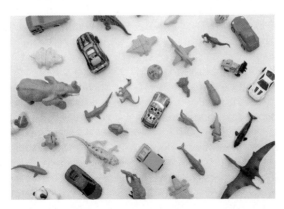

Figure 6-12 *Common items that may be choking hazards for infants and young toddlers.*
© Carol Yepes/Moment/Getty

Case Study

A 17-year-old mother has brought her 2-month-old infant into the pediatric clinic for a well-child check-up and immunizations. The infant's anthropometric measurements are taken and are plotted to be in the 60th percentile for weight and the 42nd percentile for height. The infant is asleep in the young mother's arms after just finishing a bottle of formula. The mother initially tells the nurse that her breastmilk has recently become very scant and she just started feeding the infant formula. Upon further questioning, however, the mother admits that her milk production is fine—the real issue is that she feels "stressed out" and ambivalent about breastfeeding. Although she has support to breastfeed her baby through her high school extension program for young mothers with children and encouragement at home from her mother and grandmother, several of her friends have made derogatory comments about the practice, and she feels uncomfortable about it—even though she states that "what's best for the baby is what matters." The mother also complains that breastfeeding leaves her little time for anything outside of school, and mentions that she would like to take a part-time job to improve her finances.

Case Study Questions

1. What are the benefits from breastfeeding an infant that the nurse can share with the mother?
2. Which resources are available in many communities to provide support for the teen mother of an infant?

As the Case Evolves...

Four months after their initial visit to the pediatric clinic, the teen mother and her now 6-month-old daughter are back for a well-child visit. The mother asks the pediatric nurse what the average time is for an infant to begin walking independently.

3. On average, infants walk within
   A. 10 months to 18 months of age.
   B. 12 months to 18 months of age.
   C. 9 months to 16 months of age.
   D. 11 months to 18 months of age.
4. While speaking to the nurse, the teen mother asks about the best way to encourage her infant's social and language skills. Based on Erikson's theory of psychosocial development, which of the following recommendations should the nurse make?
   A. Challenge the infant's primitive reflexes by eliciting them daily.
   B. Provide a busy board to the infant by attaching the toy to the crib rails.

C. Contact the local mothers' club and enroll the young infant into a play group of similar-age young infants.
D. Hold the infant frequently; talk and sing to the infant, smile at her, hold her close, and attend to her basic needs.

During the well-child visit for her infant, the mother asks if the child will need any shots at this visit. The nurse takes the opportunity to review the immunization schedule.

5. Which of the following immunizations should an infant receive during the first 10 months of life? (Select all that apply.)
   A. Measles, mumps, and rubella (MMR)
   B. Diphtheria, tetanus, and pertussis (DTaP)
   C. Hepatitis A and B combined
   D. Polio (IPV)
   E. Hepatitis B
   F. Rotavirus (RV)
   G. *Haemophilus influenzae* type b (Hib)
   H. Pneumococcal
   I. Influenza
   J. Varicella

The teen mother brings her 6-month-old daughter for a sick visit. The child is fussy and crying, but is afebrile and seems otherwise healthy. Her chin and fists are wet with saliva. The mother explains that she has been unable to soothe her and is worried that she is in pain, noting that neither of them got much sleep the previous night. Upon examination, the child has one newly erupted tooth and a red, swollen site on her lower gum line suggesting a second tooth is about to emerge.

6. Based on best practices for managing infant pain, which recommendations should be offered to the young mother?
   A. A single dose of infant-formulated over-the-counter ibuprofen
   B. A single dose of infant-formulated over-the-counter acetaminophen
   C. Infant-formulated ibuprofen, 1 dose every 4 hours until the second tooth erupts
   D. Infant-formulated acetaminophen, 1 dose every 4 hours until the second tooth erupts
7. Which safety concerns regarding administration of medication should the nurse proactively address with the mother of this infant with anticipatory guidance? (Select all that apply.)
   A. Concerns about accidental overdose
   B. Concerns regarding aspiration and asphyxiation
   C. Concerns regarding the child's dental health
   D. Concerns regarding developmental delay related to sleep deprivation

Chapter Summary

- Pediatric nurses must have a strong foundation in the principles of growth and development. Care of pediatric patients focuses on expected or normal growth and development from the neonate through adolescent periods.
- The infant developmental stage is marked by rapid growth in height, weight, head circumference, and body mass index. Infants are typically expected to double their birth weight by 6 months of age and triple their birth weight by 1 year. Height typically increases by 50% from birth to 1 year of age.
- The infant developmental stage is divided into three distinct periods: the neonatal period (birth to 28 days), the young infancy period (1 month to 6 months), and the older infancy period (6 months to 1 year). Each time frame has unique cognitive and motor milestones.
- Neonates experience the highest rate of mortality of all pediatric age cohorts. The majority of neonates who die do so in the first 72 hours; this outcome may be due to congenital anomalies, complications of birth, complications of prematurity, or a life-threatening condition.
- The transition from the uterus to the environment requires the infant to establish and maintain a breathing pattern.
- In terms of their development, infants are described as being in Erikson's trust versus mistrust stage, Piaget's sensorimotor stage, and Freud's oral stage.
- Infants follow a unique path of motor milestones that progress from holding their head up to walking within one year. After birth, they present with primitive reflexes (most of which disappear by four to six months) that are subsequently replaced with purposive movements.
- Safety is an extreme concern during the infant's first year of life. Infants are inquisitive and will mouth everything they can reach, fall easily, and are at risk for suffocation, aspiration, poisoning, head injuries, and drowning.
- Pediatric nurses are in a position to offer anticipatory guidance to new parents about what to expect next and how to plan for safety in all environments.

Bibliography

Blumberg, M. S., Gall, A. J., & Todd, W. D. (2014). The development of sleep-wake rhythms and the search for elemental circuits in the infant brain. *Behavioral Neuroscience, 128*(3), 250–263.

Cole, S., & Lanham, J. S. (2011, April 1). Failure to thrive: An update. *American Family Physician, 83*(7), 829–834.

Dobson, D., Lucassen, P. L. B. J., Miller, J. J., Vlieger, A. M., Prescott, P., & Lewith, G. (2012). Manipulative therapies for infantile colic. *Cochrane Database of Systematic Reviews, 12*, CD004796.

Graf Estes, K., & Bowen, S. (2013). Learning about sounds contributes to learning about words: Effects of prosody and phonotactics on infant word learning. *Journal of Experimental Child Psychology, 114*(3), 405–417.

Hockenberry, M. J., & Wilson, D. (2013). *Wong's essentials of pediatric nursing* (9th ed.). St. Louis, MO: Mosby.

Hopkins Medicine. (2015). Contact dermatitis in children. Retrieved from http://www.hopkinsmedicine.org/healthlibrary/conditions/adult/pediatrics/contact_dermatitis_in_children_90,p01679/

Hudson-Barr, D., Capper-Michel, B., Lambert, S., Palermo, T. M., Morbeto, K., & Lombardo, S. (2002). Validation of the Pain Assessment in Neonates (PAIN) scale with the Neonatal Infant Pain Scale (NIPS). *Neonatal Network, 21*(6), 15–21. doi: 10.1891/0730-0832.21.6.15

Jehan, I., Harris, H., Salat, S., Zeb, A., Mobeen, N., Pasha, O., . . . Goldenberg, R. (2009). Neonatal mortality, risk factors and causes: A prospective population-based cohort study in urban Pakistan. *Bulletin of the World Health Organization, 87*, 130–138.

Johnson, J. D., Cocker, K., & Chang, E. (2015). Infantile colic: Recognition and treatment. *American Family Physician, 92*(7), 577–582.

Krechel, S. W., & Bildner, J. (1995). CRIES: A new neonatal postoperative pain measurement score. Initial testing of validity and reliability. *Paediatric Anaesthesia, 5*(1), 53–61.

Malviya, S., Voepel-Lewis, T., Burke, C., Merkel, S., & Tait, A. R. (2006). The Revised FLACC Observational Pain Tool: Improved reliability and validity for pain assessment in children with cognitive impairment. *Pediatric Anesthesia, 16*(3), 258–265.

Mayoclinic.org. (2014). Diseases and conditions: Colic. Treatment and drugs. Retrieved from http://www.mayoclinic.org/diseases-conditions/colic/basics/definition/con-20019091

National Capital Poison Center. (2014). Poison statistics: Washington, DC metro area, 2015. Retrieved from http://www.poison.org/poison-statistics-wash-dc-metro-area

National Library of Medicine, National Institutes of Health. (2015). Apgar score. *MedlinePlus.* Retrieved from https://www.nlm.nih.gov/medlineplus/ency/article/003402.htm

Rabasco, J., Vigo, A., Vitelli, O., Noce, S., Pietropaoli, N., Evangelisti, M., & Pia Villa, M. (2016, May 10). Apparent life-threatening events could be a wake-up call for sleep disordered breathing. *Pediatric Pulmonology.* [Epub ahead of print]. doi: 10.1002/ppul.23468

Scheers, N. J., Woodard, D. W., & Thach, B. T. (2016). Crib bumpers continue to cause infant deaths: A need for a new preventive approach. *Journal of Pediatrics, 169*, 93.e1–97.e1.

Scher, A., & Cohen, D. (2015). Sleep as a mirror of developmental transitions in infancy: The case of crawling. *Monographs of the Society for Research in Child Development, 80*(1), 70–88.

Spruyt, K., Aitken, R. J., So, K., Charlton, M., Adamson, T. M., & Horne, R. S. (2008). Relationship between sleep/wake patterns, temperament and overall development in term infants over the first year of life. *Early Human Development, 84*(5), 289–296.

Task Force on Sudden Infant Death Syndrome & Moon, R. Y. (2011). SIDS and other sleep-related infant deaths: Expansion of recommendations for a safe infant sleeping environment. *Pediatrics, 128*(5), 1030–1039.

Tieder, J. S., Bonkowsky, J. L., Etzel, R. A., Franklin, W. H., Gremse, D. A., Herman, B., . . . Smith, M. B. (2016, April 25). Brief resolved unexplained events (formerly apparent life-threatening events) and evaluation of lower-risk infants. *Pediatrics, 137*(5). [Epub ahead of print]. pii: e20160590. doi: 10.1542/peds.2016-0590

World Health Organization, UNICEF. (2014). Children and poisoning. Retrieved from http://www.who.int/violence_injury_prevention/child/injury/world_report/Poisoning_english.pdf

CHAPTER 7

Caring for Toddlers

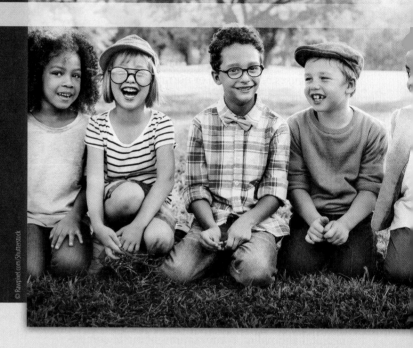

© Rawpixel.com/Shutterstock

LEARNING OBJECTIVES

1. Apply key concepts used in caring for a child in the toddler developmental stage.
2. Apply the classic psychosocial and developmental theories to children within the toddler developmental stage.
3. Assess a child with respect to the expected rates of growth and development that occur during the toddler developmental period.
4. Interpret play needs and play behaviors expected for a child in the toddler developmental period in the context of psychosocial development theories.
5. Critically evaluate common health concerns during the toddler developmental period.
6. Analyze safety concerns for the toddler at home, in a daycare program, and at play.
7. Develop helpful guidelines regarding temperament issues for parents caring for a toddler.

KEY TERMS

Autonomy
Cognitive development
Developmental theory
Moral development
Parallel play
Psychosexual development
Psychosocial development
Shame and doubt
Temperament
Tooth caries

Introduction

The toddler period includes the age range of 1 year up to the child's 3rd birthday. During this phase, children's physical growth slows down, they master locomotion, and they feel the need to express themselves as independent and autonomous. Sometimes labeled as the "terrible twos," the toddler period brings both challenges and joys. Parents watch as their infant becomes a small mobile child with developing language skills and increasingly expressive emotions. They also become acutely aware of how fast, unsafe, and in need of constant supervision their toddler is. Indeed, children of this age are inherently unsafe, as they explore their environment using all of their senses and try out new motor skills that make them prone to falls and other potential harm. Toddlers are very curious and persistent in their exploration. In turn, pediatric nurses must demonstrate excellent role modeling in safety while practicing patience and applying boundaries. Specific negotiation skills can help when assisting a toddler and his or her parents in navigating a healthcare encounter.

As toddlers grow, they demonstrate more energy, more creativity, and more sophistication in their play activities. Fine motor development of their fingers allows for greater manipulation of small objects. Yet, overall, they are clumsy and uncoordinated, making them unsafe in many situations. Parents are often in awe as they see their toddler move from crawling to cruising along furniture to independent walking to running, all in the course of a few quick months (**Figure 7-1**).

Social considerations at this age include the child's ability to understand object permanence, stranger anxiety, and the beginning of toilet training. If the family has another baby while the previous child is a toddler, the older child may display jealousy toward the new sibling or regression to earlier behaviors.

Developmental Theory

The toddler period is marked by exploration, cognitive expansion, and increasing motor activities. Toddlers learn to play on their own as they sense they are separate from their primary caregivers. This section presents the work of four theorists whose contributions to a deeper understanding of the developmental stages of childhood (i.e., to **developmental theory**) can enhance the pediatric nurse's appreciation of toddler needs and desires.

Erik Erikson's Theory of Psychosocial Development

"Autonomy versus shame and doubt" is the crisis that characterizes the toddler stage of Erik Erikson's **psychosocial development** theory (a theory of the development of personality over the life span based on social influences and environmental factors). During this stage, toddlers struggle with becoming perceptually aware of their separation from the primary caregiver. Mastery over **autonomy** (the ability to act without another person's control or influence) must occur, or otherwise subsequent feelings of **shame and doubt** (self-questioning about one's ability to handle problems) will emerge. Toddlers may display frustration as they learn that they must wait to have their needs met or gratification secured.

Parents have an integral role in assisting with autonomy by offering opportunities for toddlers to show they "can do it" or "me do it." Parents need to be encouraging and supportive, yet also provide rules, boundaries, and feedback. Children must learn that their behaviors and responses will have predictable effects on others, and they need positive feedback to develop acceptable behaviors. Egotistical thought, frequently saying "NO," loud protests, and tantrums all add to the special patience and guidance required to care for a toddler in a positive and productive way (Muscari, 2001) (**Figure 7-2**).

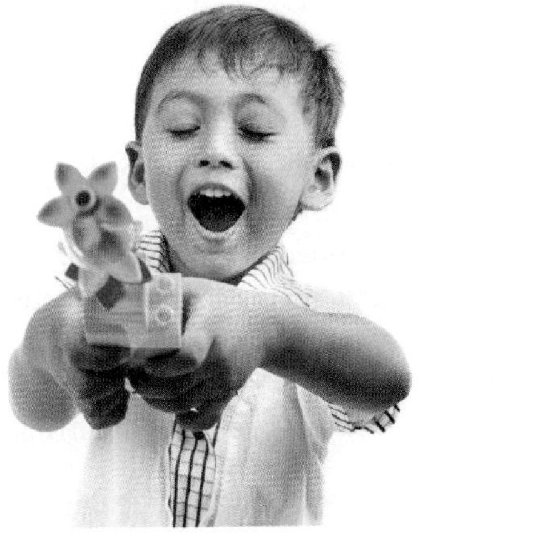

Figure 7-1 *As toddlers grow, they demonstrate more energy, more creativity, and more sophistication in their play activities.*

© Pikul Noorod/Shutterstock

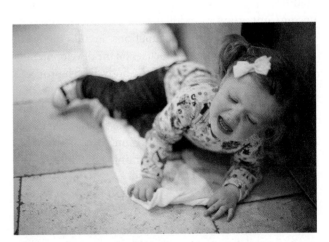

Figure 7-2 *Tantrums can add to the patience and guidance required to care for a toddler in a positive and productive way.*

© Jill Tindall/Moment/Getty

Sigmund Freud's Theory of Psychosexual Development

The toddler stage, according to Freud, is focused on the sexual centers of the buttocks and the anus. This "anal" stage is marked by the required mastery of retention and voluntary expulsion of fecal elimination. Toileting skills become important as toddlers gain ever-increasing control of their neuromuscular functions. Freud's theory of **psychosexual development** focuses on the development of libido fixed on specific areas of the body, which proceeds through five stages (oral, anal, phallic, latent, genital); it suggests that the mastery of toileting and established control of eliminative behaviors gives the toddler a sense of mastery over "letting go or holding on." **Box 7-1** provides additional information on toilet training a toddler.

Kohlberg's Theory of Moral Development

Obedience, punishment, and rewards shape the toddler period, which Kohlberg identifies as part of the preconventional stage of **moral development** (i.e., development of a sense of right and wrong, and the ability to perform moral reasoning). As the child is egocentric—without the ability to see others' points of view—negativity develops toward actions that produce punishment. Caregivers must apply consistent rules and consequences when dealing with toddlers, who may not understand the connection between their actions and the discipline. Time-outs are effective if kept short and accompanied by a quick, developmentally appropriate explanation as to why the time-out is occurring (Muscari, 2001).

Jean Piaget's Theory of Cognitive Development

Piaget's theory of **cognitive development** (i.e., development of the ability to think and reason) describes the toddler period as being marked by sensorimotor exploration and development. Toddlers are actively exploring, using their senses, and creating an understanding of their environment, and they require constant stimulation, movement, and play. Both spatial relationships and causal relationships bloom as they experience increasing interest in their environment, experiment with objects, and achieve locomotion.

Expected Growth and Development: Toddler

The period of infancy is marked by rapid growth in all aspects of the baby's body, from height to weight to head circumference. The toddler, in contrast, experiences slower growth through what are known as "spurts and lags." The toddler gains only 1.8 to 2.72 kg (4-6 lb) in weight per year, the head circumference expands by just 1.25 to 2.5 cm (0.5–1 in) per year, and height increases by only 7.5 cm (3 in) per year, or less. Most experts agree that the weight of a toddler who is 2½ years of age should be approximately 4 times (quadruple) the birth weight. Toddlers should continue to have their head circumferences measured at each well-child check-up to ensure expected head growth and confirm closure of the anterior fontanel. Notably, injuries or conditions of the brain tissue and cerebral spinal fluid can affect this measurement. Head circumference, weight, and height should be plotted on a standardized growth chart for frequent comparisons. **Table 7-1** identifies important considerations regarding toddler development.

Communication

Language development occurs rapidly in the toddler period. The toddler begins the second year with only 1 to 2 words, but ends the toddler period at the third birthday with between 300 and 500 words. Typically, the toddler uses 2- to 3-word sentences, learns to use pronouns, and states his or her first and last names by approximately 2½ years of age.

Multilingual families typically provide rich cultural experiences, but may create some challenges in language development. Residence in a household where two languages are spoken has been known to cause small delays in toddler language development. Residence in a home with three or more spoken languages can cause further delays. The toddler may demonstrate an understanding of what is said around him or her, but responses may be delayed.

The toddler stage is the point at which many developmental delays and neurologic disorders, including autism, first become apparent. Because of the direct link between a toddler's language development and experiences with positive and supporting parenting (Glascoe & Leew, 2010), the toddler's ability to communicate and any barriers to developing language skills should be assessed. Many tools are available for developmental assessment of toddlers and preschool-age children; a comprehensive review of such tools is available through the National Early Childhood Technical Assistance Center (Ringwalt, 2008).

TABLE 7-1	Toddler Development
Locomotion	› Most toddlers walk unassisted by 15–16 months or earlier
	› Bow-leggedness (tibial torsion) fades as the legs grow longer and stronger to hold the weight of the trunk
	› Toddlers will walk up stairs one step at a time by placing both feet on each stair by 2 years of age
	› Toddlers can ride a tricycle at age 3 years
Nutrition	› Toddlers require reduced calories compared to infants
	› Toddlers need 70–90 kcal/kg of body weight
	› They need two snacks per day between meals to keep blood glucose levels even
	› Milk should be limited to 24 oz per day; should be whole milk until their 2nd birthday (fat is required for brain cell growth), then skim milk is sufficient throughout childhood
	› Toddlers are at risk for iron-deficiency anemias and "milk anemias"
	› Toddlers need 1.2 g/kg of protein per day (approximately 13 g)
	› Juice should be restricted, soda and other sugary drinks should not be introduced
Sensory development	› All sensory organs are intact
	› Visual acuity is still developing
	› Acuity is thought to be 20/40–60, on average

(continues)

TABLE 7-1	Toddler Development (continued)	
Eating behaviors	›	Age group has severe choking risks; finger foods need to be chopped into small pieces for safe consumption
	›	Foods associated with a high risk of choking should be avoided (e.g., hot dogs, popcorn with kernels, carrots, hard candy and nuts)
	›	Toddlers must sit while eating to prevent aspiration and choking episodes
	›	Toddlers may demonstrate picky eating, food favorites, and hunger lags
	›	Neither manners nor sitting at the table very long should be expected
Tooth eruption	›	The first teeth that appear during infancy should be assessed by a dental professional
	›	Toddler teeth need twice-daily brushing
	›	Sugar intake should be minimized
	›	Deciduous teeth (10–14) should erupt during the toddler stage
	›	Sippy cups should replace bottles and pacifiers by the first birthday
Expected vital signs	Temperature: 37.2°C	
	Pulse: 80–110 beats/min	
	Oxygen saturation: 98–100%	
	Blood pressure: 90–105/55–70 mm Hg	
	Respiratory rate: 22–25 breaths/min	

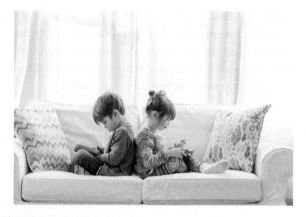

Figure 7-3 *Toddlers typically engage in parallel play.*
© Elizabethsalleebauer/RooM/Getty

Play Needs of the Toddler

The active toddler needs many play opportunities throughout each day. Children of this age are moving away from individual play, also called solitary play, in favor of **parallel play**. Toddlers will move toward each other and play near each other, but they typically end up back to back, or alongside each other, not sharing toys or craft supplies (**Figure 7-3**). Due to their developmental stage, toddlers have difficulty learning to share or being cooperative with toys or play items. For this reason, it is best to offer each toddler a separate activity. Sharing is a learned behavior that requires parental role modeling, support, and positive reinforcement.

It is typical for a toddler to be interested in a toy for a short period of time and then want to move on to another play item. Offering a variety of large, colorful, safe toys creates a successful play opportunity for the young child. Appropriate toys that are fun for this age include blocks for building or stacking, play telephones, play kitchens and workshops, large puzzles, musical instruments made for young children, and pretend medical supplies. All play items should be assessed for small parts that can be chewed off or swallowed, or are considered a choking or aspiration risk.

Health Concerns for the Toddler

The concerns described in this section are unique to the toddler period and should be kept in mind when interacting with parents of patients in this age group. Anticipatory guidance can include discussions on nutrition, respiratory concerns, prevention of skin issues, and gastrointestinal health.

UNIQUE FOR KIDS

Order of Assessments for Toddler

Toddlers will benefit from a logical and thoughtful order of physical assessment techniques. It is recommended that the nurse conduct an assessment in the following order:

1. Visual inspection of the child from head to toe and all surfaces. This can be done during a game with the child in a diaper.

(continues)

2. Auscultation of the lungs, heart, and abdomen with a warmed stethoscope and a toy for distraction.
3. Percussion of the abdomen.
4. Light palpation followed by deep palpation of the abdomen while the toddler is positioned in a comfort hold in the parent's lap.
5. Genital inspection.
6. Ear inspection (pull the pinna down and back, as the eustachian tube in a toddler is wider, shorter, and slanted compared to that in an adult). The toddler might find this to be the most distressing aspect of the assessment, so it should be performed last.

Nutrition

Toddlers are at risk for developing nutritional deficiencies. Iron-deficiency anemia is a medical diagnosis directly related to the quality of the young child's diet. Many health-care providers are now screening young toddlers for iron, hemoglobin, and hematocrit levels to assess for anemia. The **Unique for Kids: Toddler Nutrition** feature describes the toddler's nutritional needs and concerns (CDC, 2017).

UNIQUE FOR KIDS

Toddler Nutrition

- The growth spurt during the infant period slows down at the end of the first year of life. The toddler period is not marked by rapid growth, so the toddler will eat less and demonstrate a decreased appetite.
- The toddler's appetite is sporadic, is marked by "food lags and jags," and the child might be very ritualistic and opinionated as to what he or she will and will not eat. Patience is required during this time, and parents should be encouraged to keep offering a variety of small portions of foods.
- The toddler's deciduous teeth have come in, with a child of this age having an average of 14 to 20 teeth. This set of teeth enables the toddler to chew foods.
- The need to feel autonomous and demonstrate "me do" autonomy to others makes these children interested in learning to feed themselves. Parents should provide a safe spoon. The toddler often holds the spoon in one hand and picks up finger foods in the other hand.
- Transition from the bottle to the cup should take place early in the toddler period to prevent tooth decay.
- Foods during the toddler period should include whole milk until 2 years of age (brain growth needs the fat), and a full range of meats, veggies, fruits, breads, and iron-rich cereals.
- If a toddler has a lack of interest in meats or eggs or has a vegetarian diet, carbohydrates should not be served as a food alternative. Toddlers need at least 13 g of protein per day.
- Toddlers should experience food with all of the senses; providing them with a variety of colors, textures, flavors, and aromas is important.
- Foods should not be spicy, high in salt, sugary, or commercially prepared.
- Caution should be taken when microwaving foods, as the center of the food may be much hotter than the periphery.
- Family members need to recognize that toddlers cannot sit for very long. The meal time should be calm, without discipline, bribes, or rewards. Table manners cannot be mastered during the toddler period.
- To prevent the development of iron-deficiency anemia, also known as "milk anemia," the toddler should not consume more than 24 oz of milk per day. Whole milk is filling and may influence how much other foods are consumed. Milk is not considered a complete protein.

RESEARCH EVIDENCE

Iron Deficiency and Lead Poisoning

Iron-deficiency anemia is the most common nutritional disorder in the United States. Although the overall prevalence has declined since 1960, the prevalence of this disorder is increasing in the 1- to 3-year-old group. The current reported prevalence is approximately 3%. It is imperative to identify this disorder early, as it may have long-lasting consequences, such as diminished motor, mental, and behavioral functioning (Kazal, 2002).

Lead poisoning affects toddlers at roughly the same rate as iron deficiency. Risk factors for lead poisoning include low household income, living in an older home or neighborhood where exposure can come from flaking lead paint or lead-lined water intake pipes, and contact with contaminated soil. The presence of items imported from countries where use of lead is not regulated, such as toys, cosmetics, ceramics, jewelry, and other products, also can contribute to toxicity. In addition, a variety of folk remedies are known to be contaminated with lead. Symptoms of lead poisoning can include gastrointestinal problems, decreased height, delayed sexual maturation, increased **tooth caries** (breakdown of the teeth because of bacterial actions), and impaired neurologic development (e.g., behavioral changes, mental impairment, seizures).

Iron-deficiency anemia and lead poisoning are sometimes related, as iron-deficient children are at higher risk of lead toxicity should exposure occur (Warniment, Tsang, & Galazka, 2010).

Respiratory Concerns

As toddlers become more social and begin to attend preschool or other childcare environments, their exposure to infectious diseases increases. Toddlers may experience colds and other viral infections that lead to respiratory symptoms. A toddler with respiratory distress, such as the distress that can occur with the highly communicable respiratory syncytial virus, can present with loud adventitious breath sounds, persistent coughing, and mucus production. Toddlers should be evaluated for supportive care if distress is present.

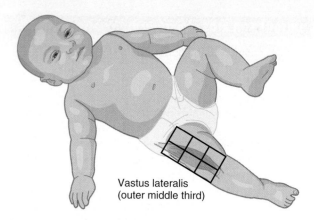

Vastus lateralis
(outer middle third)

Figure 7-4 *Vastus lateralis.*

QUALITY AND SAFETY

A toddler who presents with adventitious breath sounds should be immediately evaluated for respiratory distress. Distress can be associated with foreign objects in the airway, bronchiolitis, reactive airway disease, or asthma.

UNIQUE FOR KIDS

Therapeutic Holds for Toddlers Undergoing Procedures

Have all equipment set up and ready to go!

- Ear assessment: Seat the child in the parent's lap. Have the parent hold the child's arms down with one arm, hold the child's head against the parent's chest with ear out, and wrap a leg around the child's legs to prevent kicking.
- Vastus lateralis intramuscular (IM) injection (**Figure 7-4**): Place the child in a mummy wrap, or have the child lean back on the parent's chest while the parent holds the child's arms down and legs straight.
- Urinary catheter insertion: Have enough staff present to assist, as this procedure can take three adults to hold the child. Place a mummy wrap around the child's arms, then have one staff member at each leg to hold the child's legs open. The parent should comfort the child at the head and help to hold the child's shoulders down.
- Intravenous (IV) line insertion: Place the child in a mummy wrap, with only the extremity that will be used to insert the IV showing. The parent should be at the child's head to offer support and distraction, and hold the child's shoulders down.
- Accessing a central line/dressing change: For this sterile procedure, the child should be held against the parent's chest with arms restrained and head up and out (prevent tears from dripping on the sterile chest skin site). Two staff members and one parent may be required to perform this sterile technique on a toddler.

PHARMACOLOGY

Immunizations

During the toddler period, a child should receive the following immunizations:

1. DTaP: Administered IM, this vaccine covers three bacterial infections—diphtheria, tetanus, and pertussis. Giving acetaminophen before and 4 hours after the vaccine can reduce the incidence of immunization-related fever and tenderness with local skin reactions.
2. Measles: The first dose is given subcutaneously (SQ) in the toddler period between 12 and 15 months of age. Mild post-immunization symptoms may include fever, irritability, and transient skin rash.
3. Mumps: The mumps vaccine is given with the rubella and measles vaccine as part of the MMR vaccine.
4. Rubella: Given with mumps and measles vaccines as part of the MMR vaccine, this vaccine prevents congenital rubella syndrome.
5. Polio: Oral polio vaccine (live virus excreted in the stool for up to one month) is no longer recommended by the Centers for Disease Control and Prevention (CDC) in the United States. Inactivated polio vaccine (IPV) is exclusively recommended today.
6. Influenza: Annual influenza vaccines are recommended throughout childhood.
7. Hepatitis B: The toddler should receive the third and last dose of the hepatitis vaccine series.
8. Pneumococcal: The toddler should receive either the PCV7/Prevnar IM or the 23-valent PPV/Pneumovax, given either IM or SQ.
9. Varicella: Given as a SQ injection, this vaccine is first administered during the toddler period between 12 and 15 months and repeated at least 3 months later, but preferably between 4 and 6 years of age.

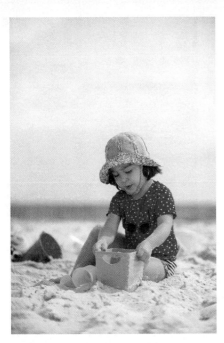

Figure 7-5 *Toddlers should wear sunscreen and a hat whenever they are playing outside.*

© Ignacio Ayestaran/Moment/Getty

Skin Issues

Toddlers are learning to be toilet trained and, therefore, are still in diapers. Frequent diaper changes are needed to prevent skin breakdown and contact dermatitis. Toddlers should wear a sunscreen with a high sun protection factor (SPF) and a hat whenever they are playing outside (**Figure 7-5**). Any rash found on a toddler should be assessed for the presence of a communicable disease such as varicella, measles, or rubeola.

Gastrointestinal Health

Toddlers can be prone to constipation; to avoid this problem, their diet should include a variety of high-fiber foods. The introduction of fruits daily and vegetables with every lunch and dinner is an educational point that the nurse should discuss with the family. Making sure the child drinks enough water is imperative. Fruit juices are discouraged due to their high fructose or sugar content and their large amount of calories. Toddlers who present with diarrhea should be put on immediate contact precautions and monitored for viral gastroenteritis.

Screening for Developmental and Neuropsychiatric Concerns

Toddlerhood is often when developmental delays and neuropsychiatric issues first appear. Developmental

delays can be relatively straightforward to identify, as developmental and speech milestones are simple to assess and have been compiled into evidence-based tools that are handy for screening (Dosman, Andrews, & Goulden, 2012; Moharir et al., 2014; Thomas, Spragins, Mazloum, Cronkhite, & Maru, 2016). Even autism spectrum disorders (ASDs) now have screening tools for children in the 18- to 24-month age bracket. The American Academy of Pediatrics recommends that "all children be screened with an ASD-specific instrument during well-child visits at ages 18 and 24 months in conjunction with ongoing developmental surveillance and broadband developmental screening" (Zwaigenbaum et al., 2015).

Nevertheless, identifying "problem" behaviors in toddlers is difficult. At this stage, many behaviors that might seem to suggest "something is wrong" are actually short-term conditions rather than long-lasting issues. A child's development is so rapid during the toddler phase that it complicates potential diagnosis; behaviors that are concerning in a slightly older child may be perfectly normal in a toddler. As Gardner and Shaw (2008) point out, "six temper tantrums a day might be bothersome but normal at 22 months, but could contribute to a diagnosis of oppositional defiant disorder (ODD) in a 4-year-old." This makes using a toddler's behavior to assess for the presence of behavioral disorders difficult for clinicians.

Nevertheless, recent research has shown that as many as 55% of children with early behavioral problems do not spontaneously outgrow their issues (Bagner, Rodríguez, Blake, Linares, & Carter, 2012), which makes early identification of children with true emotional or behavioral disturbances important. Many discussions about assessment of toddler behavior (e.g., Reynolds, 2010) focus on the need for clinicians to perform an assessment based on multiple sources of information, including the child's observable behavior, the parent–child interaction, and the child's self-perception (using an age-appropriate method).

Safety Concerns for the Toddler

Toddlers are inherently unsafe. They are very active, love to explore their environments, want to test boundaries, and will test limits often. Providing safe environments at preschool, home, outside play areas, and healthcare settings is imperative (**Box 7-2**; **Figure 7-6**). Safety sweeps should be conducted often to make sure there are no potential scenarios where injuries, falls, or drowning might take place. Toddlers should not be trusted to be alone in any environment. See **Quality and Safety: Safety Concerns for the Toddler** for safety concerns and tips.

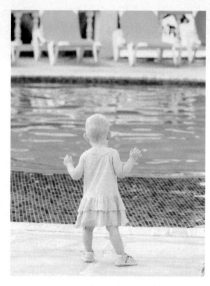

Figure 7-6 *Providing safe environments for toddlers is imperative.*
© PHB.cz (Richard Semik)/Shutterstock

11. Do not allow animals to approach toddlers, and set firm limits by not allowing the child to run up to pet unfamiliar animals. Dog bites can be devastating, and cat bites or scratches can lead to significant infections.
12. Use only approved car sets appropriate for toddlers. Never place the car seat by air bags or in the front passenger seat, and have the seat's placement inspected.
13. Prevent burns by cooking on back burners, never drinking hot beverages around the toddler, and keeping the temperature of the home water heater less than 120°F.

PHARMACOLOGY

Toddlers are very prone to ingesting toxic substances. Families should not administer the emetic ipecac unless instructed to do so by the National Poison Control Center. Provide families with the national hotline number to seek immediate advice on poisoning: (800) 222-1222 (American Association of Poison Control Centers, 2014).

Toddlers who are hospitalized have unique safety concerns. Providing a safe sleeping arrangement should be based on institutional policy; a high-top crib is the safest place for a toddler to sleep. Administering medications safely is also a major concern. **Box 7-3** provides tips on safe medication administration for children in this developmental stage.

BOX 7-3 Administering Medications to Toddlers

- Try to give the toddler two choices, such as a choice between two flavors of syrup (cherry or chocolate).
- Do not give advance warning of administration of oral medications, as the child may have a tantrum.
- Do not administer oral medications while the child is crying.
- Elevate the child to a sitting position.
- Use an oral syringe (no needle) to give medications.
- If appropriate, offer to allow the child to hold medicine cup or syringe and self-administer the medication.
- Offer the child a fluid chaser to mask the flavor.
- Use a teaspoon or tablespoon if that is what the family uses at home.
- Never store medications at the bedside; if the child is not able to take them, return the medications to the medication room.
- Always teach the parent or caregiver how to give medications safely.
- Offer a simple smile and short praise when medication administration is completed; do not bribe or reward the child with prizes or candy.
- Never tell the toddler the medication is candy.

Because toddlers are notorious for taking off their identification tags/bands, it is important that the pediatric healthcare team perform safety "time-outs" prior to any medication administration or procedure. Parents should confirm the toddler's full name, spelling, and date of birth.

Toddlers in a Hospital Crib

Toddlers should not be placed in a regular twin-sized bed unless institutional policy and practice allows for this possibility when the parents are always present. Instead, a toddler should be placed in a safe, metal, high-top crib so that there is no chance that the child will experience a fall by climbing over the crib rails. Even at a young age, children will stack objects left in their bed and use them to provide the boost needed to climb out of a crib.

Whenever a pediatric healthcare provider, or parent, has lowered the crib rails, they should put them up safely when done and then double-check that the rail lock is secure. A toddler can experience a significant injury if the rail is not hooked and the child leans on it, causing the rail to fall rapidly.

Make sure the toddler does not have access to wires, pumps, or medical devices by reaching the arms through the rail. Toddler cribs should not be close to oxygen delivery devices, electrical outlets, or suction devices. Try to arrange the location of the crib in full view from the open door.

Temperament of the Toddler

Caring for a toddler has its own joys and challenges. Each child is unique: He or she comes from a unique family background, culture, and childrearing practice, and has a unique **temperament** (the dominant disposition of an individual—an aspect of personality). Some toddlers are more easygoing; others have a difficult time with change. Some toddlers are loud and rowdy; others are quieter and more contemplative. Most toddlers throw tantrums and create battles over items or situations where they want to exert control. Some, faced with the introduction of an infant sibling, may temporarily regress to behaviors appropriate to younger children or display other behaviors (sleep disturbance, aggression) in response to the change of their status (Volling, 2012). This behavior is to be expected during this developmental stage. Parents need to be reassured that setting boundaries and limits, ignoring tantrums when safe to do so, and being patient during this time of growing "autonomy" are important.

Case Study

Kevin, a 19-month-old toddler, has been hospitalized for facial cellulitis requiring 5 days of intravenous antibiotic therapy via a peripheral saline lock line. His mother, Karen, is a single parent; in addition to Kevin, she has a 4-year-old daughter at home. Karen's parents assist the family with daily child care in their home so that Karen can maintain a part-time job.

After the admission process was completed, Karen told the staff that she would need to go home for the night to be with her other child and work early in the morning. She stated that she would call to check on her toddler throughout the time she would be away, but that realistically she would not be back to see Kevin until late in the afternoon the next day. As Karen held and kissed Kevin, she told him she was leaving, became tearful, and placed him back into the high-top crib. Kevin immediately became very distressed, crying loudly and banging his head on the bars of the crib. Karen left in tears, obviously very upset about leaving.

Case Study Questions

1. How do Kevin's behaviors fit with the concept of hospitalization for a child in the toddler developmental period?
2. Which behaviors can the pediatric staff most likely expect to see in Kevin over the next several hours?
3. Which support, distraction, and play can be offered to comfort Kevin during his hospitalization and his mother's absence?

As the Case Evolves. . .

Kevin is in a stage of development described by Piaget as "sensorimotor," characterized by exploration of the environment via sensory stimulation such as touch, sound, and color perception.

4. Which aspects of the sensorimotor stage are demonstrated in Kevin's behavior upon his mother's departure?
   A. Demonstrating anxiety during separation from the primary caregiver, often the mother
   B. Expression of fear of strangers both at home and in healthcare clinical settings
   C. Use of physical behaviors that stimulate sensory inputs to express emotions
   D. Empathy to a parent's negative emotional state

After having a tantrum over his mother's departure, Kevin lies down in his bed. A student nurse making rounds with an instructor stops by. The instructor notes that toddlers like Kevin have unique differences in their anatomy and physiology as compared to adults.

5. Which of the following statements is (are) true? (Select all that apply.)
   A. Toddlers have thin skin and easily absorb medications directly into their bloodstream.
   B. Toddlers have a narrower airway and demonstrate louder adventitious breath sounds than adults.
   C. Toddlers have greater appetites and higher metabolism rates than adults.
   D. Toddlers demonstrate the same blood pressure readings as older children.
   E. Toddlers demonstrate abdominal breathing more so than thoracic breathing.
   F. Toddlers are able to store glycogen in their livers to maintain steady blood glucose levels.

Chapter Summary

- The classic psychosocial and developmental theories support a deeper understanding of children within the toddler developmental stage.
  - Erik Erikson's theory of psychosocial development places toddlers in the stage of "autonomy versus shame and doubt."
  - Toddlers are in the "anal" stage, according to Sigmund Freud's theory of psychosexual development.
  - Kohlberg's theory of moral development suggests that toddlers are in the preconventional stage.
  - Jean Piaget's cognitive development theory describes toddlers as being in the sensorimotor exploration stage.
- Growth during the toddler developmental period slows down in comparison to infancy.
- Toddlers master higher levels of gross and fine motor movements, require fewer daily calories as compared to infants, and need only one nap. They are known for tantrums, exerting their autonomy, participating in parallel play, and expanding their language skills.
- Developmental delays may become evident in the toddler phase, but long-term behavioral issues are difficult to identify with certainty and require use of various assessment tools to pin down.
- Play behaviors expected for a child in the toddler developmental period should consider safety first, as toddlers are very curious, still place objects in their mouths, and

demonstrate choking and aspiration risks. Toys should be large, colorful, challenging, and free of small parts that can be chewed off.

Bibliography

American Association of Poison Control Centers. (2014). Poison help numbers. Retrieved from http://www.aapcc.org

Bagner, D. M., Rodríguez, G. M., Blake, C. A., Linares, D., & Carter, A. S. (2012). Assessment of behavioral and emotional problems in infancy: A systematic review. *Clinical Child and Family Psychology Review, 15*(2), 113–128.

Centers for Disease Control and Prevention. (2017, March 3). Nutrition. Retrieved from https://www.cdc.gov/nutrition

Dosman, C. F., Andrews, D., & Goulden, K. J. (2012). Evidence-based milestone ages as a framework for developmental surveillance. *Paediatrics and Child Health, 17*(10), 561–568.

Gardner, F., & Shaw, D. S. (2008). Behavioral problems of infancy and preschool children (0–5). In M. Rutter, D. Bishop, D. Pine, S. Scott, J. Stevenson, E. Taylor, & A. Thapar (Eds.), *Rutter's child and adolescent psychiatry* (5th ed., pp. 882–893). Oxford, UK: Blackwell.

Glascoe, F. P., & Leew, S. (2010). Parenting behaviors, perceptions and psychosocial risk: Impacts on young children's development. *Pediatrics, 125*(2), 313–319.

Kazal, L. (2002, October 1). Prevention of iron deficiency in infants and toddlers [Patient family handout]. *American Family Physician.*

Mahat, G., Lyons, R., & Bowen, F. (2014). Early childhood caries and the role of the pediatric nurse practitioner. *Journal for Nurse Practitioners, 10*(3), 189–193.

Moharir, M., Barnett, N., Taras, J., Cole, M., Ford-Jones, E. L., & Levin, L. (2014). Speech and language support: How physicians can identify and treat speech and language delays in the office setting. *Paediatrics and Child Health, 19*(1), 13–18.

Muscari, M. (2001). *Lippincott's review series: Pediatric nursing* (3rd ed.). Philadelphia, PA: Lippincott.

Reynolds, C. R. (2010). Behavior assessment system for children. In I. B. Weiner, & W. E. Craighead (Eds.), *Corsini encyclopedia of psychology.* Hoboken, NJ: John Wiley & Sons.

Ringwalt, S. (2008). *Developmental screening and assessment instruments with an emphasis on social and emotional development for young children ages birth through five.* Chapel Hill: University of North Carolina, FPG Child Development Institute, National Early Childhood Technical Assistance Center. Retrieved from http://www.nectac.org/~pdfs/pubs/screening.pdf

Thomas, R. E., Spragins, W., Mazloum, G., Cronkhite, M., & Maru, G. (2016). Rates of detection of developmental problems at the 18-month well-baby visit by family physicians using four evidence-based screening tools compared to usual care: A randomized controlled trial. *Child: Care, Health and Development, 42*(3), 382–393.

Volling, B. L. (2012). Family transitions following the birth of a sibling: An empirical review of changes in the firstborn's adjustment. *Psychology Bulletin, 138*(3), 497–528.

Warniment, C., Tsang, K., & Galazka, S. S. (2010). Lead poisoning in children. *American Family Physician, 81*(6), 751–757.

Yapucu Güneş, Ü., Ceylan, B., & Bayindir, P. (2016). Is the ventrogluteal site suitable for intramuscular injections in children under the age of three? *Journal of Advanced Nursing, 72*(1), 127–134.

Zwaigenbaum, L., Bauman, M. L., Fein, D., Pierce, K., Buie, T., Davis, P. A., . . . Wagner, S. (2015). Early screening of autism spectrum disorder: Recommendations for practice and research. *Pediatrics, 136*(suppl 1), S41–S59. Retrieved from http://pediatrics.aappublications.org/content/136/Supplement_1/S41.long

CHAPTER 8

Caring for Preschoolers

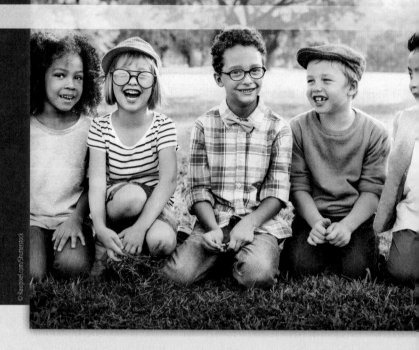

©Rawpixel.com/Shutterstock

LEARNING OBJECTIVES

1. Define and apply key concepts used in caring for a child in the preschool developmental stage.
2. Apply the classic psychosocial and developmental theories to children within the preschool developmental stage.
3. Evaluate patient growth and development in comparison to that expected for children during the preschool developmental period.
4. Assess the play needs and play behaviors of a child in the preschool developmental period.
5. Critically evaluate common health concerns during the preschool developmental period.
6. Analyze safety concerns for the preschooler at home, at preschool, and at play.
7. Apply nursing care concepts in offering anticipatory guidance for parents of a preschooler.

KEY TERMS

Associative play
Egocentric
Initiative versus guilt
Intuitive thinking
Magical thinking
Night terrors
Nightmares
Phallic–locomotion
Preconceptual thought
Preconventional
Symbolic functioning

Introduction

The preschool period includes the age range of 3 years through the end of the child's 5th year. During this phase, the preschooler's growth continues to be slow and steady. Although *growth* refers to an increase in physical size, *development* refers to an increase in skill and an increase in complexity of demonstrated tasks. The preschooler's development is characterized by an increasing ability to show more complexity in movement, cognitive processing, language, and fine motor abilities. The preschool period is also marked by participation in **magical thinking**—the idea that merely thinking about or wishing an interaction, person, or event will cause it to occur. Magical thinking in an older child or adult is considered irrational; however, for children in this stage of development, it is normal.

As preschool-age children grow, they demonstrate more graceful and coordinated movements. Fine motor development of their fingers continues, which allows for greater manipulation and progressive success in the use of writing utensils, art supplies, crafting skills, and toys that require more fine manipulation (**Figure 8-1**). Emotionally, preschool-age children have fewer tantrums and greater ability to express themselves verbally and negotiate.

Developmental Theory

The preschool period features many different transitions and changes. This section presents the work of four theorists whose contributions to a deeper understanding of the developmental stages of childhood can enhance the pediatric nurse's appreciation of the child's changing behaviors, needs, and desires.

Erik Erikson's Theory of Psychosocial Development

The preschool period is characterized by what Erikson describes as **initiative versus guilt**. In this stage, the child attempts new skills, tries out new relationships, and participates in new activities (initiative) (**Figure 8-2**). If discouraged or unsuccessful in these attempts, the child may develop a sense of self-doubt and guilt. Without mastery of this phase, the preschool-age child will not continue to demonstrate a sense of exploration, initiation, and desire for mastery of new experiences.

Preschoolers are learning how assertiveness and purposeful actions influence their environment. As they progress, they evaluate their own behavior and notice the behavior of others. This process helps to guide the development of conscience. If the child initiates actions that are met with parental disapproval, the child may develop further guilt.

Sigmund Freud's Theory of Psychosexual Development

According to Freud's theory, the preschool-age child is in the **phallic-locomotion** phase. In this stage, the child recognizes differences in the genders and shows an interest in discovery and understanding of the genital area. Freud's theory introduces four distinct experiences for the preschool-age child: penis envy, the Oedipus complex, the Electra complex, and castration anxiety (also referred to as genital mutilation anxiety). According to Freud's concept of the Electra complex, a preschool-age female child feels a psychosexual competition with the child's mother or significant female figure over her father. In opposition, the male child experiences the Oedipus complex as competition with his father figure over his mother.

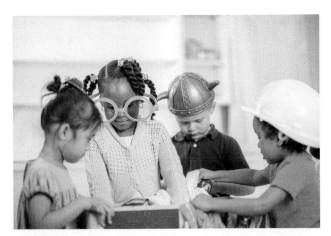

Figure 8-1 *During the preschool period, fine motor development continues, allowing for greater manipulation.*

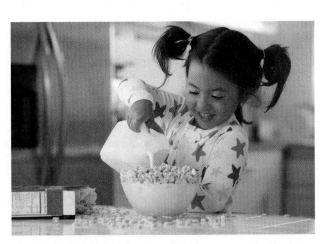

Figure 8-2 *According to Erikson, the preschool period is characterized by initiative.*

Lawrence Kohlberg's Theory of Moral Development

After beginning as a developmental psychologist, Kohlberg, a Harvard University professor, moved into the field of moral education. His well-known theory of moral development was based on Swiss psychologist Jean Piaget's work. Both Kohlberg and Piaget believed that a person develops in a progressive pattern, including a progressive development of moral reasoning. Kohlberg describes a child at the preschool level as **preconventional**, signifying that the child's moral thinking and behavior are based on concepts related to obedience and punishment (Kohlberg & Hersh, 1977). In this developmental stage, the child learns socially accept-able "normal" behavior by being compelled by the threat of punishment and rewarded by social obedience. Included in Kohlberg's theory is the notion that a child does not "jump" stages of moral reasoning, but rather progresses stage by stage through various experiences and levels (Barger, 2000).

Jean Piaget's Theory of Cognitive Development

Piaget describes the preschool period as one marked by **preconceptual thought** (inability to distinguish members of the same class). In this developmental stage, the child continues to use egocentric approaches to address the demands made by both society and the environment. According to Piaget, the preschool-age child participates in **intuitive thinking**, in which the child centers his or her thinking on one characteristic of something and then forms a judgment or makes a decision based on that single characteristic. This phase in early preschool includes the **egocentric** perspective that the world revolves around "me," but during this phase, their thoughts begin to include others.

This stage can be also be defined based on the young child's judgment of self or the environment through visual experiences. Young children thoroughly enjoy exploring their environments and rapidly develop language that allows them to describe their world and experiences to others, albeit not always truthfully, in great detail. The preschooler also learns to understand cause and effect.

Toward the middle of the preschool developmental stage, the egocentric thought process diminishes and children begin to include others' ideas and preferences into their thinking. Throughout this phase, children express their experiences in words, even if their thoughts are not based completely on reality.

Expected Growth and Development: Preschooler

During the preschool period, children experience slow and steady growth. "Spurts and lulls" in growth are still common, but overall growth in height, weight, and head circumference is slow and steady. The preschooler gains only 2.27 kg (5 lb) per year and increases in height by 7 cm (less than 3 in) per year. Average height for preschoolers is 97.5 to 112.5 cm (39–45 in) and average weight is 15.9 to 20.5 kg (35–45 lb). Development milestones for preschoolers are shown in **Table 8-1** (Centers for Disease Control and Prevention [CDC], 2014).

TABLE 8-1	Preschool Development
Locomotion	› Preschoolers are more graceful and fluid in their movements. They run, jump, and climb well and can sustain longer walks or runs than during toddlerhood. › Finger dexterity improves and can be noticed during development of skills such as buttoning clothing or learning to write one's name. By the preschooler's 5th birthday, the child will be able to dress and undress independently.
Nutrition	› A preschooler needs an average of 1200–1600 cal/day. › Pediatric nurses can use calorie need equations such as 70–90 kcal/kg/day for preschoolers (Linnard-Palmer, 2005).
Social behaviors	› Like to imitate and copy adults and others who are around them; like to play mom, dad, and teacher. › Cooperate with other children in sports, games, and classroom activities, but will cheat to win. › Enjoy describing what is coming next, such as in a book or story, in a children's film, or in real life. › Show affection for others without prompting. › Show increasing concern for others having an emotionally hard time, such as persons who are crying or feeling distressed. › Separate easily from parents in later preschool years. › Have a wide range of emotions; vacillate between cooperation and being demanding to others. › Older preschoolers are more likely to agree to a set of rules and adhere more consistently to them as pleasing adults becomes more important.
Eating behaviors	› Often copy adult eating behaviors. › Children may start the preschool period with poor manners and low mastery of utensils; by late preschool, they can use a fork and a spoon and begin to use a table knife. › Preschoolers can continue to be picky eaters and may want only their favorite foods. Remind parents to keep offering a variety of colorful and interesting foods and let them know that their child will eventually be open to eating most foods. › Involve the older preschool-age child in food selections and meal preparation as deemed safe. › Never force children to "clean their plate" or eat when they state they are full. › Provide preschoolers with three meals per day, plus morning and afternoon snacks. Unplanned snacking should be discouraged and monitored, as this habit will highly affect meal consumption. › Because preschoolers are very active, they are still at a choking risk. Preschoolers should never eat unless they are sitting down.
Tooth development	› Preschoolers typically start this developmental stage with all 20 deciduous teeth (baby teeth) and may be starting to shed the lower central incisor teeth. › Early preschoolers should be supervised when brushing their teeth no less than twice a day.
Expected vital signs	› Temperature: 36.7–37.2°C › Pulse: 90–115 beats/min › Oxygen saturation: 98–100% › Blood pressure: 85–95/50–60 mm Hg › Respiratory rate: 16–22 breaths/min
Language development	› Preschoolers enjoy talking; parents or caregivers can find themselves with very robust conversational partners, as these children's curiosity moves them to ask many questions. › Preschoolers are increasing their vocabulary; on average, they master 900–1500 words before their 5th birthday.

(continues)

TABLE 8-1	Preschool Development (*continued*)
Sleep needs	› A preschooler needs, on average, 11.5–12 hr of sleep per night.
	› The young preschooler is transitioning from having a significant nap in the afternoon as a toddler to now needing a shorter nap or just a rest period.
	› **Nightmares** (bad dreams) are very real to preschoolers; parents may need to help these children process their dreams.
	› **Night terrors** (sleep disorder characterized by screaming, intense fear, and flailing) may occur in the preschool period, with the child waking up at night with a profound emotional reaction to a dream or nightmare.
	› Preschoolers may truly believe there is a monster in their closet. Parents can leave the bedroom door open, provide a nightlight, and have a process of checking the child's room before bedtime for imaginary monsters or frightening fantasy beings (Linnard-Palmer, 2005).

Communication and Discipline

Language development flourishes during the preschool period. A typical 3-year-old will have, on average, 300 to 900 words; a 4-year-old will have 1,000 to 1,500 words; and a 5-year-old's vocabulary will increase to 1,500 to 2,100 words.

During this phase of development, children become capable of distinguishing reality from imagination and knowing limitations. Because they have not fully developed their sense of cause and effect, however, discipline for misbehavior needs to take into account what the child is and is not able to comprehend. Realistic expectations and positive, behavior-focused practices (time-outs, rewards and approval, and praise, but not lectures or denial of play, food, or affection) that are applied consistently by all caregivers are important in disciplining preschool-age children (Canadian Paediatric Society, 2004; Dosman & Andrews, 2012). Parents should be guided to avoid disciplining preschoolers using physical or corporal punishment, as these strategies have been associated with negative long-term behavioral patterns (MacKenzie, Nicklas, Waldfogel, & Brooks-Gunn, 2012).

Play Needs of the Preschooler

Preschoolers enjoy moving from the toddler style of play called parallel play to activities that are more interactive with their peers. Most preschoolers enjoy **associative play**, which includes loose rules, creativity, and pretend or dramatic play. Associative play typically starts as spontaneous with little preparation, thought, organization, or role delineation.

Preschoolers enjoy imitating adults and will have fun dressing up as adult-type characters such as a nurse, police officer, fire fighter, construction worker, dentist, doctor, business person, ballerina, and characters from movies (e.g., Disney films). They also enjoy using "play" or toy replicas of adult items, such as toy cash registers, toy medical equipment, play computers, and play structures such as kitchens, schoolrooms, and toolkits. Some children enjoy the development of an imaginary friend and will demonstrate intense conversations and interactions with their "friend." Parents need anticipatory guidance that this behavior is normal throughout the preschool period and does not represent any pathology or concerns.

Preschoolers also participate in **symbolic functioning**, in which they are able to take an item and turn it into an object of their reality. For instance, preschoolers' imaginations might lead them to make a king's crown out of a paper plate, use a towel to dress up in a royal cape, use a cardboard box as a race car, or create a classroom by setting up dolls and stuffed animals arranged as an audience (**Figure 8-3**).

UNIQUE FOR KIDS

Initiating Communication with a Preschooler

Pertinent questions to ask a preschooler to begin to establish a therapeutic and trusting rapport include the following talking tips:

1. Who is your family? Who are each of the members of your family?
2. What grade are you in? Do you like school? Tell me about your teacher…
3. Who are your friends? What do you like to do with your friends?
4. What is your funniest game? What makes you laugh at home?
5. Do you like to dress up and pretend you are someone else? Who is your favorite person to dress up as? What do you like to do when you dress up?

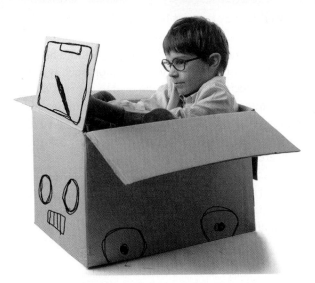

Figure 8-3 *Preschoolers also participate in symbolic functioning, in which they are able to take an item and turn it into an object of their reality.*

© Ollyy/Shutterstock

Health Concerns for the Preschooler

Nutrition

Many parents who are concerned about their preschool-age child's "picky eating" or refusal to eat are simply unaware that their child's eating habits are normal (Leung, Marchand, & Suave, 2012). Pediatric nurses should provide anticipatory guidance to parents about what to expect regarding pre-schoolers' eating behaviors and nutritional needs. Ethnicity and food security have important effects on consumption of fruits and vegetables as well as sedentary behavior, and should be taken into consideration when offering guidance (Asfour et al., 2015).

The following list presents the basic nutritional needs of preschoolers (AboutKidsHealth, 2015; Chandler, 2015):

- Preschool-age children should consume grains, lean proteins, dairy products, fruits, and vegetables daily.
- The daily calcium requirement for the preschool-age child is 1,000 mg.
- Vitamin D is very important for a young child's growing bone structure. The daily requirement for vitamin D is 600 to 1,000 IU for preschoolers be-tween 3 and 4 years of age, and 1,000 to 2,000 IU for preschoolers between 4 and 5 years of age.
- Protein intake should be approximately 0.95 g/kg of weight per day (approximately 19–21 g of protein per day in young childhood).

Dental Care

Dental health is important during this time, yet fewer preschool-age children access preventive dental care than access preventive medical care (Kim & Kaste, 2013). Preschool-age children are still dependent on their parents for their oral hygiene. Anticipatory guidance for parents includes the importance and impact of preventive dental care for primary teeth, the essential role of fluoride, and the effects of feeding practices on dental health (Chhabra & Chhabra, 2012). Nurses should also inquire whether families have access to dental care (Askelson et al., 2013) and whether a family's primary drinking water source is fluoridated.

UNIQUE FOR KIDS

Preschool Nutrition

Parents often claim that the most challenging aspect of preschoolers' diet is getting them to eat sources of protein. Many children in this age group do not like meat and will refuse or only pick at sources of protein. Nevertheless, protein is very important during this developmental stage for the production of enzymes, skin, bones, muscle tissue, hormones, and cells. A variety of sources of proteins can be offered to preschoolers:

- Lean skinless chicken
- Lean beef
- Seafood
- Eggs
- Beans
- Peas
- Soy products
- Unsalted nuts
- Seeds

PHARMACOLOGY

The Centers for Disease Control and Prevention (CDC) recommends a flu shot for all children 6 months or older, with its administration taking place early in the season when the shot becomes available. Vaccination by nasal spray (FluMist) is no longer recommended for children by the CDC, as it has been found to be ineffective (Preidt, 2016). The trivalent injectable vaccine is effective in healthy children, even those younger than 2 years; however, if a shot is administered to a child younger than 9 years, and the child has not had the flu vaccine before, two doses will be required (Blythe et al., 2014; CDC, 2015). Recent data show that involving parents in pain mitigation (via distraction or use of pain-disrupting devices) limits children's anticipatory distress, so parents or caregivers should be encouraged to participate in managing pain associated with vaccination, with guidance from the clinician as needed (Racine et al., 2016).

Safety Concerns for the Preschooler Across Settings

Preschoolers who are hospitalized have unique safety concerns (**Box 8-1**). Preschoolers should be told what is going to happen to them in a friendly, nonstressful, and non-intimidating way at the child's eye level. Rules should be explained to them and reinforced as needed. Preschoolers cannot be allowed to wander the halls if a parent or guardian is not with them in the hospital. Because they are too big for a hospital crib with rails and a topper, these children must be reminded about safety and instructed in how to use the call light. Preschoolers should never be allowed to play around hospital elevators or stairwells. (Golisano Children's Hospital, 2015).

A Child Life specialist, if available, should be asked to assist in providing choices for distraction, such as appropriate art projects, drawing, being read to, movies, computer pads, and music, which can be very helpful to pass time. Medical play offered by members of the Child Life staff can also help preschoolers understand their environment and care (**Figure 8-4**).

Preschoolers in clinic or ambulatory settings require frequent explanations of what is going on and what will be occurring shortly. It is important that the child understands that painful procedures are not a form of punishment (Khan &

BOX 8-1 Safety in Various Settings: Preschool-Age Children

Safety in the Hospital

- Encourage a parent or guardian to stay with a hospitalized preschooler at all times.
- Check frequently that the child has his or her identification wrist band on and that it remains clean, dry, and legible.
- Because a preschooler will be in a twin-size hospital bed, and not in a crib, the child should be monitored frequently, and if left alone, should be placed in a room close to the nursing station for visual monitoring.
- Do not allow a preschooler to walk around the pediatric unit alone.
- Never leave medications or medical equipment by the preschooler's hospital bed.

Safety in the Home

- Prevent poisoning by keeping all medicines and vitamins out of sight and out of reach.
- Never refer to medicine as candy.
- Prevent drowning by ensuring constant supervision around any body of water, even buckets or trash cans with standing water.
- Do not allow animals to approach preschoolers, and set firm limits on not allowing children to run up and touch or pet unfamiliar animals. Dog bites can be devastating; cat bites or scratches can lead to significant infections.
- Store all cleaning products and dangerous materials in their original containers in locked cabinets or storage compartments.
- Keep the poison control number displayed in various key areas in the home: (800) 222-1222.
- Prevent burns by keeping preschoolers safe in the kitchen. Do not allow preschoolers to assist with dangerous cooking activities. Keep matches stored away from their reach.
- Do not leave electrical equipment plugged in next to a source of water. Keep shavers, hair dryers, curling irons, and other electrical devices unplugged and stored away from sinks.
- Continue to serve only safe foods to preschoolers; prevent choking up through the age of four by not serving high-risk foods such as hot dogs, popcorn, whole grapes, raw carrots, hard candies, chewing gum, or raisins.
- Cover all electrical outlets, and remove any electrical devices from around sinks. Be clear to the preschooler about not touching electrical equipment and asking permission and help when required.
- Use safe, approved, and certified car seats for preschoolers. Check state laws on car seat requirements and follow the manufacturer's recommendations for use. Preschoolers should be in a front-facing car seat until at least 4 years of age; then, depending on state laws, the 4-year-old may be able to transition to a safe booster seat.

Safety in the Clinic

- Do not leave a preschooler alone in any area of the clinic environment.
- Visually inspect toys in the waiting area for safety and cleanliness.
- Ensure that the child does not sift through the drawers and cabinets of medical supplies kept in the clinic room.
- Do not allow the preschooler to play with medical equipment such as vital signs measurement equipment, otoscopes, or ophthalmoscopes.
- Make sure the preschool-age child does not climb up and stand on the examination table.
- Ensure that sharps containers are emptied when one-half to two-thirds full, and keep trashcans clean of soiled or infectious materials.

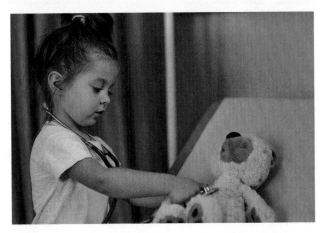

Figure 8-4 *Medical play offered by members of the Child Life staff can help preschoolers understand their environment and care.*
© gpointstudio/Shutterstock

Weisman, 2007). The pediatric nurse should allow the child to touch, handle, and play with medical equipment if safe, and all procedures should be explained immediately prior to the process (e.g., otoscope use, blood pressure checks, lab draws, immunizations and physical assessments) (**Figure 8-5**). Adequate preparation for procedures and parent participation can reduce the child's stress (Fincher, Shaw, & Ramelet, 2012; Stock, Hill, & Franz, 2012).

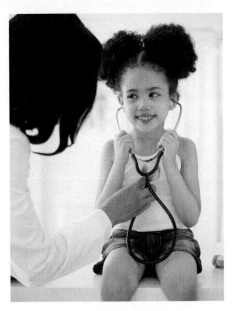

Figure 8-5 *The pediatric nurse should allow the child to touch, handle, and play with medical equipment if safe.*
© JGI/Jamie Grill/Blend Images/Getty

UNIQUE FOR KIDS

Concept of Death for a Preschooler

Preschoolers, unlike toddlers, can accept the concept of "forever," yet they will often associate death with being a temporary state, like sleep, that can be reversed. Death is often associated in the preschooler's mind with a form of punishment, and these children may take slang terms such as "scared to death" or "deathly afraid" literally. Preschoolers continue to fear separation from their parents and siblings, and they may talk about death as a frightening separation from loved ones.

FAMILY EDUCATION

Anticipatory guidance for parents should be clear about safety. Preschoolers are far more verbal than toddlers, but are not necessarily safer. Parents, preschool teachers, babysitters, and other guardians must know what a preschooler is doing at all times and often should provide direct supervision during play. Because of their desire to imitate adults, preschoolers may seek out equipment, cleaning solutions, buckets of water, and other items whose use requires preventive precautions, direct approval, and supervision. A preschooler's environment should continue to be kept safe by using cabinet locks, keeping the kitchen and stove/oven safe, supervising outdoor play, and preventing bathroom play.

Case Study

A 4-year-old girl came to the pediatric well-child clinic for an annual flu immunization. She described to the nurse as logically and clearly as she could why today was not the right day for a shot: "My legs are broken. I hid our cat from my brother, so he broke my legs. Sometimes my dad breaks his legs, so

he can't dance with me when he gets home from work so . . . my legs are broke and now I can't dance. We better wait and not get a shot today, so you don't break my arms, too." The child is rocking back and forth, folding her arms over her chest and smiling. The child's grandmother, who brought her

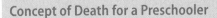

(continues)

Case Study (continued)

to the clinic, trying not to laugh, held her hand over her mouth to disguise her amusement. When the child finally finished her story, the nurse asked the grandmother if the child had received the flu shot the previous year. The grandmother stated that she had not. The nurse then asked the grandmother to distract the child with a colorful kaleidoscope toy and quickly administered the vaccine injection. The nurse explained to the grandmother and child that two doses are needed and requested a second appointment.

Case Study Questions

1. How does this child display normal and expected preschool-age thinking?
2. What is the nurse's best response to the child?
3. According to Erikson's psychosocial theory, which developmental phase is this child in? How would you describe her behavior and statements in relation to Erikson's theory?

As the Case Evolves. . .

Piaget's cognitive development theory describes common thinking and behaviors for the child in the preschool development stage.

4. Which of the following behaviors by the preschool-age child in this Case Study are characteristic of this phase of Piaget's theory entitled intuitive thought? (Select all that apply.)
   A. Expresses her thoughts in sentences
   B. Can think of two ideas at a time
   C. Egocentric thinking
   D. Includes others in her consideration of her environment
   E. Extreme literalism in word choice

The 4-year-old girl returns for a sick visit with complaints of fever of 102.5°F, sore throat, and general malaise. Upon examination, she is found to have signs of streptococcal throat infection, confirmed by a positive rapid-acting strep test. The nurse offers her mother a prescription for amoxicillin and prepares to give the child a dose of acetaminophen to help reduce her fever and relieve some of her pain.

5. When administering a bitter-tasting oral medication to a 4-year-old preschooler, which approach would be most appropriate?
   A. After explaining all of the child's choices, ask the child to decide the time and method to take the medication.
   B. Allow the child to choose between cherry flavoring and chocolate flavoring, then allow the child to self-administer the medication.
   C. Hand the medication to the parent and ask that he or she administer the medication to solicit greater acceptance.
   D. Provide the child with an auditory and visual distraction, open the child's mouth, and administer the medication.

During the sick visit, the 4-year-old girl's father notes that she likely contracted strep from one of the other children at her daycare program. He asks anxiously which other communicable diseases his daughter is likely to encounter at this phase of her life.

6. Aside from strep infections, which of the following are among the most common communicable illnesses encountered in the preschool period? (Select all that apply.)
   A. Oral thrush
   B. Impetigo
   C. Lice
   D. *Pseudomonas* infections
   E. Contact dermatitis
   F. Eczema
   G. Pyelonephritis

Chapter Summary

- The classic psychosocial and developmental theories of children within the preschool developmental stage include Erikson's stage of initiative versus guilt. According to Erikson, the preschooler attempts new skills, tries out new relationships, and participates in new activities. If discouraged or unsuccessful in these attempts, the child may develop a sense of self-doubt and guilt.
- Piaget describes the preschool period as being characterized by intuitive thought. According to his theory, the child continues to use egocentric approaches to the demands made by both society and the environment. This phase in early preschoolers includes the perspective that the world revolves around "me," but their thoughts begin to include others.
- Freud describes the phase of development in the preschool period as phallic-locomotion. In this phase, the child recognizes differences in the genders and shows an interest in the genital area. Freud's theory suggests that there are distinct experiences for the preschool-age child including penis envy, possessiveness toward the differently gendered parent (if applicable), and castration anxiety.
- Kohlberg describes the preschool child as "preconventional," with the child's moral thinking and behavior being based on the obedience and punishment realm. According to this theorist, the child learns socially acceptable "normal" behavior through being compelled

by the threat of punishment and rewarded by social obedience.

- "Spurts and lulls" are still common in preschoolers, but their overall growth in height, weight, and head circumference is slow and steady.
- Most preschoolers enjoy associative play, which is characterized by loose rules, creativity, and dramatic play or "playing pretend." Associative play typically starts as spontaneous with little preparation, thought, organization, or role delineation.
- Nutrition is a common health concern for many parents of preschool children. Picky eating may continue in this phase of development, and anticipatory guidance on appropriate, safe, healthy food choices is paramount.
- Safety concerns for the preschooler at home, preschool, hospital, and clinic center on limiting access to soiled, infected, unsafe, and dangerous materials.

Bibliography

AbouKidsHealth. (2015). Nutrition. Retrieved from http://www.aboutkidshealth.ca/En/ResourceCentres/Nutrition/Food-fundamentals/Canadas-Food-Guide/Pages/default.aspx

Asfour, L., Natale, R., Uhlhorn, S., Arheart, K. L., Haney, K., & Messiah, S. E. (2015). Ethnicity, household food security, and nutrition and activity patterns in families with preschool children. *Journal of Nutrition Education and Behavior, 47*(6), 498.e1–505.e1.

Askelson, N., Chi, D., Hanson, J., Ortiz, C., Momany, E., Kuthy, R., & Damiano, P. (2013, September). Preventive dental care utilization for preschool-aged children in Medicaid: Parents' perceptions and experiences with Medicaid dentists. *Journal of Theory and Practice of Dental Public Health, North America, 1.* Retrieved from http://www.sharmilachatterjee.com/ojs-2.3.8/index.php/JTPDPH/article/view/83

Barger, R. (2000). A summary of Lawrence Kohlberg's stages of moral development. Retrieved from http://www.csudh.edu/dearabermas/kolhberg

Blyth, C. C., Jacoby, P., Effler, P. V., Kelly, H., Smith, D. W., Robins, C., . . . Richmond, P. C.; WAIVE Study Team. (2014). Effectiveness of trivalent flu vaccine in healthy young children. *Pediatrics, 133*(5), e1218–e1225.

Canadian Paediatric Society. (2004). Effective discipline for children. *Paediatrics and Child Health, 9*(1), 37–41.

Centers for Disease Control and Prevention (CDC). (2014). Important milestones: Your child at three years. Retrieved from https://www.cdc.gov/ncbddd/actearly/milestones/milestones-3yr.html

Centers for Disease Control and Prevention (CDC). (2015). Children, the flu, and the flu vaccine. Retrieved from http://www.cdc.gov/flu/protect/children.htm

Chandler, S. (2015). How much protein should kids get in a day? *SFGate.* Retrieved from http://healthyeating.sfgate.com/much-protein-should-kid-day-6207.html

Chhabra, N., & Chhabra, A. (2012). Parental knowledge, attitudes and cultural beliefs regarding oral health and dental care of preschool. *European Archives of Paediatric Dentistry, 13,* 76.

Dosman, C., & Andrews, D. (2012). Anticipatory guidance for cognitive and social-emotional development: Birth to five years. *Paediatrics and Child Health, 17*(2), 75–80.

Fincher, W., Shaw, J., & Ramelet, A.-S. (2012). The effectiveness of a standardized preoperative preparation in reducing child and parent anxiety: A single-blind randomized controlled trial. *Journal of Clinical Nursing, 21,* 946–955.

Golisano Children's Hospital. (2015). Child safety: Toddler/preschooler safety tips. Retrieved from https://www.urmc.rochester.edu/childrens-hospital/safety/age-tips/toddler-safety.aspx

Khan, K. A., & Weisman, S. J. (2007). Nonpharmacologic pain management strategies in the pediatric emergency department. *Clinical Pediatric Emergency Medicine, 8,* 240–247.

Kim, J., & Kaste, L. M. (2013). Associations of the type of childcare with reported preventive medical and dental care utilization for 1- to 5-year-old children in the United States. *Community Dentistry and Oral Epidemiology, 41,* 432–440.

Kohlberg, L., & Hersh, R. H. (1977). Moral development: A review of the theory. *Theory into Practice, 16*(2), 53–59.

Leung, A. K. C., Marchand, V., & Suave, R. S.; Canadian Paediatric Society. (2012). The "picky eater": The toddler or preschooler who does not eat. *Paediatrics and Child Health, 17*(8), 455–457.

Linnard-Palmer, L. (2005). *PedsNotes.* Philadelphia, PA: F. A. Davis.

MacKenzie, M. J., Nicklas, E., Waldfogel, J., & Brooks-Gunn, J. (2012). Corporal punishment and child behavioral and cognitive outcomes through 5 years-of-age: Evidence from a contemporary urban birth cohort study. *Infant and Child Development, 21*(1), 3–33.

McGrath, P. (2008). My two-year-old daughter masturbates in her crib: Is this normal? Retrieved http://www.aboutkidshealth.ca/En/News/DrPat/Pages/My-two-year-old-daughter-masturbates-in-her-crib-Is-this-normal.aspx

McMurtry, C. M., Chambers, C. T., McGrath, P. J., & Asp, E. (2010). When "don't worry" communicates fear: Children's perceptions of parental reassurance and distraction during a painful medical procedure. *Pain, 150*(1), 52–58.

Preidt, R. (2016, June 23). CDC panel says FluMist nasal flu vaccine ineffective. *MedlinePlus HealthDay.* Retrieved from https://www.nlm.nih.gov/medlineplus/news/fullstory_159535.html

Racine, N. M., Pillai Riddell, R. R., Flora, D. B., Taddio, A., Garfield, H., & Greenberg, S. (2016, April 18). Predicting preschool pain-related anticipatory distress: The relative contribution of longitudinal and concurrent factors. *Pain.* doi: 10.1097/j.pain.0000000000000590

Stock, A., Hill, A., & Franz, B. E. (2012). Practical communication guide for paediatric procedures. *Emergency Medicine Australasia, 24,* 641–646.

CHAPTER 9

Caring for School-Age Children

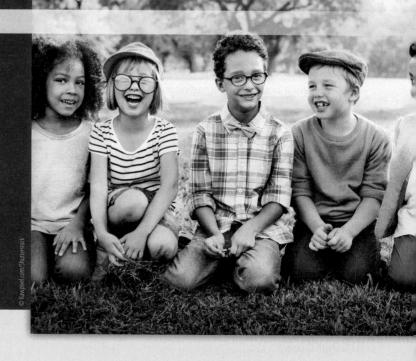

© Rawpixel.com/Shutterstock

LEARNING OBJECTIVES

1. Explore the classic psychosocial and developmental theories for children within the school-age developmental stage, including the theories developed by Erikson, Freud, Kohlberg, and Piaget.
2. Discuss expected growth and development during the school-age developmental period.
3. Compare the physical, emotional, intellectual, and social needs of the young school-age child and the older school-age child.
4. Analyze the relationships among the school-age child's play needs, play behaviors, and recreational needs in relation to the child's growth, development, and maturity.
5. Analyze the effects of the school environment and social structure on the growth, development, and safety of the school-age child.
6. Critically evaluate common health concerns during the school-age developmental period.
7. Analyze safety concerns for the latch-key school-age child and the process of being either under-supervised or unsupervised after school hours.

KEY TERMS

Abstract thinking
Concrete operations
Industry
Latch-key child
Obesity
Overweight
Precocious puberty
Prepubescence
Secondary sex characteristics
Sexual latency

Introduction

The school-age developmental period, which extends over 7 years, is the longest of the five developmental stages for children. This stage starts when the child enters kindergarten (usually age 5½ or 6) and lasts until age 13. Because of the diversity in maturation, this developmental period can be conceptualized as consisting of two distinct segments: (1) the early school-age period, in which the child is leaving the preschool developmental stage marked with dependence and magical thinking, and (2) the later school-age period, as the child begins to enter prepubescence.

Parents describe the shift from the preschool stage to the school-age stage as very powerful, as children begin to relate to their peers as much as or more than they relate to the family, and they spend more time away from the family as their social life and extracurricular activities expand and grow (**Figure 9-1**). The parenting role changes as the child demonstrates increased independence. Many describe this stage as the "easiest" in parenting, as children are mastering independent tasks and becoming accomplished in social expansion, academic work, and self-care. The school-age child even looks different than in previous stages, losing the "baby face" and growing taller and leaner with increasing coordination and independence in tasks. Many describe young school-age children (ages 6 to 10) as sweet; cooperative; eager to please parents, teachers, and others in authority such as coaches; and easy to be around (**Figure 9-2**). Similarly, many teachers describe children in the school-age stage as being more compliant with academic responsibilities including homework assignments and classroom activities.

Developmental Theory

The work of four theorists contributes to a deeper understanding of the developmental stages of childhood, enhances

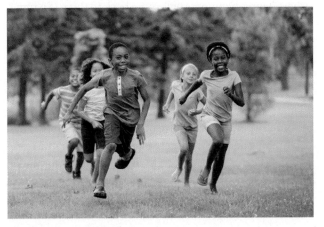

Figure 9-1 *The social life and extracurricular activities of school-age children expand and grow.*

© FatCamera/E+/Getty

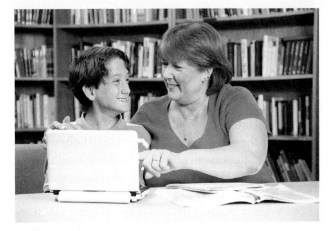

Figure 9-2 *Many describe young school-age children as easy to be around.*

© Lisa F. Young/Shutterstock

the pediatric nurse's appreciation of children's needs and desires, and allows the nurse to plan care.

Erik Erikson's Theory of Psychosocial Development

According to Erikson's theory, the school-age child is in the psychosocial stage of "industry versus inferiority." **Industry** is a feeling of competence and mastery of skills. School-age children need to master projects, academics, and actions that make them feel as though they are industrious, successful, and accomplished. If they do not master these feelings, children in this stage may develop a sense of inferiority, judging their performance against others' accomplishments and successes. The transition from preschool to elementary and middle school launches the child into a world of academic demands, recreational and sports activities, increasing household chore responsibilities, and expanding social encounters.

BEST PRACTICES

Nurses' Influence on Children's Feelings of Industry

By understanding the school-age child's need for a sense of accomplishment, engagement, and industry, the pediatric nurse interacting with a school-age child in a healthcare setting can more effectively identify opportunities to support the developmental tasks associated with this stage of development. Asking school-age children about their schooling, teachers, principal, and peers may open the door for personal disclosure. School-age children enjoy talking about their work and their current projects. While in the healthcare setting, the pediatric nurse can ask for "help" from the child through projects such as organizing pamphlets, drawing maps of the healthcare setting including where the fire extinguishers are located, or determining how many fire doors are present on the nursing unit.

Sigmund Freud's Theory of Psychosexual Development

Freud's theory focuses on the school-age child's developing sexuality and maturity. During this phase of development, children are learning to adapt to their school community and academic demands as well as determining their place in the family structure and social structure of peers. The term **sexual latency** is applied to this developmental phase to indicate the child's minimal attention to bodily details and greater attention to activities, hobbies, socialization, and schoolwork (**Figure 9-3**). Thus, parents of school-age children may find themselves having to remind children about hygiene, dental care, and other self-care practices, even if the child has mastered independent practice of these activities in the prior stage of development.

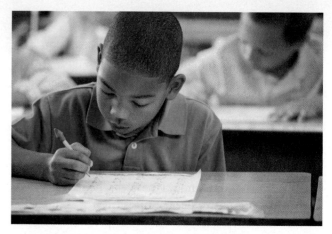

Figure 9-3 *The school-age child gives minimal attention to bodily details and greater attention to activities, hobbies, socialization, and schoolwork.*

© Ariel Skelley/Blend Images/Getty

FAMILY EDUCATION

School-Age Children and Bullying or Cyberbullying

The school-age period is a time when a child can experience the negative consequences of bullying. Even minor bullying, such as teasing, can have serious consequences for a child's sense of well-being, self-esteem, and self-concept (U.S. Department of Health and Human Services, n.d.). Adults must develop and enforce strong anti-bullying policies in classrooms and playgrounds, sports activities, after-school programs, and organizations such as Scouts. Cyberbullying is the latest form of bullying, in which the child is taunted, threatened, belittled, or teased via an electronic device. Cyberbullying behaviors can occur via social media, email, blogging, chat rooms, instant messaging, and texting; they affect between 20% and 40% of all children and adolescents (Aboujaoude, Savage, Starcevic, & Salame, 2015). According to the American Society for the Positive Care of Children (2011), bullying without resolution can lead to anxiety and depression. Data from the Centers for Disease Control and Prevention (CDC, 2014) on bullying show the gravity of the problem:

- More students are bullied in person than are cyberbullied.
- Verbal bullying is the most prevalent form of bullying.
- Bullying leads to school absences due to safety concerns.
- Psychosomatic manifestations of the stress from being bullied include chronic headaches, stomachaches, and anorexia.
- Bullying is highly related to a child's state of overweight or obesity.
- Youth with disabilities are often singled out for bullying.
- Youth identifying as lesbian, gay, or bisexual are at increased risk of bullying.

Lawrence Kohlberg's Theory of Moral Development

Moral development during the school-age period centers on the development of and respect for rules, order, and expectations. Those outside of the child are most influential in the development of the child's expectations of right and wrong, rather than the child's intrinsic self. Both feelings of guilt and fear of discipline or loss of privileges influence the child's behavior. Hockenberry and Wilson (2013) describe how the younger school-age child sometimes associates injuries, accidents, and unfortunate events with punishment. Older school-age children, by comparison, judge their behaviors and the outcomes of their behaviors as intentional—a perception that allows for the child to begin processing consequences prior to engaging in the act or behavior.

Kohlberg describes the school-age child as being in stage 2—a stage characterized by the early emergence of moral reciprocity, in which children believe that if they do what is right, they will receive good back, and if they make others happy, happiness will come back to them (Snarey & Samuelson, 2014). Nevertheless, school-age children will mentally process their desire to apply rules and order thinking depending on whether abiding by the rules will benefit them.

Jean Piaget's Theory of Cognitive Development

Piaget's theory of cognitive development describes the school-age period as the stage of **concrete operations**. Logical thinking and basic inductive reasoning about the world and life's events guide the child in processing information and developing thinking strategies. **Abstract thinking** (i.e., thinking in terms of concepts and general principles), according to Piaget, is not yet available to a child in this stage—although later researchers have disagreed with this conclusion (Keenan, Evans, & Crowley, 2016)—so children may misinterpret metaphorical phrases or analogies by taking such statements literally. At the same time, school-age children are no longer limited to the types of magical, unstructured thinking seen in preschoolers, and they have better ability to access memory and develop strategies for remembering things. Their concepts of identity and physical properties of objects are stable, and they are capable of understanding cause-and-effect relationships. By this time, they have also expanded their worldview by moving away from egocentrism, and have developed an understanding that other people may have different points of view from their own.

Expected Growth and Development

The developmental period of the school-age child is marked by slow and steady growth. This phase spans the longest portion of childhood, and the school-age child's physical, emotional, and cognitive maturity undergoes considerable changes during these years. **Table 9-1** outlines aspects of school-age development that should be noted by the pediatric nurse and explained to the child's parents or guardian.

TABLE 9-1	School-Age Development
Physical growth and development	› Grows taller and stronger and looks leaner
	› Muscle tissues replace preschool fat tissues, which changes the ratio of muscle to fat
	› Able to participate in increasing activities with physical demands
	› Becomes more coordinated in both fine and gross motor activities
	› Lung function expands, which allows for higher levels of rigorous physical activity without fatigue
	› Overall growth is slower than in earlier developmental stages but remains steady
	› Average height increase for girls and boys is 3.75–5 cm (1.5–2 in) per year
	› Average weight increase for girls and boys is 2–3 kg (4–6.5 lb) per year
	› In girls, initial signs of puberty (e.g., breast buds) may start at approximately 10 years; the peak growth spurt occurs a year later
	› In boys, initial pubertal changes occur at approximately 11 years; peak growth occurs 2 years later
	› Head circumference expansion slows significantly; growth in brain size and weight slows
	› Potential for injuries is present due to increasing sports activities, yet functionally less mature muscle mass and strength compared to adolescents
Nutrition	› Nutrition during the school-age period greatly affects physical stamina, academic performance, and overall cognitive development and functioning
	› Nutritional deficiencies or malnutrition during this time can have lasting consequences
	› The school-age child should consume fewer calories per kilogram than the preschool child did, but many more kilocalories per kilogram will be required if the child is very active in sports activities
	› On average, the early and later school-age stages require only 1500 calories for the first 20 kg of weight, with an additional 25 calories for each 1 kg over 20 kg
Sensory development	› Visual acuity is secure
	› Any deviations in vision or hearing should be identified early through screening and follow-up for intervention so the child can be academically successful
	› All other sensory organs are fully intact and functioning at the level of the adult
Cognitive development	› School-age children begin to think differently; they develop empathy and concern about others as the egocentrism of the toddler and preschool period diminishes
	› They develop greater thinking capacity and process information in a more mature way
	› They think more logically and more rationally, with increasingly abstract perceptions
	› Increased levels of attention occur; cognitive development begins to decrease impulsivity and more screened responses
	› Memory increases and expands to various areas of life in school and at home
	› By 7 years of age, the child is able to focus on multiple aspects of a given circumstance or situation, incorporating past, present, and future aspects of an event or situation

(continues)

TABLE 9-1	School-Age Development (*continued*)
Eating behaviors	› School-age children should be encouraged to eat reasonable portions of a variety of foods and to sit at the table to eat
	› Overeating is problematic for the school-age child; obesity is a national epidemic
	› Intake of processed, high-fat, or high-carbohydrate foods and beverages that have little or no nutritional value should be restricted
	› Family meals become very important in the developing structure of the family; they provide quality time for families to come together on a daily basis to develop feelings of connectedness
Dentition	› All deciduous teeth are shed to completion during this time frame, leaving permanent adult teeth
	› School-age children need consistent dental hygiene and should learn to floss daily
	› Children should be seen by a dentist for regular cleaning and tooth caries identification every 6 months
Expected vital signs	› Temperature: 36.5–37.2°C
	› Pulse: 70–110 beats/min
	› Oxygen saturation: 98–100%
	› Systolic blood pressure: 80–120 mm Hg
	› Diastolic blood pressure: 60–75 mm Hg
	› Respiratory rate: 20–30 breaths/min
Rest and sleep requirements	› Rest and sleep are highly correlated with academic performance
	› Young school-age children need 10–12 hours of uninterrupted sleep
	› Older school-age children should have no less than 10 hours of sleep
	› Stalling behaviors, sneaking social media, and using gaming or electronic technology are common concerns of bedtime; families should set and adhere to limits on these activities

FAMILY EDUCATION

Supporting the Older School-Age Child with Unique Growth Patterns

Children in this developmental stage can demonstrate wide variety in weight, height, coordination, sports abilities, social graces, and emotional stability and maturity (**Figure 9-4**). Pediatric nurses are in a unique position to provide education through anticipatory guidance for both the child and the child's family. Knowing that variations exist, and that it is normal to be taller or shorter than their peers, can be comforting for children. Explaining growth charts while discussing normal and expected variations between peers can be emotionally helpful to an older school-age child.

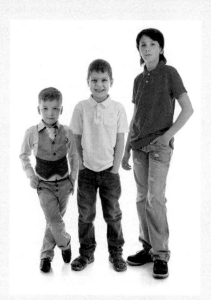

Figure 9-4 *Older school-age children can demonstrate wide variety in weight and height.*

The end of the school-age period is marked by a specific growth experience called **prepubescence**. During this phase of development, children of all sexes develop **secondary sex characteristics** over a period typically spanning 2 years, although girls usually undergo this transition earlier than boys. Specifically, due to the secretion of estrogen and testosterone, pubertal changes—that is, breast tissue development and menstruation in girls; facial hair, penile growth, testicular growth, and deepening of the voice in boys; and development of body odor, body hair, and acne in all sexes—occur at a rapid but expected rate. The end of the prepubescence period is marked by the ability of the older school-age child, or early teen, to procreate, as capacity for fertility is the hallmark of puberty.

During prepubescence, extreme body changes occur and emotional upheaval takes place owing to production of sex hormones within the child's body:

- Gonadotropin-releasing hormone (Gn-RH) is produced by the hypothalamus.
- Follicle-stimulating hormone (FSH) and luteinizing hormone (LH) are released in the presence of the Gn-RH hormone.
- Estrogen is produced in the ovaries and testosterone is produced in the testicles in response to the secretion of LH and FSH.

In the rare condition known as **precocious puberty**, prepubescence and puberty occur earlier than expected—before the age of 9 for boys and before the age of 8 for girls (Berberoğlu, 2009). Children who experience precocious puberty should be seen by an endocrinologist to discern whether some type of pathology may have produced the condition. Notably, tumors, brain abnormalities, and hormone disorders can contribute to precocious puberty and should be ruled out.

Social and Emotional Development

School-age children become more in tune with their feelings and are able to express themselves emotionally with more clarity and sophistication. Although young school-age children may continue to have fears of new situations and new people, they are beginning to demonstrate patterns of acceptance and more flexibility. Stress may continue, however, as academic demands and social pressures to win acceptance by their peers increase. Children need to have support in learning how to cope with stressors and stressful situations. School-age children listen keenly to adults talking around them and may develop concerns, fears, and stress when faced with natural or human-made disasters, crime, homicides, suicides, bullying, elements of poverty and homelessness, and other social problems.

The classroom structure can also influence a school-age child's social and emotional state. *Pro-social* behaviors must be encouraged at home and in the classroom, where demonstrated kindness, empathy, acceptance, acknowledgment, and respect for diversity can flourish. It is not uncommon for children in later-elementary classrooms to develop social hierarchies where a child is "in" or "out" of a social network. Teasing or bullying can develop if the child is deemed different, weaker, or of lower social stature. It is imperative that adults develop anti-bullying protocols and procedures to prevent bullying from occurring or escalating. In particular, instituting school-wide positive behavioral interventions and support systems has been found to be effective in reducing behavioral problems (Bradshaw, Waasdorp, & Leaf, 2012). Supervision for playground and after-school activities should continue on school grounds throughout this developmental period (**Figure 9-5**).

RESEARCH EVIDENCE

Mortality Rates in School-Age Children

According to the *National Vital Statistics Report* released by the U.S. Department of Health and Human Services (2016), 5340 school-age children die annually in the United States, or approximately 13 out of every 100,000 children. The three top causes of death in school-age children are as follows:

1. Accidents and injuries
2. Cancer
3. Intentional self-harm, such as suicide

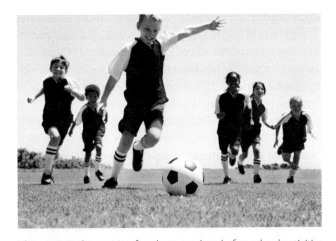

Figure 9-5 *Supervision for playground and after-school activities should continue on school grounds throughout the school-age period.*
© Squaredpixels/E+/Getty

Activities that promote safety in school-age children include the following:

- Car safety, including appropriate booster seat use and adherence to keeping limbs inside
- School bus safety and adherence to rules set forth by the state
- Bicycle safety and adherence to well-fitted helmets, use of lights at night and reflective clothing, and following the rules of the road
- Playground safety, including following the rules for specific play structures
- Gun safety and use of locks, separation of bullets from guns, and strict family rules about guns
- Water safety, swimming lessons, and compliance with rules against rough-housing, dunking, or swimming alone
- Fire safety, including teaching about matches, and safe storage of flammable fluids, chemicals, and substances
- Internet safety, including supervised use of social media sites and consistent family limits on time and search sites
- Sun and heat safety, including using sunblock, maintaining good hydration, and avoiding excessive exertion in heat
- Personal safety, including "good touch/bad touch" instruction, "stranger danger," not giving out personal information, and knowing what to do when lost in city or outdoor locations

Safety Concerns for the School-Age Child

School-age children spend increasing amounts of time away from their parents, home, and family structure. Their circle of socialization is expanding, and they are increasingly more influenced by the behavior of others—far more so than during the toddler and preschool developmental periods. This time away with varying levels of supervision poses safety risks.

The foundation of safety mindedness must be laid early in the school-age period. Interacting with other families, strangers, sports groups, and pets (especially dogs), and having transportation provided by other adults require conversations about safety starting in the beginning of the first year of this expanded developmental stage. Children as young as 6 years old must hear consistent reinforcement about street safety, fire safety, car safety, water safety, pet safety, stranger safety (including online communication), and prevention of injuries (Morrongiello, Widdifield, Munroe, & Zdzieborski, 2014).

As the school-age child grows, more opportunities for peer pressure and "dares" arise, and responding to these challenges can lead to serious consequences. Parents must understand the need to provide boundaries, specify restrictions, and instill confidence in the child to say "no" to pressures. Building on Piaget's work, child psychologist David Elkind suggested that older school-age children tend to construct "personal fables" about themselves that, in addition to emphasizing their personal uniqueness, offer a sense of invulnerability (Alberts, Elkind, & Ginsberg, 2007). Owing to their perception of immunity from threats, experimenting with new, unsafe, even potentially life-threatening behaviors may take place during this developmental stage (e.g., smoking, playing with firecrackers or matches).

Nurses are in the unique position of being able to provide sound anticipatory guidance to those adults and caregivers who provide supervision and safety for school-age children. Teaching families about health risk behaviors for this age group is essential and should include discussion about violence, tobacco, drug, alcohol, and sex prevention, as well as promotion of healthy diets and increased physical activity (Eaton et al., 2012). The following list identifies seven topics of anticipatory guidance for nurses to discuss with caregivers of school-age children:

- School behaviors such as being prepared with homework done, fed breakfast, well hydrated, dressed appropriately, on time, and with minimal absences
- Provision of healthy and safe after-school activities and supervision; minimizing time as a "**latch-key child**" (i.e., returning home after school, but not being supervised by an adult until the parent returns home from work), if possible, and walking home in groups
- Consumption of healthy meals and snacks *in healthy portions*; reduction of intake of low- and no-nutrient foods, processed foods, high-fat foods, and high-calorie foods, including fast-food items (Share with families the U.S. Department of Agriculture's [2016] MyPlate site at www.choosemyplate.gov.)
- Strict no-experimentation rules for sexual activity, smoking, truancy, shoplifting, and other illegal or concerning behaviors of the older school-age child
- Restrictions and limits on electronics, gaming, social media, and television, especially with a "homework first" rule for all children in the home; televisions and computers should be excluded from the child's bedroom (American Academy of Pediatrics, 2016)
- Prevention of injuries with consistent use of (and parental role-modeling use of) sports safety equipment, padding of knees and elbow, use of helmets, and use of mouth guards
- Consistently reinforced appropriate discipline for any infringement of family rules

Best Practices of Discipline and Consequences for School-Age Children

The true essence of childhood discipline is to teach what is right and wrong, and to reinforce the priorities of a family through appropriate and successful disciplinary actions. Discipline does not equate to punishment. School-age children thrive and develop in a positive direction when they have clearly set and reinforced boundaries and rules. How to implement discipline is considered richly set in cultural and ethnic values, however, and is considered quite controversial.

Overall, school-age children need to understand the consequences of their behaviors, and then experience those consequences on a regular and consistent basis. Discipline should be fair, developmentally appropriate, consistent in quality (e.g., not harsh one time and mild on the next occasion), and should match the behavior needing change. For example, if a child is found playing on social media or electronic games when told not to do so, the consequence may mean the loss of that privilege for a fair period of time. If a child comes home late from a social activity, the child should then be restricted from outside social activities for a period of time. The goals of discipline are to help the child learn the family's rules, keep the child safe by learning what is acceptable and what is not, help the child develop self-discipline, and help the child develop a sense of responsibility.

Data from Canadian Paediatric Society. (2004). Effective discipline for children. *Paediatrics and Child Health, 9*(1), 37–41; Department of Education. (2014). Guiding Principles: A resource guide for improving school climate and discipline. Retrieved from http://www2.ed.gov /policy/gen/guid/school-discipline/guiding-principles.pdf

TABLE 9-2	Health Screening for the School-Age Child

According to the National Institutes of Health, the following screenings should be performed for all school-age children to promote wellness and identify early deviations in health:

› Vision acuity screening (**Figure 9-6**)

› Hearing acuity screening

› Scoliosis screening

› Blood pressure screening

› Hours of sleep per night

› Immunization compliance with vaccines that are often required for school attendance, including measles, mumps, and rubella (MMR); tetanus, diphtheria, and pertussis (Tdap); varicella; and others recommended for children in this age group, such as yearly influenza vaccine, human papillomavirus (HPV) vaccine for all sexes (three doses), meningococcal conjugate vaccine, and pneumococcal vaccine (CDC, 2016)

› Lice infestations (presence of nits, larvae, and adults)

› Child abuse, including sexual, physical, and emotional abuse and neglect

› Dental health, including caries, abscesses, and gum health; presence of fluoride in the child's water supply (at least 0.6 ppm or less)

› Emotional and mental health screening for depression and anxiety

› Anthropometric measurement of height, weight, abdominal circumference (for high-risk children), and body mass index (BMI) above the 95th percentile

› Daily consumption of vitamin D (400 IU) to assist in the prevention of osteoporosis and type 1 diabetes mellitus (Riley, Locke, & Skye, 2011)

Data from HealthyChildren.org (2016). Health Screenings at School. Retrieved from https://www .healthychildren.org/English/ages-stages/gradeschool/school/Pages/Health-Screenings-at-School.aspx; American Family Physician (2011). Health Maintenance in School-aged Children: Part 1. History, Physical Examination, Screening and Immunizations. Retrieved from http://www.aafp.org/afp/2011/0315/p683 .html

Health Issues Common to the School-Age Child

In addition to awareness of developmental stages, the pediatric nurse must be aware of health conditions (including illness and injury) that are commonly seen in the school-age period. Contemporary data show that many concerns persistently arise in the school-age developmental period: epidemics of infectious diseases such as measles and pertussis related to increased rates of vaccination refusal (Phadke, Bednarczyk, Salmon, & Omer, 2016); lice infestations; food allergies; childhood obesity rates; emotional health concerns; rapidly increasing rates of diagnosis of autism (Blumberg et al., 2013), attention-deficit disorder and attention-deficit/hyperactivity disorder (Polanczyk, Willcutt, Salum, Kieling, & Rohde, 2014); and mental health issues such as depression and anxiety. **Table 9-2** summarizes the recommended wellness screenings for school-age children.

Obesity

Middle childhood is a period of slowed growth and, unfortunately, today's children have demonstrated a trend toward poor eating habits, limited exercise and outdoor activities, and increased body mass. Childhood obesity is a national epidemic with very concerning rates. The rate

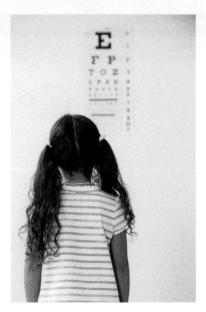

Figure 9-6 *Visual acuity screening should be performed for all school-age children.*
© KidStock/Blend Images/Getty

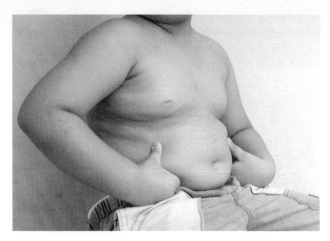

Figure 9-7 *Several health concerns are directly related to childhood obesity.*
© kwanchai.c/Shutterstock

of childhood obesity in 2011–2012 was approximately 17.7% overall among children age 6–11, although some ethnic groups had higher rates; among Hispanic children, for example, the prevalence of obesity for children and adolescents was 22.4% (CDC, 2015).

A child is considered **overweight** when he or she weighs more than is normal for the child's age group. **Obesity**, or extremely excessive weight, occurs in children when dietary intake exceeds the child's energy expenditure on a daily basis (Canoy, 2011). Obese children run a high risk of being overweight or obese as adults (CDC, 2013a). Several health concerns are directly related to childhood obesity, including type 2 diabetes, joint disorders, secondary (acquired) hypertension, high cholesterol, and sleep apnea, in addition to stigmatization and overall lower self-esteem (**Figure 9-7**).

Pediatric nursing education for families with school-age children must include topics that increase healthful eating and overall activity (such as promoting outdoor play activities) and reduce screen time. Teaching the American Cancer Society's (2016) recommendation of five to nine servings of fruits and vegetables per day, portion control, and consumption of a healthful diet that restricts sugar-rich beverages and high-carbohydrate, low-nutritional-value foods is a must to promote health in the school-age population. Many pediatricians and pediatric primary care providers do not promote "dieting" in the school-age period, but rather encourage family health through healthy eating and increased activities and exercising.

Food Allergies (Peanuts)

A major concern for parents with school-age children who have food allergies is the potential for a severe reaction at school. The number of children with peanut allergies—a growing concern across the United States—has more than doubled in the last decade or so (Sicherer, Muñoz-Furlong, Godbold, & Sampson, 2010). Roasting peanuts has been shown to increase the amounts of allergy-triggering compounds in these nuts (Kopper et al., 2005). Children with peanut allergies must be very careful at school not to be exposed to nut-based products in the classroom. Some schools protect children from exposure by implementing peanut-free classrooms and peanut-free schools.

A peanut allergy cannot be "outgrown," so children with severe allergies must carry injectable intramuscular epinephrine at all times (such as an EpiPen Jr autoinjector). If possible, a spare injector should be kept available in a secure location at the school, such as a nurse's office, and a comprehensive management plan for emergencies developed (CDC, 2013b). Emergency assistance must be called when a reaction is suspected, even after epinephrine injection has taken place, due to the risk of a biphasic reaction (or recurrence of symptoms), which affects as many as 20% of children. It is imperative that pediatric nurses are confident in teaching children and their caregivers how to identify a reaction and how to administer injectable epinephrine to reduce the chance of a full anaphylactic reaction (which is characterized by laryngeal edema, bronchoconstriction, and hypotension).

Discussion of Hand-off (Change-of-Shift Report or Multidisciplinary Rounds)

School-age children should be allowed to be present during discussions of their treatment or during rounds *if appropriate*. Because of their level of information processing, logical reasoning, and beginning abstract thinking, many, if not most, school-age children can benefit from hearing about their condition and treatment plan. For young school-age children, having a Child Life specialist present to provide support and developmentally appropriate education during and after the discussion will allow the parents and healthcare team to engage in reviewing and planning treatment for the child's medical diagnosis. This sort of participation may not be appropriate for school-age children with developmental disabilities, cognitive impairment, anxiety disorders, or emotional distress.

Case Study

Logan, a 10-year-old boy, has a diagnosis of severe asthma that requires him to have around-the-clock access to an emergency rescue inhaler of a beta-2 agonist (albuterol). Logan is very conscious of how his peers view him and hides his albuterol inhaler in his athletic socks during school hours. Because of his frequent use of oral steroids, he is currently in the 5th percentile for height and weight. Logan has experienced bullying by his male peers and often plays and eats alone during school. Upon questioning the pediatric pulmonary team, the family is told that Logan will catch up in his expected height and weight once the frequency of his oral steroid use diminishes.

Case Study Questions

1. Why does Logan feel the need to hide his rescue medications?
2. What are consequences of bullying (actual or the perception of potential) for children in the school-age period?

As the Case Evolves...

Logan has been referred for counseling because of his emotional issues related to bullying at school. During Logan's initial discussion with the counselor about his experience in school, it becomes clear that Logan is an outstanding student. He completes all his homework on time and regularly scores 100 on tests and quizzes. Logan explains to the counselor that he likes doing schoolwork because "it shows I can be good at something, no matter what those other kids say."

3. According to Erikson, a behavior commonly associated with the psychosocial developmental stage of the school-age child is:
   A. Enjoyment of repetitive tasks.
   B. Academic effort and accomplishments.
   C. Strong focus on social status with peers.
   D. Respect for rules and order.

A year after the visit, Logan's use of inhaled steroids has substantially decreased, and his parents say they expect to see an increase in his rate of growth. Upon assessing Logan's growth, the nurse notes that the 11-year-old has grown 1.5 in (3.75 cm) in the last 2 years—still well below expectations.

4. The nurse realizes that this child:
   A. Most likely has a growth hormone deficiency.
   B. Needs to catch up with his peers in average growth.
   C. Requires an immediate referral to the nutritionist.
   D. Will continue to be evaluated by anthropometrics during future visits.

Logan is learning coping skills from a counselor to help him manage both his health issues and the negative peer interactions he experiences because of his short stature. He still struggles with the fact that some children are unkind to him, even when he goes out of his way to be nice to them. He describes to his counselor helping another student with an assignment, only to have that student make fun of him later during gym class.

5. Which of the following developmental theories is linked to Logan's expectations of his peer interactions?
   A. Piaget's theory of concrete operational thinking in school-age children
   B. Erikson's theory of industry versus inferiority in school-age children
   C. Kohlberg's theory of the emergence of moral development in school-age children
   D. Freud's theory of sexual latency in school-age children

Chapter Summary

- The school-age developmental period spans 7 years, starting at the child's 6th birthday and continuing through the child's 12th year. This developmental period can be conceptualized as consisting of two distinct segments: (1) the early school-age period, in which the child is leaving the preschool developmental stage marked with dependence and magical thinking, and (2) the later school-age period, when the child enters prepubescence.

- According to Erikson's theory, the school-age child is in the psychosocial stage of "industry versus inferiority." Children of this age need the mastery of projects, academics, and actions that make them feel as though they are industrious, successful, and accomplished.

- Freud's theory describes the school-age child in the context of hidden, or latent, sexual desires and maturity. The school-age child has previously experienced the oral stage of the infant, the anal stage of the toddler, and the phallic stage of the preschooler, but now enters a period of quietness or dormancy related to sexuality.

- Moral development during the school-age period centers on the development of and respect for rules, order, and expectations. Kohlberg describes the school-age child as being in stage 2—a stage characterized by the "emergence of moral reciprocity," in which children believe that if they do right, they will receive good back, and if they make others happy, happiness will come back to them.

- Piaget's theory of cognitive development describes the school-age period as characterized by concrete operations. Logical thinking and basic inductive reasoning about the world and life's events guide the child in processing information and developing thinking strategies.

- The end of the school-age period is marked by a specific growth experience called prepubescence, during which the child develops secondary sex characteristics. Prepubescence typically takes place over a two-year time frame in both boys and girls.

- Healthcare concerns for the school-age child include epidemics of infectious diseases such as measles and pertussis, lice infestations, food allergies, and childhood obesity rates. Emotional health concerns include increasing rates of autism, attention-deficit disorder and attention-deficit/hyperactivity disorder diagnoses, mental health issues such as depression and anxiety, and bullying.

Bibliography

Aboujaoude, E., Savage, M. W., Starcevic, V., & Salame, W. O. (2015). Cyberbullying: Review of an old problem gone viral. *Journal of Adolescent Health, 57*(1), 10–18.

Alberts, A., Elkind, D., & Ginsberg, S. (2007). The personal fable and risk-taking in early adolescents. *Journal of Youth and Adolescence, 36*(1), 71–76.

American Academy of Pediatrics. (2016). Media and children. Retrieved from https://www.aap.org/en-us/advocacy-and-policy/aap-health-initiatives/Pages/Media-and-Children.aspx

American Cancer Society. (2016). Nutritional guidelines for reducing your risk of cancer: February module. Retrieved from https://www.cancer.org/acs/groups/content/@highplains/documents/document/04februaryupdatedpdf.pdf

American Society for the Positive Care of Children. (2011). Bullying statistics and information. Retrieved from http://americanspcc.org/bullying/statistics-and-information/

Berberoğlu, M. (2009). Precocious puberty and normal variant puberty: Definition, etiology, diagnosis and current management. *Journal of Clinical Research in Pediatric Endocrinology, 1*(4), 164–174.

Blumberg, S. J., Bramlett, M. D., Kogan, M. D., Schieve, L. A., Jones, J. R., & Lu, M. C. (2013). Changes in prevalence of parent-reported autism spectrum disorder in school-aged U.S. children: 2007 to 2011-2012. *National Health Statistics Report, 65*, 1–11ff.

Bradshaw, C. P., Waasdorp, T. E., & Leaf, P. J. (2012). Effects of school-wide positive behavioral interventions and supports on child behavior problems. *Pediatrics, 130*(5), e1136–e1145.

Canadian Paediatric Society. (2004). Effective discipline for children. *Paediatrics and Child Health, 9*(1), 37–41.

Canoy, D. (2011). Obesity in children. *BMJ Clinical Evidence, 2011*, 0325.

Centers for Disease Control and Prevention (CDC). (2013a). Make a difference at your school. *Chronic Disease, 31*. Retrieved from http://digitalcommons.hsc.unt.edu/disease/31

Centers for Disease Control and Prevention (CDC). (2013b). *Voluntary guidelines for managing food allergies in schools and early care and education programs.* Washington, DC: U.S. Department of Health and Human Services.

Centers for Disease Control and Prevention (CDC). (2014). Bullying surveillance among youths: Uniform definitions for public health and recommended data elements. Version 1.0. Retrieved from https://www.cdc.gov/violenceprevention/pdf/bullying-definitions-final-a.pdf

Centers for Disease Control and Prevention (CDC). (2015). Childhood obesity facts. Retrieved from http://www.cdc.gov/healthyschools/obesity/facts.htm

Centers for Disease Control and Prevention (CDC). (2016). Recommended immunization schedule for children and adolescents aged 18 years or younger, United States, 2017. Retrieved from http://www.cdc.gov/vaccines/schedules/hcp/child-adolescent.html

Eaton, D. K., Kann, L., Kinchen, S., Shanklin, S., Flint, K. H., Hawkins, J., . . . Wechsler, H.; Centers for Disease Control and Prevention. (2012). Youth risk behavior surveillance, United States, 2011. Youth Risk Surveillance System. PMID:22673000

HealthyChildren.org. (2016). Health screenings at school. Retrieved from https://www.healthychildren.org/English/ages-stages/gradeschool/school/Pages/Health-Screenings-at-School.aspx

Hockenberry, M., & Wilson, D. (2013). *Wong's essentials of pediatric nursing* (9th ed.). St. Louis, MO: Elsevier Mosby.

Keenan, T., Evans, S., & Crowley, K. (2016). *An introduction to child development* (3rd ed.). Los Angeles, CA: Sage.

Kopper, R. A., Odum, N. J., Sen, M., Helm, R. M., Stanley, J. S., & Burks, A. W. (2005). Peanut protein allergens: The effect of roasting on solubility and allergenicity. *International Archives of Allergy and Immunology, 136*(1), 16–22.

Morrongiello, B. A., Widdifield, R., Munroe, K., & Zdzieborski, D. (2014). Parents teaching young children home safety rules: Implications for childhood injury risk. *Journal of Applied Developmental Psychology, 35*(3), 254–261.

Phadke, V. K., Bednarczyk, R. A., Salmon, D. A., & Omer, S. B. (2016). Association between vaccine refusal and vaccine-preventable diseases in the United States: A review of measles and pertussis. *Journal of the American Medical Association, 315*(11), 1149–1158.

Polanczyk, G. V., Willcutt, E. G., Salum, G. A., Kieling, C., & Rohde, L. A. (2014). ADHD prevalence estimates across three decades: An updated systematic review and meta-regression analysis. *International Journal of Epidemiology, 43*(2), 434–442.

Riley, M., Locke, A. B., & Skye, E. P. (2011). Health maintenance in school-aged children: Part 1. History, physical examination, screening and immunizations. *American Family Physician, 83*(6), 683–688. Retrieved from http://www.aafp.org/afp/2011/0315/p683.html

Sicherer, S. H., Muñoz-Furlong, A., Godbold, J. H., & Sampson, H. A. (2010). US prevalence of self-reported peanut, tree nut, and sesame allergy: 11-year follow-up. *Journal of Allergy and Clinical Immunology, 125*(6), 1322–1326.

Snarey, J., & Samuelson, P. (2014). Lawrence Kohlberg's revolutionary ideas: Moral education in the cognitive-developmental tradition. In L. Nucci, D. Narvaez, & T. Krettenauer (Eds.), *Handbook of moral and character education* (2nd ed., pp. 136–144). New York, NY: Routledge.

U.S. Department of Agriculture. (2016). MyPlate MyWins: Dietary guidelines for Americans 2015-2020. Retrieved from http://www.choosemyplate.gov

U.S. Department of Education. (2014). Guiding principles: A resource guide for improving school climate and discipline. Retrieved from http://www2.ed.gov/policy/gen/guid/school-discipline/guiding-principles.pdf

U.S. Department of Health and Human Services. (n.d.). Facts about bullying. Retrieved from https://www.stopbullying.gov/media/facts/index.html#state

U.S. Department of Health and Human Services, National Center for Health Statistics, Centers for Disease Control and Prevention. (2016). Deaths: Final data of 2013. *National Vital Statistics Reports, 64*(20). Retrieved from https://www.cdc.gov/nchs/data/nvsr/nvsr64/nvsr64_02.pdf

CHAPTER 10

Caring for Adolescents

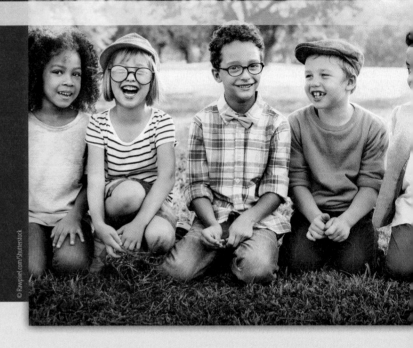

© Rawpixel.com/Shutterstock

LEARNING OBJECTIVES

1. Apply key nursing concepts in caring for a child in the adolescent developmental stage.
2. Apply the classic psychosocial and developmental theories to children in the adolescent developmental stage.
3. Analyze growth and development against expected norms during the adolescent developmental period.
4. Assess recreational needs and behaviors expected for an adolescent.
5. Critically evaluate common health concerns during the adolescent developmental period.
6. Analyze safety concerns for the adolescent at school, work, and home, and in social interactions.
7. Assess independence, autonomy, and emotional issues, and provide helpful guidelines for parents raising a teenager.

KEY TERMS

Adolescence
Anemia
Body image
Primary sex characteristics
Puberty
Secondary sex characteristics
Tanner stages

Introduction

The adolescent developmental period marks the transition from childhood to physiological adulthood. **Adolescence** begins at the onset of puberty—usually begins anywhere from age 11 to 13—and lasts through approximately age 18. It is considered the time period from the emergence of secondary sex characteristics through the cessation of growth (in height). Most care providers distinguish between three distinct adolescent phases: early (approximately 11–13 years of age), middle (13–15 years of age), and late (15–18 years of age).

During these developmental phases, individuals experience tremendous physical growth, as well as cognitive, emotional, and sexual maturation. Emerging feelings of independence and a move toward relating more to their peers than to their family (**Figure 10-1**) can lead adolescents to make decisions that highly influence their overall health and wellness. For instance, choices about food and meals, experimentation with expression of sexuality, independence in learning and mastering driving, and experiences with peer pressure can cause a teen to make suboptimal choices that have lasting consequences. Conformity is also a strong drive during adolescence and may lead the teen away from the family's cultural, religious, and ethnic practices.

The adolescent developmental period is also associated with increased incidence of unintentional injuries, unintended pregnancies, and a higher risk for participating in violent behaviors (Casey, Jones, & Hare, 2008). Although teens appear to be growing more independent, they are very interested in the opinions and behaviors of the adults in their lives (**Figure 10-2**). It may appear that teens are aloof or rebellious toward their parents' guidelines, rules, priorities, and opinions, but teens are actually listening and

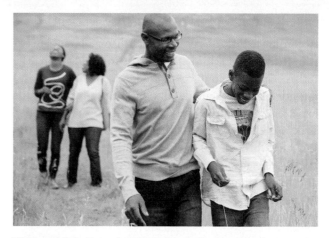

Figure 10-2 *Even though feelings of independence increase, adolescents are very interested in the opinions and behaviors of the adults in their lives.*
© Hero Images/Getty

making choices about whether to incorporate the views of their parents (and other adults in their lives) into their own thought processes.

Contemporary teens face great pressures and stressors during this developmental period. Pediatric nurses, across all settings, can be influential in reinforcing healthy behaviors, encouraging positive relationships with those in authority, and educating teens on safety precautions in their choices and decisions.

Developmental Theory

The adolescent period is marked by rapid physical growth, intellectual curiosity, emergence of sexual drives, and vacillating emotions. Based on its portrayal in many forms of current media, adolescence appears to be a tumultuous period of sex, drug and alcohol use, injuries, gang life, and other self-destructive behaviors. In reality, most adolescents in the United States do well in academics, graduate from high school, and move on to have productive lives. They are attached to their families, seek opportunities to serve their communities, and generally do not succumb to the pressures so often portrayed in the media, such as eating disorders, gang violence, teen pregnancy, sexually transmitted infections, alcoholism, and drug use. The adolescent period is a time of experimentation, but the majority of U.S. teens balance experimentation with success in school, social life, and family life.

The following subsections present the work of four theorists whose contributions to a deeper understanding of the developmental stages of childhood and adolescence can enhance the pediatric nurse's appreciation of those stages. This body of work includes Erikson's psychosocial theory, Piaget's cognitive development theory, Freud's psychosexual theory, and Kohlberg's theory of moral development.

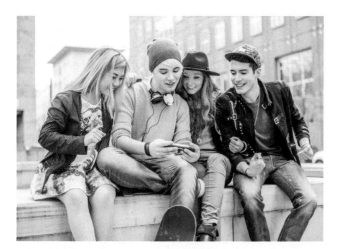

Figure 10-1 *Adolescents experience emerging feelings of independence and movement toward relating more to their peers than their family.*
© oneinchpunch/Shutterstock

Erik Erikson's Theory of Psychosocial Development

According to Erikson's psychosocial theory, the adolescent is in the stage of self-identity versus role confusion. The "crisis" (internal conflict) that adolescents must resolve is to determine their identity, or who they are, versus experiencing confusion about their role or self-identity. Erikson's theory suggests that successful navigation of this stage through self-awareness and self-understanding allows teens to share themselves with others, feel healthy, and feel well adjusted. Ultimately, the teen can relate to and associate with others without losing the knowledge of or being uncertain about who he or she is.

Jean Piaget's Theory of Cognitive Development

Piaget's cognitive theory describes the teen's mental processing as the stage of formal operations. Here, the teen has achieved deductive reasoning, propositional thought, and higher processing of complex information than in previous developmental stages. Formal operations are defined as both the mental ability to determine a very likely outcome and the processing of concrete, tangible, and intangible circumstances. Abstract thinking develops during the teen years, which allows the adolescent to process difficult concepts.

Sigmund Freud's Theory of Psychosexual Development

Freud's theory of psychosexual personality development describes the period of adolescence as being characterized by a sexual drive or sexual instinct that Freud called "genital." In this phase, the central "conflict" the teen must master and surpass is associated with the penis or vagina, and with sexual intercourse. The teen may experiment with his or her sexuality. A successful resolution of the conflict is marked by the teen's ability to experience an intimate relationship with another once adolescence is over (McLeod, 2008) (**Figure 10-3**).

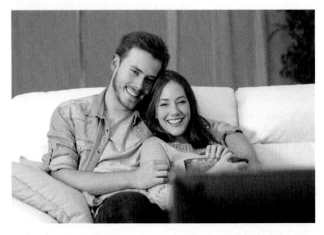

Figure 10-3 *An adolescent may experiment with his or her sexuality and may develop intimate, loving relationships.*

Lawrence Kohlberg's Theory of Moral Development

According to Kohlberg, the teen is experiencing conventional morality. In this stage of development, the adolescent moves beyond the previous focus on obedience, punishment, and the perception that there is just one right view (the focus of the school-age child) and begins to internalize adult standards of moral thinking, behaviors, and actions. The main focus for the teen is to understand the principles of good personal relationships; being seen as a good person becomes a priority. Another focus is on the maintenance of social order, including wider social justice issues, and obeying rules. At the conclusion of this developmental period, the principle of authority is internalized (McLeod, 2013; Oswalt, 2010).

Expected Growth and Development: Adolescent

Adolescence is marked by rapid growth in height, weight, hair growth and distribution, adipose distribution, and maturation of the sexual organs. In addition, this period is defined by somatic maturity, reproductive capacity and psychosocial maturity. Most female teens will gain 1 to 3 inches in height each year during early to middle adolescence, while male teens will gain 2 to 4 inches each year throughout the adolescent time frame. Females typically stop gaining height around their 16th year, whereas most males will experience a significant linear growth spurt in height around their 13th year that may continue through late adolescence, although the rate of growth may slow after age 17 (Rogol, Clark, & Roemmich, 2000; Rogol, Roemmich, & Clark, 2002). Growth spurts are regulated by the release of gonadotropins, leptin, sex steroids, and growth hormones (Rogol et al., 2002). Teens' nutrition—that is, energy intake in calories as well as nutrients—will influence their rate of growth. Adolescent growth patterns are unique to each individual, however, and families need to understand that in the majority of cases when concern arises regarding delayed growth, maturation, and puberty, patience is all that is required.

It is important to continue to compare adolescent growth to national standardized growth charts to see previous trends and current status. (See the appendices for examples of growth charts that extend through adolescence.) **Table 10-1** outlines expected development milestones for adolescents.

The experience of puberty is central to the adolescent period. Prepubescence refers to the first signs of sexual/reproductive development through sexual maturation. **Puberty** is defined as the period in which sexual maturation is completed, so that a teen is able to reproduce.

TABLE 10-1 Adolescent Development

Physical growth	› Females: Overall weight gain averages 6.8–24 kg (15–55 lb)
	› Females: Overall height increase averages 5–21 cm (2–8 in)
	› Males: Overall weight gain averages 6.8–30 kg (15–66 lb)
	› Males: Overall height increase averages 10–31 cm (4–12 in) (Rogol et al., 2000, 2002)
Nutrition	› Teens' caloric needs depend on their level of activity (sports and exercise) and can range from 1800 to 2500 calories per day; averages are 45–70 kcal/kg of weight per day (Gidding et al., 2006)
	› Although all are important, iron, calcium, and protein are especially important nutrients for healthy growth during adolescence; daily calcium needs are approximately 2200 mg, daily protein needs are 46–44 g, and daily iron requirements are 8–18 mg, depending on gender and age
Motor milestones	› Fine motor skills: Easily manipulates complicated objects. Demonstrates high skill level via video games and computer technology. Precision with hand–eye coordination and dexterity in intricate tasks improved. Artistic endeavors further hone skills.
	› Gross motor skills: Increasing endurance, coordination and speed. Hones skills in areas of personal interest.
Eating behaviors	› Adolescents should be encouraged to eat 3 meals per day
	› Eating behaviors include consumption of high-fat and high-salt fast foods; teens need to be encouraged to balance fast food with nutritional meals
	› Evening family meals (sit-down togetherness) remain important (**Figure 10-4**)
Dentition	› Teens need to have their teeth cleaned every 6 months, should brush at least twice a day, and should floss daily
	› Consumption of high-sugar-content foods such as sodas and candy should be limited
Expected vital signs	› Temperature: 97.4–99.6°F, average 98.6°F
	› Heart rate: 60–100 beats/min
	› Oxygen saturation: 98–100%
	› Blood pressure: 110–135/65–85 mm Hg
	› Respiratory rate: 12–18 breaths/min
	› Pain assessments: Use an adolescent pain perception tool, or numerical tool, and administer minimally with each set of vital signs or more frequently if hospitalized with pain experiences
Sensory	› Teen's sensory development is complete
	› Teens develop many preferences based on sensory experiences
	› Teens should have their vision and hearing checked if any concerns in academic performance arise
Sleep needs	› Teens need 9–10 hr of sleep each night
	› Teens frequently sleep longer when they can; their bodies need extra sleep to perform the internal work needed for rapid growth spurts (Ruffin, 2009)
Physical exercise needs	› Most teenage girls get less physical exercise than teen boys
	› Given that high school students have as little as 3–4 hr of physical education per week, on average, promoting exercise outside of school is important
	› Physical exercise provides the release of endorphins from the brain, which helps with stress reduction, improved body image, increased self-esteem, and healthy sleep patterns (Chulani & Gordon, 2014)

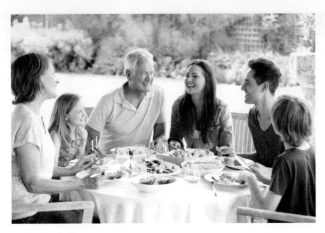

Figure 10-4 *Family meals encourage closeness.*

© Monkey Business Images/Shutterstock

This phase is marked by development of both **primary sex characteristics** (maturation of testes, ovaries, and external genitalia) and **secondary sex characteristics** (development of pubic hair and underarm hair, breast development, facial hair and voice changes in males, increased production of skin oils, and distribution of fat). The age at which menses typically starts currently ranges from 10 to 15 years, with the average being about 12 years 5 months (American College of Obstetricians and Gynecologists, 2015). Nocturnal emissions—that is, first ejaculation, also called "wet dreams"—typically occur for teen boys during early puberty.

The **Tanner stages** of sexual maturity are commonly used to distinguish between the phases of puberty. The Tanner stages describe the maturity phases of pubic hair growth and distribution, breast changes during puberty, and penile enlargement. **Figure 10-5** illustrates the Tanner stages.

BEST PRACTICES

Assessment and Education of Sexuality and Sexual Activity

Pediatric nurses need to be confident in initiating conversations with teens about topics of sexuality and sexual activity. The nurse is often seen as a safe person to talk to, with whom to discuss choices made or choices currently being contemplated, and from whom to receive straightforward and accurate education. The pediatric nurse working with teens should keep in mind the following points:

- Gain trust and encourage the teen to "open up" by acknowledging that the teen may feel awkward.
- Know that preparation will promote safety and that talking to teens about sex does not encourage sexual activity.

- Be honest, straightforward, and willing to discuss any topic from abstinence or birth control to anal sex—*whatever the teen brings up should be discussed*.
- Acknowledge that peer pressure is real, but emphasize that it should not influence the teen's decisions.
- Do not make an assumption about what teens know, as they may act as if they know a great deal but have many questions needing answers.
- Discuss the influence of the media and musical lyrics on sexuality.
- Clarify that sexual activity needing precautions against sexually transmitted infections (STIs) is not limited to vaginal/penis penetration.
- Educate teens that masturbation is normal and a healthy part of growing up.
- Encourage teens to have a comprehensive physical exam that includes genital assessment, breast assessment, and demonstration of breast self-exam and testicular self-exams.

Data from Monasterio, E., Combs, N., Warner, L., Larsen-Fleming, M., & St. Andrews, A. (2010). *Sexual health: An adolescent provider toolkit*. San Francisco, CA: Adolescent Health Working Group. Retrieved from https://partnerships.ucsf.edu/sites/partnerships.ucsf.edu/files/images/SexualHealthToolkit2010BW.pdf

---

Communicating with Teens

Communicating with teenagers is not always easy. Establishing a rapport with a teen often requires skill. One way to successfully establish rapport is to ask simple questions about friends, family, in-school and after-school activities, where teens see themselves in three to five years, and how they feel about a certain current event. Once eye contact and a pleasant rapport are established, the pediatric nurse can explain that the conversation is considered private and confidential, unless abuse is suspected. Teenagers often see the pediatric nurse as a safe person to whom they can ask very personal questions, disclose health concerns, solicit guidance on topics of sexuality, and receive honest, open, and accurate education.

Each state in the United States has its own laws concerning the provision of assessments, distribution or prescriptions of birth control, and treatment for sexually transmitted infections (STIs). Currently, 21 states explicitly allow children younger than age 18 (minors) to consent to and obtain contraceptive services without parental permission (Contracept.org, 2015); pediatric nurses must know the state laws governing this care where they are practicing.

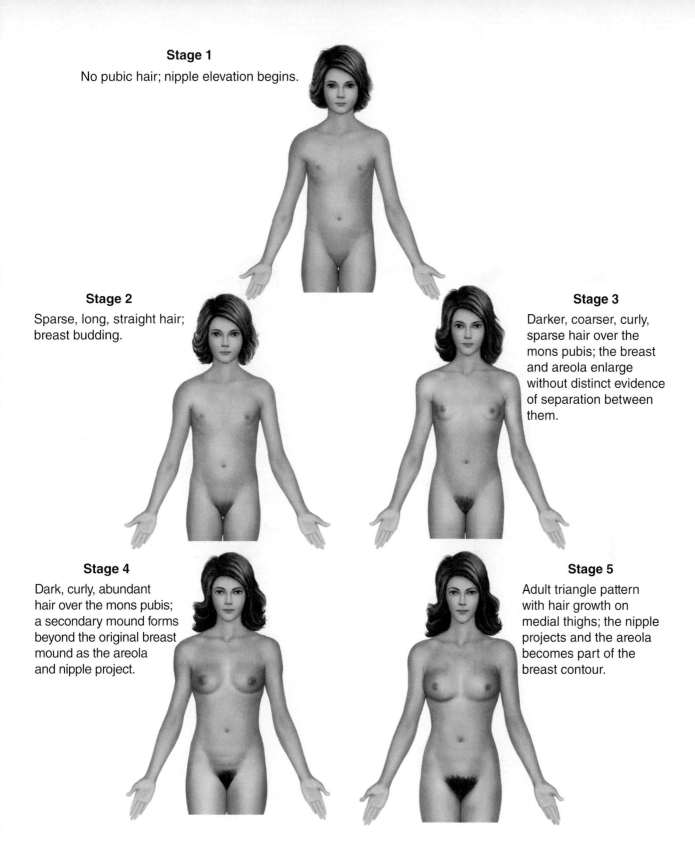

Stage 1

No pubic hair; nipple elevation begins.

Stage 2

Sparse, long, straight hair; breast budding.

Stage 3

Darker, coarser, curly, sparse hair over the mons pubis; the breast and areola enlarge without distinct evidence of separation between them.

Stage 4

Dark, curly, abundant hair over the mons pubis; a secondary mound forms beyond the original breast mound as the areola and nipple project.

Stage 5

Adult triangle pattern with hair growth on medial thighs; the nipple projects and the areola becomes part of the breast contour.

Figure 10-5 *Tanner stages of sexual maturity.* (continues)

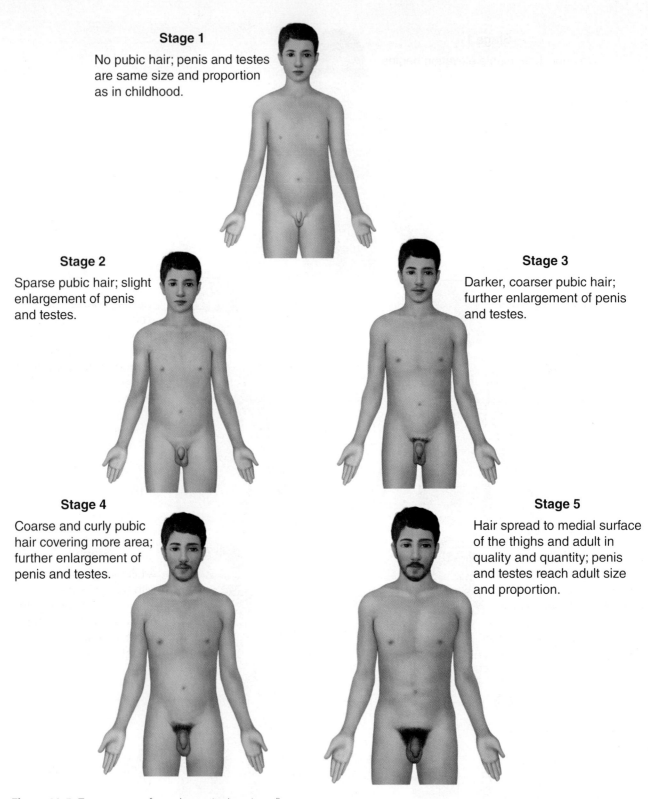

Stage 1

No pubic hair; penis and testes are same size and proportion as in childhood.

Stage 2

Sparse pubic hair; slight enlargement of penis and testes.

Stage 3

Darker, coarser pubic hair; further enlargement of penis and testes.

Stage 4

Coarse and curly pubic hair covering more area; further enlargement of penis and testes.

Stage 5

Hair spread to medial surface of the thighs and adult in quality and quantity; penis and testes reach adult size and proportion.

Figure 10-5 *Tanner stages of sexual maturity.* (continued)

Concentration levels and active listening skills increase during the adolescent years, such that teens are better able to learn and follow instructions than school-age children. The average teen has 50,000 words in his or her vocabulary (Ward, 2014). Some teens are very shy, whereas others are verbose in their communication styles. Overall, teens demonstrate increasingly more abstract thinking and can communicate with increasing complexity of thoughts and ideas.

Play and Recreation Needs of the Adolescent

Most teenagers enjoy peer-related play and recreation. Participation in team sports is common among this age cohort (**Figure 10-6**), youth groups are popular, and clubs are attractive to many teens. As teens typically desire more independence from parents and family, guiding teens to healthy, positive, and appropriate activities can enhance their emotional development.

Pediatric nurses caring for hospitalized teens need to plan for distraction, play, and recreation. Managing patients in the teen period requires thoughtful planning and consultation with a Child Life specialist. Some teens have their own laptop computers, homework, and cell phones. Others are open to engaging socially with other hospitalized teens and agree to participate in activities such as beading, card making, crafting, movie watching, and electronic video gaming. Regardless of how mature a teen might seem to an external audience, planning for recreation and distraction is an important part of this patient's healing process.

Health Concerns for the Teenager

Many health concerns are unique to the adolescent developmental period. Owing to their increasing independence and increased time spent with peers rather than family, adolescents are at higher risk for experiencing health concerns based on poor eating patterns, high-risk behaviors and choices, and their growing, changing, and maturing bodies. Adolescent health concerns increase when assessment, diagnosis, and treatment of common health conditions are delayed; thus, it is important to continue to provide anticipatory guidance during the teen years. **Table 10-2**

TABLE 10-2	Appropriate Medical Screening for Teens

› High blood pressure

› Obesity and overweight

› Eating disorders

› Depression

› Hyperlipidemia

› Use of drugs and/or alcohol

› Sexually transmitted infections (if sexually active)

› Tuberculin skin testing

› Use of protective devices such as helmets, seat belts, and sports gear

› First visit to gynecologist for females; learning how to perform testicular self-exam for males

› Need for immunizations—by 13 years of age, the teen should have a complete set of immunizations:

- Hepatitis B vaccine (HBV)
- Hepatitis A vaccine (HAV)
- Human papillomavirus (HPV)
- Measles, mumps, and rubella (MMR)
- Meningococcal vaccine
- Inactivated polio
- Tetanus, diphtheria, and acellular pertussis (Tdap) booster in adolescence, followed by tetanus and diphtheria booster every 10 years
- Varicella vaccine

Data from KidsHealth.org. (2015). What to expect in the doctor's office. Retrieved from http://kidshealth.org/en/parents/medical-care-13-18.html

identifies appropriate screenings during this period. A few of the common health conditions of the adolescent developmental period are described next.

Nutrition

Adolescents are at risk for nutritional deficiencies. They are growing rapidly, have large appetites, and tend to crave fast foods that are high in calories, sugars, fat, and sodium. Many teens seem to be "always hungry"; indeed, it is common to hear the phrase "hollow leg syndrome," meaning they eat amounts of food beyond what is expected. Although growth spurts require increased protein and caloric intake, many teens skip meals, snack throughout the day, and then eat nutritious meals infrequently. Heavy homework demands, socialization, and peer activities surrounding fast foods commonly affect the teen's proper eating habits.

Eating disorders are also a common concern during the adolescent period. Eating disorders can be devastating, in

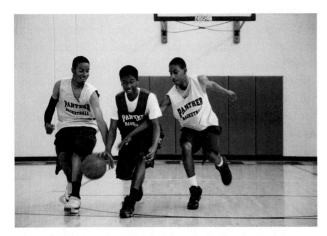

Figure 10-6 *Participation in team sports or other peer-related play is common among adolescents.*

© Hill Street Studios/Blend Images/Getty

that they can cause significant health problems and early death (Franko et al., 2013; Smink, van Hoeken, & Hoek, 2012). The most common eating disorders in the adolescent stage are binge-eating, bulimia nervosa, and anorexia nervosa. According to recent research, genetics, biological factors, personality traits, pursuit of perfection, anxiety, and societal pressures (including becoming a star athlete) can all contribute to the development of eating disorders (Keel & Forney, 2013). Pediatric nurses are in an excellent position to talk to teens about healthful eating, **body image** (i.e., a person's perception of the attractiveness of his or her own body), and self-esteem, and to screen for signs of eating disorders.

Anemia

Teenagers, especially girls, are at risk for developing **anemia**, a condition in which the blood lacks adequate numbers of red blood cells or hemoglobin. Risk factors include iron-poor nutrition, heavy menses, and chronic illnesses (National Heart, Lung and Blood Institute [NHLBI], 2014; Sekhar, Murray-Kolb, Kunselman, & Paul, 2015). Teenagers who become pregnant are at a higher risk for iron-deficiency anemia due to their need for twice as much oral iron intake as their nonpregnant peers (NHLBI, 2014). Teenagers who complain of fatigue, loss of energy, shortness of breath, dizziness, leg cramps, insomnia, and loss of energy should be further assessed for anemia. If the nurse notices pallor, pica, koilonychias (nails curved upward; spoon nails), mouth sores, or tachycardia, the teen should have a complete blood cell count performed. Iron, folic acid, and vitamin B$_{12}$ are all required for red blood cell (RBC) production; while they can take several weeks to work, supplements of these nutrients can be administered if the etiology of the anemia is determined to be poor nutrition and low dietary iron consumption. Females between 9 and 13 years of age should consume 8 mg of iron per day, whereas females between 14 and 18 years of age should consume 14 to 18 mg of iron per day (15 mg per day is the Recommended Daily Allowance [RDA] of iron). Pregnant teens need 27 mg of iron daily. Male teens need between 11 and 15 mg (11 mg RDA) of iron per day (NHLBI, 2014).

Acne

Body image is a major concern for many teens, which explains why the experience of acne may be profoundly distressing during the teen years. During the adolescent period, hormones are released that increase the production of sebum from the oil-producing tissues called sebaceous glands. This process may lead to two forms of acne: inflammatory and non-inflammatory. Inflammatory acne includes papules, pustules, and cysts—that is, large infected, clogged pores. Non-inflammatory acne includes open comedones (blackheads) and closed comedones (whiteheads); comedones are clogged oil glands (sebaceous glands). Whiteheads form as a result of an infection accompanied by an accumulation of white blood cells or pus. The bacteria that most commonly cause teen acne are *Propionibacterium acnes*.

Pediatric nurses can be of assistance to adolescents who are experiencing significant acne by providing education on skin hygiene (wash with mild soap at least twice a day), cleansing solutions with salicylic acid or benzoyl peroxide, and nutrition. Nurses can also dispel myths about the causes of acne: Acne is related more to the developmental period and hormone production, and less to conditions such as consuming certain foods or being in greasy work environments such as employment in fast-food restaurants.

Alcohol and Drug Experimentation

Teens commonly experiment with drugs and alcohol, and this experimentation may have serious ramifications. Harmful drinking increases risky behaviors such as unprotected sexual encounters and leads to a reduction of self-control behaviors. Significant injuries, such as those associated with violence and accidents, and early death experienced during adolescence can be linked to experimentation with substances (World Health Organization [WHO], 2014).

Screening for substance experimentation and abuse during health check-ups, followed by referral for mental health assistance as needed, can save lives. For instance, screening for marijuana use is important, as 6.5% of high school seniors have been reported to use this substance on an almost daily basis (National Institute on Drug Abuse [NIDA], 2016).

Mental Health

Depression is the most common contributing factor to disability, illnesses, and suicide during adolescence (WHO, 2014). Poor self-esteem, feeling devalued, bullying, poverty, and humiliation all negatively influence adolescent mental health conditions and concerns. Early screening for the symptoms of depression can provide the pediatric nurse with a foundation for referral and rapid interventions for teens at risk for depression, anxiety, or other mental health issues.

Sexuality/Pregnancy and Sexually Transmitted Infections

As of 2013, the rate of pregnancy and childbirth in the teen years had declined by 57% from its peak in 1991; overall sexual activity had likewise declined significantly (Martinez & Abma, 2015). Today's high school students report less sexual activity than the previous generation, and they have lower rates of teen abortions, teen pregnancy, and teen births. Nevertheless, several problematic trends persist. High school students report that 22% of the time, alcohol or drugs were involved in their last sexual experience (Hanes, 2012). An estimated 1 of every 6 boys (17%) and 1 of every 4 girls (25%) are sexually abused before the age of 18, with 35.8% of teen rapes occurring in persons between 12 and 17 years of age (U.S. Department of Justice, 2012).

Pediatric nurses are well positioned to provide confidential assessments, screening, and education for teens concerning abstinence, protection from STIs and pregnancy, and violence. Given that only 66% of males and 53% of females in the adolescent period report using condoms during their last sexual encounter (Martinez & Abma, 2015), nurses have the imperative to educate, support, and direct teens in safer sex practices.

RESEARCH EVIDENCE

Encouraging Testing for HIV in Teens

Recent research has disclosed that only 13% of adolescents have ever been tested for human immunodeficiency virus (HIV) infection, and only approximately 20% of gay adolescent males get HIV testing, despite the fact that 80% of new diagnoses in the 13–24 age range are gay and bisexual males. According to the Centers for Disease Control and Prevention (CDC), the proportion of schools requiring instruction on HIV prevention as an element of education dropped from 64% in 2000 to 41% in 2014. When a trusting relationship is established and a male teenager discloses to the nurse that he has experimented with homosexual sexual activity, or when either a male or female teen discloses any high-risk sexual activity, the nurse should discuss and encourage HIV testing.

Data from Centers for Disease Control and Prevention (CDC). (2016). HIV among youth. Retrieved from http://www.cdc.gov/hiv/group /age/youth; Martinez, G. M., & Abma, J. C. (2015). *Sexual activity, contraceptive use, and childbearing of teenagers aged 15–19 in the United States*. NCHS Data Brief, no 209. Hyattsville, MD: National Center for Health Statistics; Preidt, R. (2015, August 26). Only 1 in 5 gay teen boys get HIV tested. *U.S. News and World Report*. Retrieved from http://health.usnews.com/health-news/articles/2015/08/26 /only-1-in-5-gay-teen-boys-get-hiv-test

Unintentional Injuries

According to the CDC's (2010) National Center for Health Statistics, at least 16,375 adolescents in the United States die each year due to unintentional injuries. These injuries are linked to bodily harm as an outcome of poor decision making, motor vehicle crashes, homicide, suicide, and violence. Accidents currently are responsible for half of all teen deaths, with motor vehicle crashes being the number one cause of teen deaths. Male teens are at far greater risk (three times as much as female teens) for injuries, accidents, and death. Adolescent death rates are directly linked to age: For each year of adolescent development, there is a 32% average increase in deaths (CDC, 2010). **Table 10-3** identifies important teen safety tips.

TABLE 10-3   Safety in Various Settings: Adolescents
Safety in the Hospital
› Allow independence while maintaining safety.
› Provide realistic choices and allow for teens to take control of their care while maintaining safety and adhering to institutional policy.
› Teens should not leave the floor without permission from staff and a parent or legal guardian.
› All visitors for a teen should check in with the nursing station.
› Encourage distressed or angry teenagers to share their feelings; refer them to a social worker or Child Life specialist as needed to diffuse the situation.
Safety in the Home
› Keep narcotics and other potential recreational-use drugs locked up.
› Talk to the teenager about family rules of no parties in the absence of parents or adults.
› Provide instructions to teens about family curfews, limits, and boundaries.
› Discuss rules about activities around bodies of water, while swimming, and during pool use.
› Create a contract concerning use of the family car; require seat belts to be worn at all times.
Safety in the Clinic
› Have a second person with the nurse if conducting examinations on genitals or breasts.
› Ask teens if they want their parents to come into the clinic examination room; provide privacy and confidentiality as allowed by institutional policy and state law.
Safety in School Settings
› Promote the use of sports safety equipment.
› Encourage cleaning of sports equipment to prevent bacterial and fungal infections.

Increased Emotional Reactivity

During adolescence, with the change in their social environment, the majority of most teens' time is spent with peers rather than with family members. During this time, conflicts are common between the teen and his or her parents. It is common for teens to defend their behaviors and choices, hide consequences for as long as possible, and argue with parents and adults concerning boundaries, chores, expectations for homework, and time away from home. Many adolescents experience an "increased emotional reactivity," in which their emotional state is pronounced, their responses are exaggerated, their voices become loud, and their behaviors, in response to adult feedback or attempts at control, become oppositional. Much of this can be explained by their need and desire to become independent, trusted, and viewed as more of an adult than a child.

The pediatric nurse needs to provide parents with anticipatory guidance that conflicts with their teens are normal and to be expected. Guidelines for parents include understanding this period so that conflicts, verbal assaults, and the need for demonstrative independence are limited; holding strong to communicating family values and priorities; and continuing to express to the teen the need for family time. As difficult as it may be at times, teens often respond to a call for quality family time and considerations for special occasions that bring family members together. Parents need to be encouraged to view the adolescent period as transitional and temporary.

UNIQUE FOR KIDS

Neurobiological and Cognitive Explanations for Adolescent Behavior

Research has demonstrated that neural mechanisms within the brain leave adolescents vulnerable to a "heightened responsiveness to incentives and socioemotional contexts" (Casey et al., 2008). Recent investigations involving brain imaging have demonstrated that impulse control is immature during the teen years, as compared to during adulthood. Scientists have found that impulsivity, which can lead teens to make risky decisions, diminishes with age as the prefrontal cortex develops. According to Casey, Jones, and Hare (2008), prefrontal cortical control systems need maturation before a teen can override the propensity to make inappropriate choices that lead to risky behaviors.

PHARMACOLOGY

Parents and Teenage Drug Use

Parents need to perform environmental sweeps in the home to identify access to high-risk over-the-counter medications and prescription drugs they may have on hand. Locking drugs up from access, even from older teens, can prevent dangers.

According to the National Institute on Drug Abuse (2016), the following over-the-counter drugs and prescription drugs were often taken for recreational purposes in 2015:

- Pain control medications such as hydrocodone (Vicodin) and oxycodone (OxyContin)
- Sleep assistance drugs such as Lunesta and Ambien
- Simulant drugs such as methylphenidate (Ritalin) and amphetamine (Adderall)
- Antianxiety medications such as diazepam (Valium) and lorazepam (Ativan)
- Marijuana (prescription or "card holders")
- Cough syrups and tablets containing dextromethorphan
- Bath salts containing synthetic cathinones

BEST PRACTICES

Administering Medications to Teenagers

- Teach teens, using straightforward and clear language, about the medications they are on and why they are taking them and for how long.
- Talk to teens about the "rights of safe medication administration," so they are involved with their safety.
- Try to give teenagers responsibility for their medication administration times.
- Most teenagers can swallow pills, but provide an alternative formulation if they are unable to do so.
- Teach teens about the importance of the medication, based on the understanding that teens might hide their medications from their peers or be unwilling to take medications during the day or at school where peers may cause them to be embarrassed or be teased—they do not want to look "different" from their peers.
- Discuss compliance and adherence, as teens who are responsible for medication administration may feel "invincible" and choose not to take their medications if they do not feel they need them.

Case Study

Danielle, a 15-year-old girl, has been contemplating starting birth control pills. Although she has not yet become sexually active, she talks to her peers about the experience of sex and decides that being prepared and preventing pregnancy are very important to her. She conducts a search on the Internet to find out about the various forms of birth control and learns that the pill is effective but does not prevent sexually transmitted infections.

After a few weeks, Danielle decides to go to the afternoon teen clinic offered by the public health department. She obtains 3 months of a low-dose estrogen pill, but decides not to start right away. She hides the pills in her room for a later date. She decides not to discuss her thought processes with her parents because she worries how they will respond. Her greatest concern in her decision-making process is whether, and when, to start the pill. She is concerned about the side effects that she has heard about from her peers, such as weight gain. Knowing that a conversation with the district school nurse is confidential, Danielle stops in the nurse's office open hours at her school and asks for advice.

Case Study Questions

1. What are the top-priority questions the school nurse should ask Danielle about her situation?
2. Which common side effects of low-dose estrogen birth control pills should be discussed with Danielle?
3. How does Danielle's developmental stage of adolescence influence her decision-making pattern?
4. Which education can the school nurse provide Danielle to help her decide her next actions?

As the Case Evolves...

Danielle confides to the nurse that it is likely she will have sex with her boyfriend at some point in the next few months. She is unsure whether she wants a sexual relationship right now, but wants to "be prepared" by obtaining birth control. She explains to the nurse that her parents are highly religious and would never permit her to take birth control pills, and that they would try to forbid her relationship with her boyfriend if they knew sex was under discussion.

5. Which of Danielle's behaviors demonstrate(s) a classic developmental milestone(s) for an adolescent? (Select all that apply.)
   A. Danielle's efforts to keep her relationship secret from her parents because she fears their judgment.
   B. Danielle's effort to take control of her sexual and reproductive capacity.
   C. Danielle's rebellion against her parents' beliefs and authority.
   D. Danielle's ambivalence about becoming sexually active.
6. In the discussion with Danielle about her birth control pills, the nurse must take into account Danielle's developmental phase. According to Sigmund Freud's psychosexual theory, which of the following characteristics are present during adolescence? (Select all that apply.)
   A. Phallic (masturbation) exploration
   B. Sexual latency
   C. Anal fixation
   D. Oral aggressiveness
   E. Genital fixation
7. The nurse working with Danielle identifies her as being in the middle adolescent developmental phase. Which of the following behaviors is associated with middle adolescence?
   A. Reestablishes relationship with family and achieves independence
   B. The concept of here and now is most important in the teen's thinking
   C. Sexual interest begins
   D. Struggles for autonomy, rebels, and demands privacy

Chapter Summary

- Adolescence is considered the period from the beginning of secondary sex characteristics development, through the end of the period of rapid growth in height and complete development of reproductive maturity (development of primary sex characteristics).
- Most care providers distinguish between three distinct adolescent phases: early (approximately 11–13 years of age),

middle (13–15 years of age), and late (15–18 years of age). During these developmental phases, teens experience tremendous physical growth, along with cognitive, emotional, and sexual maturation mixed with intellectual curiosity, emergence of their sexual drives, and vacillating emotions.
- Emerging feelings of independence and a move toward relating more to their peers than to their family can lead

adolescents to make decisions that highly influence their overall health and wellness.

- In Erik Erikson's psychosocial theory, adolescence is associated with the developmental phase of self-identity versus role confusion; Jean Piaget's cognitive development theory describes teens' mental processing model as formal operations; Sigmund Freud's theory of psychosexual development suggests that teens are focused on the sexual drive (the "genital" sexual instinct); and Lawrence Kohlberg's theory of moral development proposes that teens are experiencing conventional morality.

- A teen's nutrition (i.e., energy intake in calories as well as nutrients) is the most significant determinant of the teen's growth. Adolescent growth patterns are unique to each individual, and families need to understand that in the majority of cases involving concerns about delayed growth, maturation, and puberty, patience is all that is required.

- Health concerns unique to the teenager include poor nutrition, eating disorders, anemia, body image concerns, acne, alcohol and drug experimentation, mental health issues, sexuality, pregnancy, and sexually transmitted infections.

Bibliography

American College of Obstetricians and Gynecologists. (2015). Menstruation in girls and adolescents: Using the menstrual cycle as a vital sign. Committee Opinion No. 651. *Obstetrics and Gynecology, 126,* e143–e146.

Casey, B. J., Jones, R. M., & Hare, T. (2008). The adolescent brain. *Annals of the New York Academy of Sciences, 1124,* 111–126.

Centers for Disease Control and Prevention (CDC). (2010). *Mortality among teenagers aged 12–19 years: United States.* NCHS Data Brief, number 37, May 2010. Retrieved from http://www.cdc.gov/nchs/data/databriefs/db37.htm

Centers for Disease Control and Prevention (CDC). (2016). HIV among youth. Retrieved from http://www.cdc.gov/hiv/group/age/youth

Chulani, V., & Gordon, L. (2014). Adolescent growth and development. *Primary Care: Clinics in Office Practice, 41*(2014), 465–487.

Contracept.org. (2015). Minors access to contraceptive health care: State policies in brief, AGI, Dec 1st, 2005. Retrieved from http://www.contracept.org/minorsaccess.php

Franko, D. L., Keshaviah, A., Eddy, K. T., Krishna, M., Davis, M. C., Keel, P. K., & Herzog, D. B. (2013). A longitudinal investigation of mortality in anorexia nervosa and bulimia nervosa. *American Journal of Psychiatry, 170,* 917–925.

Gidding, S. S., Dennison, B. A., Birch, L. L, Daniels, S. R., Gilman, M. W., Lichtenstein, A. H., . . . Van Horn, L. (2006). Dietary recommendations for children and adolescents: A guide for practitioners. *Pediatrics, 117*(2), 544–559.

Hanes, M. (2012, September). Effects and consequences of underage drinking. *Juvenile Justice Bulletin.* Retrieved from http://www.ojjdp.gov/pubs/237145.pdf

Keel, P. K., & Forney, K. J. (2013). Psychosocial risk factors for eating disorders. *International Journal of Eating Disorders, 46,* 433–439.

KidsHealth.org. (2015). What to expect in the doctor's office. Retrieved from http://kidshealth.org/en/parents/medical-care-13-18.html

Martinez, G. M., & Abma, J. C. (2015). *Sexual activity, contraceptive use, and childbearing of teenagers aged 15–19 in the United States.* NCHS Data Brief, no 209. Hyattsville, MD: National Center for Health Statistics.

McLeod, S. A. (2008). Psychosexual stages. Retrieved from http://www.simplypsychology.org/psychosexual.html

McLeod, S. A. (2013). Kohlberg. Retrieved from http://www.simplypsychology.org/kohlberg.html

Monasterio, E., Combs, N., Warner, L., Larsen-Fleming, M., & St. Andrews, A. (2010). *Sexual health: An adolescent provider toolkit.* San Francisco, CA: Adolescent Health Working Group. Retrieved from https://partnerships.ucsf.edu/sites/partnerships.ucsf.edu/files/images/SexualHealthToolkit2010BW.pdf

National Heart, Lung and Blood Institute (NHLBI). (2014). Who is at risk for iron-deficiency anemia. Retrieved from http://www.nhlbi.nih.gov/health/health-topics/topics/ida/atrisk

National Institute on Drug Abuse (NIDA). (2016). Monitoring the Future survey: High school and youth trends. Retrieved from https://www.drugabuse.gov/publications/drugfacts/high-school-youth-trends

Oswalt, A. (2010). Jean Piaget's theory of cognitive development. American Addiction Center. Retrieved from https://www.mentalhelp.net/articles/moral-development-piaget-s-theory

Preidt, R. (2015, August 26). Only 1 in 5 gay teen boys get HIV tested. *U.S. News and World Report.* Retrieved from http://health.usnews.com/health-news/articles/2015/08/26/only-1-in-5-gay-teen-boys-get-hiv-test

Rogol, A. D., Clark, P. A., & Roemmich, J. (2000). Growth and pubertal development in children and adolescents: Effects of diet and physical activity. *American Journal of Clinical Nutrition, 72,* 521s–528s.

Rogol, A., Roemmich, J., & Clark, P. (2002). Growth at puberty. *Journal of Adolescent Health, 31,* 192–200.Ruffin, N. (2009). Adolescent growth and development. Virginia Cooperative Extension. Publication 350-850. Retrieved from https://www.pubs.ext.vt.edu/350/350-850/350-850.html

Sekhar, D. L., Murray-Kolb, L. E., Kunselman, A. R., & Paul, I. M. (2015). Identifying factors predicting iron deficiency in United States adolescent females using the ferritin and the body iron models. *Clinical Nutrition, 10*(3), e118–e123.

Smink, F. R. E., van Hoeken, D., & Hoek, H. W. (2012). Epidemiology of eating disorders: Incidence, prevalence and mortality rates. *Current Psychiatry Reports, 14,* 406.

U.S. Department of Justice. (2012). National Sex Offender Public Website: Facts and statistics. Retrieved from https://www.nsopw.gov/en-US/Education/FactsStatistics

Ward, S. (2014). *Pediatric nursing care: Best evidence-based practice.* Philadelphia, PA: F. A. Davis.

World Health Organization (WHO). (2014). *Adolescents: Health risk and solutions.* Fact Sheet No. 345. Retrieved from http://www.who.int/mediacentre/factsheets/fs345/en/

CHAPTER 11

Symptom Management Across Childhood

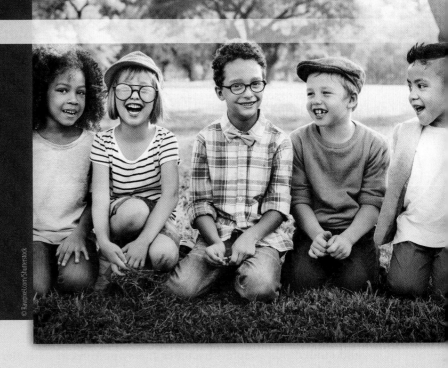

© Rawpixel.com/Shutterstock

LEARNING OBJECTIVES

1. Apply key concepts in caring for a child experiencing symptoms associated with discomfort, fatigue, nausea, respiratory distress, sleep disturbances, and emotional distress.
2. Apply the principles of pain pathophysiology experienced by children across the developmental period.
3. Apply the components of the University of California, San Francisco School of Nursing's symptom management model to understand symptom experience, symptom management strategies, and outcomes.
4. Evaluate the need for interdisciplinary teamwork to best manage children's symptoms.
5. Differentiate assessments used for symptoms across the developmental period.
6. Create a comprehensive care plan for children with discomfort, nausea, fatigue, dyspnea, and sleep disturbances.
7. Examine medical diagnostics and medical treatments used to manage symptoms in children.
8. Differentiate the level of nursing care needed based on differing clinical settings to assist children and their families in the assessment and management of discomfort.
9. Critique components of family education needed to provide symptom assessment and management for children with varying medical diagnoses and conditions.

KEY TERMS

Allodynia
Breakthrough pain
Discomfort
Emetogenic
Fatigue
Idiopathic pain
Narcotic
Nausea
Neuropathic pain
Pain
Pain assessment tools
Pain threshold
Respiratory distress
Sleep disturbances

Introduction

For most pediatric patients and their caregivers, the experience of disease symptoms is the principal factor that causes them to seek care. The majority of hospitalizations and clinic visits for medical and nursing care are associated with the presence of symptoms requiring evaluation, treatment, and management. Symptom management is a large part of the holistic role of the nurse within all healthcare settings. Untreated symptoms can have severe consequences for the child's social, emotional, developmental, academic, and home life. Special attention to the assessment, treatment, and continued management of symptoms is a critical responsibility of the practicing professional nurse.

Although pain appears to be the symptom that has garnered the most attention in the literature and in practice, the assessment, treatment, and continued management of other symptoms requires consideration and study. This chapter discusses the symptoms of pain, discomfort, fatigue, nausea, dyspnea, and sleep disturbances.

Model of Symptom Management

One contribution to the understanding of the experience of symptoms has come from the model of symptom management developed by the faculty at the University of California, San Francisco (UCSF) School of Nursing's Center for System Management (Dodd et al., 2001; Linder, 2010). In the UCSF model, the focus is placed on the nurse's understanding of the six symptoms of discomfort, dyspnea, nausea, emotional distress, fatigue, and sleep disturbances. The model depicts the close relationships between the person's demographics, sociological, physiological, psychological, and developmental aspects of symptom experiences (**Figure 11-1**). It weaves together the importance of symptom experiences, symptom management strategies, and outcomes. Outcomes are described in terms of a person's functional status, emotional status, self-care, quality of life, and other factors. When applied to children, the UCSF model allows the pediatric nurse to better comprehend the complexities of symptom management while understanding the uniqueness of the child, his or her environment, and his or her sense of well-being.

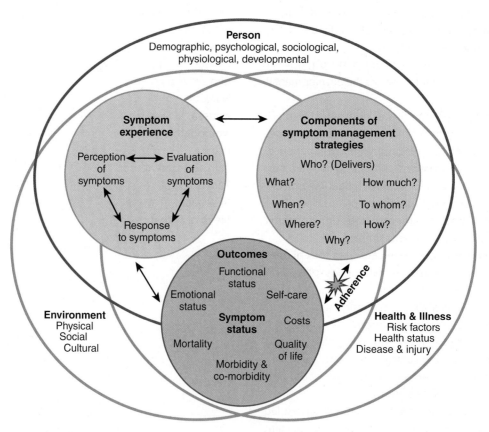

Figure 11-1 *University of California, San Francisco (UCSF) School of Nursing's Symptom Management Model.*

Reproduced from Dodd, M., Janson, S., Facione, N., Faucett, J., Froelicher, E. S., Humphreys, J., . . . Taylor, D. (2001). Advancing the science of symptom management. *Journal of Advanced Nursing, 33(5)*, 668-676.

Teamwork

Regardless of the healthcare setting, teamwork is needed to provide a comprehensive treatment plan for a child's symptoms. Interdisciplinary groups can use a variety of professional perspectives to best determine the etiology of a child's symptom(s). From there, the team can diagnose the underlying pathology, determine how to assist the child in a developmentally appropriate way, and determine how best to treat and manage the experience. Nurses, physicians, physical therapists, occupational therapists, pharmacists, child psychologists, social workers, and family members need to collaborate in defining the priorities when helping a child cope with symptoms. This collaborative care of the child's symptoms should begin immediately and continue during treatment.

The pediatric nurse, applying the principles of family-centered care, must serve as the primary advocate for the child. This advocacy role provides navigation and guidance for the comprehensive symptom management approach.

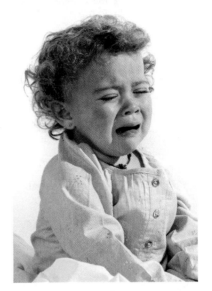

Figure 11-2 *The experience of pain is highly influenced by a child's psychology and state of health.*

Pain

Pain is the most feared of all symptoms and can cause both the child and the family tremendous distress. The experience of pain is unique for each child, and is influenced by the child's individual cognitive, cultural, affective, behavioral, and spiritual personal aspects. Understanding the definition of pain is important and is the first step in appreciating the child's pain experience. According to the International Association for the Study of Pain (2014), **pain** is a unique experience for each person that may be defined as "[a]n unpleasant sensory and emotional experience associated with actual or potential tissue damage, or described in terms of such damage." Pain typically starts with a noxious stimulus (a precipitator of pain) and launches the process of the pain experience, which is highly influenced by the child's physiology and state of health (**Figure 11-2**).

Pain Physiology

Typically, pain occurs when an injury from chemical, thermal, pressure, or mechanical stimuli causes activation of the free nerve endings (nociceptors) located within tissues. Chemical substances released when tissues are damaged or injured activate the nerve endings and send signals via afferent fibers to the dorsal horn of the spinal cord (**Figure 11-3**). From the dorsal horn, the message is then carried to the brain for interpretation. The chemical substances released during this process include prostaglandins, serotonin, bradykinins, histamine, and substance P. Two fibers are involved in this transmission of stimuli: A-delta fibers, which send messages of sharp pain, and unmyelinated C fibers, which send signals for aching, diffuse and burning sensations.

Pain Experiences

A person's **pain threshold** is defined as the minimal sensory stimulus that is perceived as a source of discomfort or pain. A child's pain threshold is unique and variable. Some children have high pain thresholds and can experience or tolerate potentially painful stimuli before perceived pain begins. Others have very low pain thresholds and perceive a pain experience with even low-level stimuli. The challenge for the pediatric nurse is to understand this principle, apply it to the assessment and management of pain, and not pass judgment or be deterred from adequate and competent pain management regardless of how children express their pain. This expression includes how severe the pain experience is for each child, and how low a pain threshold may be to require nursing intervention. **Table 11-1** identifies the various types of pain that may be distinguished.

Pediatric nurses must be aggressive in applying principles of pain assessment and management to prevent the undertreatment of pain and discomfort. Undertreated pain leads to consequences that influence healing. A child with undertreated pain may experience short-term (immediate) and long-term sequelae.

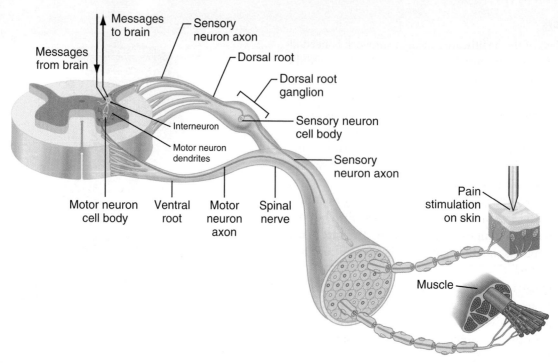

Figure 11-3 *The pathway of pain.*

Immediate Responses
- Decreased oxygen saturation readings
- Rapid shallow breathing that can lead to a state of alkalosis
- Inadequate lung expansion, contributing to atelectasis
- Increased heart rate and heart rate variability
- Increased systolic blood pressure
- Diaphoresis
- Guarding with decreased movements
- Restlessness preventing restfulness
- Decrease in peripheral blood flow to the skin
- Delayed wound healing
- Increased metabolic rate (especially in newborns and young infants with minimal stored resources or energy)
- Increased loss of fluids and electrolytes
- Impaired gastrointestinal function, anorexia, and nausea
- Increased metabolic caloric consumption
- Prolonged hypoglycemia or—with adrenal activation and secretion of stress hormones—prolonged hyperglycemia
- Mistrust in the child's environment
- Feelings of anxiety, stress, and sadness

Long-Term Consequences
- Impaired inflammatory responses
- Decreased immune system function
- Poor motor performance
- Hypersensitivity to continued pain or new sources of discomfort
- Poor adaptive behavior, learning disorders, and cognitive defects
- Temperament changes and long-term psychosocial problems

Pain Assessment

The assessment of a child's pain is crucial for the development of a holistic nursing care plan (**Figure 11-4**). The location and severity of the pain are important factors, but so are the circumstances surrounding the pain experience. Pain is a unique human experience, yet some physical cues are consistent across the various developmental stages (**Table 11-2**).

When faced with a child experiencing pain, the assessment should start with background information. The nurse should ask the following questions:

- What are child's previous experiences with pain?
- How did the child find relief? Which specific pain interventions have worked in the past for the child?
- How does the child display symptoms of pain? Is the child verbal about pain or does the child become quiet?
- If verbal, which words does the child currently use to express pain?
- What are the child's experiences with non-narcotic and narcotic pain control medications?

TABLE 11-1 Types of Pain Experiences

Acute pain: Often has a sudden onset; associated with trauma, injury, surgical wounds, and severe inflammation.

Chronic pain: Pain that persists for months, may progress, and is often resistant to traditional or standard pain medical treatments.

Episodic pain: Recurring pain that comes in intervals, such as acute episodic pain associated with sickle cell anemia's acute vaso-occlusive episodes. Episodic pain can be unpredictable and debilitating.

Idiopathic pain: Pain described or experienced by a child even in the presence of no identifiable pathological condition that would contribute to the source of the discomfort.

Breakthrough pain: The experience of continued and increasing pain above the child's baseline pain experience. Also, pain that emerges during a period of symptom management and may be associated with new activity or increased movement.

Neuropathic pain: Persistent discomfort that is experienced in the presence of structural damage, lesions or disease, or nerve cell dysfunction or injury within the central or peripheral nervous system (somatosensory). Neuropathic pain, which can be described as a sensory dysfunction, may be expressed in the following ways:

› Hyperalgesia (increased pain response to stimuli that do not normally cause a child pain)

› Hypoalgesia (diminished pain response to normally painful stimuli)

› Paresthesia (abnormal sensations experienced after exposure to stimuli, such as tingling, stinging, and numbness)

› Hyperesthesia (increased sensitivity to stimuli)

› Hypoesthesia (decreased sensitivity to stimuli)

Nociceptive pain: Pain that arises from tissues other than nerve tissue or cells and caused by the activation of nociceptors (sensory receptor of the peripheral nervous system).

Somatic pain: Pain caused by activation of the nociceptors in surface tissues such as the child's skin and mucosa, or deep tissues such as the child's muscles, connective tissues, bones and joints.

› Nociceptive superficial somatic: Pain in the anus, urethra, skin, nose, and mucosa of the mouth

› Nociceptive deep somatic: Pain in the bones, joints, connective tissues, and muscles

Visceral pain: Pain caused by the activation of the nociceptors in visceral tissues. The viscera include the child's internal organs of the abdomen and thoracic region.

› Nociceptive visceral: Pain in the liver, pancreas, pleura, and peritoneum

Allodynia: A pain experience due to a type of stimulus that normally does not induce or provoke pain

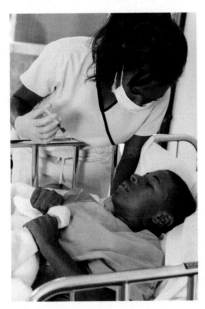

Figure 11-4 *The assessment of a child's pain is crucial for the development of a holistic nursing care plan.*

© Juanmonino/E+/Getty Images

QUALITY AND SAFETY

The Joint Commission requires documentation of pain assessment, interventions implemented for a pain experience, evaluation of all interventions implemented, and documentation of reassessment of pain at regular intervals appropriate for each patient's pain experience.

Data from Baker, D. W. (2016). Joint Commission statement on pain management. Retrieved from https://www.jointcommission.org/topics/pain_management.aspx; The Joint Commission. (2010). *Approaches to pain management: An essential guide for clinicians* (2nd ed). Oakbrook Terrace, IL: Joint Commission Resources.

Pain assessment tools are critical to adequately managing pain for children. Many effective, reliable, and valid tools are available for use in children spanning the developmental period. The nurse should take into consideration three types of assessments:

- Biophysical assessments of pain through vital signs measurement and oxygen saturation findings

TABLE 11-2 Developmental Aspects of Pain Expression

Pain may be expressed through common physical or behavioral findings in each of the developmental periods:

› **Fetus:** Fetuses who are at least 8 weeks' gestational age respond to touch. After 20 weeks' gestation, a fetus will recoil from a painful stimulus (Gupta, Kilby, & Cooper, 2008).

› **Infant:** Infants display pain by crying, drawing eyebrows together, squeezing eyes shut, open and rectangle-shaped look to the mouth, and quivering chin. Body tension, fist clenching, arching, and flailing are other indicators of pain.

› **Toddler:** Owing to their limited verbal skills, toddlers will display pain through grimacing, limb movement, grasping onto an object or their caregiver, crying, groaning, and moaning.

› **Preschooler:** Given their expanding verbal skills, most preschoolers can use a 4- to 5-item discrimination scale such as the Wong-Baker FACES Pain Rating Scale. They demonstrate pain though crying, whimpering, grasping onto an object or person, limb movement, and distinct facial features including eye squeezing, flared nostrils, furrowed forehead, and mouth stretching.

› **School age:** Most school-age children verbalize their pain experience as well as expressing themselves nonverbally. These children display facial expressions of pain, crying, and body movements of thrashing, leg movement, or recoiling. Developmental regression may occur with pain experiences. The FACES Scale, Visual Analogue Scale, numeric scales, and Adolescent Pediatric Pain Scale have all been used in this age group successfully, although the last two instruments require a more advanced comprehension of numeric values and vocabulary than are typically found in children younger than age 10.

› **Adolescent:** When in front of peers, adolescents may hide or minimize their pain symptom display. Teens are typically very verbal about their pain and communicate in detail various aspects of the pain experience. They may show pain through facial features and body posturing. They may be tearful or act stoically. Pain assessment is often best accomplished using the Adolescent Pediatric Pain Scale, as it allows for a more nuanced expression of a teenager's experience.

Data from Srouji, R., Ratnapalan, S., & Schneeweiss, S. (2010). Pain in children: Assessment and nonpharmacological management. *International Journal of Pediatrics*, vol. 2010, Article ID 474838. http://dx.doi.org/10.1155/2010/474838

- Subjective pain assessment tools, which allow the child to express his or her experience of pain
- Objective pain assessment tools, which rely on the clinical judgment of the nurse to determine the level of pain the child is experiencing

Biophysical Assessments

Vital signs do not always adequately convey the level of pain a child is experiencing. The child's autonomic nervous system may be activated during a painful event and may—or may not—cause fluctuations in vital signs. Because research has demonstrated that vital signs changes occur with the application of a nociceptive procedure, experts suggest that measurement of vital signs be used as part of a full pain assessment (Arbour, Choiniere, Topolovec-Vranic, Loiselle, & Gelinas, 2014). The pediatric nurse performing the pain assessment should be aware of how vital signs generally reflect the experience of pain:

- Heart rate: Heart rate becomes elevated with an acute pain experience or an exacerbation of chronic pain.
- Respiratory rate: Typically, pediatric respirations will be faster and more shallow with acute pain.

- Systolic blood pressure: During a pain episode, a child's systolic blood pressure will increase.
- Temperature: Although a child's temperature will not fluctuate with pain, the child may demonstrate diaphoresis and elevated temperature if experiencing pain associated with infectious processes, with these effects then contributing to the child's overall discomfort.
- Oxygen saturation: During acute pain episodes and changes in breathing patterns, a child's oxygen saturation measurement may decrease.

Subjective Tools

Subjective tools—that is, tools that can be used to obtain the child's own assessment of his or her pain experience—have been validated and deemed reliable across childhood from the young preschool period onward. For children who do not have cognitive impairments or changes in their level of consciousness, and who are able to express themselves verbally, the administration of subjective tools has been shown to be of great value in pediatric pain management. Subjective tool use can begin in the early years of the preschool developmental period.

Wong-Baker FACES® Pain Rating Scale

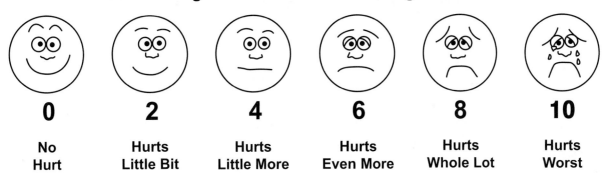

0	2	4	6	8	10
No Hurt	**Hurts Little Bit**	**Hurts Little More**	**Hurts Even More**	**Hurts Whole Lot**	**Hurts Worst**

Figure 11-5 *Wong-Baker FACES Pain Rating Scale.*

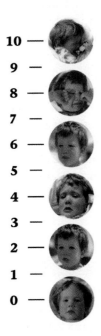

Figure 11-6 *Oucher Scale.*

Preschoolers

Appropriate tools for assessing pain in preschoolers include the Wong-Baker FACES Scale and the Oucher Scale.

- Wong-Baker FACES Pain Rating Scale (**Figure 11-5**): A series of six drawings of a simple face character that expresses a range of facial features, from smiling (no pain) to crying intensely (score of 10).
- Oucher Scale (**Figure 11-6**): A series of six photographs of children appearing to experience increasing levels of pain. Children are asked to select the face that most closely matches their current pain

experience. The tool comes in a variety of ethnicities to more closely resemble the child. Each photograph is associated with a numerical value with scores ranging from 0 to 10.

School-Age Children

Appropriate pain assessment tools for school-age children include the Wong-Baker FACES Scale, the Numeric Rating Scale, the Visual Analogue Scale, and the poker chip pain assessment tool.

- Numeric Rating Scale (**Figure 11-7**): This scale is used when a child is developmentally able to understand and apply numerical values; it is generally not used in children younger than age 8 because they often lack the ability to grasp the significance of the numbers as applied to pain experience (von Baeyer, 2006). Rating can be done via a verbalization of the numbers "zero to ten" or by presenting the child with a scale of numbers.
- Visual Analogue Scale (VAS; **Figure 11-8**): The child is presented with a 100-mm line on a paper or card, with "no pain" written at one end of the line and "worst possible pain" written at the other end. The patient is asked to draw a perpendicular line according to where his or her pain falls. The nurse then uses a 100-mm ruler to determine the final pain scale value; numbers range from zero to 100. The VAS can also be presented as a "pain thermometer" concept. It shows good sensitivity and validity for most children from approximately age 7 and older (Srouji, Ratnapalan, & Schneeweiss, 2010; von Baeyer, 2006). Given a choice, though, many children prefer using the FACES Scale over a VAS measurement (von Baeyer, 2006).

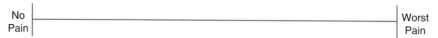

0	1	2	3	4	5	6	7	8	9	10
No Pain					Moderate Pain					Worst Pain

Figure 11-7 *Numerical Rating Scale.*

No Pain ├───┤ Worst Pain

Figure 11-8 *Visual Analogue Scale (VAS).*

- Poker chip tool: Most commonly, the nurse provides the child with a stack of five poker chips of the same color, spreads them out in a row, and communicates that they represent "pieces of hurt" (Srouji et al., 2010; von Baeyer, 2006). The child then chooses the number of chips to represent his or her pain, from zero chips (no pain) to five chips (representing the most intense pain the child can imagine). Some institutions have used a more sophisticated process of color-coding the chips to represent various degrees of pain intensity.

Adolescents

Appropriate pain assessment tools include the Numeric Rating Scale, the Visual Analogue Scale, and the Adolescent Pediatric Pain Tool.

The Adolescent Pediatric Pain Tool provides the opportunity for older children and teenagers to communicate to the healthcare team member a number of aspects or dimensions of their pain experience. The tool consists of three categories: (1) a body diagram that allows the child to point to an anatomic location; (2) a word–graphic rating scale, usually consisting of a line with anchor points that identify a pain spectrum ranging from "no pain" to "worst possible pain"; and (3) a selection of words that allows the child to choose descriptions of the nature of the pain (e.g., burning, stinging, aching, throbbing) and its timing (e.g., always, sometimes, at night, during the day). These descriptors were identified in a three-phase research process involving more than 1200 children, both healthy and hospitalized, ranging in age from 8 to 17. The first two phases identified words that were useful and meaningful to the children, while the third phase validated the reliability of the pain descriptors selected (Fernandes, De Campos, Batalha, Perdigão, & Jacob, 2014; Srouji et al., 2010).

UNIQUE FOR KIDS

Assessing Pain in the Adolescent: Essential Components

Due to their age, most teens will have had a life experience of a painful stimulus and, therefore, can benchmark a current pain experience against their previous pain experiences. Teens want to express themselves in regard to pain in terms of onset, location, duration, severity, and described sensory experience. Time is required to conduct a holistic assessment of a teenager's pain, and nurses should allow sufficient time for this interaction. Administering a pain scale tool that allows the older child to draw where the pain is, use shading to show severity, use descriptive words to articulate the type of pain and sensations, and use words denoting both chronology and intensity typically works well for most developmentally intact adolescents.

The maturity of an adolescent is both a benefit and a drawback to the provider. On the one hand, teens are capable of providing more detailed and nuanced information than younger children. On the other hand, their developmental phase—which emphasizes differentiating themselves from parental and other forms of authority—may diminish their willingness to speak openly with healthcare providers about their experiences (Murphy, 2011), particularly if the nature of the pain is highly sensitive (e.g., genitourinary tract pain) or if they fear disclosure of their condition to the parent. Parental assessment of pain often differs from the teen's own assessment (Vetter, Bridgewater, Ascherman, Madan-Swain, & McGwin, 2014). Offering a pain assessment tool that is intended for younger children (e.g., the Wong-Baker FACES Scale) may be counterproductive, as the teen may feel disrespected or patronized and, in turn, become uncommunicative. Try to provide an opportunity to complete a thorough pain assessment in privacy so the teen feels respected and can engage in open discussion without worry about responses from family, peers, or other patients.

Objective Tools

Objective pain tools allow the nurse to identify behaviors in infants and young children that are expressions of pain. These tools are very helpful in assessment and management of preverbal or nonverbal children's pain. The following demonstrate examples of various objective tools used in pediatric pain management.

Neonates

- Neonatal Infant Pain Scale (NIPS): Face, cry, breathing pattern, movement of arms and legs, and state of arousal
- Neonatal Facial Coding System (NFCS): Brow, eye squeeze, furrow, kips, stretched mouth, lip purse, taut tongue, and chin quiver
- CRIES Scale: Crying, requires oxygen, increased vital signs, expression, and sleeplessness

Toddlers

- Toddler–Preschooler Postoperative Pain Scale (TPPPS): Assesses pain in children who are between 1 and 5 years of age by looking at verbal cues, facial expressions, and body movement.
- FLACC Behavioral Pain Assessment Scale (**Figure 11-9**): Face, legs, activity, cry, and consolability. This scale can be used for pediatric patients, ages 2 months to 7 years, who are unable to verbally express their pain experience.

Pharmacologic Pain Control

The generally accepted method of controlling a child's pain is by applying a pain scale score to determine dosing of a non-narcotic or **narcotic** (i.e., opioid) pain medication. For instance, a medical order for pain medication may take the form of a scale. If the child's pain level is less than 2 or 3 on the scale, the provider may elect to prescribe a non-narcotic medication such as ibuprofen or acetaminophen. A pain scale score of 3 to 5 may allow

UNIQUE FOR KIDS

Myths About Pain in Children

Although state-of-the-science guidelines for assessment and management of pain in children can be found in the literature, children, especially infants, continue to be under-medicated for pain—even in situations, such as postoperative care, where pain is anticipated (Birnie et al., 2014; Stevens et al., 2011). Management of children's pain during procedures remains inadequate (Bice, Gunther, & Wyatt, 2014). Unfortunately, myths and misconceptions that developed in the 19th and 20th centuries continue to permeate comprehensive care of children experiencing pain (Rodkey & Riddell, 2013):

- Neonates do not experience pain due to physiological immaturity and, therefore, do not require pain medications.
- Children, in general, do not experience pain of the same intensity, duration, or significance as adults.
- Young children cannot express the location or intensity of their pain.
- Memory of pain in children is less than memory of pain in adults.
- Children always tell the truth about pain.
- Biophysical displays of pain through vital signs do not demonstrate pain experiences in children.
- Children are at high risk to develop addiction to narcotic pain control measures.
- If a child is playing, no pain or insignificant pain is present.

Categories	Scoring		
	0	**1**	**2**
Face	No particular expression or smile	Occasional grimace or frown, withdrawn, disinterested	Frequent to constant frown, quivering chin, clenched jaw
Legs	Normal position or relaxed	Uneasy, restless, tense	Kicking or legs drawn up
Activity	Lying quietly, normal position, moves easily	Squirming, shifting back and forth, tense	Arched, rigid, or jerking
Cry	No cry (awake or asleep)	Moans or whimpers; occasional complaint	Crying steadily, screams or sobs, frequent complaints
Consolability	Content, relaxed	Reassured by occasional touching, hugging, or being talked to; distractible	Difficult to console or comfort

Note: Each of the five categories Face (F), Legs (L), Activity (A), Cry (C), and Consolability (C) is scored from 0–2, which results in a total score between 0 and 10.

Figure 11-9 *FLACC Behavioral Pain Assessment Scale.*

TABLE 11-3 Medications Used for Pain Control in Children

Non-Opioid Medications for Pain

› Choline magnesium trisalicylate: 25 mg/kg PO every 12 hours

› Acetaminophen: 10–15 mg/kg PO every 4–6 hours

› Ibuprofen: 5–10 mg/kg PO every 6 hours

› Naproxen: 5–10 mg/kg PO every 12 hours

› Ketorolac: 1 mg/kg IV loading dose, followed by 0.5 mg/kg up to 30 mg IV maximum in children every 6 hours, for no more than 5 days

Narcotic Medications for Pain

› Fentanyl: 5–15 mcg/kg PO or 0.5–2 mcg/kg every 1–2 hours

› Hydromorphone: 0.03–0.08 mg/kg PO every 4 hours, or 0.01–0.015 mg/kg IV every 3–4 hours

› Levophanol: 0.04 mg/kg PO every 6–8 hours, or 0.02 mg/kg IV every 6–8 hours

› Methadone: 0.1–0.2 mg/kg PO every 12–36 hours, or 0.1–0.2 mg/kg every 12–36 hours

› Morphine: 0.05–0.1 mg/kg IV every 2–4 hours, or 0.3 mg/kg PO every 3–4 hours

› Oxycodone: 0.1–0.2 mg/kg PO every 3–4 hours

› Tramadol: 1–2 mg/kg PO every 4–6 hours (investigational)

the child to receive a lower-intensity narcotic medication such as tramadol (Benini & Barbi, 2014; Food and Drug Administration, 2015) or low-dose morphine (Wong, Lau, Palozzi, & Campbell, 2012); these options have replaced codeine as the analgesic of choice for some providers due to safety concerns. Although frequently used for mild to moderate pain in children, codeine use has been associated with a number of pediatric deaths (Thompson, 2016). Pain scored as 6 or greater is generally treated with standard opioid analgesia. Thus, selection of the appropriate pharmacologic pain control treatment is based on the child's subjective pain scale score, along with the nurse's objective pain scale score on behalf of the child.

Table 11-3 lists medications that are commonly used to treat mild to severe pain in children.

RESEARCH EVIDENCE

Children who have developmental delays are at risk for poor pain assessment and pain control. According to Gilbert-MacLeod, Craig, Rocha, and Mathias (2000), developmentally delayed children may display a lower-intensity pain distress response to a pain stimulus compared to children without developmental delays. Some developmentally delayed children in these researchers' study showed no physical or emotional response to a painful stimulus or procedure. The researchers also found that developmentally delayed children have a lower incidence of participating in "help-seeking" after a painful experience. This lack of response and failure to show the classic displays of discomfort and pain that pediatric nurses rely on for assessments can place a developmentally delayed child at risk for poor management.

QUALITY AND SAFETY

Assessments and Interventions for Respiratory Depression with Narcotic Pain Control

The development of respiratory depression in children who receive narcotics for pain control, also known as opioid-induced respiratory depression (OIRD), is both rare and unpredictable. If dosed within the safe dose range for a narcotic medication and given the medication only at the recommended time intervals, a child in pain should not be expected to experience any respiratory depression. Clinical symptoms of OIRD include unresponsiveness, progressive decreasing respiratory rate with shallow breathing, and small pupils. Fatalities are possible in children with OIRD due to airway obstruction by the child's tongue. Nurses must be able to identify patients who are at risk for opioid-induced respiratory depression and advancing sedation (Jarzyna et al., 2011). Confounding factors include renal impairment, frequency of medication dosage times, sensory deafferentation (Dahan, Overdyk, Smith, Aarts, & Niesters, 2013), obesity, respiratory disorders and pulmonary diseases, female sex, and breathing disorders during sleep (Overdyk et al., 2014).

Because OIRD can be fatal, and due to the unpredictability of its occurrence, recommendations for managing children who are receiving narcotic pain control in hospital settings include continuous monitoring of respiratory rate and oxygen saturations. OIRD is most often associated with morphine use and typically occurs in the pediatric postoperative period. Interventions to reverse narcotic agents in the presence of respiratory depression include naloxone (10 mcg/kg mixed with saline to yield 0.5 mcg/kg every 1 to 2 minutes).

PHARMACOLOGY

Meperidine (Demerol) is rarely administered to children due to its toxic metabolite, normeperidine. Meperidine is metabolized via the CYP450 pathway to normeperidine, which is considered a nonactive metabolite that has half the

(continues)

potency of meperidine but three times the toxicity. Norme-peridine can build up in the child's system with prolonged use and cause neurologic side effects such as shaking, tremors, anxiety, hyperreflexia, mood changes, hallucinations, and seizures. These toxic outcomes can occur within only 24 hours of dosing with meperidine (DePriest, Puet, Holt, Roberts, & Cone, 2015).

Nonpharmacologic Pain Control

Research has shown that "closing the pain gate" by inhibiting pain impulses being carried to the brain is effective in managing many sources of pain. Application of ice, pressure, or massage can cause the A-beta fibers to reduce or inhibit transmission of pain stimuli through the substantia gelatinosa, which is located in the dorsal horn of the spinal cord. This helps in blocking messages to the brain. Other complementary pain-reducing or pain-relieving interventions that have been successfully applied to children include the following options:

- Distraction via sensory stimulation (auditory, visual, olfactory) through reading, music, and arts
- Hypnosis to facilitate awareness, concentration away from pain stimuli, and an increased state of relaxation
- Guided imagery to provide progressive muscle relaxation or focused concentration on pleasant mental images such as the ocean, hiking, playing, or dancing
- Breathing techniques to relax and reduce anxiety
- Sucrose solutions (typically 1 to 2 mL of 24% sucrose solution) administered just before a painful procedure
- Holding and rocking a young child

Nursing Diagnoses for Pain

The over-arching nursing diagnosis associated with discomfort and pain is impaired comfort. NANDA International (2012) provides a framework in which to create a care plan using the nursing process. In this framework, which was first developed by Lynda Juall Carpenito, pain diagnoses are divided into acute and chronic types:

- Pain
- Acute pain related to injury, trauma, or surgical manipulation
- Chronic pain related to inflammation

According to Carpenito (2013), the framework encompasses "perceived lack of ease, relief, and transcendence in physical, psychospiritual, environmental, cultural and social dimensions."

Medical Treatments for Pain

Interdisciplinary teams can work together to create a plan of pain control for a child who will be exposed to a painful procedure or surgical manipulation. The medical model of pain control includes the following interventions, among others:

- Local injected anesthetics containing lidocaine buffered by sodium bicarbonate or bupivacaine
- Regional pain management delivered via epidural injections
- Nerve blocks, such as needle-injected anesthetics to nerves surrounding the tissues involved in the painful site
- Patient-controlled analgesia providing a basal rate plus patient-controlled dosing of narcotics (**Figure 11-10**)
- Topical cutaneous interventions such as vapo-coolant sprays, EMLA cream (eutectic mixture of local anesthetics), anesthetic patches containing lidocaine and tetracaine, and needle-free powder lidocaine delivery systems
- Transcutaneous electrical nerve stimulation (TENS)

Nursing Care for Pain

Nursing care for a child with **discomfort** (lack of comfort or ease) or pain should be guided by principles of the nursing process. After performing subjective and objective assessments of the pain, the nurse focuses on establishing goals for pain control and interventions that concentrate on pain alleviation. Ultimately, the goal is to remove or reduce the cause of the discomfort or pain. The following interventions may be administered following a thorough pain assessment using the principles of anticipation and proactive nursing care:

- Use topical cream anesthetics such as EMLA before starting intravenous (IV) infusions or giving injections (not on young infants).

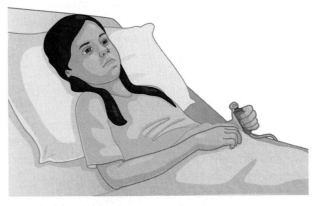

Figure 11-10 *A pain control plan for a child may include patient-controlled analgesia.*

- Believe children about their pain: Pain is a symptom that occurs whenever a child says it does. Take all reports of pain seriously and intervene appropriately.
- Listen carefully to a child's communication and description of the pain experience, regardless of the child's developmental stage or ability to express himself or herself.
- Expect variations in children of similar ages, as pain thresholds vary with developmental stages, diagnoses, and surgical procedures.
- Inquire about previous pain experiences and ways of coping that were successful.
- Involve parents and caregivers in pain assessment and interventions.
- Understand that fatigue, anxiety, and fear can increase a child's sensitivity to pain.
- Use a variety of words to describe pain; take into account the child's developmental level and the words the family uses. Ask the parents which words they use (ouch, ouchie, booboo, owie, hurtie); write the words on a card and keep the card at the bedside. Document these preferences for the interdisciplinary team.
- Use a team approach for pain control, including Child Life specialists.
- Assess the effectiveness of pain interventions within 1 hour; document the findings.
- Provide ongoing education and support for parents or guardians.
- Explain to parents that addiction to narcotics in the presence of pain is a rare phenomenon.
- Understand the potential side effects of narcotics administration, including gastrointestinal distress, nausea, constipation, intense itching, and sedation. Educate parents on what to expect.

Nausea

Children typically have many experiences with **nausea** (upset stomach, which may be followed by vomiting) throughout their childhood. Children encounter many potential etiologies of gastrointestinal (GI) distress. For example, acute viral gastroenteritis, food allergies, intolerance to foods, food poisoning, motion sickness, severe abdominal pain, overeating, intestinal blockages or obstructions, and medications such as oral antibiotics, chemotherapy, and anesthesia may all potentially trigger nausea. Nausea may resolve on its own, but for some children, antinausea medications are required for elimination or control of this symptom. The experience of nausea is both troubling to the child and family and concerning for the nurse caring for the child. Put simply, the experience of nausea makes a child miserable.

Nausea may be caused by any number of noxious stimuli that affect the vomiting center either directly or indirectly. The vomiting center, which is located in the medulla oblongata, comprises both the nucleus of the tractus solitaries and the reticular formation. When it is activated, electrical messages are sent via the fifth, seventh, ninth, 10th, and 12th cranial nerves to the GI tract, and sympathetic and vagal nerve messages to the lower GI tract. Chemicals can have an immediate direct effect on the vomiting center in the brain, or indirect stimulation can occur in one of four areas: the gastrointestinal system, the chemoreceptor trigger zone, the vestibular region, or the cerebral cortex and thalamus. The chemoreceptor trigger zone is easily permeated by nausea-inducing chemicals and irritants because it is not surrounded by the tightly constructed capillaries and protective endothelium associated with the blood–brain barrier. When this zone is stimulated, reverse peristalsis occurs, sending the intestinal contents from the lower small intestine to the upper small intestine, and then into the stomach. During vomiting, the esophageal sphincter relaxes, sending the stomach contents up to the child's mouth (Becker, 2010).

The act of vomiting, or emesis, is a clinical sign of nausea, and may be accompanied by retching. As it is a strong muscular event, a child may retch without passing gastric contents.

Nausea is common in the postoperative period. Though this phenomenon is known as postoperative nausea and vomiting (PONV), the experience of nausea may precede the act of vomiting, or vomiting may occur without first experiencing nausea. The pediatric nurse should expect and plan for the assessment and treatment of PONV.

Assessment of Nausea

The pediatric nurse should assess the child's level of described nausea. For children with a grasp of "more" and "less" in a numeric sense, a 0 to 10 numeric scale can be used to describe the intensity of the nausea. With nonverbal children, the nurse has added challenges in assessing nausea. A quiet child, holding the stomach, with closed eyes, lying still on one side or curled in a fetal position, may indicate nausea. It is important that the nurse take into account the reason for the young child's unexpected behaviors and assume that nausea is present before the child begins to retch or vomit.

After assessment of the severity of the nausea, the pediatric nurse should discern the cause of this symptom. Causes may be emotional, physical, or a result of medical treatment. A variety of **emetogenic** (vomiting-inducing) medications are administered in healthcare settings, and their administration must be identified—the need for repeated dosing will require antiemetics to be offered either as premedications or around the clock (ATC). Medications that can cause nausea in children include inhaled anesthetics, chemotherapy, opioids administered for pain, and several antibiotics.

Nursing Diagnoses for Nausea

As noted earlier, nausea may be related to stimulation of the vomiting center. In addition, it may reflect fluid imbalance owing to lack of oral intake of fluids.

Medical Treatments for Nausea

Antiemetics, which block receptors on the cells of the vomiting center, are the medical cornerstone for the control or alleviation of nausea. If the emetogenic trigger is vestibular in nature (such as in motion sickness), medications are given that block histamine and acetylcholine. If the trigger is linked to use of opioids or anesthetics, antiemetics that block dopamine will be most effective. In the vomiting center itself, serotonin antagonists are most effective. In addition, anxiolytics may be useful in children who have repeated emetogenic experiences such as chemotherapy and endure anticipatory nausea and vomiting (Becker, 2010).

Common antiemetic medications administered to children include the following agents:

- Serotonin antagonists such as ondansetron (Zofran)
- Tricyclic antidepressants such as promethazine (Phenergan) (not recommended for children younger than age 2)
- Phenothiazine such as prochlorperazine (Compazine) (not recommended for children younger than age 2)
- Antihistamines such as diphenhydramine (Benadryl) (indicated for motion sickness)
- Gut motility stimulators such as metoclopramide (Reglan)
- Corticosteroids such as dexamethasone (Decadron)
- Anticholinergic agents approved for pediatric use

Nursing Care for Nausea

Children need to be soothed and cared for when they are experiencing the misery of nausea. It may be better to refrain from offering food and drink until the sensation subsides. Antinausea medications should be administered if ordered, and the cause of the nausea must be identified. The child should be placed in a semi-Fowler's or side-lying position in case the nausea is accompanied with vomiting, which carries a risk of aspiration (**Figure 11-11**). The child should remain in a cool, quiet, low-stimulation environment. Encourage stress reduction behaviors such as deep breathing, relaxation, and sleep. When a child is vomiting, follow-up oral care is important to protect the integrity of the teeth.

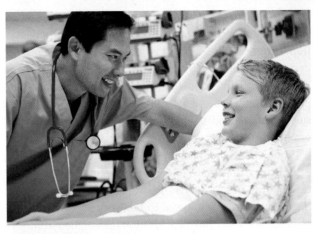

Figure 11-11 *A child with nausea should be placed in a semi-Fowler's (pictured here) or side-lying position in case the nausea is accompanied with vomiting, which carries a risk of aspiration.*

When the nausea has resolved and there has been no vomiting for several hours, introduce fluids and foods slowly. Chilled fluids may be tolerated well by older children. Many children enjoy small ice chips after a period of nausea and vomiting. Small servings of low-fat, visually appealing foods without strong aromas may help the child begin to eat again.

The pediatric nurse must assess for complications of prolonged nausea and vomiting. Monitor for blood in the vomit (hematemesis), dehydration, and the presence of debilitating abdominal pain and cramping. Report any passage of fecal material in the vomit.

Fatigue

Fatigue is a complicated human experience and is actually considered quite common across the lifespan. The experience of fatigue can provoke a frustrating and disruptive daily state that affects a child's ability to function, eat well, sleep well, play, interact and socialize, and perform activities of daily living.

In children, **fatigue** is often described as a state of being tired, exhausted, wearied, or unmotivated, with poor energy and poor concentration. Fatigue may also be associated with hyperthermia or fever. Children may report having significantly reduced ability or capacity to perform daily work, play, and interactions with others. Regardless of the expansive research that exists on fatigue in children, however, there is no single well-accepted definition of this phenomenon. Instead, the child's personality, culture, social support, family network, physical environment, and health state all combine to make the experience of fatigue unique. More generally, fatigue can be conceived as a continuum from unpleasant to mildly distressing to severely disabling.

Fatigue can cause severe functional impairment that affects both the child's education and his or her socialization. Fatigue at the level that is considered disabling is the primary reason for children's prolonged absences from academic settings (Fowler, Duthie, Thapar, & Farmer, 2005). Fatigue can be associated with mental health issues, medical treatments for acute and chronic illnesses, or physiological disruptions such as anemia, or it can exist without a psychological or physiological etiology.

It is very important that the child expresses his or her experiences and sensations associated with fatigue so that interventions can be initiated and individualized. The pediatric nurse should look objectively at the fatigue symptoms presented and, when the child is able, encourage the child to provide a subjective description of the fatigue experience. The healthcare team then needs to look at the greater health context in which fatigue has developed, including illness, disease, and comorbidity with mental health disorders.

Fatigue has unique sensations that are described differently by children in each developmental stage. Among verbal children, fatigue has been described as a physical sensation, alternating and sometimes merging with mental tiredness. Many school-age and adolescent children indicate that their primary means to alleviate fatigue comes from pacing—that is, a balance of resting periods and play or distractions (Goudsmit, Nijs, Jason, & Wallman, 2012).

According to the Centers for Disease Control and Prevention (CDC), the definition of chronic fatigue syndrome—now formally called myalgic encephalomyelitis/chronic fatigue syndrome (ME/CFS)—includes fatigue at a level that diminishes the patient's functional status, exists for 6 months or longer, and is associated with four or more of the following clinical symptoms: (1) poor concentration and memory; (2) sleep that does not provide a sense of refreshment; (3) severe post-exercise malaise; (4) muscle and joint pain; and (5) signs of illness such as sore throat, headache, and tender lymph nodes (CDC, 2012; Fukuda et al., 1994). In children, however, ME/CFS symptoms often differ from the standard syndrome in adults, and may include abdominal pain and rashes; symptoms in children also vary more on a day-to-day basis compared to symptoms in adults (Jason, Barker, & Brown, 2012). To be formally diagnosed with ME/CFS, children must meet the standard criteria for adults as well as exhibit additional symptoms such as two or more neurocognitive manifestations and at least one of the following: autonomic manifestations, neuroendocrine manifestations, or immune manifestations (Jason et al., 2012; Jason et al., 2006).

Assessment of Fatigue

The pediatric nurse has the challenge of assessing the degree or severity of a child's fatigue experience. Fatigue can be situational, acute, chronic, or disabling. Assessment of a child's state of depression should go hand in hand with the assessment of fatigue. One lens through which to view fatigue is to consider whether the experience is primary or secondary. Primary fatigue is associated directly with a mental health issue or a physical disorder. By comparison, secondary fatigue is associated with a progression or worsening of symptoms owing to a disease state, medical treatment, or surgical intervention.

UNIQUE FOR KIDS

The Underpinnings of Fatigue

Fatigue has been associated with the following specific disease states and conditions:

- Hematologic issues such as anemia
- Infections that influence the child's metabolism
- States of prolonged inflammation
- Cancer
- Poor nutrition
- Prolonged bed rest, lack of exercise, and immobility
- Dehydration
- Obesity
- Depression
- Trauma
- Pain experiences
- Stress, grief, and anxiety
- Sleep disorders including sleep apnea
- Neurologic and immunologic conditions such as ME/CFS, AIDS, autoimmune diseases, and fibromyalgia
- Prolonged use of fatigue-inducing medications

Data from Morris, G., Berk, M., Walder, K., & Maes, M. (2015). Central pathways causing fatigue in neuro-inflammatory and autoimmune illnesses. *BMC Medicine, 13*, 28; Fragkandrea, I., Nixon, J. A., & Panagopoulou, P. (2013). Signs and symptoms of childhood cancer: A guide for early recognition. *American Family Physician, 88*, 185–192; Sánchez-Rodríguez, E., & Miró, J. (2015). The assessment of fatigue in children with chronic pain: A review of existing measures. *European Journal of Psychological Assessment, 31*(2): 75–82; Sacheck, J. M., Rasmussen, H. M., Hall, M. M., Kafka, T., Blumberg, J. B., & Economos, C. D. (2014). The association between pregame snacks and exercise intensity, stress, and fatigue in children. *Pediatric Exercise Science, 26*, 159–167; Viner, R. M., Clark, C., Taylor, S. J. C., Bhui, K., Klineberg, E., Head, J., . . . Stansfeld, S. A. (2008). Longitudinal risk factors for persistent fatigue in adolescents. *Archives of Pediatrics and Adolescent Medicine, 162*(5), 469–475.

Fatigue assessments should include the following elements:

- Overall functional status, including mobility and sleep patterns
- Ability to participate in activities of daily living (ADLs), including self-care, hygiene, hydration, and nutrition

- Impact on the child's academic life and ability to engage in school activities and homework
- Impact on the child's social life, including degree of ability to socialize and interest in socializing
- Severity of the fatigue's disruption of the family's daily activities and interactions
- When appropriate, laboratory analyses: complete blood cell count (CBC), comprehensive chemistry panel (CMP), liver panel, thyroid function tests, and inflammatory markers such as erythrocyte sedimentation rate (ESR) and C-reactive protein (CRP)

Nursing Diagnoses for Fatigue

The nurse may make any of the following diagnoses in a pediatric patient with fatigue:

- Fatigue
- Exercise intolerance
- Inability to complete ADLs

Medical Treatments for Fatigue

The best approach to treating fatigue depends on the etiology of the fatigue experience. If the child has anemia related to cancer treatment, poor nutrition, or a hematologic/cardiovascular disorder, treatment may include the infusion of blood products. If the fatigue is associated with a specific pathology, such as a prolonged infection or an extended healing process required for an extensive surgical procedure, the medical treatments should focus on the administration of care to expedite healing. Consultation with a nutritionist, physical therapist, and occupational therapist may be warranted to develop a comprehensive plan for fatigue treatment. Unfortunately, for some children, their fatigue experience may not have a medical treatment.

Nursing Care for Fatigue

Implementing holistic practices when providing support to a child and his or her family is essential. After a comprehensive health history and assessment, the nurse should assist the child to balance energy expenditures with rest and energy conservation. Attaining and maintaining adequate nutrition, hydration, sleep patterns, exercise, and play/recreation opportunities should be the focus of nursing care. Understanding the underlying cause of the fatigue, such as electrolyte imbalances, malnutrition, anemia, mental health disorders, pain, or poor sleep quality, will allow for the development of a unique and individualized nursing care plan.

Dyspnea

The symptoms of dyspnea can be very frightening and uncomfortable. Feeling breathless, feeling as though one cannot

calmly catch one's breath, feeling as if one is not getting enough air, and feeling like one is suffocating are descriptive phrases used by children who have this experience. Children who have chronic lung disease may have repeated experiences with dyspnea. Asthma, severe bronchiolitis, cystic fibrosis, severe obesity, and acute respiratory distress syndrome may be pathological underpinnings to the symptom of dyspnea. Mental health disorders such as anxiety, depression, and panic attacks may also leave the child feeling dyspneic.

Assessment of Dyspnea

Typical assessments of this symptom include objective indicators of dyspnea severity. If the child is tripoding; unable to lie down or get comfortable; unable to speak, drink, or eat; and looking fatigued, the nurse should implement immediate interventions while anticipating **respiratory distress** (difficulty in breathing), respiratory failure, and possibly respiratory arrest. Assessment should include the following steps:

- Taking a complete set of vital signs, oxygen saturations, and arterial or capillary blood gases as indicated
- Soliciting a health history for underlying pathologies such as asthma or other chronic lung diseases
- Observing overall color, as well as for the presence of cyanosis, dehydration, and poor perfusion
- Observing the child's ability to speak, positioning, and work of breathing, including use of accessory muscles, presence of retractions, and adventitious breath sounds

In mild cases, the child may be able to participate in the use of an assessment tool for dyspnea. Verbal descriptions may include the use of words such as "mild," "moderate," and "severe." The child may be able to respond to questions based on a 0 to 10 scale denoting severity. Older children may also be able to use the Visual Analogue Scale (VAS) to identify the perceived severity of their symptom experience.

Nursing Diagnoses for Dyspnea

Potential diagnoses for pediatric patients with dyspnea include the following conditions:

- Ineffective airway clearance
- Ineffective breathing pattern
- Impaired gas exchange
- Fear
- Anxiety
- Ineffective individualized coping

Medical Treatments for Dyspnea

A dyspneic child may require immediate respiratory support via oxygen, humidified air, inhaled bronchodilators, steroids, diuretics, antibiotics, and suctioning. The child should be placed in a position of comfort that also maximizes respiratory function and chest expansion. The child may desire to sit straight up or maintain a leaning-forward stance. Diagnostics may be ordered to determine the etiology of the dyspnea before further medical treatments are initiated.

Nursing Care for Dyspnea

The child experiencing significant dyspnea may feel panicky. In fact, both the child and the family may be quite frightened. The child will benefit from a calm and trusting relationship with the pediatric nurse who focuses attention on immediate assessment, relaxation, and symptom resolution. Providing support, medical treatments, and nursing interventions for dyspnea will allow the child to calm down and feel less anxious.

While medical management is under way, the pediatric nurse can gently rub the child's arm, stroke the child's back gently, and provide appropriate distraction. Being present and communicating that the team is here to help and interventions are under way may be powerfully soothing to the frightened child.

Sleep Disturbances

A variety of circumstances can cause a child to experience **sleep disturbances**—that is, conditions that impair the ability to sleep well on a regular basis (**Table 11-4**). If a child is experiencing any of the other symptoms discussed earlier in this chapter, it is very likely that the child will also have disrupted sleep or poor sleep quality. Discomfort, fatigue, dyspnea, nausea, and emotional distress can all influence how well a child falls asleep and stays asleep. Many medications can influence sleep, and most conditions for which a child would be hospitalized or seek healthcare services have the potential to influence sleep quality. Children with sleep disorders, or those often associated with pathologies, are at risk for further health detriments. For example, academic performance is closely tied to the quality and quantity of a child's sleep (Abraham & Scaria, 2015; Diaz et al., 2016). Children with sleep disturbances are more prone to accidents, injuries, behavioral issues, mood disorders, memory problems, and overall learning difficulties (Berger, Miller, Seifer, Cares, & LeBourgeois, 2012; Boto et al., 2012).

Research has shown that children who have sleep disorders also have significant behavioral and medical morbidity. The most concerning morbidities relate to severe sleep-disordered breathing, including arrhythmias, heart failure, and even death. Milder sleep disorders have been associated with lower cognitive functioning, poor weight

TABLE 11-4 Types or Causes of Sleep Disturbances in Children
› Insomnia
› Sleep terrors
› Sleep walking
› Sleep deprivation over time
› Pain or discomfort
› Fear
› Bedtime resistance
› Infectious respiratory conditions
› Non-infectious respiratory conditions such as asthma and chronic bronchitis
› Obstructive sleep apnea and/or snoring (e.g., due to enlarged tonsils or adenoids)
› Headaches
› Difficulty falling back to sleep
› Mental health issues
› Autistic spectrum disorders
› Obesity
› Restless leg syndrome
› Co-sleeping or communal sleeping quarters

management, learning disabilities, mood disorders, anxiety disorders, depression, and emotional lability (Anders & Eigen, 1997; Angriman, Cortese, & Bruni, 2016; Hedger Archbold, Pituch, Panahi, & Chervin, 2002; Dahl, 1996; Stanford Health Care, 2015).

Sleep disorders can be classified into two distinct categories. *Dyssomnias* involve difficulty initiating or maintaining sleep; they include sleep-onset problems, inadequate total sleep hours, poor sleep hygiene, sleep apnea, and significant snoring. *Parasomnias* involve difficulty with the sleep–wake transition; in these disorders, the child experiences nightmares, sleepwalking, night terrors, or abnormal motor movements. Other conditions such as cataplexy (sudden weakening of muscles associated with narcolepsy) and automatic behavior symptoms (being half-asleep, then waking up with no memory of activities performed during this time) can be associated with narcolepsy, a condition characterized by a reduced quantity of hypocretin in the brain (Stanford Health Care, 2015).

Assessment of Sleep Disturbances

The pediatric healthcare team should conduct a thorough assessment of children who demonstrate signs and symptoms of, or report, sleep disturbances. Ask the child or caregiver the following questions:

1. How many hours of sleep does the child average per night? What hour is the child's bedtime? Does the child consistently go to bed at this hour?
2. Which activities does the child participate in during evening hours and right before bed?
3. Which current health issues does the child have? Is there a documented mental health or cognitive health concern?
4. Does the child have difficulty falling asleep? Staying asleep? Going back to sleep once awake during the night?
5. Does the child sleep during the day or take naps? Does the child fall asleep during the day?
6. Does the child snore? Does the child have any acute or chronic airway health issues?
7. How would you describe the environment in which the child typically sleeps?
8. Are you aware of any stressors or emotional issues facing the child at this time, such as bullying, homework issues, or social issues of concern?

Nursing Diagnoses for Sleep Disturbances

Nursing diagnoses for children with sleep disturbances include insomnia and sleep pattern disturbance.

Medical Treatments for Sleep Disturbances

Medical treatment for children with sleep disturbances typically depends on the underlying pathology, emotional problems, stressors, or mental health issues. Sleep evaluation, evaluation by an ear/nose/throat (ENT) specialist, and sleep apnea assessment may be suggested. Only rarely are children prescribed or offered sleeping pills—though melatonin has been used successfully in the treatment of sleep disturbances in children, especially those with chronic insomnia (Paavonen, 2004). Most medical treatment plans for children with sleep disturbances include behavioral modification, positive reinforcement, limits setting, sleep expectations setting, and, if needed, psychological evaluation, counseling, and referral to a sleep specialist.

Nursing Care for Sleep Disturbances

Pediatric nurses are in an excellent position to educate children and families about proper sleep hygiene (good sleep habits). The entire family should become aware of the detrimental effects of poor sleep quality and quantity. Suggestions for improving a child's sleep include the following:

- Reevaluate the child's sleep arrangements. Remove any stimuli that could delay bedtime or wake the child during the night. There should be no TV in the child's room, and the family should set and enforce rules concerning screen time in the evening. Music should not be played during a child's sleep time. Cell phones, computers, and laptops should be turned off or removed from the child's room.
- Assess the lighting in the child's room. Make sure the room is dark, but provide a nightlight if requested.
- Create a comforting, relaxing, and anticipated bedtime ritual. This ritual may take as long as 15 to 60 minutes. A young child could be quietly read to; an older child could be given the opportunity to lie in bed and talk about his or her day.
- Use relaxation breathing techniques, guided imagery, or other forms of relaxation while in bed.
- Do not allow a child to have caffeinated beverages in the evening. Avoid large meals close to bedtime.
- Insist on the child sleeping in his or her own bed. If the child has been allowed to fall asleep in another bed, on the couch, or elsewhere, break this habit by setting limits, being assertive, and being consistent.
- Consider naturopathic sleep aids such as melatonin supplements, chamomile tea, lemon balm, and lavender oil or a lavender sleep sachet. A warm bath before bedtime can be very soothing.
- Take into account the child's developmental stage. For instance, an infant should not be allowed to fall asleep in the parent's arms, but rather should be placed in the crib when demonstrating sleepiness. Toddlers may need rigid bedtime rituals and have great trouble falling to sleep if the ritual is

not followed or is shortened for convenience. Preschoolers may verbalize fears of the dark, presence of monsters, or ghosts. They should be allowed to express themselves and shown that no such entity is physically present. School-aged children and teens may sneak social media and conversations with friends before bedtime.

- Talk to the child about the importance of sleep. Teach the child about the detrimental factors associated with sleep disturbances. Praise the child for participating in efforts to improve his or her sleep.

Cultural Influences on Symptom Management

Much research has addressed the behaviors, values, faith, preferences, and customs of different cultures. Within the multicultural healthcare environment, it is helpful for members of the pediatric healthcare team to understand that culture can influence both a child's expressions of pain and other symptoms and the culturally acceptable interventions for symptom management. For instance, drug metabolism may differ in people of certain ethnicities, such that some individuals may experience more pain because pain-relieving drugs wear off more quickly than in persons of other ethnicities. As an example, 30% of Hong Kong Chinese, 9% of Europeans, and 1% of Arabs lack the enzyme that converts codeine into its active form of morphine (Williams, Hatch, & Howard, 2011).

Language barriers have been shown to be responsible for parents of children under-reporting and even misinterpreting their child's pain (Weiner, McConnell, Latella, & Ludi, 2013). Fear of the authority associated with licensed healthcare providers, called power distance, can influence whether a family reports their child's health condition or symptoms. Cultural influences may also affect sleep disturbances, as in situations where co-sleeping or communal sleeping quarters, or practices regarding the use of swings and breastfeeding to soothe infants, are a cultural value (Anuntaseree et al., 2008).

Another misconception by healthcare workers encountering patients from different cultures is the assumption that all people from the same culture are the same in their beliefs, values, cultural expressions, and cultural behaviors, and that cultural customs regarding pain expressions and management are superficial and frivolous. Results from a 2012 study showed that patients who were non-white had significantly lower pain scores documented than patients who were white (Ortega, Velden, Lin, & Reid, 2012). Mistakes based on cultural misunderstandings can negatively impact communication, compliance, adherence, satisfaction, and, ultimately, adequate pain control in the pediatric population. Nurses must be vigilant about learning and understanding how cultural factors influence symptom experiences in their pediatric patients.

Case Study

A 3-month-old infant was admitted to the pediatric unit with a 2-day history of fever. The mother had an uncomplicated vaginal delivery and did not present with any evidence of illness at the time of her delivery or subsequently. The child was admitted through the emergency department (ED). Blood cultures, urine cultures, lumbar puncture, and nasal swab for respiratory syncytial virus (RSV) and influenza A and B were all performed in the ED prior to the patient's admission to the pediatric unit. The hospitalist conducted a thorough assessment of the infant and determined that that child had clinical signs of meningitis, including mild nuchal rigidity and evidence of headache and neck discomfort.

The infant has been settled into her room, both parents are present and are tearful, and the infant is now on contact and droplet precautions.

Case Study Questions

1. Considering the infant's age and developmental stage, which pain assessment tools would be appropriate for the nurse to use?
2. Of the various types of pain, which would the nurse suspect the infant is experiencing?
3. What education can be provided to the family to support the child's pain assessments, management, and evaluation?

(continues)

Case Study (continued)

As the Case Evolves. . .

The child in this case study is assessed and diagnosed based on symptoms of fever and evidence of headache and neck discomfort.

4. Which of the following represents "evidence" of pain symptoms in this child?
   A. Quiet moaning and whimpering
   B. Excessive sleepiness and slow heartbeat and respirations
   C. Crying, flailing, furrowed brow, and fist clenching
   D. Lack of facial expression and withdrawal

When the infant is admitted into the hospital with meningitis, her parents are distraught and confused. They ask anxiously whether their daughter is experiencing significant pain, and what, if anything, can be done about it.

5. Which of the following statements is the most appropriate response?
   A. "Infants don't experience pain the way adults do, so while your daughter may have some pain, the priority is giving her supportive care so she gets over her illness."
   B. "Yes, your daughter is experiencing pain, but most pain medications aren't safe for infants her age, so we're going to focus on curing her illness as quickly as possible."

   C. "Our options for medications are limited because of your daughter's age, but we can use other methods to soothe her pain, such as massage."
   D. "The best therapy for your daughter's pain is her parents' concern."

The infant has been diagnosed with bacterial meningitis. She is started on combined chloramphenicol and ampicillin. Within 2 hours of the first dose, the mother, who has been sitting with the infant in her room, alerts the nursing staff that her daughter is "spitting up." Upon entering the room, the nurse notes that the infant is not merely spitting up, but is projectile vomiting.

6. What is the most likely reason for this change in the child's condition and the most appropriate response by the nursing staff?
   A. Acid reflux due to the antibiotic medication; provide liquid probiotic therapy.
   B. Nausea/vomiting possibly secondary to beta-lactam allergy; alert the treating physician of the need to discontinue chloramphenicol/ampicillin and initiate ceftriaxone.
   C. Nausea as a secondary symptom of meningitis; administer liquid or sublingual ondansetron.
   D. Nausea/vomiting possibly secondary to increased intracranial pressure; obtain computed tomography (CT) or magnetic resonance imaging (MRI).

Chapter Summary

- Symptom management is part of the holistic role of the nurse across all healthcare settings.
- Untreated symptoms, such as pain, discomfort, fatigue, nausea, dyspnea, and sleep disturbances, can have severe consequences for a child's social, emotional, developmental, academic, and home life.
- The experience of pain is unique for each patient.
- Nurses must address pain assessment and pain management to prevent undertreatment of pain. Undertreated pain can lead to short- and long-term sequelae.
- Subjective pain assessment tools are available for children in each developmental stage, including the Wong-Baker FACES Pain Rating Scale, the Numeric Rating Scale, and the Visual Analogue Scale.
- Nursing care for pain includes subjective and objective assessment, establishment of goals for pain control, and interventions for pain alleviation.

- Nausea has many potential etiologies, but is most commonly experienced in the postoperative period. Nausea may or may not be accompanied by vomiting. Nursing care for pediatric patients with nausea includes antinausea medications, stress reduction, a low-stimulation environment, and placing the child in a side-lying position.
- Fatigue can impact a child's ability to eat or sleep well, play, socialize, and perform activities of daily living. The pediatric nurse must assess the severity of a child's fatigue experience and determine whether it is primary or secondary, acute or chronic, situational, or disabling.
- Nursing care for children experiencing fatigue focuses on attaining and maintaining adequate nutrition, hydration, sleep patterns, exercise, and balance of energy expenditure with energy conservation.
- Children who have chronic lung disease (e.g., asthma, severe bronchiolitis, cystic fibrosis, severe obesity, and acute respiratory distress syndrome) may have repeated experiences with dyspnea. Mental health disorders such

as anxiety, depression, and panic attacks may also leave the child feeling dyspneic.

- ◆ Providing support, medical treatments, and nursing interventions for dyspnea will allow the child to calm down and feel less anxious.
- ◆ Children with sleep disorders, or those often associated with pathologies, are at risk for further health detriments, including accidents, injuries, behavioral issues, mood disorders, memory problems, and overall learning difficulties.
- ◆ Most medical treatment plans for children with sleep disturbances include behavioral modification, positive reinforcement, limits setting, sleep expectations setting, and, if needed, psychological evaluation, counseling, and referral to a sleep specialist. In addition, pediatric nurses are in an excellent position to educate children and families about proper sleep hygiene.
- ◆ Mistakes based on cultural misunderstandings can negatively impact communication, compliance, adherence, satisfaction, and, ultimately, adequate pain control in the pediatric population. Nurses must be vigilant about learning and understanding how cultural factors influence symptom experiences in their pediatric patients.

Bibliography

Abraham, J., & Scaria, J. (2015). Influence of sleep in academic performance: An integrated review of the literature. *IOSR Journal of Nursing and Health Science, 4*, 78–81.

Anders, T. F., & Eigen, H. (1997). Pediatric sleep disorders: A review of the past 10 years. *Journal of the American Academy of Child Adolescent Psychiatry, 36*(1997), 9–20.

Angriman, M., Cortese, S., & Bruni, O. (2016, July 1). Somatic and neuropsychiatric comorbidities in pediatric restless legs syndrome: A systematic review of the literature. *Sleep Medicine Review.* [Epub ahead of print]. pii: S1087-0792(16)30060-0. doi: 10.1016/j.smrv.2016.06.008

Anuntaseree, W., Mo-suwan, L., Vasiknanonte, P., Kuasirikul, S., Ma-a-lee A., & Choprapawan, C. (2008). Night waking in Thai infants at 3 months of age: Association between parental practices and infant sleep. *Sleep Medicine, 9*(5), 564–571.

Arbour, C., Choiniere, M., Topolovec-Vranic, J., Loiselle, C. G., & Gelinas, C. (2014). Can fluctuations in vital signs be used for pain assessment in critically ill patients with traumatic brain injury? *Pain Research and Treatment, 2014*, Article 175794.

Baker, D. W. (2016). Joint Commission statement on pain management. Retrieved from https://www.jointcommission.org/topics/pain_management.aspx

Becker, D. E. (2010). Nausea, vomiting and hiccups: A review of mechanisms and treatment. *Anesthesia Progress, 57*(4), 150–157.

Benini, F., & Barbi, E. (2014). Doing without codeine: Why and what are the alternatives? *Italian Journal of Pediatrics, 40*, 16.

Berger, R. H., Miller, A. L., Seifer, R., Cares, S. R., & LeBourgeois, M. K. (2012). Acute sleep restriction effects on emotion responses in 30- to 36-month-old children. *Journal of Sleep Research, 21*(3), 235–246.

Bice, A. A., Gunther, M., & Wyatt, T. (2014). Increasing nursing treatment for pediatric procedural pain. *Pain Management Nursing, 15*, 365–379.

Birnie, K. A., Chambers, C. T., Fernandez, C. V., Forgeron, P. A., Latimer, M. A., McGrath, P. J., . . . Finley, G. A. (2014). Hospitalized children continue to report undertreated and preventable pain. *Pain Research and Management, 19*, 198–204.

Boto, L. R., Crispim, J. N., de Melo, I. S., Juvandes, C., Rodrigues, T., Azeredo, P., & Ferreira, R. (2012). Sleep deprivation and accidental fall risk in children. *Sleep Medicine, 13*, 88–95.

Carpenito, L. J. (2013). *Handbook of nursing diagnosis* (14th ed.). Philadelphia, PA: Wolters Kluwer/Lippincott Williams & Wilkins.

Centers for Disease Control and Prevention (CDC). (2012). Chronic fatigue syndrome (CFS): CFS case definition. Retrieved from http://www.cdc.gov/cfs/case-definition/index.html

Dahan, A., Overdyk, F., Smith, T., Aarts, L., & Niesters, M. (2013). Pharmacovigilance: A review of opioid-induced respiratory depression in chronic pain patients. *Pain Physician, 16*(2), E85–E94.

Dahl, R. E. (1996). The impact of inadequate sleep on children's daytime cognitive function. *Seminars in Pediatric Neurology, 3*(1996), 44–50.

DePriest, A. Z., Puet, B. L., Holt, A. C., Roberts, A., & Cone, E. J. (2015). Metabolism and disposition of prescription opioids: A review. *Forensic Science Review, 27,* 115–145.

Diaz, A., Berger, R., Valiente, C., Eisenberg, N., VanSchyndel, S. K., Tao, C., . . . Southworth, J. (2016, March 1). Children's sleep and academic achievement. *International Journal of Behavioral Development.* [Epub ahead of print]. doi: 10.1177/0165025416635284

Dodd, M., Janson, S., Facione, N., Faucett, J., Froelicher, E. S., Humphreys, J., . . . Taylor, D. (2001). Advancing the science of symptom management. *Journal of Advanced Nursing, 33*(5), 668–676.

Fernandes, A. M., De Campos, C., Batalha, L., Perdigão, A., & Jacob, E. (2014). Pain assessment using the Adolescent Pediatric Pain Tool: A systematic review. *Pain Research and Management, 19*(4), 212–218.

Food and Drug Administration. (2015). FDA drug safety communication: FDA evaluating the risks of using the pain medicine tramadol in children aged 17 and younger. Retrieved from http://www.fda.gov/Drugs/DrugSafety/ucm462991.htm

Fowler, T., Duthie, P., Thapar, A., & Farmer, A. (2005). The definition of disabling fatigue in children and adolescents. *BNC Family Practice, 6*, 33.

Fragkandrea, I., Nixon, J. A., & Panagopoulou, P. (2013). Signs and symptoms of childhood cancer: A guide for early recognition. *American Family Physician, 88*, 185–192.

Fukuda, K., Straus, S. E., Hickie, I., Sharpe, M. C., Dobbins, J. G., & Komaroff, A. (1994). The chronic fatigue syndrome: A comprehensive approach to its definition and study. International Chronic Fatigue Syndrome Study Group. *Annals of Internal Medicine, 121*, 953–959.

Gilbert-MacLeod, C. A., Craig, K. D., Rocha, E. M., & Mathias, M. D. (2000). Everyday pain responses in children with and without developmental delays. *Journal of Pediatric Psychology, 25*(5), 301–308.

Goudsmit, E. M., Nijs, J., Jason, L. A., & Wallman, K. E. (2012). Pacing as a strategy to improve energy management in myalgic encephalomyelitis/chronic fatigue syndrome: A consensus document. *Disability and Rehabilitation, 34*, 1140–1147.

Gupta, R., Kilby, M., & Cooper, G. (2008). Fetal surgery and anesthetic implications. *Continuing Education in Anesthesia, Critical Care and Pain, 8*(2), 71–75.

Hedger Archbold, K., Pituch, K. J., Panahi, P., & Chervin, R. D. (2002). Symptoms of sleep disturbances among children at two general pediatric clinics. *Journal of Pediatrics, 140*(1), 97–102.

International Association for the Study of Pain. (2014). IASP taxonomy. Retrieved from http://www.iasp-pain.org/Taxonomy

Jarzyna, D., Jungquist, C. R., Pasero, C., Willens, J. S., Nisbet, A., Oakes, L., . . . Polomano, R. C. (2011). American Society of Pain Management Nursing guidelines on monitoring for opioid-induced sedation and respiratory depression. *Pain Management in Nursing, 12*(3), 118–145.e10. doi: 10.1016/j.pmn.2011.06.008

Jason, L. A., Barker, K., & Brown, A. (2012). Pediatric myalgic encephalomyelitis/chronic fatigue syndrome. *Reviews in Health Care, 3*(4), 257–270.

Jason, L. A., Bell, D. S., Rowe, K., Elke, L. S., Jordan, K., Lapp, C., . . . De Meirleir, K. (2006). A pediatric case definition for myalgic encephalomyelitis and chronic fatigue syndrome. *Journal of Chronic Fatigue Syndrome, 13*(2/3), 1–44.

Joint Commission. (2010). *Approaches to pain management: An essential guide for clinicians* (2nd ed.). Oakbrook Terrace, IL: Joint Commission Resources.

Linder, L. (2010). Analysis of the UCSF symptom management theory: Implications for pediatric oncology nursing. *Journal of Pediatric Oncology Nursing, 27*(6), 316–324.

Mindel, J. A., & Owens, J. A. (2015). *A clinical guide to pediatric sleep: Diagnosis and management of sleep problems* (3rd ed.). Philadelphia, PA: Wolters Kluwer.

Morris, G., Berk, M., Walder, K., & Maes, M. (2015). Central pathways causing fatigue in neuro-inflammatory and autoimmune illnesses. *BMC Medicine, 13*, 28.

Murphy, M. (2011). The adolescent interview. In: M. A. Goldstein, ed., *The MassGeneral Hospital for Children adolescent medicine handbook*. Boston, MA: Springer Science+Business Media.

NANDA International. (2012). *Nursing diagnoses: Definitions and classifications 2012-2014.* Ames, IA: Wiley-Blackwell.

Ortega, H. W., Velden, H. V., Lin, C. W., & Reid, S. (2012). Ethnicity and reported pain scores among children with long bone fractures requiring emergency care. *Pediatric Emergency Care, 28*(11), 1–4.

Overdyk, F., Dahan, A., Roozekrans, M., van der Schrier, R., Aarts, L., & Niesters, M. (2014). Opioid-induced respiratory depression in the acute care setting: A compendium of case reports. *Pain Management, 4*(4), 317–325.

Paavonen, E. J. (2004). Effectiveness of melatonin in the treatment of sleep disturbances in children with Asperger disorder. *Journal of Child and Adolescent Psychopharmacy, 13*(1), 83–95.

Rodkey, E. N., & Riddell, R. P. (2013). The infancy of infant pain research: The experimental origins of infant pain denial. *Journal of Pain, 14*, 338–350.

Sacheck, J. M., Rasmussen, H. M., Hall, M. M., Kafka, T., Blumberg, J. B., & Economos, C. D. (2014). The association between pregame snacks and exercise intensity, stress, and fatigue in children. *Pediatric Exercise Science, 26*, 159–167.

Sánchez-Rodríguez, E., & Miró, J. (2015). The assessment of fatigue in children with chronic pain: A review of existing measures. *European Journal of Psychological Assessment, 31*(2), 75–82.

Srouji, R., Ratnapalan, S., & Schneeweiss, S. (2010). Pain in children: Assessment and nonpharmacological management. *International Journal of Pediatrics, 2010*, Article 474838.

Stanford Health Care. (2015). Pediatric sleep disorders. Retrieved from https://stanfordhealthcare.org/medical-conditions/sleep/pediatric-sleep-disorders.html

Stevens, B. J., Abbott, L. K., Yamada, J., Harrison, D., Stinson, J., Taddio, A., . . . Finley, G. A. (2011). Epidemiology and management of painful procedures in children in Canadian hospitals. *Canadian Medical Association Journal, 183*(7), E403–E410.

Thompson, D. (2016). Codeine not safe for kids, pediatricians warn. Retrieved from http://www.webmd.com/children/news/20160919/codeine-not-safe-for-kids-pediatricians-warn#1

Vetter, T. R., Bridgewater, C. L., Ascherman, L. I., Madan-Swain, A., & McGwin, G. L. (2014). Patient versus parental perceptions about pain and disability in children and adolescents with a variety of chronic pain conditions. *Pain Research and Management, 19*(1), 7–14.

Viner, R. M., Clark, C., Taylor, S. J. C., Bhui, K., Klineberg, E., Head, J., . . . Stansfeld, S. A. (2008). Longitudinal risk factors for persistent fatigue in adolescents. *Archives of Pediatrics and Adolescent Medicine, 162*(5), 469–475.

von Baeyer, C. L. (2006). Children's self-reports of pain intensity: Scale selection, limitations and interpretation. *Pain Research and Management, 11*(3), 157–162.

Weiner, L., McConnell, D. G., Latella, L., & Ludi, E. (2013). Cultural and religious considerations in pediatric palliative care. *Palliative and Supportive Care, 11*, 47–67.

Williams, D. G., Hatch, D. J. & Howard, R. F. (2011). Codeine phosphate in pediatric medicine. *British Journal of Anesthetics, 86*, 413–421.

Wong, C., Lau, E., Palozzi, L., & Campbell, F. (2012). Pain management in children: Part 2: A transition from codeine to morphine for moderate to severe pain in children. *Canadian Pharmacists Journal, 145*, 276–279.

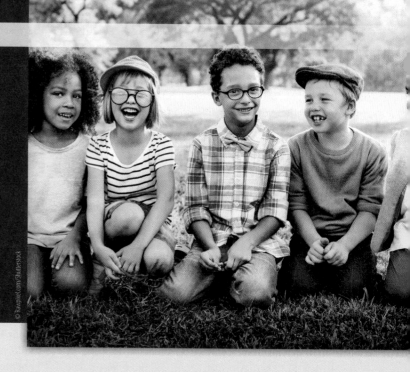

UNIT V

Caring for Families in Need

CHAPTER 12

Caring for Families Under Stress

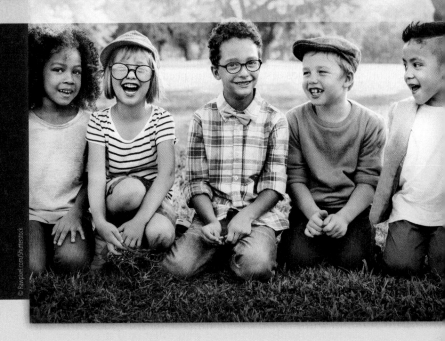

© Rawpixel.com/Shutterstock

LEARNING OBJECTIVES

1. Integrate family stress theory and concepts into family-centered care.
2. Analyze the physical, physiological, and emotional aspects of stress.
3. Identify and address the common symptoms of stress experienced across childhood developmental stages and across family members.
4. Apply the components of Hans Selye's stress theory to patient care.
5. Apply interventions and strategies for identifying and reducing the experience of stress for families.

KEY TERMS

Coping
Cortisol
Distress
Epinephrine
Neurochemicals
Norepinephrine
Stress
Stressors

Introduction

According to the Centers for Disease Control and Prevention (CDC, 2015a), everyone, across the lifespan, experiences periods of stress, and most need help in assessing and managing stress so that they can cope with threatening or disturbing situations. Various models of familial stress have been proposed, including models focusing on the impact of economic factors on family coping (e.g., the Family Stress Model developed by Conger et al. [2002]); models addressing the family's ability to adjust and adapt to stress (e.g., the FAAR model developed by Patterson [1988]); and social-ecological models that look at individuals in the context of their immediate relationships, the community, and society as a whole (CDC, 2015b). These models all offer perspectives that nurses can use in their assessment of families under stress.

With the current demands placed on families, it is not uncommon to have a family under stress while in the care of a pediatric healthcare team. Regardless of the clinical setting, a family can present with situational stress from the child's current illness or injury, or family members be experiencing many **stressors** (i.e., stimuli that create stress) associated with the family's life and society's demands.

Myriad causes of stress exist in contemporary society. Some stressors relate to the chaos of daily life, especially when a family is trying to juggle the demands of work, home, school, child care, traffic, and commutes (American Psychological Association [APA], 2010). Other common family stressors include marital relationships, childrearing and discipline, health issues, elder care, and finances. Individual family members may also experience stress from personal concerns. With the current rates of unemployment, debt, substance abuse, domestic violence, and crime, it is not uncommon to encounter family groups or individual family members experiencing significant stress that affects their ability to balance life's demands (**Figure 12-1**). The caregiver of a child—be it a parent, grandparent, or guardian—may present with severe stress symptoms requiring intervention; the child may, in turn, identify with the caregiver's stress and experience secondary stress as a result (APA, 2010).

This chapter provides guidelines for assisting a family that is experiencing stress. Stress-related tools and assessments are described, as well as interventions and communication tips to assist in working with a family under stress (**Figure 12-2**).

UNIQUE FOR KIDS

According to the National Child Traumatic Stress Network (2015), children can experience a wide variety of traumatic stressors:

- Community violence where the child is a witness or a victim
- Domestic violence or intimate-partner violence
- Early childhood trauma (from birth to 6 years of age), such as the loss of a parent
- School violence, which includes a range of stressful situations, such as aggression, bullying, and violence
- Physical abuse, sexual abuse, and neglect
- Medical trauma, in which the child is exposed to surgery, treatments, and painful procedures
- Complex trauma, if the child is exposed to prolonged events or multiple events
- Traumatic grief
- Natural disasters such as tornadoes, earthquakes, fires, hurricanes, and floods

Definitions of Stress

The experience of stress is inevitable for all people, regardless of age. Although daily life can bring numerous challenges, the physiological reaction known as **stress** is felt when the challenges experienced exceed one's ability to control and manage one's environment. When stress is not managed or becomes chronic, it turns into **distress**,

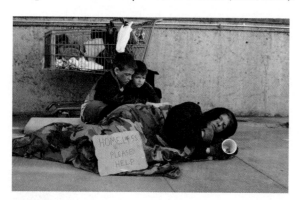

Figure 12-1

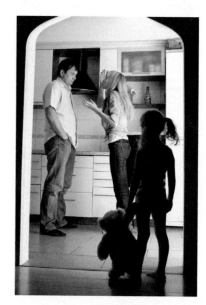

Figure 12-2 *Nurses will encounter families under stress.*

a condition in which one feels the effect of stress beyond emotional reactions and the body begins to respond to the stressful stimuli.

Stress is generally defined as a three-step process: (1) the encounter of a stressful stimulus, (2) a response to that stressful stimulus, and (3) the process of adjustment and interactions between the person feeling stress and the stressful stimuli. Stress provokes a series of responses—developmental, neurochemical, and emotional. Although some stress is normal, excessive stress is detrimental to one's health, both in the short and long terms (Felitti, 2009; Felitti et al., 1998; Gilbert et al., 2015).

Stress can provoke the adrenal glands to release certain **neurochemicals** (stress hormones), which cause a number of physiological symptoms. During periods of significant stress, the body releases **epinephrine** and **norepinephrine** from the adrenal medulla (the inner portion of the adrenal gland), as well as **cortisol** from the adrenal cortex (the outer portion of the adrenal gland). The release of these stress hormones leads to the following symptoms:

- Tachycardia
- Tachypnea
- Vasoconstriction
- Elevated blood pressure
- Muscle tension (when prolonged, it can lead to tension headaches)
- Clammy hands
- Gastrointestinal disturbances

Stress can be classified into three major types:

- Positive stress—for example, when a child encounters a new experience, but it brings few or only minor changes in emotions, hormonal response, or heart rate change
- Tolerable stress—for example, when a child has a more intense experience such as a family death or an accident and the child adapts
- Toxic stress—where the stressor is severe, intense, and sustained, leading to a prolonged stress activation (e.g., physical or sexual abuse, or witnessing abuse of the child's parent)

Findings from the Adverse Childhood Experiences (ACE) study suggest that toxic stress causes profound alterations in brain structure and functioning, particularly if the events occur during the developmental period (Anda et al., 2006). This kind of stress affects immune system function and reduces learning and memory, leading to cognitive deficits and impairment (DeBellis & Zisk, 2014). Prolonged and toxic levels of stress have been known to damage a child's hippocampus—the part of the brain where memory, learning, and cognitive processing occur (Audage & Middlebrooks, 2008).

Recognizing Stress in Families and Individuals

A certain amount of stress experienced by families is inevitable. When a child is ill or injured, however, a family's stress level can increase exponentially. The pediatric nurse must realize that stress will inevitably happen, so it is *how* the family and each family member handle stress that is critically important. The various models of family stress can offer different perspectives on causes of stress and assist the nurse in identifying underlying issues and offering strategies for reducing them or improving **coping**—that is, skills for handling stressful events, stressful circumstances, and stressors. Both individual family members and the family as a whole must develop effective coping skills.

FAMILY EDUCATION

Often, children across the developmental period will model their parents' behaviors. This modeling can include behaviors related to managing stress—both healthy coping behaviors and unhealthy coping behaviors. If parents deal with stress in unhealthy ways such as overeating, engaging in substance use, and performing other high-risk behaviors, they may inadvertently encourage those behaviors in their children. Conversely, parents who cope with stress in healthy ways can promote better adjustment and happiness for the entire family. Parents need anticipatory guidance that children watch and listen to their parents and often model their own decisions and behaviors after those of their role models.

RESEARCH EVIDENCE

The American Psychological Association (2010) conducted an online survey of families, in conjunction with Harris Interactive, and found that obese parents are much more likely than those who are within a normal weight range to have children who are obese. The researchers discovered that overweight children are more likely than normal-weight children to report that their parents are often worried and stressed. These research findings can help pediatric healthcare teams assist families who have weight issues to identify stressors and seek appropriate means to identify stress, reduce stress, and participate in healthy eating and increased physical activity.

Reactions to stress may differ in each of the developmental stages (Cohen, 2002). Infants demonstrate stress by being irritable, becoming fearful, and demonstrating increased crying and gastrointestinal distress. Children younger than age 3 may react to stress by being aggressive or demonstrating regressive behaviors. Children in the preschool period may show stress by acting out, being fearful of separation or abandonment, and having increased nightmares. School-age children will manifest stress by poor school performance, aggression, and increased acting-out behaviors. Adolescents who experience significant stress can exhibit poor self-esteem, delinquency, high-risk behaviors, and problems in relationships. Knowing the relationship between the various developmental stages and the expression of stress can assist a pediatric nurse in anticipating behaviors and intervening rapidly. For example, nursing interventions to reduce the impact of traumatic events can include teaching coping skills or self-soothing techniques such as meditation or therapeutic play, guiding parent–child dialogue in reviewing the traumatic incident, or advocating to correct problematic or unsafe practices (Mulvihill, 2007) (**Figure 12-3**).

UNIQUE FOR KIDS

According to the U.S Department of Health and Human Services (Audage & Middlebrooks, 2008), children who experience prolonged stress, but lack the ability to cope with that stress, can experience significant short-term and long-term health effects. Notably, childhood stress has been linked to alcoholism, eating disorders, heart disease, depression, and other chronic disorders later in life.

FAMILY EDUCATION

The two most common reactions to stress encountered in children are regression of behavior to a lower developmental period or stage and a change in behavior recognizable to the child's parents or significant adults in their lives (DeBord, 2014).

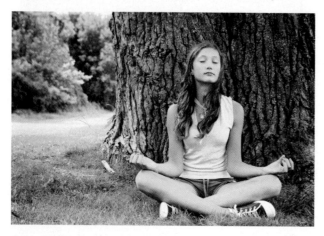

Figure 12-3 *Nursing interventions to reduce the impact of traumatic events can include teaching self-soothing techniques such as meditation.*
© Pinkcandy/Shutterstock

Symptoms of Stress

Stress is the body's reaction to harmful situations, either real or perceived. Written in 1956, Hans Selye's general adaptation syndrome (GAS) theory describes the stress response of an organism as occurring in three stages (Szabo, Tache & Somogyi, 2012). In the first stage, known as "alarm," the body's physiology changes as the body attempts to mobilize to compensate for the stressful event (the "flight or fight" response). This first stage is considered the arousal stage, as the body releases hormones (epinephrine, norepinephrine, and cortisol) into the bloodstream. In the second stage, known as "resistance," the body continues to compensate at peak capacity as it tries to adapt to the stressor. The final stage, "exhaustion," causes the body's natural defenses to break down, such that the body becomes susceptible to illness, tissue damage, ulcers, high blood pressure, and chronic health conditions directly linked to an impaired immune function.

Symptoms of stress may vary widely for individual family members according to the type and duration of exposure to a stressor or multiple stressors. Although stressors for children can be very different than the stressors experienced by adult family members, the impact of stress can nonetheless be damaging to the body and mind. Prolonged or chronic stress can lead directly to illness. Individuals under severe or chronic stress may report or display some of the following conditions (APA, 2016; CDC, 2015b; Dufton, Dunn, Slosky, & Compas, 2011).

- Fight-or-flight responses of tachycardia, tachypnea, tight muscles, headaches, and increased blood pressure
- Feelings of fatigue and low energy
- Emotional reactions such as crying, anger, sadness, frustration, helplessness, tension, and irritability
- Difficulty making decisions or having clear thinking processes
- Difficulty falling asleep, interrupted sleep, insomnia, hypersomnia (especially in adolescents), and bizarre and disturbing dreams
- Jaw pain, tooth pain, and grinding of teeth
- Hair loss
- Intestinal disturbances such as abdominal pain, nausea, diarrhea, and constipation
- Menstrual cramps and difficult menstrual periods
- Muscle twitching, aches, muscle and nerve pains, and eyelid spasms
- Acne development and other cutaneous reactions to stress, including rashes and areas of inflammation

- Physiologic or somatic responses such as recurrent stomachache or headache
- Development of colds and other common viral infections associated with a lower immune response (i.e., lowered immune system response)
- Changes in weight—weight loss or weight gain
- In situations of severe, chronic, long-term stress, development of a chronic illness such as asthma, diabetes, hypertension, and arthritis

The family unit may be experiencing stress due to daily demands (APA, 2010; Walsh, 2013). In such circumstances, it is not uncommon for families to report the following behaviors (APA, 2010):

- Being "too busy" or lacking time to spend quality time together enjoying one another's company and eating meals together at an unrushed pace
- Turning to sedentary and often solitary behaviors such as watching television, using a computer, listening to music, or playing video games (**Figure 12-4**)
- Behaviors such as yelling, arguing, and complaining, or "venting" about problems that other family members cannot solve or address
- Experiencing a sense of frustration with other family members that may then develop into a sense of guilt
- Family members feeling—but not expressing— worry or stress; irritability and lack of motivation
- Alcohol use, use of drugs, eating disturbances (overeating or skipping meals), sleeping, self-harm, or extra work responsibilities or other activities to remove an individual family member from dealing with the stress experienced by the family
- Awareness of parental stress by children that translates into sadness or worry

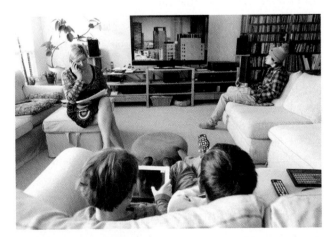

Figure 12-4 *It is not uncommon for families to report turning to solitary behaviors such as watching television, using a computer, listening to music, or playing video games.*

© Fertnig/E+/Getty Images

In contrast, less stressed families seem to find time to enjoy and support one another, display more flexibility, have reasonable expectations, communicate regularly with one another, set priorities, and view stress as a challenge that is both temporary and controllable. As a pediatric nurse, it is important to communicate to families that it is never too late to learn effective coping strategies (APA, 2015).

BEST PRACTICES

Hostile and Aggressive Behaviors

Emotional reactions to stress can trigger a person to display hostile and aggressive behaviors. When a person with limited coping abilities becomes emotionally distressed, anger can surface. Fear, harm to other people and property, personal injury, feeling persecuted, perceiving a loss, shock, denial, and guilt are all human responses to stress.

When a child, parent, or any adult in a healthcare environment begins to display hostile or aggressive behaviors, the pediatric healthcare team must mobilize to work together to handle the situation before harm occurs. A single healthcare professional should never try to handle a hostile, aggressive, and potentially violent person on his or her own, and use of a third person not initially involved in the confrontation can often help de-escalate the situation (Su, 2010). Keeping calm, keeping a safe distance, respectfully acknowledging the emotions, suspending personal responses, being supportive, and using a quiet and soothing voice while offering help can potentially diffuse the escalating hostility (Richmond et al., 2012; Sheldon & Foust, 2014).

Care teams should practice how to respond to these kinds of scenarios via simulated hostile, aggressive, and violent patient situations. Knowing how to maintain personal safety and safety of others, as well as practicing how to interact with a hostile person, can keep a team ready to respond. In addition, knowing how to call for help from the institutional security department or a response team is imperative for maintaining a safe environment for staff, patients, and families.

Interventions for Stress

The role of the pediatric nurse for families experiencing stress centers on securing a state of immediate safety. If a family in stress presents to a pediatric healthcare setting, the primary assessment should include an immediate sweep for safety and health concerns; if any are present, the safety concerns should be minimized. For instance, if a family and child presents with evidence of trauma, violence, current drug or alcohol use, or severe neglect or abuse, the team's focus would be on securing a safe environment for the child. Once the child is in a state of safety, the next priority would be to assess the severity and symptoms of the child's and family's stress and then provide interventions.

Nurses should work directly with parents or guardians, if appropriate, to provide a child with support to help the child cope. According to the CDC (2015a) and Kidshealth. org (2015), ideas for adults to help children cope with stress include the following:

- Ensure the child's safety, and emphasize to the child that steps are being taken for this purpose.
- Acknowledge that the child seems bothered by something by expressing concern and stating that you want to help the child.
- Listen carefully to the concern expressed by the child and restate the perceived emotion or concern back to the child to ensure clarity of the issue at hand.
- Encourage children to talk, draw, or engage in play to express their fears or concerns, and provide understanding and reassurance in response to these expressions.
- Monitor for concerning behaviors and promote healthy behaviors.
- Promote self care and connecting with others.
- Help a child maintain his or her normal routine in terms of sleep, eating, school attendance, chores, and participation in social events or after-school activities.
- Help the child find ways to cope by talking together about ideas to reduce the stressful event or situation.
- Spend time with the child in play, sports, long walks, or cuddling on the couch (**Figure 12-5**).
- Seek resources and referrals for psychological support and interventions if needed.

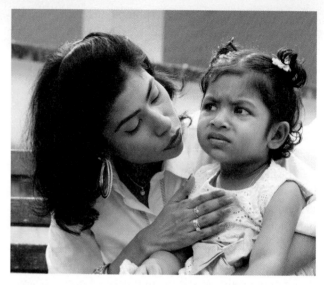

Figure 12-5 *Ideas for adults to help children cope with stress include spending time holding a child in a soothing way.*
© szefei/Shutterstock

FAMILY EDUCATION

According to the American Psychological Association (2015), family members who do not deny or avoid dealing with stress, but rather acknowledge a child's stress, take action on the source of the stress, and zero in on the problem, tend to report lower levels of depression and anxiety.

Resources for Stress

The pediatric healthcare team should provide information and referrals if a family unit, individual members, or a child is experiencing continued stress and poor health or behavioral outcomes due to the stress experience. The following list provides resources that can be shared with families.

- National Child Traumatic Stress Network: www .nctsn.org
- Disaster Distress Helpline: 1-800-985-5990
- Youth Mental Health Line: 1-888-568-1112
- Child-Help USA, Coping with Stress: 1-800-422-4453
- National Suicide Prevention Lifeline: 1-800-273-TALK
- National Suicide Prevention Lifeline in Spanish: 1-888-628-9454

Principles of Family-Centered Care and Stress

When a child is hospitalized, the family may experience moderate to severe stress. Applying the principles of family-centered care (FCC) can provide a structure of support by focusing

BEST PRACTICES

When families are experiencing multiple stressors to the point of feeling overwhelmed, working with trusted friends, family members, healthcare providers, clergy, and counselors can be quite helpful. The following five ideas may promote a healthier approach to stressful circumstances:

- Evaluate the source or cause of the stress. Who is it affecting—the entire family or individuals?
- Evaluate one's lifestyle. Is it healthy and balanced, or does it produce feelings of being overwhelmed?
- Talk to others, including extended family members, friends, clergy, counselors, or mental health professionals.
- Create healthy behaviors, including quality sleep behaviors, healthy eating behaviors, and laughter.
- Make healthy choices and encourage other family members to join in.

on the promotion of well-being. Within the philosophy of family-centered care, one premise is that the family is a constant in the child's life (Neal, Frost, Kuhn, Green, & Gance-Cleveland, 2007). Families should be informed of the status of their child's health as well as all treatment decisions, interventions, and short- or long-term plans. Including the family in change-of-shift reports, walking rounds, patient conferences, and treatment decisions may reduce the stress felt when a child is hospitalized. Incorporating the FCC principles of empowerment and enabling may also reduce the stress felt by family members. Bear in mind that children observe and respond to stress in their parents and other family members, so addressing caregivers' stress will, in turn, have an impact on the child's stress level.

Ensuring consistent, supportive, and clear communication; answering all of the family's questions; and providing culturally sensitive care are other measures that may help reduce a family's stress. When parents are engaged in collaboration with the healthcare team and are supported in helping their child cope with illness, injury, and hospitalization, the parent–child relationship deepens (Saleeba, 2008). Making sure that all healthcare team members understand the health literacy level of the family members (and the primary decision maker), and provide health information at the level of complexity that is understood, can also assist in reducing stress.

Caring for the holistic healthcare needs of the child is a paramount concern for the pediatric nurse. Providing opportunities for rest, relaxation, play, medical play, nutrition, pain management, and sibling involvement can help a child through a stressful health encounter.

PHARMACOLOGY

The state of being hospitalized and having an injury, illness, or surgical procedure can cause significant stress for children. In fact, children who experience a serious medical condition may develop a peptic stress ulcer secondary to their condition (Revelz, Guerrero-Lozano, Camacho, Yara, & Mosquera, 2010). Despite limited evidence supporting this practice, many primary care providers choose to order the use of prophylactic antiulcer medications, such as histamine blockers for acid suppression, to prevent a child from developing an ulcer (Kliegman, Stanton, St. Geme, & Schor, 2016). Oral stress ulcer-prevention medications such as Prilosec (omeprazole), Protonix (pantoprazole), Prevacid (lansoprazole), Pepcid (famotidine), and Zantac (ranitidine) may be ordered for this purpose.

Case Study

A family of five has been living in their car in the San Francisco Bay area for the last year. The oldest child, a 10-year-old boy, suffers from the effects of cold weather, stress, and poor nutrition. This child has been experiencing frequent and severe asthma attacks that have required two emergency room visits and one hospitalization in the last 6 months. During the current emergency room visit, the pediatric healthcare team identifies a direct relationship between the cold weather and the patient's asthma exacerbations. While discussing their concerns with the parents, the family appears very distraught and the mother is tearful while she holds her youngest child, a 2-year-old girl.

Case Study Questions

1. Homelessness affected 1.5 million children in the United States in 2010 (Substance Abuse and Mental Health Services Administration, 2015). What are common stressors facing homeless families?
2. Which types of stress responses would a pediatric nurse expect to see in a family living in their car in a large urban area?

3. What is the relationship between exacerbations of chronic illness and the stressors facing a homeless child?

As the case evolves...

The 10-year-old patient is found to have symptoms of pneumonia as well as asthma and is admitted. While waiting for the boy's room assignment to take place, the father takes the family's other school-age child—a boy, age 8—out to the lobby, while the mother stays at the sick boy's bedside with her 2-year-old daughter. Nursing staff note that the parents appear to have an argument prior to the father's departure with the middle child; shortly thereafter, the mother is seen wiping her eyes surreptitiously.

4. Which of the following descriptions accurately summarizes the type of stress in this case and the appropriate short- and long-term interventions that nursing staff should take?
   A. The family is experiencing situational stress related to their son's illness, but they appear to be coping reasonably well, dividing responsibilities among them so that they can continue caring for their other

(continues)

Case Study *(continued)*

children during the crisis. A degree of conflict under such circumstances is normal. Nursing staff can help in the short term by offering access to distractions for the children via Child Life services. No long-term interventions other than treatment of the sick child are needed.

B. The family is experiencing situational stress related to their son's illness and the parents are having trouble coping. For short-term assistance, nursing staff should contact Child Life services to assist with the younger children so that the parents can focus on the sick child. For long-term intervention, staff should offer counseling for the parents via an affiliated licensed clinical social worker or a chaplain, if the family prefers.

C. The family is experiencing toxic stress due to their economic hardships. For short-term assistance, nursing staff should refer the parents to a patient advocate

to help them obtain financial assistance in paying for their son's care. As a long-term intervention, a referral to a free health clinic to help them obtain better primary care at no cost is appropriate.

D. The parents are experiencing a combination of serious situational, relationship, and economic stresses that creates a toxic stress environment for their children. Short-term interventions may include referral of the other children to Child Life services (to reduce the demands on the parents during the situational stress) and referral of the parents to both a social worker/chaplain to help them improve their coping under severe stress and a patient advocate to work with them on obtaining financial assistance for care. Long-term intervention in a complex and difficult case such as this warrants referral to local or state social services to address a multitude of health, economic, and housing concerns.

Chapter Summary

- The physical, psychological and emotional aspects of stress are complex and unique for each individual. Children are prone to demonstrate stress responses when faced with minor or significant health concerns and when interacting with healthcare settings.

- Families need to know that stress is common, and that they may need assistance from healthcare providers or professionals to cope with stress related to a child's illness.

- The pediatric nurse must recognize the common symptoms of stress experienced across childhood developmental stages and across family members. Common symptoms include fight-or-flight responses, fatigue and low energy, emotional reactions, difficulty making decisions, sleep disturbances, intestinal disturbances, changes in weight and eating habits, and acute or chronic health conditions.

- Hans Selye's general adaptation syndrome theory describes the stress response of an organism as occurring in three stages: "fight or flight," "resistance," and "exhaustion." During the stress response, the body's natural defenses break down, such that the body becomes susceptible to illness, tissue damage, ulcers, high blood pressure, and chronic health conditions directly linked to an impaired immune function.

- The pediatric nurse and other members of the pediatric healthcare team should work together to identify stress in families and children. Once the causative factors are

identified, the team should help children cope with the stressors and their individual stress responses.

- Ideas for helping children cope with stress include maintaining normal routines with sleeping, eating, school attendance, chores, and participation in social events or after-school activities; encouraging children to talk and express themselves; and promoting healthy behaviors and connection with others.

- If the child and family's stress levels need further intervention, the pediatric healthcare team should provide referrals and/or encourage the family to seek resources for support.

Bibliography

American Psychological Association (APA). (2010). Stress in America findings. Retrieved from https://www.apa.org/news/press/releases/stress/2010/national-report.pdf

American Psychological Association (APA). (2015). Managing stress for a healthy family. Retrieved from http://www.apa.org/helpcenter/managing-stress.aspx

American Psychological Association (APA). (2016). Stress effects on the body. Retrieved from http://www.apa.org/helpcenter/stress-body.aspx

Anda, R. F., Felitti, V. J., Walker, J., Whitfield, C. L., Bremner, J. D., Perry, B. D., . . . Giles, W. H. (2006). The enduring effects of abuse and related adverse experiences in childhood: A convergence of evidence from neurobiology and epidemiology. *European Archives of Psychiatry and Clinical Neuroscience, 56*(3), 174–186.

Audage, N. C., & Middlebrooks, J. S. (2008). *The effects of childhood stress on health across the lifespan* [Pamphlet]. Atlanta, GA:

U.S. Department of Health and Human Services, Center for Disease Control and Prevention, National Center for Injury Prevention and Control.

Centers for Disease Control and Prevention (CDC). (2015a). Violence prevention: Coping with stress. Retrieved from http://www.cdc.gov/violenceprevention/pub/coping_with_stress_tips.html

Centers for Disease Control and Prevention. (2015b). Violence prevention: The social-ecological model: A framework for prevention. Retrieved from http://www.cdc.gov/violenceprevention/overview/social-ecologicalmodel.html

Cohen, G. J. (2002). Helping children and families deal with divorce and separation. *Pediatrics, 110*(5), 1–16.

Conger, R. D., McLoyd, V. C., Wallace, L. E., Sun, Y., Simons, R. L., & Brody, G. H. (2002). Economic pressure in African American families: A replication and extension of the family stress model. *Developmental Psychology, 38,* 179–193.

DeBellis, M. D., & Zisk, A. A. B. (2014). The biological effects of childhood trauma. *Child and Adolescent Psychiatric Clinics of North America, 23*(2), 185–222.

DeBord, K. Y. (2014). *Helping children cope with stress.* North Carolina State University & A&T State University Cooperative Extension Service. Retrieved from https://content.ces.ncsu.edu/helping-children-cope-with-stress

Dufton, L. M., Dunn, M. J., Slosky, L. S., & Compas, B. E. (2011). Self-reported and laboratory-based responses to stress in children with recurrent pain and anxiety. *Journal of Pediatric Psychology, 36*(1), 95–105.

Felitti, V. J. (2009). Adverse childhood experiences and adult health. *Academic Pediatrics, 9,* 131–132.

Felitti, V. J., Anda, R. F., Nordenberg, D., Williamson, D. F., Spitz, A. M., Edwards, V., . . . Marks, J. S. (1998). Relationship of childhood abuse and household dysfunction to many of the leading causes of death in adults: The Adverse Childhood Experiences (ACE) study. *American Journal of Preventive Medicine, 14,* 245–258.

Gilbert, L. K., Breiding, M. J., Merrick, M. T., Parks, S. E., Thompson, W. W., Dhingra, S. S., & Ford, D. C. (2015). Childhood adversity and adult chronic disease: An update from ten states and the District of Columbia, 2010. *American Journal of Preventive Medicine, 48*(3), 345–349.

Kidshealth.org. (2015). Helping kids cope with stress. Retrieved from http://kidshealth.org/parent/positive/talk/stress_coping.html

Kliegman, R. M., Stanton, B. F., St. Geme, J. W., & Schor, N. F. (Eds.). (2016). *Nelson textbook of pediatrics.* Philadelphia, PA: Elsevier.

Mulvihill, D. (2007). Nursing care of children after a traumatic incident. *Issues in Comprehensive Pediatric Nursing, 30*(1-2), 15–28.

National Child Traumatic Stress Network. (2015). Types of traumatic stress. Retrieved from http://www.nctsn.org/trauma-types

Neal, A., Frost, M., Kuhn, J., Green, A., & Gance-Cleveland, B. (2007). Family centered care within an infant-toddler unit. *Pediatric Nursing, 33*(6), 481–485.

Patterson, J. M. (1988). Families experiencing stress: I. The Family Adjustment and Adaptation Response Model: II. Applying the FAAR Model to health-related issues for intervention and research. *Family Systems Medicine, 6*(2), 202–237.

Revelz, L., Guerrero-Lozano, R., Camacho, A., Yara, L., & Mosquera, P. A. (2010). Stress ulcer, gastritis, and gastrointestinal bleeding prophylaxis in critically ill pediatric patients: A systematic review. *Pediatric Critical Care Medicine, 11*(1), 124–132.

Richmond, J. S., Berlin, J. S., Fishkind, A. B., Holloman, G. H., Zeller, S. L., & Wilson, M. P. (2012). Verbal de-escalation of the agitated patient: Consensus statement of the American Association for Emergency Psychiatry Project BETA De-escalation Workgroup. *Western Journal of Emergency Medicine, 13*(1), 17–25.

Saleeba, A. (2008). The importance of family-centered care in pediatric nursing. University of Connecticut Digital Commons @ UConn, School of Nursing Scholarly Works. Retrieved from http://digitalcommons.uconn.edu/son_articles

Sandor, S., Tache, Y., & Somogyi, A. The legacy of Hans Selye and the origins of stress research: A retrospective 75 years after his landmark brief "letter" to the editor of *Nature. Stress, 15*(5), 472–478.

Sheldon, L. K., & Foust, J. B. (2014). *Communication for nurses: Talking with patients* (3rd ed.). Burlington, MA: Jones & Bartlett Learning.

Su, I. (2010, April 12). De-escalating the aggressive patient. *Medscape.* Retrieved from http://www.medscape.com/viewarticle/719791

Substance Abuse and Mental Health Services Administration. (2015). Homelessness Resource Center: Current statistics on the prevalence and characteristics of people experiencing homelessness in the United States. Retrieved from https://www.samhsa.gov/homelessness-housing

Walsh, F. (2013). Community-based practice applications of a family resilience framework. In D. C. Becvar (Ed.), *Handbook of family resilience* (pp. 65–82). New York, NY: Springer Science+Business Media.

CHAPTER 13

Caring for an Abused Child

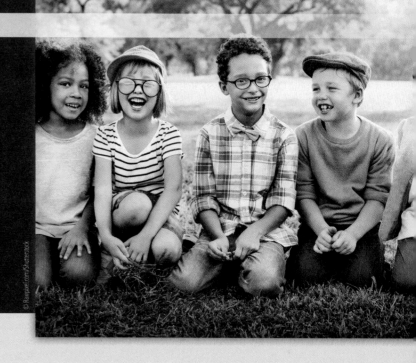

© Rawpixel.com/Shutterstock

LEARNING OBJECTIVES

1. Apply key nursing concepts in caring for a child with actual or suspected maltreatment.
2. Evaluate assessment techniques, history taking, and reporting methods when actual or suspected child maltreatment is identified.
3. Analyze the social, emotional, and developmental factors associated with the development of child maltreatment.
4. Practice in accordance with the legal aspects of child abuse, including reporting laws, child abuse forms submission, documentation, mandatory reporting, and court appearances.
5. Discuss the six types of child maltreatment (physical abuse, physical neglect, emotional abuse, emotional neglect, verbal abuse, and sexual abuse), including the physical and emotional consequences of each.
6. Analyze the consequences of child maltreatment for each of the developmental stages.

KEY TERMS

Abuse
Child maltreatment
Child Protective Services
Cycle of abuse
Extensor surfaces
Good faith
Mandatory reporter
Munchausen syndrome by proxy
Neglect
Reasonable suspicion

Introduction

Child maltreatment is a widespread and complex social issue that remains one of the greatest social concerns across the world. According to the Centers for Disease Control and Prevention (CDC, 2016b), **child maltreatment** comprises "any act or series of acts of commission or omission by a parent or other caregiver (e.g., clergy, coach, teacher) that results in harm, potential for harm, or threat of harm to a child." Child abuse crosses all cultures, races, ethnicities, religions, socioeconomic statuses, parental age groups, individuals with or without previous parenting experience, and geographic locations. Considered highly detrimental to the development and well-being of a child, the many forms of maltreatment can have lifelong consequences.

Members of the pediatric healthcare team are in a unique position to identify abuse and, therefore, provide a safety net for the child. A child might enter the healthcare environment for treatment of abuse-related sequelae, such as an infection superimposed on an intentional burn, or gastrointestinal upset from poisoning; or the child might enter for an unrelated reason, such as pneumonia, where lung radiographs identify broken ribs in various stages of healing. Regardless of the child's age, gender, race, culture, social status, or location, healthcare providers must be aware of the signs of abuse and know what to do to provide safety to the child (**Figure 13-1**).

Pediatric nurses have enormous responsibilities as front-line caregivers who often are the first to suspect a child has been abused. Because the pediatric nurse spends the most time with the child and family, he or she is a **mandatory reporter** and has the responsibility to participate in the assessment of maltreatment, report suspected maltreatment to authorities (usually, an agency such as Child Protective Services and police), and protect the child from further harm. Novice nurses should tap into the experience and judgment of experienced nurses to help confirm any suspicions or concerns, as injury without maltreatment due to a fall or other trauma is not uncommon, especially in small children as they begin to walk (Flaherty et al., 2014). Without immediate identification, protection, and interventions, child maltreatment can be perpetual, accelerating, and potentially fatal.

Principles of childrearing and child care may be dictated by a family's cultural group and cultural norms. What is accepted in one cultural group may be considered a reportable act of child abuse in another group. For example, "female circumcision" (i.e., female genital mutilation) is illegal in the United States and many other countries, but is considered culturally acceptable and even desirable in other parts of the world (CDC, 2016c; World Health Organization, 2014). Despite the ban on this practice, the CDC (2016c) has reported its incidence to be on the rise in the United States due to immigration from regions where this

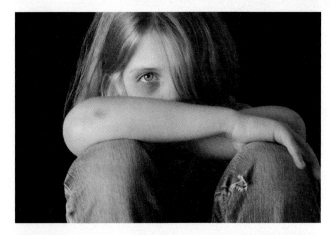

Figure 13-1 *Healthcare providers must be aware of the signs of abuse and know what to do to provide safety to the child.*
© nautilus_shell_studios/iStock/Getty Images

practice is considered acceptable. Less extreme examples include the debate over corporal punishment, such as spanking or "whipping" a child with a stick or belt; this practice is considered acceptable among some groups, but has been found by numerous studies to carry long-term psychological impacts for the child (Gershoff, 2013).

One challenge for pediatric healthcare professionals is to determine which child discipline and childrearing practices are concerning, neglectful, or abusive. The Child Abuse Prevention and Treatment Act (CAPTA), originally signed into law in 1974 and since reauthorized, defines child abuse as "any recent act or failure to act on the part of a parent or caretaker, which results in death, serious physical or emotional harm, sexual abuse, or exploitation, or an act or failure to act which presents an imminent risk of serious harm" (National Child Abuse and Neglect Training and Publications Project, 2014).

Further challenges for healthcare professionals include determining the seriousness of the injury. For instance, bruising, a very typical childhood condition, is considered very normal and is frequently associated with active play and exploration. A challenge for healthcare professionals is to determine at what point should bruising be considered abuse. A typical bruise is red, purple, blueish, black, or yellow as the area of blood vessel trauma is healing. The evaluation of an area of cutaneous trauma should include the child's age, medical history, developmental level, and, most importantly, the stated history or circumstances surrounding the bruise. For instance, a bruise in a child under 9 months of age, located on soft tissue not associated with a bony prominence, under the eyes, on the neck or trunk, or in various stages of healing should raise suspicion (Tomkia, 2010).

Unrealistic parental expectations of a child and the inability of a child to behave in a developmentally inappropriate way or conform to the parents' wishes have both been shown to

Reducing Abuse Through Family Education

Pediatric nurses can contribute to the reduction of child maltreatment by creating and implementing family education opportunities. Promoting educational opportunities for middle school and high school students to learn about family dynamics, self-care, safety in dating, therapeutic communication, acceptable discipline, stress reduction, and healthy relationships can be highly beneficial in developing foundations for good relationships and good parenting later in life. Local organizations that provide guidance in safe and appropriate care of children, teach appropriate child discipline, and offer safety nets for families to secure needed resources to reduce stress can also be of great assistance in reducing child maltreatment rates. For example, providing courses in "never shaking your baby" can save lives by reducing rates of shaken baby syndrome and abusive head trauma.

Nurses should also be aware of, and teach families about, the **cycle of abuse**—a pattern of behavior in which children who experience child maltreatment grow up and abuse their own children—to help them understand how abuse suffered in childhood affects adulthood:

- Thirty percent of abused children will grow up to abuse their own children (American Society for the Positive Care of Children, 2014).
- Eighty percent of children who were abused will meet the criteria for at least one psychological/psychiatric disorder.

Clearly, the impact of this disorder can last a lifetime.

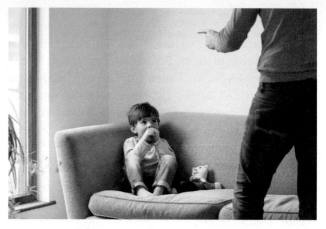

Figure 13-2 *A parent's expectations that a young child will behave at a level above his or her developmental capacity may contribute to an abusive situation.*
© SolStock/E+/Getty Images

contribute to an abusive situation. A parent's expectations that a very young child will behave on a level above his or her developmental capacity, or a parent's expectations that a young child will do chores beyond his or her cognitive, emotional, or physical development, may contribute to an abusive situation and are considered risk factors (Krug, Dahlberg, Mercy, Zwi, & Lozano, 2002) (**Figure 13-2**). Other child-associated risk factors associated with maltreatment include the following:

- Children with a chronic health issue that imposes demands exceeding the parent's ability to cope
- Children younger than three years of age
- Children with difficult or demanding temperaments
- Children who were unplanned or whose births were unexpected

Incidence and Prevalence of Child Maltreatment

The CDC (2016b) provides a breakdown of the various forms of child maltreatment into categories representing acts of commission (**abuse**—that is, physical abuse, sexual abuse, and psychological abuse) and acts of omission (**neglect**—that is, physical neglect, emotional neglect, medical/dental neglect, educational neglect, and failure to supervise). The overall percentages for the incidences of these forms of abuse add up to more than 100%, as it is common for a child to suffer multiple types of maltreatment (CDC, 2016a):

- Neglect: 52% of child maltreatment cases
- Physical abuse: 24%
- Sexual abuse: 12%
- Other (abandonment, school truancy, congenital drug addiction, and more): 16%

Child victims of abuse who have the highest incidence rates are infants across the first year of life (21% of cases). In 2012, female children accounted for 51% and male children accounted for 49%. The reported three top ethnicities for child abuse include Caucasian (44.0%), Hispanic (21.8%), and African-American (21%). Approximately 13% of reported pediatric abuse cases are concerning children with disabilities (U.S. Department of Health and Human Services, Administration for Children and Families, 2012).

Facts for the Pediatric Nurse to Consider When Assessing a Possibly Abused Child

According to the American Academy on Pediatrics' Committee on Child Abuse and Neglect, the following evidence-based tips can be used to distinguish accidental traumatic injuries from abuse injuries (Flaherty et al., 2014):

- Bruises and fractures are the most common injuries in children who have suffered physical abuse. Bruising in a child who is not yet mobile or bruises in unusual locations (ears, neck, back of the legs, or trunk) should raise suspicion for abuse.

(continues)

- Age of the child, location and type of injury, and discrepancies in history can help distinguish abuse.
- Eighty percent of abuse-related fractures occur in children younger than 18 months. In children younger than 1 year who are not yet starting to walk, 25% of fractures are due to abuse. This includes long-bone fractures that are not generally considered suspicious in older (ambulatory) children.
- The most common fracture pattern found in abused children is a single long-bone diaphyseal fracture. The following fractures have moderate to high specificity for abuse:
  - High: rib fractures (presence is 95% predictive of abuse in children younger than 3 years)
  - High: classic metaphyseal lesions (in first year of life)
  - High: complex or bilateral skull fractures
  - High: fractures of different ages or stages of healing*
  - Moderate: epiphyseal separations
  - Moderate: vertebral body fractures
  - Moderate: digital fractures
- Long bone fractures (other than classic metaphyseal lesions), linear skull fractures, clavicle fractures, and isolated subperiosteal new bone formation are unlikely to indicate child abuse.
- Family history, evaluation of siblings, and lab values for serum calcium, phosphorus, and alkaline phosphatase should be assessed to assist with supporting or ruling out an abuse determination.
  - Providers should ask themselves whether the injury is consistent with the described history of the injury or circumstances stated that caused the injury or evidence.
  - Inconsistent, vague history, history that contradicts the nature of the injury, or a significant (more than 96 hours) delay in seeking care can offer clues toward abuse.
  - Approximately one-third of caregivers in abuse situations will give a false history of a high-impact accident (e.g., car crash or fall from height). Others omit history or give inconsistent history.
  - Most caregivers in non-abuse situations describe a low-impact fall from stairs or rough play with a sibling.

*Bone fragility due to prematurity, osteomyelitis, or syndromes such as osteogenesis imperfecta should be ruled out.

Data from Flaherty, E. G., Perez-Rossello, J. M., Levine, M. A., Hennrikus, W. L., & American Academy of Pediatrics Committee on Child Abuse and Neglect, Section on Radiology, Section on Endocrinology, and Section on Orthopaedics, and the Society for Pediatric Radiology. (2014). Evaluating children with fractures for child physical abuse. *Pediatrics, 133*(2), e477–e489.

Forms of Child Maltreatment

Child maltreatment can present in one or more of six distinct forms. It is not uncommon for a child to suffer more than one form of maltreatment during a particular developmental period. Forms of maltreatment are categorized as follows:

- Physical abuse
  - Examples include hitting, slapping, burning, choking, poisoning, kicking, and shaking. Injury that causes lasting erythema is considered abuse in many states.
  - Physical abuse can include repeated injuries to any of the child's systems, including the integumentary, reproductive, skeletal, peripheral nervous, or central nervous system.
  - Unlawful corporal punishment is considered physical abuse.
- Physical neglect
  - Examples include not providing for a child's nutrition, warmth, clothing, housing, health care, supervision, and education.
  - Evidence of physical neglect in a child can include very poor personal hygiene, poor academic performance from deep hunger, and untreated medical conditions.
  - Dental neglect such as untreated caries or abscesses (significant pain) is a form of child abuse and is rarely the only form of neglect found in a child with untreated dental issues (Bradbury-Jones, Innes, Evans, Ballantyne, & Taylor, 2013).
- Emotional abuse
  - Examples include belittling, ridiculing, degrading, or failing to provide a supportive environment in which the child can emotionally thrive.
  - Other examples of emotional abuse include threats, humiliation, blame, name-calling, and a persistent state of being ridiculed.
- Emotional neglect
  - Examples include neglecting a child's emotions, not attending to the child's psychological needs, or ignoring a child's emotional needs.
- Verbal abuse
  - Examples include using aggressive, demanding, detrimental, and demeaning forms of communication as the primary method of engaging a child.
- Sexual abuse
  - Examples include actual or threats of sexual abuse such as fondling, forced kissing, penetration, oral copulation, anal intercourse, and vaginal intercourse.
  - Sexual abuse may also include sexual exploitation of a child, pornographic photography of a child, exposing a child to pornography, or genital exhibitionism in front of a child.
  - Evidence of sexual abuse in children may include yeast infections, sexually transmitted infections, bruising to the genitalia, bleeding from the rectum or anus area, abdominal discomfort or pain, and acting out explicit sexual behaviors. Behaviors

such as self-harm, depression, nightmares, or regression may also suggest sexual abuse.

- Battered-child syndrome
  - ◆ A complex term, first described in 1962, used to denote a clinical condition where a child has experienced or received serious physical abuse or neglect leading to permanent injury (Kempe, 1962).

UNIQUE FOR KIDS

Whenever a pediatric nurse is first assessing a young child, he or she should examine all surfaces of the child's skin. Basic abuse assessments should be performed on all children during health screenings, at wellness appointments, or when a family is seeking medical treatment for a health concern or issue. The nurse should keep in mind that approximately 25% of children (702,000 children in 2014 alone confirmed by child protective agencies) are abused (CDC, 2016a); thus, all children should be assessed for indicators of maltreatment such as the following:

- Burns (young children with immersion burns such as sock or glove burns, and older child with scalding burns from hot liquids being thrown) (**Figure 13-3**)
- Bite marks (double horseshoe, doughnut, or oval shaped) (**Figure 13-4**)
- Lacerations and abrasions ("U" or "C" shaped, such as a whipping injury) (**Figure 13-5**)
- Bruises and contusions (especially on the face, buttocks, back, or genitals, with a clear impression such as a handprint or a loop mark on a body curve)
- Evidence of neglect, such as failure to thrive, malnourishment, poor hygiene, and neglected medical conditions
- Evidence of emotional neglect, emotional abuse, and verbal abuse, including aversion to touch, withdrawal, inappropriate aggression (e.g., defiant or argumentative behavior), hyperactivity, somatic symptoms such as stomachache or headache, or nonverbal behaviors such as twitching, pulling hair, rigidity/tensing, self-soothing movements such as rocking or stroking, or physical disengagement*

* These behaviors may also indicate reluctance to disclose physical abuse to investigators (Katz et al., 2012).

Data from Al Odhayani, A., Watson, W. J., & Watson, L. (2013). Behavioural consequences of child abuse. *Canadian Family Physician, 59*(8), 831–836; Centers for Disease Control and Prevention. (2016a). Child abuse and neglect: Consequences. Retrieved from https://www.cdc.gov/violenceprevention/childmaltreatment/consequences.html; Katz, C., Hershkowitz, I., Malloy, L. C., Lamb, M. E., Atabaki, A., & Spinder, S. (2012). Non-verbal behavior of children who disclose or do not disclose child abuse in investigative interviews. *Child Abuse & Neglect, 36*, 12–20; Naughton, A. M., Maguire, S. A., Mann, M. K., Lumb, R. C., Tempest, V., Gracias, S., & Kemp, A. M. (2013). Emotional, behavioral, and developmental features indicative of neglect or emotional abuse in preschool children: A systematic review. *JAMA Pediatrics, 167*(8), 769–775.

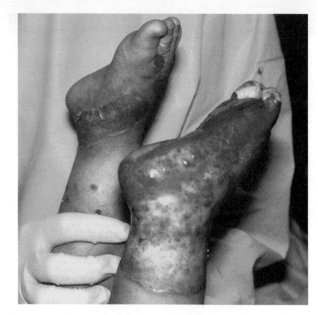

Figure 13-3 *An immersion (sock) burn.*

Courtesy of Ronald Dieckmann, MD

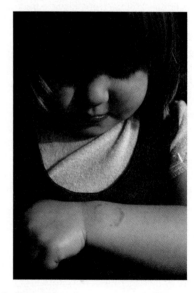

Figure 13-4 *Bite marks.*

ian west/Alamy Stock Photo

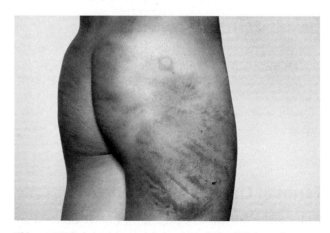

Figure 13-5 *Lacerations and abrasions ("U" or "C" shaped).*

© Biophoto Associates/Science Source

Ways to Approach the Topic of Potential Maltreatment with Children in Various Developmental Stages

The pediatric nurse does not assess for child maltreatment alone; rather, the entire pediatric healthcare team will be involved with the assessment and reporting of a suspected or actual case of abuse. The pediatric nurse, who is often trusted by the child and the family, is a good source of information in suspected maltreatment cases.

Infants

Infants are in Erikson's stage of "trust versus mistrust." Building caring and trustful relationships in which infants' needs are met and they feel safe is paramount. Infants have no way to communicate abuse, so the nurse must use objective data to discern if an infant is experiencing abuse. Growth charts may reveal evidence of failure to thrive (repeated plots of anthropometrics below the 5th percentile). Physical exams should include assessing for bruising, fractures, and marks made by implements.

Toddlers

Toddlers are very emotional beings, who are in Erikson's stage of "autonomy versus shame and doubt." Abused children in this developmental stage may show delays in motor and language development, and may act out aggressively toward peers with anger or violence.

Preschoolers

Preschool-age children are in Erikson's developmental stage of "initiative versus guilt." Children with suspected abuse should be engaged through simple play situations such as dolls to allow them to reenact or demonstrate their emotions through the use of medical play dolls.

School-Age Children

School-age children are in Erikson's stage of "industry versus inferiority." Abused children in this stage may become depressed, socially isolated, unfocused on schoolwork and academic demands, distracted, overactive, and aggressive. A deep sense of inferiority may also develop in abused school-age children.

Adolescents

Teens should be seeking and learning who they are, what they want in life, and what their overall identity is. According to Erikson, adolescents are in the developmental stage of "identity versus role confusion." Abused and neglected teens may become truants; may demonstrate depression, withdrawal, and disengagement; or may engage in high-risk behaviors that can lead to unlawful behavior and delinquency.

Assessing for Child Maltreatment

As noted in the Unique for Kids feature, certain injuries raise the suspicion of child maltreatment—but nurses must also recognize both that children can and do get hurt in the normal course of their daily activities without maltreatment being present, and that some forms of abuse are physically invisible. Similarly, specific disease states (osteogenesis imperfecta, osteomyelitis, and other forms of brittle bone or bruising disorders), markings (Mongolian spots), and other injuries (e.g., straddle injuries to the genitals in a child who fell on a bicycle crossbar) can mimic maltreatment even when none is present. In addition, some cultural practices might appear to be maltreatment when they are, in fact, considered healing practices to some cultures—for example, cupping, gua sha/coining, and moxibustion (Lilly & Kundu, 2012) (**Figure 13-6**). Misdiagnosis of child maltreatment can cause significant stress for a family and misdirect resources that should be reserved for true cases of child maltreatment. The difficulty for the nurse, then, is identifying those signals that point to abuse being present while ruling out other causes of injuries or psychiatric issues.

Becoming a Sexual Abuse Forensic Nurse

Forensic nursing—a relatively new specialty area recognized by the American Nurses Association (ANA)—is defined as the "application of nursing science to public or legal proceedings." Nurses who become forensic specialists provide assistance in collecting evidence and identifying perpetrators of violent crimes. Forensic nurses may be requested to provide legal opinions and testify in court. The goal of this specialty is to develop healthcare expertise that provides skills to assist in establishing legal causation and responsibility for violent and traumatic injuries. Education required to become a forensic nurse can be found in four areas: (1) continuing education courses; (2) certification programs offered by universities; (3) elective courses offered within graduate or undergraduate programs; and (4) graduate studies programs with a core forensic nursing curriculum. See the website of the International Association of Forensic Nurses (IAFN; www.iafn.org) or American Forensic Nurses (www.amrn.com) for more information.

As with any patient, the first step in the patient assessment is to identify the nature and severity of the injury. It is crucial that the patient's physical well-being be managed *before* any steps are taken to determine whether child maltreatment has occurred. In life-threatening situations such as a skull fracture, internal bleeding or compromised airway/circulation, stabilizing the patient takes precedence over gathering information for reporting, even when the history offers clear evidence of maltreatment. In taking the

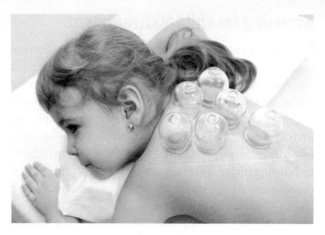

Figure 13-6 *Some cultural practices, such as cupping, might appear to be maltreatment when they are, in fact, considered healing practices to some cultures.*

Peter Banos/Alamy Stock Photo

history from the child's caregiver, the American Academy of Pediatrics notes that "the best approach is to allow the parent or other caregiver to provide a narrative without interruptions, so that the history is not influenced by the clinician's questions or interpretations" (Christian, 2015). Doing so allows the nurse to assess the caregiver's behavior as well.

FAMILY EDUCATION

Never, Ever Shake an Infant!

Serious head trauma occurs when an infant is shaken. Shaken baby syndrome (also called abusive head trauma) is defined as a constellation of signs and symptoms that result when an infant or young child is violently shaken with coup/contrecoup forces. The violent shaking can lead to seizures, stupor, coma, and death. The traumatized brain tissue is injured through damage to and destruction of blood vessels, increased intracranial pressure, brain tissue hypoxia, and retinal hemorrhages. Outcomes for infants subjected to shaken baby syndrome range from mild learning and behavioral issues to persistent vegetative state to death.

Parents must be repeatedly educated on the importance of never shaking their infant.

With a stable patient, it is important to obtain a history of how the injury occurred or, in the event of a psychiatric or mental health crisis, what may have preceded the change in the child's behavior. Be aware that caregivers may not necessarily know the specifics of some incidents; for example, a child who has been sexually assaulted outside the home may be too fearful, shamed, or confused to explain to the parent what happened (particularly if the assailant is someone known to them, such as a family member or the other parent). In such situations, the caregiver's own expressions of concern, worry, fear, or similar emotions will likely support the proposition that he or she is truly ignorant of the nature of the incident.

In assessing injuries, the nurse should bear in mind which kinds of forces and activities would appropriately produce the injury. For example, bruising in school-age or ambulatory preschool/toddler-age children is normal, but such bruises will generally occur on **extensor surfaces**—that is, surfaces of muscles that move a body part, such as elbows, knees, shins, and forehead. Bruises should be considered suspicious for child maltreatment if they occur in locations other than where a child might land after falling, such as the back, upper arms, upper legs, abdomen, buttocks, or ear (Blair, Clauss, & Meredith, 2011), particularly if the explanation for the injury is inconsistent with its presentation (e.g., a caregiver claims the child fell down a flight of stairs but bruises appear only on the child's torso and not on the legs, knees, or arms). In children age 4 and younger, findings predictive of maltreatment include bruising on the torso, ear, or neck for a child and bruising in any region for an infant younger than 4 months (Pierce, Kaczor, Aldrige, O'Flynn, & Lorenz, 2010).

In many cases, however, the nature of the injury or complaint may mask the presence of maltreatment. The following signs should raise suspicion and prompt nurses to examine or question the patient or caregiver more thoroughly:

- Vague, inconsistent, or absent explanation of how an injury occurred
- Significant (more than 96 hours) delay in seeking care for a significant illness or injury
- Distracted, irritable, or uninterested affect in the caregiver
- Unexplained injuries to the genitals or presence of sexually transmitted disease symptoms in a child or sexually immature adolescent
- Underweight or subnormal height, evidence of malnutrition, significantly unkempt appearance (dirty, ill-fitting clothes and matted hair), or verbal expression of extreme hunger
- Seizure in an afebrile child with no history of seizure

In contrast, other aspects of the child's presentation and history may allay suspicions of maltreatment:

- Documented history of a disorder leading to frequent bruising, brittle bones, or other symptoms that might otherwise be concerning
- Appropriate display of affection, concern, and engagement by the caregiver, reciprocated (when possible) by the child
- History of ailment or injury that is consistent with the presentation
- Appropriateness of the complaint to the patient's age and developmental stage (e.g., multiple bruises

on a 4-month-old's extensor surfaces would be considered suspicious, but the same bruises would be considered normal in a 14-month-old)

If a healthcare practitioner develops **reasonable suspicion** of child maltreatment, he or she is mandated to report it. Most laws indicate that when a healthcare professional, or other mandatory reporter, suspects abuse either by visual evidence or "gut feelings," "bells going off," or "being uncomfortable" with the child's emotional and physical presentation, reporting should take place. It is in the best interest of all concerned to ensure that physical examination, history taking, and documentation are thorough and complete if maltreatment is suspected (Blair et al., 2011).

BEST PRACTICES

Talking to a Family About Suspected Child Abuse

Suspected child abuse is an emotionally difficult issue for the pediatric healthcare team. Having a "time-out" or a huddle about the case can provide support and confidence for the provider when the team agrees a suspicion of abuse is warranted. The following are a few opening lines a nurse can use with the family to introduce this topic:

- "I have concerns that someone may have hurt your child."
- "I am required by law to report what I am worried about in your child. . ."
- "Let's talk for a moment away from your child so I can express a concern I am seeing."
- "It is our priority to provide safety for you and your child. We have a concern that your child has not been provided safety. . ."

RESEARCH EVIDENCE

Unusual Cases of Child Abuse: Munchausen Syndrome by Proxy

Munchausen syndrome by proxy (MSBP)—sometimes called medical child abuse—is a rare, sometimes fatal form of child maltreatment in which a caregiver (often the mother, and sometimes with healthcare education or experience) fabricates, exaggerates, or induces the symptoms of a medical condition in a child as a way of getting attention. The caregiver may describe symptoms that cannot be observed clinically and that occur only when the child is alone with the abuser. Often the child appears well despite the caregiver's insistence that he or she is ill. Alternatively, the perpetrator may cause the child harm—for example, suffocating or choking a young child or force-feeding the child with a harmful substance—and seek assistance claiming the ailment was mysterious or accidental.

As a result of the unnecessary, sometimes painful, and potentially harmful medical care that they experience, the children of these abusers are subjected to both physical and emotional trauma. MSBP cases result in increased hospitalizations, leading to significant child morbidity and, in some cases, mortality. Nursing staff should be aware of this syndrome in cases where a child has a history of multiple, repeated complaints of unknown etiology. One clear warning sign is that the abuser does not demonstrate a normal level of concern about the child's hospitalization and subsequent diagnostic exams and procedures, yet seeks to stay in contact with the child at all times and refuses to leave the child alone (Lasher & Sheridan, 2013).

Data from Boyd, Ritchie, & Likhari, 2014; Depauw, Loas, & Delhaye, 2015; Gehlawat, Gehlawat, Singh, & Gupta, 2015; Grace & Jagannathan, 2015; Lasher & Sheridan, 2013; Roesler, 2015.

Legal Aspects of Care for an Abused Child

The legal aspects of caring for children who have been suspected or found to have been experiencing abuse vary in different states. It is imperative that all pediatric healthcare professionals learn the relevant laws of the state in which they practice. State laws will outline when a report must take place, with most requiring reporting within 24 hours of the determination of suspected child abuse at the latest. Reports can be started verbally but must be followed up within the 24-hour period with a written report. The privacy protections of the Health Insurance Portability and Accountability Act (HIPAA) do not apply to child abuse and neglect reporting, so the nurse must provide comprehensive information about the child's condition, contact information, and pertinent medical records. Some states require that the reporter contact both the law enforcement agency and **Child Protective Services** (CPS).

QUALITY AND SAFETY

Reporting of child abuse cases, either suspected or confirmed, that are considered high priority are stipulated to occur within 24 hours of encountering the abused child. Early and rapid reporting saves lives and reduces further harm (U.S. Department of Health and Human Services, Administration for Children and Families, 2014).

The reporter of child abuse must be available for further inquiry or clarification of information. Most institutions have developed a plan and mechanism through which to make a report. The institutional social worker, nursing administrator, and emergency room team can all be of assistance to help with the report and make sure local and state laws are followed. The consequences of not reporting can be severe, ranging from loss of license to practice to hefty fines and/or jail time. Both a mandatory reporter and a volunteer reporter of child abuse will be immune from liability if the report is made in **good faith**—that is, out of genuine belief that maltreatment is present, rather than for some other rationale—and with reasonable suspicion. Nevertheless, because of the potential for a child maltreatment case to end in a court case or trial (often many years after the incident that led to reporting), thorough documentation is essential.

BEST PRACTICES

Dealing with Doubts About Abuse

If a pediatric nurse is not sure that what is being seen or heard is considered abuse, it is better to seek the help of experienced professionals than to not report. Good-faith suspicion or reasonable belief is enough to warrant reporting child abuse. Most states require that a report be made when the reporter "in his or her official capacity, suspects or has reason to believe that a child has been abused or neglected."

Data from U.S. Department of Health and Human Services, Children's Bureau. (2015). Mandatory reporters of child abuse and neglect. Retrieved from https://www.childwelfare.gov/pubPDFs/manda.pdf

RESEARCH EVIDENCE

Health care professionals make approximately three-fifths (58%) of all child neglect and abuse reports annually. It is imperative that the pediatric nurse is educated, prepared, and confident in making a report so that children who are abused can be identified early and quickly (U.S. Department of Health and Human Services, Administration for Children and Families, 2014).

Reporting in Various Clinical Settings

Child abuse may be identified when a child enters the healthcare arena. The child may be brought in by the abuser or a caregiver willingly; once the parent or caregiver realizes he or she is under suspicion for maltreatment, however, that person may leave the healthcare facility with the child. This behavior, which is called leaving against medical advice (AMA), can place the child in great jeopardy. The police, sheriff, or other law enforcement representative must be contacted immediately in such a case.

Hospitals

Acute care hospitals that provide care to children within emergency departments, inpatient units, or pediatric critical care units will have policies and procedures that specify how to use teamwork to confirm suspicions of child abuse. The benefits of this structure include having access to experienced pediatric providers, social workers, and nursing administrators, and, often, having established relationships with local authorities and Child Protective Services. The pediatric nurse who suspects child abuse within a hospital setting never has to work independently on the case.

Schools

School nurses will be informed about their school district's child abuse screening and reporting policies. Child abuse that is suspected by a classroom teacher, administrative assistant, or school administrator might be communicated to the school nurse to seek the nurse's involvement and assistance with follow-through. Because the child is not in a healthcare arena, the school nurse needs to use skills in interviewing the child, working with the teachers to craft a report to CPS and being supportive of the child to reduce fears and anxiety.

Clinics

Ambulatory care settings that provide health care to children should have policies and practices for how evidence is collected, how interviews take place with family members, and how personnel fill out a child abuse report. Having a file readily available with contact information for local CPS and law enforcement agencies would be helpful. Running practice scenarios can help the team be more confident and ready when a case occurs.

BEST PRACTICES

The healthcare team should work together to provide the abused child with the following support:

- *Stabilization.* The child's physical and emotional state needs to be stabilized. Immediate care should be provided to diagnose and treat any conditions associated with the abuse. The team must provide early identification and treatment of physical harm (e.g., head trauma, neurologic stabilization, setting fractures, and stopping bleeding) as a first priority.
- *Protection from harm.* Preventing further harm to the child may require a police hold and hospital or institutional security involvement. Temporary medical foster care may be required and will be set up through the assistance of the social worker and CPS advocate.
- *History taking.* Inconsistencies between the signs and symptoms of the injury and the parental/child history or description of abuse must be determined.
- *Data collection and documentation.* Specimens, such as semen, blood, urine, and human hairs from the child's body, may need to be taken, and X-rays and other diagnostics may need to be performed. Photographs may be required, in which case strict policies must be followed—including use of only approved equipment, not personal cell phone cameras.

Preventing Child Maltreatment

Because of the serious nature of child abuse, and its potentially long-lasting consequences for the victim of abuse throughout childhood and spanning into adulthood, the goal for care in regard to child maltreatment centers on prevention. Neglect, which is the most common form of child maltreatment, is often difficult to identify in its early stages, as stressors related to unemployment and economic crises may have contributed to families not being able to provide for the needs of their child. Purposive neglect, as a form of punishment, must be identified early before serious consequences occur for the child. Prevention is the key to avoiding the long-term effects of abuse and neglect, but it is also complex. Preventing fatal consequences of child abuse is paramount. Fatalities associated with child abuse are associated with significant head and abdominal injuries (Bensel, Rheinberger, & Radbill, 1997).

RESEARCH EVIDENCE

Common Signs of Neglect

- Failure to thrive
- Clothing that is dirty, ragged, ill fitting, or inappropriate for weather conditions, particularly in a child whose family is not experiencing economic hardship
- Consistently poor hygiene, including poor oral health
- Frequently is hungry or hoards and steals food
- Flinching or shying away from touch; inappropriate friendliness with strangers, in contrast to lack of emotional intimacy with caregivers
- Extremes of behavior (e.g., withdrawal, aggression, passivity, hyperactivity)
- Developmentally inappropriate maturity or immaturity (e.g., thumbsucking or tantrums in an older child)
- Absent from school frequently, often without parental excuse

Data from DePanfilis, D. (2006). *Child neglect: A guide for prevention, assessment, and intervention.* Washington, DC: U.S. Department of Health and Human Services. Retrieved from https://www.childwelfare.gov/pubPDFs/neglect.pdf

According to the CDC, many effective programs currently exist to help prevent child maltreatment. Early identification programs such as Child–Parent Centers are funded especially to provide education for parents and guardians. One study by Reynolds and Roberston (2003) found that young children whose families participated in this type of program (Title 1 Child–Parent Center) had a 52% reduction in child maltreatment rates. Knowing when to respond to a child's physical and emotional needs, providing appropriate discipline, and good communication skills are all part of positive parenting strategies (CDC, 2016a). Notably, programs that set out to improve parent–child relationships, and those that provide social support and role modeling, have successfully reduced the incidence of child abuse (Poole, Seal, & Taylor, 2014).

Early reporting is the very essence of prevention of further harm. If a pediatric healthcare team member suspects a child is being maltreated or is under threat of being maltreated, that professional should call the National Child Abuse Hotline at 1-800-4-A-Child (1-800-422-4453).

Case Study

A Caucasian male infant with Down syndrome, age 11 months, was admitted to the pediatric unit of a large urban hospital for weight loss, inconsolable crying, and fever that his parents say has been occurring for 2 days. The pediatric healthcare team collected laboratory specimens related to the fever, including a complete blood count (CBC), urinalysis with culture, chemistry 17 panel, and lumbar puncture. All of the results came back negative for a source of infection. The infant continues to cry during all aspects of care; when asked, his mother states that this is normal behavior for the

(continues)

Case Study *(continued)*

child, whom she describes as "difficult." When changing a diaper, the nurse notes increasing crying with any leg movement. The nurse requests an order for a STAT radiograph, which identifies bilateral spiral femur fractures. The local Child Protective Services agency is notified, and the child is rapidly put on a police hold. The primary caregivers—the parents—are not allowed to visit until a further investigation is conducted.

Case Study Questions

1. What is the role of Child Protective Services? How do you contact your local branch?
2. What are the typical steps of securing state guardianship for a maltreated child?
3. Who was responsible for reporting the suspected child maltreatment in this case?

As the Case Evolves. . .

4. Which of the following characteristics of this child are risk factors associated with the development and occurrence of child abuse? (Select all that apply.)
   A. Age younger than 3 years
   B. Male gender
   C. Presence of a chronic health condition
   D. Caucasian race
   E. "Difficult" temperament

Upon being informed of the fractures found on the radiograph, the parents offer the explanation that their child is a "climber" who may have fallen from his crib at some point during the past few days, causing the fractures.

5. Which of the following aspects of the history in this Case Study suggest reasonable suspicion of child abuse? (Select all that apply.)
   A. The child's caregivers delayed seeking help for more than 24 hours despite the child's fever
   B. The child's injuries are inconsistent with the explanation given
   C. Long-bone injuries in children younger than 1 year of age have high specificity for abuse
   D. Presence of fever and weight loss accompanying the fracture

Chapter Summary

- The pediatric nurse provides insight, oversight, and team contributions to the assessment and validation of actual or suspected maltreatment. The pediatric healthcare team uses comprehensive and holistic assessment techniques, medical diagnostics, and thorough history taking to provide information for law enforcement agencies as they investigate maltreatment.
- Assessing for and reporting actual or suspected child maltreatment is a legal responsibility for all healthcare providers who interact with and care for children.
- Numerous social, emotional, and developmental factors are associated with the experience of child maltreatment. Victims of child maltreatment can suffer lifelong psychological and psychiatric mental health issues.
- It is imperative that a pediatric nurse study and understand the legal aspects of child maltreatment, including state and federal reporting laws, child abuse forms submission, documentation of evidence of suspected maltreatment, and the possibility of mandatory court appearances and testimony.
- The pediatric nurse is responsible for acting on any suspicion, assessment findings, or confirmed diagnostics that would demonstrate any type of maltreatment. A member of the pediatric healthcare team who fails to

report suspected or actual child abuse can be subject to heavy fines, suspension or loss of license, and/or jail time.
- There are six types of child maltreatment: physical abuse, physical neglect, emotional abuse, emotional neglect, verbal abuse, and sexual abuse. It is not uncommon for an abused child to be experiencing more than one type of maltreatment.
- Consequences of child maltreatment can be found in each of the developmental stages. Understanding childhood development within the framework of a developmental theory, such as Erikson's theory, can help the nurse assess the suspicion or evidence of child abuse.

Bibliography

Al Odhayani, A., Watson, W. J., & Watson, L. (2013). Behavioural consequences of child abuse. *Canadian Family Physician, 59*(8), 831–836.

American Society for the Positive Care of Children. (2014). Advocacy for children's rights protects children from abuse. Retrieved from http://americanspcc.org/advocacy

Bensel, T., Rheinberger, M., & Radbill, S. (1997). Children in a world of violence: The roots of child maltreatment. In M. Helfer, R. Kempe, & R. Drugman (Eds.), *The battered child* (pp. 3–28, 59–80). Chicago, IL: University of Chicago Press.

Blair, L., Clauss, E., & Meredith, M. (2011). Child abuse: Discovering the horrifying truth. *Journal of Emergency Medical Services, 36*(10), 62–67; quiz 68.

Boyd, A. S., Ritchie, C., & Likhari, S. (2014). Munchausen syndrome and Munchausen syndrome by proxy in dermatology. *Journal of the American Academy of Dermatology, 71*(2), 376–381.

Bradbury-Jones, C., Innes, N., Evans, D., Ballantyne, F., & Taylor, J. (2013). Dental neglect as a marker of broader neglect: A qualitative investigation of public health nurses' assessments of oral health in preschool children. *BMC Public Health, 13,* 370.

Centers for Disease Control and Prevention (CDC). (2016a). Child abuse and neglect: Consequences. Retrieved from https://www.cdc .gov/violenceprevention/childmaltreatment/consequences.html

Centers for Disease Control and Prevention (CDC). (2016b). Child abuse and neglect: Definitions. Retrieved from https://www .cdc.gov/violenceprevention/childmaltreatment/definitions .html

Centers for Disease Control and Prevention (CDC). (2016c). Female genital cutting. Retrieved from https://www.cdc.gov /immigrantrefugeehealth/guidelines/domestic/general/discussion /female-genital-cutting.html

Christian, C. W.; Committee on Child Abuse and Neglect, American Academy of Pediatrics. (2015). The evaluation of suspected child physical abuse. *Pediatrics, 135*(5), e1337–e1354.

DePanfilis, D. (2006). *Child neglect: A guide for prevention, assessment, and intervention.* Washington, DC: U.S. Department of Health and Human Services. Retrieved from https://www.childwelfare .gov/pubPDFs/neglect.pdf

Depauw, A., Loas, G., & Delhaye, M. (2015). Munchausen by proxy syndrome. *Revue Medicale de Bruxelles, 36*(3), 152–157.

Flaherty, E. G., Perez-Rossello, J. M., Levine, M. A., Hennrikus, W. L., & American Academy of Pediatrics Committee on Child Abuse and Neglect, Section on Radiology, Section on Endocrinology, Section on Orthopaedics, Society for Pediatric Radiology. (2014). Evaluating children with fractures for child physical abuse. *Pediatrics, 133*(2), e477–e489.

Gehlawat, P., Gehlawat, V. K., Singh, P., & Gupta, R. (2015). Munchausen syndrome by proxy: An alarming face of child abuse. *Indian Journal of Psychological Medicine, 37*(1), 90–92.

Gershoff, E. T. (2013). Spanking and child development: We know enough now to stop hitting our children. *Child Development Perspectives, 7*(3), 133–137.

Grace, E., & Jagannathan, N. (2015). Munchausen syndrome by proxy: A form of child abuse. *International Journal of Child and Adolescent Health, 8*(3 suppl), 259–263.

Katz, C., Hershkowitz, I., Malloy, L. C., Lamb, M. E., Atabaki, A., & Spinder, S. (2012). Non-verbal behavior of children who disclose or do not disclose child abuse in investigative interviews. *Child Abuse and Neglect, 36,* 12–20.

Kempe, C. H. (1962). The battered child syndrome. *Journal of the American Medical Association, 181,* 17–24.

Krug, E. A., Dahlberg, L. L., Mercy, J. A., Zwi, A. B., & Lozano, R. (Eds.). (2002). *World report on violence and health.* Geneva, Switzerland: World Health Organization.

Lasher, L. J., & Sheridan, M. S. (2013). *Munchausen by proxy: Identification, intervention, and case management.* New York, NY: Routledge.

Lilly, E., & Kundu, R. V. (2012). Dermatoses secondary to Asian cultural practices. *International Journal of Dermatology, 51,* 372–382.

National Child Abuse and Neglect Training and Publications Project. (2014). *The Child Abuse Prevention and Treatment Act: 40 years of safeguarding America's children.* Washington, DC: U.S. Department of Health and Human Services, Children's Bureau.

Naughton, A. M., Maguire, S. A., Mann, M. K., Lumb, R. C., Tempest, V., Gracias, S., & Kemp, A. M. (2013). Emotional, behavioral, and developmental features indicative of neglect or emotional abuse in preschool children: A systematic review. *JAMA Pediatrics, 167*(8), 769–775.

Pierce, M. C., Kaczor, K., Aldrige, S., O'Flynn, J., & Lorenz, D. J. (2010). Bruising characteristics discriminating physical child abuse from accidental trauma. *Pediatrics, 125*(4), 861.

Poole, M. K., Seal, D. W., & Taylor, C. A. (2014). A systematic review of universal campaigns targeting child physical abuse prevention. *Health Education Research, 29*(3), 388–432.

Reynolds, A. J., & Roberston, D. L. (2003). School-based early intervention and later child maltreatment in the Chicago Longitudinal Study. *Child Development, 7491,* 3–26.

Roesler, T. A. (2015). Medical child abuse/Munchausen by proxy. *The Encyclopedia of Clinical Psychology.* Retrieved from http:// onlinelibrary.wiley.com/doi/10.1002/9781118625392.wbecp087/full

Tomkia, S. (2010). Bruises in children: Normal or child abuse? *Journal of Pediatric Health Care, 24*(4), 216–221.

U.S. Department of Health and Human Services, Administration for Children and Families (2012). Child maltreatment 2012. Retrieved from http://www.acf.hhs.gov/sites/default/files/cb/cm2012.pdf

U.S. Department of Health and Human Services, Administration for Children and Families (2014). Reporting child abuse and neglect. Retrieved from https://childwelfare.gov/responding/reporting.cfm

U.S. Department of Health and Human Services, Children's Bureau. (2015). Mandatory reporters of child abuse and neglect. Retrieved from https://www.childwelfare.gov/pubPDFs/manda.pdf

World Health Organization. (2014). Global status report on violence prevention. Retrieved from http://www.who.int /violence_injury_prevention/violence/status_report/2014/en/

UNIT VI

Concept-Based Care in Pediatrics

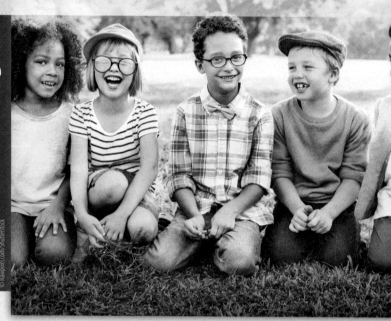

© Rawpixel.com/Shutterstock

CHAPTER 14

Gastrointestinal Elimination

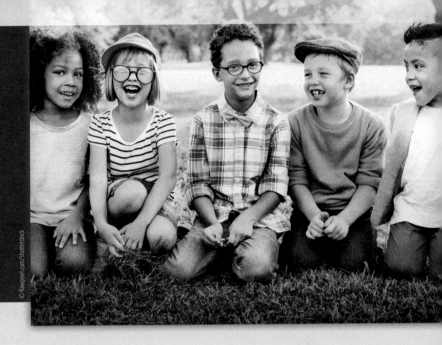

© Rawpixel.com/Shutterstock

LEARNING OBJECTIVES

1. Apply key nursing concepts used in caring for a child with an elimination disorder or condition.
2. Analyze observed behaviors against the expected patterns of elimination across childhood in a clinical setting.
3. Apply developmental perspectives to children who have elimination disorders.
4. Analyze safety concerns for the child with an elimination disorder, including dehydration and electrolyte imbalances.
5. Assess for complications associated with common structural disorders within the gastrointestinal system, including hernias and anorectal malformations.
6. Critically evaluate common health concerns within the concept of gastrointestinal elimination obstructive disorders, including intussusception, Hirschsprung disease, and hypertrophic pyloric stenosis.
7. Critically evaluate common health concerns within the concept of gastrointestinal elimination inflammatory disorders, including appendicitis and celiac disease.
8. Assess for signs distinguishing the two inflammatory bowel diseases of Crohn disease and ulcerative colitis.
9. Analyze care practices needed for safe care of a newborn who presents with hyperbilirubinemia.

KEY TERMS

Acute diarrhea
Anorectal malformations
Chronic diarrhea
Constipation
Crohn disease
Dehydration
Hernia
Hirschsprung disease
Hyperbilirubinemia
Hypertonic
Hypertrophic pyloric stenosis
Hypotonic
Intussusception
Isotonic
Kernicterus
Reflux
Ulcerative colitis
Vomiting

Introduction

The gastrointestinal (GI) system, extending from the mouth to the anus, provides the child with nutrition, fluid balance, and elimination. This system comprises the organs of digestion along with several accessory organs—the liver, pancreas, and gallbladder. Disorders of the GI system relate specifically to a disruption of the absorption or elimination function. Disorders are generally categorized as either primary (congenital or acquired) or secondary. Furthermore, disorders of the GI system are organized into three major and distinct areas: obstructive disorders, infectious/inflammatory disorders, and structural disorders. Many GI disorders disrupt children's nutritional intake and put them at risk for malnutrition, delayed growth and development, and failure to thrive. A pediatric healthcare team approach is needed to assist families through the early identification, diagnostic exams, and treatments for disorders of the gastrointestinal system, as many of these disorders require lengthy treatment regimens and some are lifelong diagnoses.

The development of the GI system begins in the fourth fetal week of gestation. As part of this development, the intestinal lining forms multiple layers, including the epithelium, mucosa with goblet mucus-producing cells, submucosa, circular muscular layer, longitudinal muscular layer, and serosa (intraperitoneal) and adventitia (retroperitoneal) (**Figure 14-1**). An intact mucosa layer is critical to lubricate the intestines and prevent first the infant and then the child from damage caused by normal digestive enzymes.

One critical aspect of the development of the newborn's host defenses is the colonization of the intestinal tract with bacteria (especially *Bacteroides*) that produce vitamin K.

Owing to their immature host defenses, newborns have a higher (though rare) risk of bleeding due to their innately low levels of vitamin K, which is required for coagulation processes. This bleeding disorder—which is vitamin K deficiency bleeding (VKDB)—is most concerning if the newborn experiences bleeding into the brain or intestines. Only very small quantities of vitamin K are required for adequate blood coagulation, however, and development of a vitamin K deficiency is unlikely once bacteria have colonized the infant's intestine and during the remainder of the life span. Only severe dietary deficiencies, such as those associated with cystic fibrosis, are apt to trigger the need for vitamin K administration. Neonates remain at the greatest risk for this condition due to their endogenous (low intestinal colonization) and exogenous (poor placental provisions) deficiencies (Lippi & Franchini, 2011).

Gastrointestinal System Function Across Childhood

The GI tract, also called the alimentary canal, is a lengthy tube beginning at the mouth and ending at the anus. This tract is responsible for the functions of swallowing, digesting, secreting digestive enzymes, absorbing a variety of nutrients, absorbing and secreting body fluids, and elimination. Each developmental stage has challenges and expectations for mastery related to growth and development of the GI system.

- *Newborns (birth to 28 days):* The newborn must master how to suck reflexively, swallow, digest, and absorb and eliminate nutrition and fluids. Newborns do not have saliva, nor do they initially produce adequate digestive enzymes (i.e., amylase, lipase, and trypsin) until they reach 4 months of age. Infants do not swallow voluntarily until they are 6 weeks old. The lower GI tract is relatively shorter in the newborn and early infancy period; due to the decreased intestinal surface area available to reabsorb water, newborns have more watery and looser stools compared to older children.
- *Infants (1 month to 1 year):* Through coordinated and voluntary swallowing, the infant must learn to pace feeding and not choke. The infant learns to eat new foods, progressing from a breast milk or formula-exclusive diet to the addition of iron-fortified cereals (maternal-derived iron stores are depleted by 6 months of age), to the addition of first vegetables, then fruits, then proteins.
- *Toddlers:* The young toddler has the challenge of becoming ready for and then mastering bowel control (toilet training) by controlling his or her elimination at will. Each child has his or her own

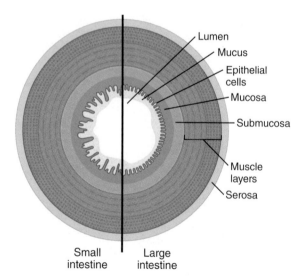

Figure 14-1 *The layers of GI mucosa.*

time frame for toilet training, but most children master bowel control by age 3 years. The age range is wide, however—from 1 to 5 years. Mastery of bowel control is typically required before a young child attends preschool. Toddlers have slowed growth patterns and require fewer calories than they did during infancy. They may appear finicky and experience food "jags" or "lags."

- *Preschoolers:* By the end of the preschool period, the child's intestinal tract is mature and produces adult-like stools. This is also a time of slower growth and development, along with fewer calorie needs.
- *School age and older:* It is not until the 6th year of life that a child has adequate amounts and full strength of hydrochloric acid in the stomach. The GI tract is fully mature and the child may pass one stool a day that is fully formed.

Assessment of the Gastrointestinal System

The assessment of the pediatric GI system begins with a pertinent family health history, then progresses to questions related to GI illnesses, surgeries, injuries, or accidents. Physical assessment includes height; weight; abdominal circumference (measure at the end of a respiratory expiration, with a tape placed horizontally at the tip of the iliac crest, snug but not tight); hydration status, including mucous membrane moisture, turgor, and presence of tears; and quality of the child's peripheral pulses.

The sequence of physical assessment in this system is important. Notably, if the child is experiencing acute pain, palpation should be performed last. The nurse should begin with a visual assessment of the child's abdomen, noting whether it is concave or convex. Next, the nurse should measure the circumference of the abdomen, followed by auscultation, percussion, and finally light to deep palpation. At the bedside, the pediatric nurse should weigh all diapers produced by newborns and toddlers (**Figure 14-2**).

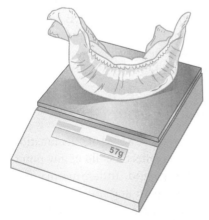

Figure 14-2 *The pediatric nurse should weigh all diapers produced by newborns and toddlers.*

The weight of the dry diaper is subtracted from the weight of the soiled diaper for accurate measurement of output.

To assess the GI tract, the pediatric healthcare team can use a variety of tools and diagnostics, including barium enemas to visualize the entire large intestine, upper GI radiography, small bowel follow-through to view the upper intestines, cholangiography to examine the gallbladder, and liver biopsy to investigate disease and neoplasm. Additional assessments include serum chemistry, liver and lipid profiles, erythrocyte sedimentation rate (ESR), C-reactive protein (CRP), stool examination for ova and parasites, presence of elevated white blood cell (WBC) count, reducing substances, and stool culture for specific pathogens. Fecal fat may be collected to rule out fat metabolism disorders.

Pain in the Gastrointestinal System

Abdominal pain is considered the number one complaint across childhood. Most abdominal pain has no known etiology and resolves without intervention. Nevertheless, abdominal pain during childhood is real and needs to be evaluated. Stress during childhood, including school difficulties, peer pressure, social interactions, and family dynamics, can lead a child to complain of stomachaches.

To evaluate a child's pain, the nurse should obtain a thorough health history and description of the chief complaint, including its timing, influencing factors, triggers, and severity. Pediatric pain tools should be used to ascertain the location and severity of the pain. Subjective pain tools such as the FACES tool, objective pain tools such as the Objective Pain Score (Tandon et al., 2016), and physiological measurements of vital signs should all be used to assess a child's complaint of abdominal pain.

QUALITY AND SAFETY

If an acute condition is suspected, such as appendicitis, active bleeding, or intestinal rupture, the pediatric nurse should not perform palpation due to the possibility of inflicting further trauma. For instance, if a child presents with a suspected ruptured appendix, a sign can be hung on the child's crib or bed stating "Do Not Palpate Child's Abdomen" until final confirmation has been established.

Nursing Care of a Child with a Gastrointestinal System Disorder

Many GI system disorders affecting nutrition and elimination require lengthy and complex management. Some disorders require several surgeries to establish normal or near-normal function. Congenital disorders such as anorectal malformations can require early surgical interventions and pose risks for complications. Some GI disorders cause complications in the genitourinary system (rectal-vaginal fistulas) and the respiratory system (tracheal-esophageal atresia). A child with a serious biliary atresia may suffer failure to thrive and develop severe complications including need for liver transplantation.

Older children with GI system disorders may be very emotionally vulnerable owing to the presence of a condition affecting the elimination tract. A disorder that causes acute diarrhea or constipation, or requires a structural diversion such as an ostomy, may lead the child to experience low self-esteem and poor body image. It is imperative that the pediatric nurse demonstrate no evidence of judgment or negativity and be supportive and caring.

Dehydration

Many disorders related to elimination cause a child to become dehydrated, a condition in which fluid loss exceeds fluid intake. **Dehydration** can be assessed by determining a child's loss of weight compared to weight prior to the illness:

- *Mild* dehydration is defined as a weight of 5% or less in infants and a 3% to 4% weight loss in children.
- *Moderate* dehydration is defined as 10% weight loss in infants and 6% to 8% weight loss in children.
- *Severe* dehydration is defined as 15% weight loss in infants and 10% weight loss in children.

Several measurement tools are available for assessing dehydration—the World Health Organization (WHO) scale, the Gorelick scale, and the Clinical Dehydration Scale (CDS), to name a few (Pringle et al., 2011). Efforts to validate them have produced mixed results. In general, however, four factors are most likely to predict dehydration well: delayed capillary refill time (more than 2 seconds suggests dehydration), skin turgor, abnormal respiratory pattern, and a generally ill appearance characterized by lack of moisture in the mucous membranes. Presence of at least two of these signs suggests a fluid deficit of 5% or greater, particularly if they are observed in combination of caregiver reports of lower-than-normal tear production or the presence of vomiting or diarrhea (Canavan & Arant, 2009).

In general, three types of dehydration are distinguished:

- **Isotonic:**
  - Equal loss of water and sodium occurs; serum sodium is normal (130–150 mEq/L).
  - The majority of the fluid lost is extracellular.
  - Hypovolemic shock can occur.
- **Hypotonic:**
  - The child's electrolyte loss exceeds the water loss; serum sodium is less than 130 mEq/L.
  - The majority of fluid shifts are extracellular to intracellular.

- **Hypertonic:**
  - The child's body water loss is greater than the electrolyte loss; serum sodium is more than 150 mEq/L.
  - The majority of fluid shifts are intracellular to extracellular.

PHARMACOLOGY

Oral rehydration, as described later in the "Acute Diarrhea" section, is the first choice in most situations. If oral rehydration is not an option, however, rehydrate children with isotonic and hypotonic dehydration relatively rapidly with fluid boluses of 0.9% normal saline (NS) and ongoing intravenous fluids (IVF). *Do not use this technique to rapidly replace fluids in case of hypertonic dehydration*, as it can lead to severe and even fatal cerebral edema.

Structural Disorders

Structural disorders include those that affect the physical structures of the GI system. Disorders that interfere with profusion, absorption, and elimination can be found anywhere along the alimentary tract. Examples of structural disorders are presented in **Table 14-1**.

FAMILY EDUCATION

The pediatric healthcare team and the parents can use the ESSR method for feeding an infant with a cleft palate: Enlarged nipple, Stimulate suck by gently rubbing the nipple on the infant's lower lip, Swallow, Rest.

Obstructive Disorders

Pediatric GI obstructive disorders prevent a child from having normal and expected patterns of elimination. Some of these disorders are so severe that no food passes from the stomach to the small intestine and no stool passes through the intestines. Several common obstructive orders are profiled in **Table 14-2**.

Inflammatory Disorders

Disorders that produce a level of inflammation that causes tissue damage can affect a child at any point during the developmental period. Inflammatory disorders can cause significant pain and are associated with serious complications, including infection and sepsis. Examples of common inflammatory disorders in children can be found in **Table 14-3**.

TABLE 14-1   Structural Disorders

Hernia

Diagnosis: A diaphragmatic **hernia** is a protrusion of abdominal contents (intestines) through an opening in the diaphragm muscle. Its etiology is a congenital disorder of the transverse septum and inability of the pleuroperitoneal folds to fully develop in utero. In general, the intestines and abdominal structures enter the thoracic cavity. Other hernias, such umbilical and inguinal, are caused by weakened abdominal musculature that leads to tissue and intestinal protrusion (**Figure 14-3**).

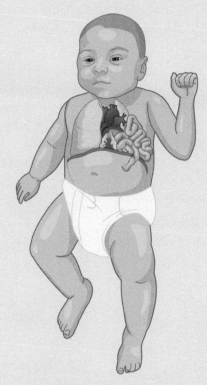

Figure 14-3 *A diaphragmatic hernia.*

Risk Factors: There are no known risk factors for the development of hernias. With diaphragmatic hernias, the fetus is at risk for impaired lung growth, and the newborn is at risk for respiratory compromise.

Treatment: Surgery is required for repair of most hernias, although some small umbilical hernias resolve spontaneously. The type of nursing care needed depends on the type of hernia and its extent as well as the impacts on other affected organs (e.g., the lungs and heart in diaphragmatic hernia, the intestines in inguinal hernia). Most hernias are addressed as soon as possible to avoid complications, so family education related to risks and benefits of surgery will be needed (Hatfield, 2014).

Anorectal Malformations: Imperforate Anus

Diagnosis: Anorectal malformations include congenital absence of a patent anorectal canal, a severe narrowing of the anal canal, or the presence of only a fistula (external to the peritoneum). An immediate assessment of patency is performed when a malformation has been identified during the immediate post-birth time frame or if the newborn fails to pass meconium stool.

Risk Factors: Because this condition is associated with many congenital syndromes, a geneticist may be contacted to rule out other conditions.

Treatment: Treatment consists of surgical repair. In some infants, the blockage is a thin membrane that can be repaired immediately. If the defect is more significant, the child may have a colostomy performed as an initial measure, with a more extensive surgical repair being planned when the child reaches 3 to 5 months of age. In such cases, the family will need education on colostomy care (Hatfield, 2014).

(continues)

TABLE 14-1 Structural Disorders *(continued)*

Gastroesophageal Reflux (GER)

Diagnosis: Regurgitation (**reflux**) of gastric contents into the esophagus due to the incompetence or relaxation of the lower esophageal sphincter causes the child to experience pain. When the condition progresses to esophageal tissue damage (esophagitis) due to the low pH of the gastric acid, the condition is called gastrointestinal reflux disease (GERD). Other possible GERD symptoms include nausea, chest pain, tooth erosion, halitosis, and respiratory complications from stomach acid entering into the lungs (pneumonia, laryngitis, asthma, hoarseness) (National Institute of Diabetes and Digestive and Kidney Diseases, 2015).

Risk Factors: Risk factors for the development of GER include prematurity and delayed maturation of the lower esophageal neuromuscular function.

Treatment: Most GER will resolve on its own. If tissue damage occurs and GERD is developing, the child will need surgical interventions (Nissen fundoplication, in which the gastric fundus is wrapped around the distal esophagus structure to remove the damaged tissue; **Figure 14-4**). Postsurgical nursing care includes maintaining the integrity of suture lines and preventing and managing pain, nausea, and vomiting. Caregivers should receive education in the 2 weeks following surgery regarding home care so as to avoid complications (Hazan, Gamarra, Stawick, & Maas, 2009).

The infant with GER or GERD may benefit from smaller, more frequent feedings and positioning prone with the head elevated after feeds.

Medications given for GI reflux include the following agents:

› Histamine blockers such as ranitidine and famotidine

› Proton-pump inhibitors such as lansoprazole and omeprazole

› Prokinetic agents to rapidly empty the stomach

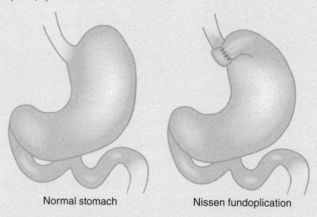

Normal stomach   Nissen fundoplication

Figure 14-4 *Nissen fundoplication.*

Cleft Lip/Cleft Palate

Diagnosis: Cleft lip and cleft palate are two distinctly different disorders that arise during fetal development at different times. Cleft lip arises in the 7th week of gestation when facial tissue fails to join completely; it can involve a small notch in the upper lip or can extend to complete separation from the lip to the nose (**Figure 14-5**). Cleft palate arises in the 9th week of gestation; it consists of cleft in the soft palate, in the hard palate, or extending through both (**Figure 14-6**). Diagnosis of these two conditions is made via visual inspection of the neonate.

Risk Factors: The prevalence of cleft lip is approximately 1 per 1000 live births. It is much more common in boys than in girls, and is correlated with hereditary, teratogenic, and environmental factors. Cleft palate is less common, occurring in 1 in every 2500 live births.

TABLE 14-1 Structural Disorders (*continued*)

Treatment: Surgery is required for both cleft lip and cleft palate. Nursing care focuses on assessing for problems with feeding and the development of respiratory complications, as aspiration and choking are common in children with these disorders. Postoperative care includes carefully maintaining the integrity of the suture lines, which will include a Logan bow (**Figure 14-7**). The use of elbow restraints is often recommended, although there is no evidence of their benefit (Huth, Petersen, & Lehman, 2013); however, no pacifiers, fingers, straws, spoons or any utensils can be used in the postoperative period for at least 7 days.

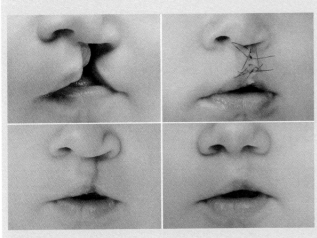

Figure 14-5 *Cleft lip.*
© malost/Shutterstock

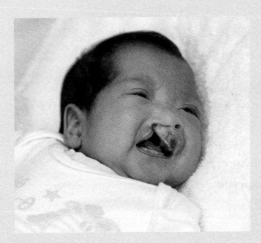

Figure 14-6 *Cleft palate.*
© PeopleImages/E+/Getty

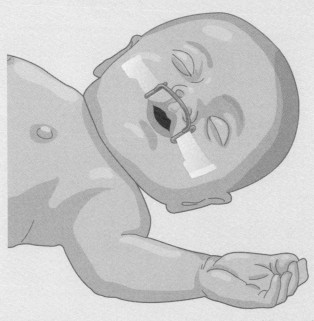

Figure 14-7 *A Logan bow is used to help maintain integrity of the suture lines.*

TABLE 14-2   Obstructive Disorders

Hypertrophic Pyloric Stenosis

Diagnosis: Hyphertrophic pyloric stenosis is the enlargement of the circular areas of muscle that surround the pyloric valve; this hypertrophy blocks gastric emptying. After reaching approximately 3 weeks of age, the infant will present with increasing vomiting, which progresses to (potentially blood-tinged) projectile vomiting. The pediatric healthcare team may also identify the hypertrophic tissue mass as an olive-shaped mass in the right upper abdominal quadrant. The child may present with visible peristalsis in the abdomen after eating and may also have dehydration and failure to thrive. The child may be very fussy, colicky, hungry after vomiting, distended, and in distress. Most vomiting occurs immediately after eating. Metabolic alkalosis may be present due to loss of hydrochloric acid.

Risk Factors: There are no known risk factors for this condition.

Treatment: Surgical intervention is required to reduce the muscular hypertrophied tissue. In a pyloromyotomy, the muscle is typically split with an incision along the anterior pylorus muscle. Preoperative care should include correction of fluid deficits and electrolyte imbalance, as these steps have been found to improve outcomes and reduce hospital stays (Wetherill, Melling, Rhodes, Wilkinson, & Kenny, 2015). Postoperative care includes monitoring of vital signs, lab values, and respiratory and hydration status, while assessing wound healing of surgical or laparoscopic incisions. If oral food intake has not resumed before discharge, parents will need education and written feeding instructions (James, Nelson, & Ashwill, 2013).

Intussusception

Diagnosis: The diagnosis of **intussusception** is made when a child presents with an acute abdomen and radiographs demonstrate an invagination or telescoping of a segment of bowel into a section just distal. Children may present with acute abdominal pain that causes them to pull their knees to their chest as the pain comes and goes every 15-20 minutes lasting longer with time (Mayo Clinic, 2016). This process usually occurs at the junction of the ileum with the lower colon. The most common age for clinical presentation of intussusception is between 5 months and 3 years, with 60% of patients being younger than 1 year at diagnosis. Children may present with classic symptoms of bloody mucus stool (also referred to as red "currant jelly" stool) due to the obstructive nature of the process, dehydration, pain, distention, and vomiting (**Figure 14-8**).

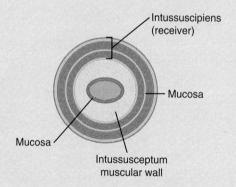

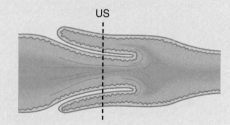

Figure 14-8 *Intussusception.*

TABLE 14-2   Obstructive Disorders (*continued*)

Risk Factors: Risk factors include age (young children), gender (more common in boys) family history, and prior history of intussusceptions. The child may have experienced hyperactive peristalsis in the proximal portion of the bowel structure, with overly inactive peristalsis in the distal intestinal segment. Both cystic fibrosis and celiac disease are risk factors for intussusception, although most cases have no known risk factors and the cause is unknown.

Treatment: Treatment focuses on reducing the telescoping or invagination of the bowel, often with a barium enema or hydrostatic (water) enema. Ultrasound is typically used to determine the presence of this condition as well as the success of the reduction. Intussusception can cause severe edema and cut off blood supply, leading to ischemia and tissue death in the bowel, which in turn requires emergency medical care. Care prior to therapeutic reduction should include assessment for dehydration, shock, and sepsis; fever, tachycardia, respiratory distress, and alterations in consciousness or blood pressure being high-priority indicators of sepsis. Postreduction nursing care includes initiation of clear fluids and gradual reintroduction of normal diet, along with monitoring for signs of success of the procedure, including passage of stool without blood and resumption of normal activities without pain. Failure of reduction requires the child (and family) to be prepared for surgical intervention. Caregivers should be educated about signs of recurrence, as intussusception recurs in approximately 10% of successful reductions and 2% to 5% of patients who undergo surgical correction (James et al., 2013).

Hirschsprung Disease (Congenital Aganglionic Megacolon)

Diagnosis: Hirschsprung disease is a structural anomaly of the lower segment of the large intestine and rectum. Its formal name of congenital aganglionic megacolon reflects its presentation (Hatfield, 2014): The condition is characterized by a lack of ganglion cells (nerve tissue) in the rectum and lower colon that prevents peristalsis (hence "aganglionic"). This segment of the bowel is narrower than it should be, which causes the section of bowel above it to become enlarged and filled with gas and fecal matter (hence "megacolon"). Definitive diagnosis is made via rectal tissue biopsy, which will identify a lack of nerve tissue (**Figure 14-9**). Affected children will pass ribbon-like, foul-smelling stools. A key indicator of this condition is the lack of passage of stool in the newborn within 2 days.

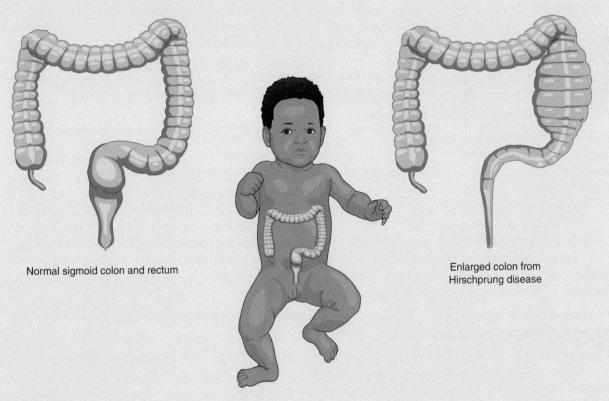

Normal sigmoid colon and rectum

Enlarged colon from Hirschprung disease

Figure 14-9 *Features of Hirschprung disease compared to the normal sigmoid colon and rectum.*

(continues)

TABLE 14-2 Obstructive Disorders (*continued*)

Risk Factors: There are no known risk factors for congenital Hirschsprung disease.

Treatment: Treatment for this condition is surgery. Either the surgeon will perform a double-barrel colostomy to cut the aganglionic section out and allow the megacolon time to heal and decrease in size, followed by a re-anastomosis, or the child will have a rectal pull-through procedure in which the aganglionic segment of bowel is removed (D'Cunha Burkardt, Graham, Short, & Frykman, 2013). Although children used to have multiple staged surgeries, single-stage surgeries involving a resection and pull-through via laparoscopic procedures is now more frequently performed (Huang, Tolley, Blakely, & Langham, 2013). Nursing assessments focus on nutritional deficits, constipation, and coping capacity of the family confronted with a serious illness in the newborn (Hatfield, 2014). If the aganglionic portion extends to the small intestine, an ileostomy will be performed and the child may need sodium supplementation due to the loss of liquid stool through the ileostomy (O'Neil, Teitelbaum, & Harris, 2014). Postoperative nursing goals include maintaining fluid balance and skin integrity, pain management, and preparing the family for home care of the child (Hatfield, 2014).

TABLE 14-3 Inflammatory Disorders

Appendicitis

Diagnosis: Appendicitis is the inflammation and infection of the appendix's vermiform, a small lymphoid tissue sac located at the end of the cecum. The inflammation and infection result from obstruction of the opening of the lumen by hardened fecal material, microbes, parasites, or foreign bodies. The subsequent accumulation of mucus causes the structure to become distended; venous engorgement occurs and pressure increases. Appendicitis can progress to rupture and peritonitis. The child may present with the classic pain picture: local right lower quadrant pain at McBurney's point (just anterior and proximal to the lower ascending colon).

Risk Factors: There are no known risk factors for appendicitis.

Treatment: Treatment for appendicitis may be antibiotics, with or without surgery. A sudden relief of the persistent pain may mean the appendix has ruptured. If antibiotic therapy is used, nursing care includes management of caregiver anxiety (which will likely be considerable) as well as management of the patient's pain and fever. Monitor for dehydration and sudden cessation of pain (which often means rupture and increased risk of complications). If surgery is indicated, relieving fear, managing pain, and maintaining fluid balance are primary preoperative goals; postoperative recovery is generally without incident, but caregivers should be educated about home care and signs of complications such as peritonitis (Hatfield, 2014).

Celiac Disease (Gluten-Sensitivity Enteropathy)

Diagnosis: In celiac disease (a condition that is becoming more common), the child has a gluten-sensitive enteropathy that leads to malabsorption due to an immune-mediated enteropathy (inflammation of tissues and gastric/intestinal villi atrophy). The child cannot digest glutenin, gliadin, or proteins from wheat, barley, rye, and sometimes oats. The child may present with steatorrhea (fatty, bulky, greasy, and malodorous stools), distention, abdominal pain, anemia, and growth delay. During a celiac crisis, the child may present with severe diarrhea, dehydration, metabolic acidosis, and electrolyte disturbances. Extra-intestinal manifestations may include osteoporosis, arthralgia, peripheral neuropathies, cardiomyopathy, and anemia. The condition is considered an autoimmune disorder requiring multiple screening tools via biopsies and seriological tests (Ryan & Grossman, 2011). A diagnosis is made by a 72-hour fecal fat collection and lab analysis of total immunoglobulin A (IgA), antigliadin antibody (AGA), and reticulin antibody levels. A biopsy of mucosal tissue for an assessment of villi atrophy and flat surfaces is diagnostic.

Risk Factors: Both environmental factors and an inherited predisposition are risk factors for celiac disease. Children also may have an abnormal immunologic reaction.

Treatment: Lifelong dietary modifications are the most important consideration in treating celiac disease. Diets considered "gluten-free" can still incorporate grains, such as rice, corn, 100% cornmeal (some commercial "cornmeal" preparations contain wheat products), and gluten-free wheat flour. Note that some nonfood products, such as cosmetics or medications, may include gluten. Caregivers should be instructed in how to examine labels and avoid gluten-containing products, as the child with celiac disease must adhere to gluten avoidance guidelines. Long-term compliance with a gluten-free diet can be assessed by following a child's celiac disease-related antibodies (serological testing) (Nachman et al., 2011). Children may need mineral and vitamin supplements such as A, D, E, and K vitamins, as well as iron and folic acid.

TABLE 14-3   Inflammatory Disorders *(continued)*

Crohn Disease

Diagnosis: A child with **Crohn disease** (inflammation of all layers of the GI mucosa, affecting any portion of the GI tract) will experience increased hyperemia in the GI mucosa, easy bleeding of the intestinal wall, and ulceration of the GI tract (any part). The child may present with diarrhea, weight loss, bloody stools, abdominal pain, anemia, dehydration, and fever. Diagnosis is made by mucosal biopsy during a colonoscopy, stool analysis for blood, and blood analysis for complete blood count (CBC), ESR, albumin and total protein. The typical presentation of ulcers associated with Crohn disease consists of "skip" lesions with normal tissue found on either side. As the disease progresses, ulcers merge to form star-shaped "stellate" ulcers; in advanced disease, a "cobblestone" appearance is present (Richards, 2015). Some children with acute disease have extra-intestinal manifestations such as joint swelling, joint pain, rashes, mouth sores, inflammation of the eyes, kidney stones, inflamed pancreas, bone disease, and abnormal liver function tests.

Risk Factors: There is no exact etiology or known risk factors for Crohn disease.

Treatment: Children with an acute episode of Crohn disease will need rest, fluids, and anti-inflammatory medications. In severe conditions, a partial colectomy may be required to surgically remove the ulcerated bowel tissue; this procedure has been found to be curative for some children with Crohn disease. Children with malnutrition symptoms may be placed on IV total parenteral nutrition (TPN) and lipids. Changes in diet are required, including eliminating consumption of foods that are associated with increasing ulcerations and discomfort—specifically, sharp cheeses; highly spiced foods; salted, blackened, or smoked meats; raw fruits; raw vegetables; and fried foods.

Ulcerative Colitis

Diagnosis: Unlike Crohn disease, **ulcerative colitis** (UC) is localized to the colon (i.e., inflammation of the colonic mucosa). Children with UC present with urgent diarrhea, weight loss, bloody stools, abdominal pain, anemia, dehydration, and fever. Diagnosis is made by mucosal biopsy during a colonoscopy, stool analysis for blood, and blood analysis for CBC, ESR, albumin, and total protein. The classic presentation of ulcerative colitis consists of continuous ulcers (not skip lesions, as in Crohn disease), with only the innermost layer of the bowel mucosa being affected; lesions generally start proximal to the rectum and extend up into the bowel over time (Hindryckx, Jairath, & D'Haens, 2016). Children with acute exacerbations can have as many as 10 stools per day. Extra-intestinal manifestations of ulcerative colitis can include joint pain, rashes, and abnormal liver function tests.

Risk Factors: There is no exact etiology or known risk factors for ulcerative colitis.

Treatment: Children with an acute episode of ulcerative colitis will need rest, fluids, and anti-inflammatory medications. In severe cases, a partial colectomy may be required to surgically remove the ulcerated bowel tissue. Children with malnutrition symptoms may be placed on IV TPN and lipids. Changes in diet are required, including eliminating consumption of foods that are associated with increasing ulcerations and discomfort—specifically, sharp cheeses; highly spiced foods; salted, blackened, or smoked meats; raw fruits; raw vegetables; and fried foods.

PHARMACOLOGY

Medications Used to Treat Chronic Inflammation of the GI Tract

Drugs used to treat inflammatory bowel disease are categorized into three types:

- Mild symptoms: aminosalicylates
  - Mesalamine (Asacol, Lialda, Rowasa, Canasa)
  - Sulfasalazine (Azulfidine)
- Moderate symptoms: corticosteroids
  - Prednisolone (Orapred)
  - Prednisone (Sterapred)
- Severe symptoms: immunomodulators
  - Infliximab infusion (Remicade)

Functional Disorders

Common functional disorders of the GI system include diarrhea, vomiting, and constipation. These disorders can be mild, requiring support that can be provided at home, or they can be significant enough to cause moderate dehydration, leading to the need for interventions in the clinic setting, or severe dehydration, requiring hospitalization and monitoring. Constipation can be either mild or severe enough to require further diagnosis for the etiology and medical treatment.

Acute Diarrhea

Diagnosis

Acute diarrhea has many potential causes, including exposure to infectious agents such as bacteria, viruses, or parasites. Antibiotic use and the presence of an upper respiratory infection or a urinary tract infection may cause acute diarrhea in some children. Infectious gastroenteritis, also called acute gastroenteritis (AGE), can cause significant dehydration. Pathogens implicated in acute diarrhea include rotavirus, *Escherichia coli*, *Clostridium difficile*, *Salmonella enterica*, and *Giardia lamblia*. Signs and symptoms of acute diarrhea include the following manifestations:

- Increased intestinal motility and rapid emptying, leading to frequent loose or liquid stools that may be foul smelling
- Dry, pale skin with poor turgor (tenting of skin) and dry mucous membranes due to loss of water
- Weakness associated with electrolyte imbalances (sodium and potassium)
- Decreased urine output
- Change in vital signs including tachycardia; tachypnea can occur with severe dehydration causing acidosis, and hypotension can occur with severe dehydration
- Increased thirst
- Acid-base imbalances, including alkalosis due to buffered bicarbonate loss

Risk Factors

Children who have traveled, attend daycare centers, live in substandard housing lacking proper sanitation, have been exposed to a causative agent, or have poor hand hygiene are at risk for acute diarrhea. **Chronic diarrhea** is typically associated with malabsorption syndrome, lactose intolerance, inflammatory bowel disease, and food allergens.

Treatment

Treatment for acute diarrhea should start prior to a definitive diagnosis if the child is becoming dehydrated from frequent loose or watery stools. Oral rehydration therapy should be initiated or, if the child unable to take oral fluids, IV replacement therapy should be started. Administration of oral rehydrating solution (ORS) should begin at a rate of 40 to 50 mL/kg per 24 hours, with an additional replacement for each diarrheal stool given at 10 mL/kg. Medications will be specific for the etiology of the acute diarrhea isolated in stool cultures. Commonly used medications include metronidazole (Flagyl) and sulfamethoxazole-trimethoprim (Bactrim or Septra). Oral fluids should not contain sugar. Fruit juices, sodas, gelatin, or any fluids with caffeine should be avoided.

UNIQUE FOR KIDS

Introducing Fluids and Foods in a Child with a Diagnosis of Diarrhea or Vomiting

Children with vomiting can benefit from an NPO (nil per os, meaning "nothing by mouth") status until vomiting stops for a period of time. In young children with diarrhea, breastfeeding should be continued if possible.

An electrolyte-based oral rehydration fluid such as Pedialyte is often used first in children with vomiting or diarrhea. If tolerated, favorite fluids can be mixed with oral rehydration fluids; in infancy, the rehydration fluids can be mixed with formula or breast milk. Products such as Pedialyte also come in gelatin and popsicles. After oral fluids are established, the BRATTY diet can be introduced (though it remains controversial due to its low nutritional value):

- Bananas
- Rice cereal or dry cereal of choice (e.g., Cheerios)
- Applesauce without added sugar (sugar can cause fluid to enter the bowel, increasing diarrhea)
- Toast without butter
- Tea: caffeine-free herbal varieties (e.g., chamomile)
- Yogurt: plain or with low-sugar fruit flavors

Constipation

Diagnosis

Constipation is a term used to denote the infrequent and difficult passage of stool. Each child has a unique stooling pattern, so it is imperative to ask the family to describe the child's normal stooling process. Constipation is typically diagnosed when a child has difficulty passing a series of small, hard stools while experiencing abdominal pain and possibly cramping.

Risk Factors

Children who have limited daily fluid intake, sedentary lifestyles, and poor fiber intake are at risk for developing constipation. Other risk factors can include the consumption of foods known to cause hardened stool, such as excessive dairy products. Severe and chronic constipation may be associated with lead poisoning, underactive thyroid function, celiac disease, and abnormal serum calcium levels (Tabbers et al., 2014).

Treatment

Dietary changes to increase fiber are considered first in children with constipation. These changes include increased intake of fresh fruits, dried fruits, vegetables, whole high-fiber grains, and oral fluids. If these measures are not successful in relieving constipation, the next step is to administer medications that increase water release (stool softeners) into the bowel, followed by the use of enemas to assist in the expelling of the hard stool, followed by laxatives that increase peristalsis.

Vomiting

Diagnosis

Vomiting—the forceful expulsion of gastric contents through the mouth—is very common in young children. It is quite often self-limiting, with rapid resolution.

Risk Factors

Factors associated with vomiting include infectious disease, toxic material ingestion, allergy, obstruction, or increased intracranial pressure (ICP). Vomiting can also be psychogenic in nature. When vomiting is also associated with fever and diarrhea, an acute infectious process should be ruled out.

Treatment

Treatment for vomiting is typically not needed unless the experience persists, leading to complications such as dehydration, electrolyte imbalances, aspiration and, with extensive vomiting, malnutrition or failure to thrive.

Other Disorders Affecting Elimination

Hyperbilirubinemia

Hyperbilirubinemia, or jaundice, refers to a yellow discoloration of the skin caused by the deposition of unconjugated bilirubin in the skin. Bilirubin is an oily substance that must be processed by the liver (conjugated) and excreted by the kidneys; it plays a role in the breakdown of red blood cells. Adequate serum protein is required to transport bilirubin from the body to the liver, where it is transformed into a water-soluble substance and eliminated in the urine or feces.

Diagnosis

Serum bilirubin levels are taken during the newborn period via laboratory analysis of blood obtained from a heel stick. Normal expected levels are less than 5 mg/dL for newborns; the diagnosis of hyperbilirubinemia is made when the serum level reaches or exceeds 15 mg/dL (Porter & Dennis, 2002). Both direct bilirubin levels (bilirubin that is bound to serum protein and can be excreted) and indirect bilirubin levels (bilirubin that is circulating in blood) may be drawn.

Risk Factors

Jaundice in the newborn period is common. There are four types of jaundice:

- *Breastfeeding jaundice:* This type occurs when a newborn's total intake of breast milk is insufficient to provide enough protein to transport bilirubin. The incidence is between 5% and 10% of all newborns.
- *Physiological jaundice:* The most common type of jaundice, this condition affects as many as 50% of all newborns. In physiological jaundice, the immature liver is unable to process the quantity of bilirubin transported. Jaundice first appears in the second or third day of life and decreases and disappears by the end of the first to second week of life.
- *Breast milk jaundice:* This type of jaundice is relatively rare, accounting for less than 1% of all cases. In this condition, a substance found in the mother's milk causes an increased uptake of bilirubin back into the infant's bloodstream from the intestines, where it is being secreted. Levels are typically not harmful, but the jaundice can persist for 3 to 11 weeks.
- *Blood group (Rh or ABO) incompatibility:* The sudden and severe hemolysis associated with blood group incompatibility causes the most severe form of jaundice.

PHARMACOLOGY

To prevent severe hyperbilirubinemia associated with blood group incompatibility, the mother should receive a Rhogam intramuscular (IM) injection within 72 hours of delivery. This preventive medication will stop the formation of antibodies that could cause severe harm, or death, from subsequent pregnancies.

Treatment

The application of fluorescent light (420-448 nm) to the neonate's exposed body surface area assists in the breakdown of bilirubin, which is then transported to the liver (**Figure 14-10**). The baby's skin absorbs light of this wavelength, which then changes the chemistry of bilirubin by oxidizing it into biliverdin (water soluble) for transport and direct excretion. Treatment can be stopped once serum bilirubin levels demonstrate a trending down (without rebound) or when the level is less than 10 mg/dL.

BEST PRACTICES

Maintenance of Phototherapy: Skills Required

The following nursing skills are associated with the care of a child with hyperbilirubinemia requiring phototherapy:

- Immediate placement upon admission to the pediatric unit
- Assessment of phototherapy light intensity
- Securing eye protection to prevent retina damage from the phototherapy
- Frequent assessment for dehydration, as infants may require 10% to 20% more fluid
- Monitoring length of breastfeeding episodes—should be no more than 30 minutes every 3 hours or on demand
- Educating the family on the rationale for phototherapy, to increase compliance
- Educating the family on the potential need for serial heel sticks to monitor for serum bilirubin levels, often every 12 to 24 hours or more frequently as ordered

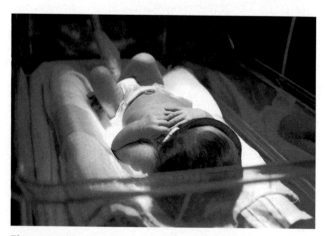

Figure 14-10 *A newborn under bili lights for hyperbilirubinemia.*

Prevention of Neurotoxicity: Kernicterus

Kernicterus is a condition in which the neonate's bilirubin levels are high enough to become absorbed by the brain tissue, potentially causing severe brain damage. Early-stage symptoms of kernicterus include poor feeding, lethargy, and hypotonia. Mid-stage symptoms include high-pitched cry, abnormal arching and posturing (opisthotonus), and eventually visual (strabismus and upgazing) and hearing impairment or loss, also known as auditory neuropathy (Shapiro, 2005). The infant may develop fevers and convulsions (Kenner & Lott, 2013). Progression leads to more serious brain damage. An infant at risk for kernicterus will need rapid phototherapy with bili lights or a biliblanket that can be increased to double or triple lights. Exchange transfusions may be required in infants with severely high bilirubin levels.

Failure to Thrive

Failure to thrive (FTT) is not considered an actual medical diagnosis, but rather a condition secondary to a medical or emotional/affective disorder. It is a serious complication of gastrointestinal disorders and diseases, and is associated with high morbidity and mortality rates.

Diagnosing and Managing Failure to Thrive

A child who presents with two or more (or consistent) growth plot points below the 5th percentile should be evaluated for the complexities of failure to thrive. The healthcare team should track weight-for-length, weight-for-age, and length-for-age, as well as head circumference and abdominal circumference while assessing for FTT (Dubowitz & Black, 2010). It takes a team approach involving several healthcare professionals to assist a child with FTT, given the wide range of health and psychosocial situations that can contribute to this condition (Iwaniec, 2004).

Two major categories of FTT are distinguished: organic, in which a pathological cause can be identified, and non-organic, in which no anatomic, functional, or pathological etiology is identified. Many children have mixed etiologies (Homan, 2016) because organic factors can trigger non-organic factors, such as familial stress. Assessment for organic factors includes a workup for pathological conditions that could decrease the absorption or metabolism of nutrients and calories. Assessment for non-organic FTT includes evaluation of the child and family for educational levels, financial challenges, family or individual stressors, mental health issues, child abuse, and other affective influences leading to poor nutrition, decreased intake, or intentional or unintentional neglect (Homan, 2016).

Case Study

The nurse is meeting a 4-year-old East Indian child for the first time; the child is being admitted for his monthly Remicade (infliximab) infusion for his chronic Crohn disease. In the past, the family has been cared for by a different GI team in a rural area of Northern California. Due to the chronic nature of his symptoms, his progressive and alarming weight loss, and his delayed growth and development, the child is now being admitted to a large urban hospital that has a GI specialty team. The hospital is more than a 3-hour drive from the family's home. The father is visibly upset by the hospitalization and his separation from other family members. The child's expected length of stay is 3 days, during which he will receive his infusion treatment, a bowel tissue biopsy, and full nutritional workup.

Case Study Questions

1. What is the relationship between inflammatory GI disorders, growth disorders, and low weight-for-age for children with Crohn disease?

2. What are classic symptoms of severe chronic Crohn disease?
3. What will the pediatric healthcare team and nutritionist ask the family about the child's diet?
4. Are there any nursing concerns or special infusion guidelines for an infliximab infusion?

As the Case Evolves...

This child has been experiencing interrupted treatment for Crohn disease and is now undergoing an initial intake at the facility of his new healthcare team.

5. Which of the following assessments should the intake encompass? (Select all that apply.)
   A. A complete review of the child's health history, including vaccination coverage and growth charts, as well as family history
   B. Barium enema and GI series, along with serum chemistry, liver and lipid profiles, erythrocyte sedimentation rate (ESR), and C-reactive protein

(continues)

Case Study *(continued)*

C. Physical assessment including height, weight, and abdominal circumference; hydration status including mucous membrane moisture, turgor, and presence of tears; and quality of the child's peripheral pulses

D. Colonoscopy and biopsy to confirm Crohn diagnosis

The child has undergone a physical assessment and complete history. Among the physical findings are significant underweight for age and length (lowest 5% of cohort), mild dehydration, and aphthous ulcers in the mouth. The child's parents state that the ulcers seem painful and make their child reluctant to eat. Based on the records from his previous visit, the child has lost approximately 1 kg and now weighs a little more than 13 kg. During history taking, the father again expresses his unhappiness at the lack of consistent care his child has received and the fact that obtaining comprehensive care requires extended travel. He states that he is concerned the treatment could affect his job, which he says he needs "desperately."

6. Which of the following statements best describes this case?

A. The child is at risk of failure to thrive.

B. The child is experiencing non-organic failure to thrive.

C. The child is experiencing organic failure to thrive.

D. The child is experiencing organic failure to thrive, with the possibility of inorganic contributing factors.

Chapter Summary

- Expected patterns of elimination across childhood vary widely. Each child has a unique pattern of growth, development, and elimination.

- The development of the GI system begins in the 4th fetal week of gestation. The intestinal lining includes multiple layers: the epithelium, mucosa with goblet mucus-producing cells, submucosa, circular muscular layer, longitudinal muscular layer, and serosa (intraperitoneal) or adventitia (retroperitoneal).

- One of the critical aspects of the development of the newborn's host defenses is the intestinal tract's colonization with bacteria (especially *Bacteroides*) that produce vitamin K. Newborns have a higher (but rare) risk of bleeding due to their innately low stores of vitamin K, which is required for coagulation processes.

- Many disorders related to elimination can cause a child to become dehydrated. Mild dehydration is defined as a weight loss of 5% or less in infants and a 3% to 4% weight loss in children; moderate dehydration is defined as a 10% weight loss in infants and a 6% to 8% weight loss in children; and severe dehydration is defined as a 15% weight loss in infants and a 10% weight loss in children. There are three types of dehydration: isotonic, hypotonic, and hypertonic.

- Common health concerns and disorders within the GI system include structural disorders, obstructive disorders, inflammatory disorders, and functional disorders.

- Pediatric structural gastrointestinal disorders include hernias, anorectal malformations, gastroesophageal reflux, cleft lip, and cleft palate.

- Pediatric gastrointestinal obstructive disorders include hypertrophic pyloric stenosis, intussusception, and Hirschsprung disease.

- Pediatric gastrointestinal inflammatory disorders include appendicitis, celiac disease, Crohn disease, and ulcerative colitis.

- The most common pediatric gastrointestinal functional disorders are diarrhea, vomiting, and constipation. Other disorders affecting elimination include hyperbilirubinemia and failure to thrive.

Bibliography

Canavan, A., & Arant, B. S. (2009). Diagnosis and management of dehydration in children. *American Family Physician, 80,* 692–696.

D'Cunha Burkardt, D., Graham, J. M., Jr., Short, S. S., & Frykman, P. K. (2013). Advances in Hirschsprung disease genetics and treatment strategies: An update for the primary care pediatrician. *Clinical Pediatrics, 53,* 71–81.

Dubowitz, H., & Black, M. (2010). Failure to thrive. *Epocrates.* Retrieved from https://online.epocrates.com/noFrame/showPage.do?method=diseases&MonographId=747&ActiveSectionId=11

Hatfield, N. T. (2014). *Introductory maternity and pediatric nursing* (3rd ed.). Philadelphia, PA: Wolters Kluwer Lippincott Williams & Wilkins.

Hazan, T. B., Gamarra, F. N., Stawick, L., & Maas, L. C. (2009). Nissen fundoplication and gastrointestinal-related complications: A guide for the primary care physician. *Southern Medical Journal, 102*(10), 1041–1045.

Hindryckx, P., Jairath, V., & D'Haens, G. (2016, September 1). Acute severe ulcerative colitis: From pathophysiology to clinical management. *Nature Reviews Gastroenterology and Hepatology.* [Epub ahead of print]. doi:10.1038/nrgastro.2016.116

Homan, G. J. (2016). Failure to thrive: A practical guide. *American Family Physician, 94*(4), 295–299.

Huang, E. Y., Tolley, E. A., Blakely, M. L., & Langham, M. R. (2013). Changes in hospital utilization and management of Hirschsprung disease: Analysis using the Kids' Inpatient Database. *Annals of Surgery, 257,* 371–375.

Huth, J., Petersen, J. D., & Lehman, J. A. (2013). The use of postoperative restraints in children after cleft lip or cleft palate repair: A preliminary report. *ISRN Plastic Surgery, 2013*, 540717. http://dx.doi.org/10.5402/2013/540717

Iwaniec, D. (2004). *Children who fail to thrive: A practice guide.* Chichester, UK: John Wiley & Sons.

James, S. R., Nelson, K., & Ashwill, J. (2013). *Nursing care of children: Principles and practice* (4th ed.). St. Louis, MO: Elsevier Saunders.

Kenner, C., & Lott, J. W. (2013). *Comprehensive neonatal nursing care* (5th ed.). New York, NY: Springer.

Lippi, G., & Franchini, M. (2011). Vitamin K in neonates: Facts and myths. *Blood Transfusion, 9*(1), 4–9.

Mayo Clinic. (2016). Intussusception. Symptoms and causes. Retrieved from http://www.mayoclinic.org/diseases-conditions/intussusception/symptoms-causes/dxc-20166963

Nachman, F., Sugai, E., Vazquez, H., Gonzalez, A., Andrenacci, P., Niveloni, S., . . . Bai, J. C. (2011). Serological tests for celiac disease as indicators of long-term compliance with gluten-free diet. *European Journal of Gastroenterology and Hepatology, 23*(6), 473–480.

National Institute of Diabetes and Digestive and Kidney Diseases. (2015). Definition and facts for GER and GERD in children and teens. Retrieved from https://www.niddk.nih.gov/health-information/digestive-diseases/acid-reflux-ger-gerd-children-teens

O'Neil, M., Teitelbaum, D. H., & Harris, M. B. (2014). Total body sodium depletion and poor weight gain in children and young adults with an ileostomy: A case series. *Nutrition in Clinical Practice, 29*, 397–401.

Porter, M., & Dennis, B. (2002). Hyperbilirubinemia in the term newborn. *American Family Physician, 65*(4), 599–607.

Pringle, K., Shah, S. P., Umulisa, I., Munyaneza, R. B. M., Dushimiyimana, J. M., Stegmann, K., . . . Levine, A. C. (2011). Comparing the accuracy of the three popular clinical dehydration scales in children with diarrhea. *International Journal of Emergency Medicine, 4*(1), 58. doi: 10.1186/1865-1380-458

Richards, C. J. (2015). Pathological considerations in Crohn's disease. In A. Rajesh & R. Sinha (Eds.), *Crohn's disease: Current concepts* (pp. 11–19). New York, NY: Springer.

Ryan, M., & Grossman, S. (2011). Celiac disease: Implications for patient management. *Gastroenterology Nursing, 34*(3), 225–228.

Shapiro, S. (2005). Definition of clinical spectrum of kernicterus and bilirubin-induced neurological dysfunction (BIND). *Journal of Perinatology, 25*(1), 54–59.

Tabbers, M. M., DiLorenzo, C., Berger, M. Y., Faure, C., Langendam, M. W., Nurko, S., . . . Benninga, M. A. (2014). Evaluation and treatment of functional constipation in infants and children: Evidence-based recommendations from ESPGHAN and NASPGHAN. *Journal of Pediatric Gastroenterology and Nutrition, 58*, 258–274.

Tandon, M., Singh, A., Saluja, V., Dhankhar, M., Pandey, C. K., & Jain, P. (2016). Validation of a new "objective pain score" vs. "numeric rating scale" for the evaluation of acute pain: A comparative study. *Anesthesiology and Pain Medicine, 6*(1), e32101.

Wetherill, C. V., Melling, J. D., Rhodes, H. L., Wilkinson, D. J., & Kenny, S. E. (2015). Implementation of a care pathway for infantile hypertrophic pyloric stenosis reduces length of stay and increases parent satisfaction. *International Journal of Care Coordination, 18*, 78–84.

Youssef, N. N., Langseder, A. L., Verga, B. J., Mones, R. L., & Rosh, J. R. (2005). Chronic childhood constipation is associated with impaired quality of life: A case-controlled study. *Journal of Pediatric Gastroenterology and Nutrition, 41*, 56–60.

CHAPTER 15

Metabolism

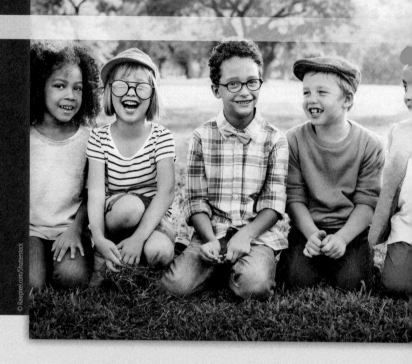

© Rawpixel.com/Shutterstock

LEARNING OBJECTIVES

1. Apply nursing concepts to care for a child with a metabolic disorder or condition.
2. Evaluate the functioning of the metabolic pathways and biochemical processes in the body.
3. Identify deviations associated with pathological changes or genetic mutations in enzyme function associated with carbohydrates, proteins, and lipids.
4. Distinguish between the various endocrine metabolic disorders, including the complications associated with hypersecretion and hyposecretion of various endocrine glands.
5. Understand the differences between genetic-based, congenital, and acquired metabolic disorders discovered during the developmental period.
6. Analyze the various assessment techniques used to identify metabolic disorders in children.
7. Evaluate the impact of a growth disorder on the physical development and emotional well-being of a child.
8. Create a nursing care plan for a child newly diagnosed with insulin-dependent diabetes mellitus.
9. Formulate a deeper understanding of specific metabolic disorders during the childhood developmental period, including diabetes, growth disorders, inborn errors of metabolism, and metabolic disorders associated with endocrine dysfunction.

KEY TERMS

Addison syndrome
Cushing syndrome
Enzyme
Galactosemia
Graves's disease
Hormones
Inborn error of metabolism
Maple syrup urine disease
Metabolic pathway
Metabolism
Phenylketonuria (PKU)
Precocious puberty

Introduction

A metabolic condition is characterized by a defect or disruption in the biochemical process of a **metabolic pathway**. The major metabolic pathways in the body comprise the complex mechanisms of carbohydrate, lipid, and protein synthesis or catabolism, as well as the production, secretion, and mechanism of action of various hormones; collectively, the chemical reactions that occur via these pathways are termed **metabolism**. A genetic defect in any part of this complex biochemical process leads to a metabolic condition referred to as an **inborn error of metabolism** or a hormonal imbalance. Such conditions can be mild or severe, and have the potential to disrupt expected growth, development, and mental processing. Some conditions, if left untreated, may be fatal.

Endocrine Dysfunction

The human body relies on a complex and integral system of checks and balances. **Hormones**, which are released by the glands in minute quantities into the bloodstream, are substances that serve as chemical messengers in the body. The fine balance of hormone secretion allows the body to receive messages concerning fluid and electrolyte balance, growth, energy production and consumption, sexual organ development, and rapid responses to stressful or dangerous stimuli. Any disruption to the complex endocrine system—whether it is caused by familial or genetic factors or is acquired due to an injury, trauma, or other factors—has a huge impact on the growing child's physiological balance and well-being.

Pediatric metabolic disorders are rare, with an average overall incidence rate of fewer than 1 case per 1 million population for extremely rare conditions, 1 case per 250,000 population for very rare conditions (e.g., maple syrup urine disease), and 1 case per 6000 to 60,000 population for more common but still relatively rare conditions (e.g., phenylketonuria, galactosemia). Although more than 1000 inherited disorders of metabolism have been identified to date, and more than 1400 metabolic disorders in general, the incidence of these conditions is relatively small.

In all U.S. states, newborn screening for at least 26 metabolic disorders is required. Some states require between 30 and 50 tests for inborn errors of metabolism, with repeat confirmatory testing being performed if the initial values are positive. Tandem mass spectrometry is widely used for this purpose because it is sensitive enough to detect many errors and requires only a minimal volume of blood for testing; the sample is usually drawn via a heel stick before the newborn leaves the hospital (**Figure 15-1**). Aggressive screening of all newborns allows for early identification

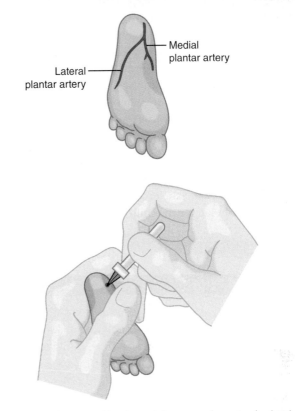

Figure 15-1 *Drawing a blood sample from a newborn via a heel stick.*

and treatment before the infant displays symptoms and experiences multisystem harm from a metabolic disorder. Clinical findings of hypoglycemia, hyperammonemia, and metabolic acidosis should be treated rapidly to ensure the child's safety before the results of metabolic screening tests are finalized (Raghuveer, Garg, & Graf, 2006).

The majority of inborn errors of metabolism are genetically linked and inherited through autosomal recessive genes. Most of these disorders are associated with particular ethnicities, such that their prevalence is greater within those populations. Families from particular ethnic groups with higher incidence of a metabolic disorder should be screened for the associated errors; in addition, any family with a history of a metabolic disorder should be offered an expanded version of the standard metabolic screening mandated by the state.

The physiologic effects of these disorders can be organized into three distinct groups:

- Disorders that disrupt synthesis or catabolism of complex molecules not related to food intake, including metabolic disorders associated with intracellular transport, intracellular processing, and lysosomal disorders
- Disorders that lead to a deficiency of energy production, including disorders affecting the liver, brain, myocardium, or muscles' ability to utilize or produce energy

- Disorders that cause a progressive or acute accumulation of toxic compounds, such as phenylketonuria, **maple syrup urine disease** (an autosomal recessive metabolic disorder that results in accumulation of three amino acids and their keto acids, which cause the urine to have a sweet odor), or intolerances of certain sugars such as galactosemia

Due to the severity of the child's response to a metabolic disorder, including severe toxicity, it is imperative that the pediatric nurse assist the healthcare team in assuring early identification of a metabolic error and maintain an effective management plan for the child's condition.

RESEARCH EVIDENCE

Research demonstrates that reduced morbidity and mortality rates, as well as increased positive overall outcomes, for children with metabolic disorders start with accurate and timely screening for biological markers of all newborns, prompt identification of symptoms (commonly, tachypnea, lethargy, vomiting, poor feeding and seizures), and rapid initiation of therapy (Raghuveer et al., 2006).

To better understand the concerns associated with metabolic disorders in childhood, reviewing the three metabolic pathways is helpful (**Table 15-1**). Carbohydrates, proteins, and lipids are critical for a child's growth, development, energy expenditure, and overall health. A disruption in any of the metabolic pathways involving these three substances produces extreme defects.

Assessment of Metabolic Disorders in the Neonatal Period

Newborns who present with inborn errors of metabolism need immediate assessments and diagnostics to confirm the existence of a metabolic pathway disorder. A delay in diagnosis can lead to toxic effects of the defect, causing both short-term and long-term cellular damage. **Table 15-2** provides examples of the most common (although still rare) inborn errors of metabolism, as well as inherited conditions of metabolism and acquired metabolic disorders that do not necessarily show up in newborns.

The neonatal and pediatric healthcare team must be aware of the most common signs and symptoms associated with metabolic disorders. Symptoms of a metabolic disorder can present acutely in the neonatal period, including poor sucking; lethargy; respiratory distress; hypotonia; gastrointestinal (GI) distress including diarrhea, vomiting, and dehydration; and seizures. Neonates who suffer metabolic disorders of toxic metabolite accumulation can become symptomatic within hours of birth to a few days of life. Approximately two-thirds of the metabolic disorders seen in newborns are congenital and present at birth, although symptoms may not manifest for several weeks. The remaining one-third of newborn presentations involve late-onset metabolic disorders.

The neonatal team must differentiate symptoms of a metabolic disorder from those of other neonatal conditions such as infection or sepsis. Conditions that could mimic a metabolic disorder include the following:

- Dysmorphic features
- Liver disease
- Muscle weakness, cramping, and hypotonia

TABLE 15-1	Metabolic Pathways	
Substance	**Process**	**Imperative**
Proteins	Amino acids undergo gluconeogenesis to pyruvate, which produces acetyl-CoA. In the Krebs cycle, ATP is formed from acetyl-CoA to produce energy.	Without protein gluconeogenesis, the child cannot grow, heal tissues, or have organ function.
Lipids	Lipids provide glycerol, triglycerides, and fatty acids. Through lipogenesis and oxidation, acetyl-CoA is produced. In the Krebs cycle, acetyl-CoA is transformed into ATP to provide energy.	Without lipogenesis and the production of acetyl-CoA, ketone bodies form, which leads to toxicity.
Carbohydrates	Carbohydrates provide glucose. Glycogen is produced in the liver via glycogenesis and made available for the body's use through glycogenolysis (breakdown and availability for immediate use). Through glycogenolysis, the metabolic pathway transforms acetyl-CoA into ATP, and then ATP into energy.	Stored glucose in the form of glycogen is imperative for the child's body to have access to an immediate source of energy for cellular functions.

Abbreviations: Acetyl-CoA = acetyl coenzyme A, ATP = adenosine triphosphate.

TABLE 15-2 Metabolic Disorders: Examples

Type of Defect	Examples	Pediatric Considerations
Inborn errors of metabolism	› Phenylketonuria › Galactosemia › Medium chain acetyl-CoA dehydrogenase (MCAD) deficiency › Maple syrup urine disease (MSUD) › Congenital hypothyroidism	› Present at birth; should be identified early in neonatal period › Corrective action and treatments must begin immediately › Family education on diet modification, drug therapy, and complications must begin immediately and be reinforced periodically › Congenital hypothyroidism detection requires high index of suspicion; reserves of maternal thyroxine can mask symptoms for as long as 4 months (Sinha & Bauer, 2014). The incidence of congenital hypothyroidism is increasing (Allen & Fomenko, 2011).
Inherited defects of metabolism	› Familial central diabetes insipidus, in which the hypothalamus no longer secretes adequate ADH › Familial hypothyroidism, which causes a reduction in thyroid hormone production and secretion › Hereditary fructose intolerance › Sickle cell anemia	› Diabetes insipidus may or may not be present at birth; symptoms of polydipsia, polyuria, and nocturia mimic diabetes mellitus, but urinalysis will show no glucosuria or ketonuria and urine will be dilute › Some children with familial hypothyroidism initially present with thyrotoxicity, but it is transient (Sinha & Bauer, 2014) › Overall incidence of sickle cell trait is approximately 1.5%, but incidence among African Americans is approximately 7.3%
Acquired errors of metabolism	› Severe diabetes insipidus related to head trauma, brain tumors, central nervous system dysfunction, or a neurosurgical procedure near the pituitary gland › Diabetes mellitus from autoimmune dysfunction (type 1) and destruction of beta cells of the pancreas › Diabetes mellitus from loss of cellular response to insulin (type 2) › Growth hormone deficiency acquired from brain injury, brain tumors, or radiation exposure	› Most of these conditions are not acquired in the neonatal period, although some may develop in infancy › Pediatric healthcare team members must be knowledgeable about the clinical signs of symptoms of acquired metabolic disorders so treatment can begin immediately and harm reduced

Abbreviations: Acetyl-CoA = acetyl coenzyme A, ADH = antidiuretic hormone.

- Gastrointestinal symptoms of malabsorption, vomiting, diarrhea, and anorexia
- Failure to thrive
- Developmental delay
- Movement disorders including cerebral palsy
- Lethargy and coma
- Metabolic acidosis
- Hypoglycemia
- Ophthalmic abnormalities
- Sudden infant death syndrome (SIDS)

Late-onset metabolic disorders—most of which develop in preschool, school-age, or adolescent children—include disorders of energy production and disorders of toxic accumulation. Even when these disorders develop in infancy, they may remain asymptomatic for months or years. With a late-onset metabolic disorder, a viral infection or other fever-related or diarrhea-related pathology may start the process leading to presentation.

Medical Management and Treatment for Inborn Errors of Metabolism

Types of Treatments

The ability to medically manage a child with an inborn error of metabolism is based on either (1) preventing the progressive deterioration (chronicity) associated with the disorder through use of medications or diet therapy or (2) counteracting the disturbance in biochemical processing, thereby preventing acute decompensation. Treatment typically involves four types of interventions:

- Altering the child's nutrition to remove a diet component causing toxic accumulations
- Providing large doses of vitamins to induce metabolism in such disorders as maple syrup urine disease (administering thiamine) or oxidation defects (administering riboflavin)
- Toxin removal by way of hemofiltration, hemodialysis, or peritoneal dialysis (such as removing toxic levels of ammonia associated with urea cycle defects)
- Providing a simulated alternative metabolic pathway via drug therapy (such as the administration of sodium benzoate for urea cycle errors)

If the infant or child has an acute and life-threatening condition associated with a metabolic dysfunction or disorder, immediate emergency management may be required. This may include a rapid admission to a pediatric intensive care unit and ventilation of the child if metabolic acidosis is severe enough to affect breathing (**Figure 15-2**). Further emergency management may include correcting electrolyte imbalances, correcting metabolic acidosis, rehydration, total parenteral nutrition (TPN), and suppression of toxic metabolite production via drug therapy (**Table 15-3**).

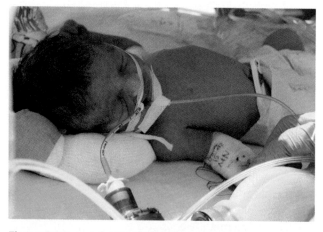

Figure 15-2 *An infant in a NICU with ventilation.*
© guvendemir/iStock/Getty Images

TABLE 15-3	Drug Therapy for Inborn Errors of Metabolism

Amino Acid Errors

› Example: Nonketonic hyperglycemia

› Drug therapy: Sodium benzoate, ketamine, dextromethorphan

Urea Cycle Errors

› Example: Carbamoyl phosphate synthetase deficiency

› Drug therapy: IV sodium benzoate, arginine, carglumic acid

Organic Acidemia Errors

› Example: Methylmalonic acidema

› Drug therapy: L-Carnitine, cobalamin

Lysosomal Storage Errors

› Example: Gaucher disease

› Drug therapy: Miglustat, alglucerase

Nursing Care

Besides immediately reporting any suspicious neonatal or infant behaviors associated with an error or pathology of the metabolic pathways, the primary responsibility of the nurse is to educate the family about all aspects of the child's lifelong care. Essential elements of that education include communicating and confirming an understanding of the complexity of the disorder on a level that aligns with the family's level of health literacy. Because each adult has his or her own way of learning, several teaching techniques should be implemented. Using a variety of teaching methods—including verbal explanations, written materials, and video education tools—will help to confirm the caregiver's understanding of the needed dietary modifications, medication adherence, and clinical signs of complications. For instance, when teaching a family about the pathology of Gaucher syndrome, the family needs to understand the disorder itself, how to safely and accurately administer drug therapy to provide the missing metabolic **enzyme** (a substance that catalyzes a chemical reaction, but is itself unchanged by the reaction), which periodic laboratory analyses and diagnostics are needed for surveillance, and which symptoms are associated with progressive disease and need to be reported to the healthcare team.

Metabolic Concept Exemplars

Given that so many metabolic conditions exist, but most are rarely encountered, the pediatric nurse should become familiar with those metabolic disorders that are more commonly seen. Exemplars for this chapter include two inborn errors of metabolism—phenylketonuria and galactosemia—as well as the endocrine dysfunction of diabetes mellitus.

Phenylketonuria

Phenylketonuria (PKU) is an inborn error of metabolism that has an incidence rate of 1 case per 15,000 live births (Raghuveer et al., 2006). Children with PKU lack the enzyme phenylalanine hydroxylase and therefore are unable to convert phenylalanine—an essential amino acid consumed in the diet that is typically used for protein synthesis—to tyrosine in the liver. This autosomal recessive genetic disorder involves a defect in metabolism of amino acids that leads to the accumulation of toxic metabolites called phenylketones. When plasma concentrations of phenylketones reach 20 mg/dL, they spill into the urine, which is the finding that gives this disorder its name. The phenylketones themselves are not what cause central nervous system (CNS) symptoms and eventual neurologic damage; rather, it is the accumulation of phenylalanine (hyperphenylalaninemia) that damages brain tissue and, ultimately, produces cognitive impairment.

Excessive vomiting may be a first clinical sign of PKU. Without identification of this disorder, medical management, and health education, the child with PKU may experience learning disabilities, hyperactivity, developmental delay, and, in the older child, intellectual disability, behavior problems, seizures, and other neurological and psychiatric disorders (Mayo Clinic, 2014).

Medical Management

The primary medical management trajectory for a diagnosis of PKU is early identification of the pathology and then dietary removal of foods that contain phenylalanine—that is, elimination of most meats, dairy, nuts, and legumes from the diet, as well as restriction of portions of starches such as potatoes, corn, and bread (Arnold & Steiner, 2014) (**Figure 15-3**). Avoiding foods and medications containing the sweetener aspartame (L-aspartylphenylalanine) is

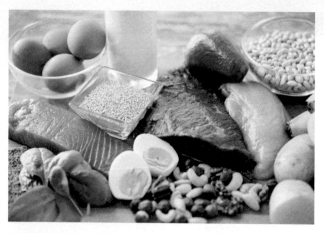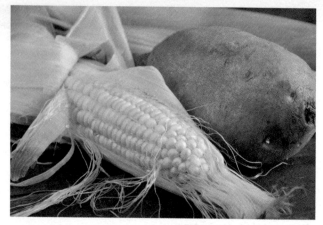

Figure 15-3 *Foods that children with PKU must avoid include most meats, dairy, nuts, and legumes, as well as restriction of portions of starches such as potatoes, corn, and bread.*

imperative to prevent severe health complications; most of these items are "diet" or "low-carb" formulations, so parents should read product labels carefully. Baby formulas, formulas required for older children, and premade infant foods must also be phenylalanine free.

Nursing Care

Because PKU is treated through dietary restrictions alone, family education is the key to astute nursing care. Teaching the family and caregivers of a child with PKU to avoid food or drinks containing phenylalanine is of primary importance. The nurse should initiate an immediate referral to a nutritionist to assist in the education and reinforcement of information throughout childhood.

Special bottle-feeding formulas are available for children with PKU. Older children should adhere to a diet that is low in milk and dairy products, meat, chicken, fish, nuts, beans, eggs, and high-protein foods. This diet must be followed for life. Processed foods to avoid include the following items:

- High-protein formulas (infants with PKU require a specialized infant formula)
- Artificial sweeteners containing phenylalanine (e.g., aspartame [Equal])
- "Sugar-free" juices or carbonated beverages, including flavored waters, that contain phenylalanine in the form of aspartame
- Processed foods prepared with phenylalanine
- Candy, sweets, ice cream, or other "diet foods" that contain phenylalanine

Screening for potential inborn errors of metabolism is important for the early identification of PKU. The accumulation of toxins associated with phenylalaninemia affecting the neurologic system occurs slowly, causing only a gradual presentation of clinical symptoms. For most accurate results, newborns should be screened within the first 24 to 48 hours of life after a protein feeding.

Galactosemia

Galactosemia is an inborn error of metabolism that occurs when a child is unable to convert galactose, a simple carbohydrate found in dairy products and milk, to glucose-1-phosphate. A deficiency in the enzyme galactose-1-phosphate uridyl transferase leads to the accumulation of galactose. Symptoms of the defect begin to present within the first few days of life after the consumption of milk feeds. They include vomiting, diarrhea, jaundice, hypoglycemia, and liver dysfunction, progressing to cataract formation, abnormal clotting, failure to thrive, and eventually cognitive impairment.

Medical Management

The only medical treatment for galactosemia is the elimination of galactose (usually present as the disaccharide lactose, which is composed of glucose and galactose and is the major carbohydrate in milk) from the diet. Infants need to be fed soy-based formula, as galactose is present even in breast milk (**Figure 15-4**).

Nursing Care

The pediatric nurse must be knowledgeable about the clinical signs and symptoms of galactosemia. Being able to identify key indicators early can preserve mental functioning and save lives. High levels of galactose due to a reduction or absence of enzymes required for metabolizing galactose requires monitoring for abnormal results on liver and kidney function tests. Identifying early signs of pediatric lens disorder is imperative, as the accumulation of the toxic metabolite puts children at increased risk for cataracts. Overall, children with galactosemia have lower

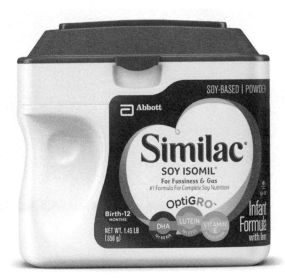

Figure 15-4 *Soy-based infant formula.*

Reprinted with permission from Abbott Laboratories, Inc.

intelligence quotients (IQ) as compared to healthy peers (Saunders, 2016). Reporting signs of jaundice, poor feeding tolerance, mental slowness, and delayed physical growth and development is required for holistic management of this condition.

Metabolic Endocrine Glands

Endocrine glands are distinct groups of tissues that produce hormones that are secreted directly into the bloodstream, rather than through a duct. Hormones, which are naturally secreted in miniscule quantities, have very specific functions and act on specific target receptors; the hormone–receptor complex is often referred to as a control center. Hormone signals influence the equilibrium, stability, and homeostasis of the human body and regulate many specific metabolic functions. Children need a healthy endocrine system to maintain the expected growth and development pattern and ensure appropriate organ and tissue function (**Figure 15-5**).

The target cells' ability to respond to the associated hormone depends on the presence and adequacy of cellular membrane receptors that bind with the hormone substance. Receptors are considered dynamic, as they can change and adapt to the needs of the cells; they respond to high levels or low levels of secreted hormones. Cellular membrane receptors react to the chemical messenger hormones, while the liver degrades hormones and the kidneys secrete hormones as needed to ensure precise regulation of the body's functions.

The stimulation of an endocrine gland that leads to its release of a hormone depends on the gland's activation by an appropriate message. These messages take the form of either other hormones or signals from humoral or neural

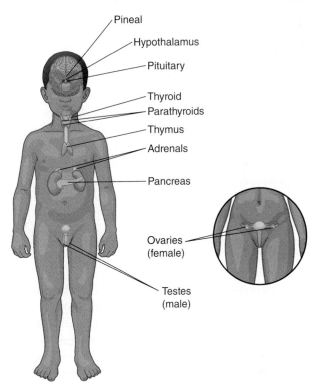

Figure 15-5 *The metabolic endocrine glands.*

sources. Both positive and negative feedback loops are imperative to maintain appropriate hormone release, target cell activation, cellular function, and turn-off mechanisms. Three factors influence this process:

- *Permissiveness:* The need for a second hormone to be present for a target cell receptor to respond to a hormone
- *Synergism:* The need for two or more hormones to work together to produce a positive effect within a target cell
- *Antagonism:* The means by which a hormone reverses the effect of another hormone, when both hormones are present within the same target cell

In some instances, sets of specific hormones regulate particular functions. For example, two pancreatic hormones, insulin and glucagon, maintain stable blood glucose levels via antagonism. The interaction of two other hormones—thyroid-stimulating hormone (TSH), which is released by the pituitary gland, and the prohormone thyroxine (T_4), which is released by the thyroid gland itself—produces a third hormone, triiodothyronine (T_3), that is required for the regulation of cellular metabolism. Some hormonal interactions can be detrimental to health under certain conditions. For example, both growth hormone, which is produced by the pituitary gland, and cortisol, an adrenal gland hormone produced in response to stress, can exacerbate insulin resistance in a child with diabetes.

Metabolic Endocrine Gland Dysfunction

When the endocrine system experiences a dysfunction, the metabolism of the child's entire body can be disrupted. A child may be born with an endocrine disorder, or he or she may develop an endocrine condition based on other pathologies, infections, toxic exposures, or injuries. Rapid identification and immediate treatment to correct hyposecretion or hypersecretion of essential hormones is critical. The following are examples of disorders associated with endocrine dysfunction (see **Table 15-4** for others):

- Gigantism: Caused by an over-secretion of growth hormone (GH) in children. It leads to excessive linear bone growth.
- Dwarfism (pituitary): Caused by the inadequate secretion of growth hormone (**Figure 15-6**).
- Diabetes insipidus: Caused by the reduced secretion of antidiuretic hormone (arginine vasopressin) produced in the hypothalmus. It may initially be confused with diabetes mellitus, as some of the

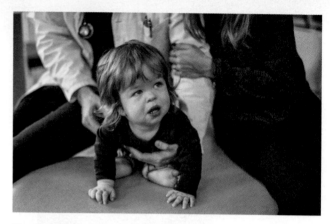

Figure 15-6 *A child with dwarfism.*
© pixelaway/Shutterstock

presenting symptoms (polyuria, nocturia, polydipsia) are similar (Babey, Kopp, & Robertson, 2011).
- Syndrome of inappropriate antidiuretic hormone (SIADH): Caused by the excessive secretion of antidiuretic hormone (severely reduced urine production, high urine specific gravity) by the pituitary gland.

TABLE 15-4   Identification, Medical Management, and Family Education for Endocrine Disorders

Cushing Syndrome

Cushing syndrome, which is rare in children, is caused by hypersecretion of the adrenal hormone cortisol. Most often, it is caused by a tumor in the pituitary, which stimulates production of the precursor to cortisol, or in the adrenal gland itself. In the presence of excess cortisol, a child experiences decreased lineal growth, development of obesity, very poor wound healing, ecchymosis, osteoporosis, weakness, poor glucose tolerance, and muscle atrophy. Medical treatment includes either drugs that inhibit cortisol production or removal of the tumor if one is present and operable.

Addison Syndrome

Addison syndrome is caused by reduced production and secretion of the hormones of the adrenal gland. Reduced levels of cortisol (a steroid hormone that regulates blood glucose and suppresses inflammatory responses) and aldosterone (a steroid hormone that controls and manages potassium and sodium) lead to poor stress responses, poor healing, severe abdominal pain, hypotension, kidney failure, and shock. Some children feel better and respond within 1 to 2 days of drug therapy.

Graves's Disease (Thyrotoxicosis)

Mostly found in adolescent females, **Graves's disease** is an immune-mediated disorder associated with hyperthyroidism and caused by stimulated B-lymphocyte immunoglobulins that bind to the thyroid hormone–releasing receptors, mimicking the action of thyroid-stimulating hormone (TSH). Increased production and release of the thyroid hormones T_3 and T_4 cause the child to have an enlarged thyroid, increased heart rate and blood pressure, widened pulse pressure, palpitations, nervousness, irritability, tremors, diarrhea, heat intolerance, profound perspiration, weight loss, exophthalmoses (protrusion of the eyes within the eye sockets, also known as Graves's ophthalmopathy), and poor sleep quality. Medical management includes drugs to suppress thyrotropic levels and decrease thyroid hormone secretion of free thyroxine (FT_4) and triiodothyronine (T_3). Surgical resection of the enlarged thyroid and beta blockers for cardiac consequences may be required as well (Bauer, 2016; Levitsky & Sinha, 2013).

Thyroid Storm

A rare phenomenon in which a child's thyroid produces dangerously large quantities of thyroid hormone, leading to high fever with dehydration, severe tachycardia, diarrhea, shock, and death if not disrupted. The child should be admitted to the pediatric intensive care unit for rapid IV fluids, steroids and antithyroid medications to stop the phenomenon, beta blockers, and close observation.

- Graves's disease (hyperthyroidism): Caused by the excessive secretion of thyroid hormones, generally due to immune system dysfunction.
- Diabetes mellitus: Caused by the inadequate secretion of insulin (type 1) or resistance or insensitivity to insulin (type 2).
- Hashimoto thyroiditis (chronic lymphocytic thyroiditis; hypothyroidism): Caused by an autoimmune disorder, which leads to inadequate secretion of thyroid hormones.
- Congenital hypothyroidism: Caused by malformation of the thyroid gland *or* an inborn error of metabolism that prevents an anatomically normal thyroid from producing thyroid hormone.
- Hypoparathyroidism: Inadequate production of parathyroid hormone in the parathyroid gland, resulting in hypocalcemia. It may be related to deficiency of magnesium or vitamin D.
- Hyperparathyroidism: Gland dysfunction resulting in extreme bone wasting.

Diabetes Mellitus

A common endocrine disorder encountered in pediatric healthcare settings is diabetes mellitus. Diabetes mellitus (which differs from diabetes insipidus) comprises a group of glucose transport disorders in which the primary transport hormone, insulin, is unable to transport glucose across cellular membranes, either because too little insulin is present to accomplish the process or because cell membranes have fewer than normal insulin receptors and so are unresponsive to insulin's signals ("insulin resistance").

Type 1 diabetes, previously called juvenile diabetes, is an autoimmune-generated destruction of the beta cells of the pancreas, causing inadequate production of insulin so that insulin replacement therapy is required. The autoimmune attack on the beta cells is thought to be triggered by viral or environmental factors (Knip & Simell, 2012), sometimes in combination with a genetic predisposition for autoimmunity. Children with type 1 diabetes present with weight loss, polyuria, nocturia, polydipsia, irritability, and dehydration.

Type 2 diabetes occurs when the child's cells develop an insensitivity to the effects of insulin; this insensitivity occurs as a result of genetic predisposition, lifestyle factors that promote insulin resistance (e.g., sedentary lifestyle coupled with an imbalanced diet), or a combination of the two. With type 2 diabetes, children can present with normal weight or obesity, but the symptom set of weight loss, polyuria, nocturia, polydipsia and so forth is similar to that seen in children with type 1 diabetes. Distinguishing the two types generally depends on family history: Most children who develop type 2 diabetes have a strong family history of the disease, whereas those who develop type 1 frequently do not.

Type 1 diabetes is associated with lifelong dependency on self-administered insulin therapy, while type 2 diabetes requires dietary modification, lifestyle modification, weight management, and sometimes the addition of oral antihyperglycemic medications. Approximately 1 in 600 children (1.93 per 1000) present with type 1 diabetes in the United States with a 21.1% increase over an 8 year time period (Dabelea et al., 2014). The average age of diagnosis of type 2 diabetes in children is 10 to 14 years, whereas children tend to be younger when they are diagnosed with type 1 disease. Sometimes, children whose type 2 diabetes was initially well controlled via oral medication can progress to needing insulin therapy. Type 2 diabetes incidence is increasing in the United States as well as worldwide. Between 20–50% of new cases of diabetes in children are new-onset type 1 (Dabelea et al., 2014). Diagnosis of diabetes can be confirmed through three tests: abnormal results of fasting or random plasma glucose levels, hemoglobin A1c levels, or an oral glucose tolerance test (Laffel & Svoren, 2011).

UNIQUE FOR KIDS

Type 1 Diabetes Mellitus

Type 1 diabetes is associated with younger age, genetic predisposition to autoimmunity, and environmental factors (such as infection) that produce an autoimmune attack on the beta cells, leading to their destruction. Owing to the decrease in the insulin-producing beta cells, other cells in the body are unable to obtain adequate glucose for energy, and the starvation response of fatty acid breakdown begins as the body seeks an alternative source of energy. Breakdown of fatty acids produces ketone bodies as a by-product, and these begin to accumulate in the blood along with glucose. The presence of these ketone bodies puts the child in an acidotic state.

Children with type 1 diabetes can present with polyuria, polydipsia, polyphagia, weakness, flushed or dry skin, changes in visual acuity, mental slowness and confusion, and weight loss (thin appearance). They may also demonstrate poor wound healing, yeast infections, dehydration, and hypotension. Laboratory analysis will show high serum blood glucose levels, low specific gravity with diuresis or high specific gravity with severe dehydration, electrolyte imbalances, ketones in the

urine, elevated triglycerides, osmotic diuresis and glycosuria, and elevated fasting blood glucose levels. Suboptimal vitamin D values are a common finding as well, although their contribution to the development of the disorder is as yet unclear.

Type 2 Diabetes Mellitus

Typically associated with older age and history of exposure to gestational diabetes, type 2 diabetes is becoming more common in children. In this endocrine disorder, insulin is produced in the child's pancreas, but the body does not use it properly (insulin resistance). People of certain races and ethnicities are at increased risk for type 2 disease, including Native Americans, African Americans, Latinos, and Hispanic Americans. Factors associated with a diagnosis of type 2 diabetes in children include family history, physical inactivity, overweight or obesity, prediabetes, gestational diabetes, race, hypertension, abnormal cholesterol lab values, and a history of hyperglycemia (American Diabetes Association, 2016).

Medical Management of Type 1 Diabetes

The entire pediatric healthcare team should be involved with the medical management of a child with diabetes and the family, parents, and caregivers. A pediatric endocrinologist, Child Life specialist, social worker, nutritionist, child psychologist, pharmacist, primary care medical staff, Certified Diabetic Nurse Educator, and pediatric nursing staff can all contribute to the establishment of a management team. The child's school must be notified, and the clinicians should work with the family to create a medical management plan (identified as a "504 Plan" under the Americans with Disabilities Act) to establish a strong relationship with the school nurse or other staff members to cover any issues related to blood glucose checking and insulin administration during school hours. Teachers should be taught the symptoms of hypoglycemia and know how to call for help if the child becomes symptomatic during classroom time. The successful care of a child with type 1 diabetes truly takes a village.

It is imperative to assist the family in managing a child's diabetes so that as the child grows into young adulthood and adulthood, there is a lesser chance of the development of severe complications of the disease. Heart disease, blindness, stroke, kidney failure, and nontraumatic lower-limb amputations are all consequences of diabetes in later years (National Center for Chronic Disease Prevention and Health Promotion, 2011).

Initially, medical management begins with the stabilization of a child who often presents to the healthcare arena in diabetic ketoacidosis (DKA), a life-threatening condition characterized by high blood glucose levels, dehydration, electrolyte imbalance, and metabolic acidosis. Children who are newly diagnosed with diabetes need to be carefully managed during the initial episode of DKA and any subsequent episodes of DKA (although the patient and caregivers should be educated so that such episodes can be avoided at all costs). **Box 15-1** summarizes stabilization of a child with an initial presentation of DKA.

After this critical period, medical management focuses on establishing an appropriate daily dosing of rapid-acting insulin complemented with extended-release insulin therapy (**Figure 15-7**). The child's fluctuating blood glucose levels need to be managed with each meal and snack, as well as over the course of the entire day. To ensure a constant rate of insulin infusion over a 24-hour period, which provides a "basal" rate of delivery, many children wear an insulin pump around the clock; this device administers rapid-acting insulin based on a complex set of calculations that take into account the child's daily insulin needs (usually based on weight), fluctuations in measured blood glucose levels, and carbohydrate intake, with the last being calculated for meal-specific dosing by the pump's internal computer. Even young children (early school age) can successfully manage their glucose with insulin pumps.

Every 3 to 6 months, the child's serum hemoglobin A_{1c} (HbA_{1c}) level should be checked to reassess the insulin regimen and troubleshoot changes in the child's needs. HbA_{1c} levels are an assessment of the percentage of hemoglobin that is glycosylated—that is, has a glucose molecule attached to it—which gives an average value of blood glucose over the preceding 3 months (90 days). Higher levels of HbA_{1c} are associated with microvascular and macrovascular complications. In a nondiabetic adult, one would expect this value to be between 5% and 6%; in diabetic children, ideal ranges are 7.5% to 8.5% for children younger than 6 years, less than 8% for children between 6 and 12 years of age, and less than 7.5% for children between 13 and 18 years of age. HbA_{1c} values consistently above the child's average for age in consecutive tests indicate a need for clinicians to identify factors contributing to hyperglycemia, including poor adherence to carbohydrate counting, blood glucose testing (**Figure 15-8**), and insulin administration; however, a transient uptick in HbA_{1c} in a child previously within average range could simply indicate a growth spurt or stress, as growth and stress hormones contribute to insulin resistance.

Annual screening for autoimmune thyroid disease and celiac disease are also recommended for children with type 1 diabetes, as these disorders are more common in people with type 1 diabetes than in the general population (Glastras et al., 2005).

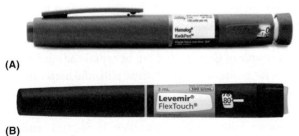

(A)

(B)

Figure 15-7 *Types of insulin: (A) Humalog KwikPen; (B) Levemir FlexTouch.*

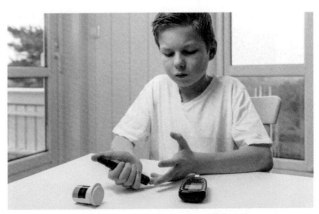

Figure 15-8 *A young child checking his blood glucose via finger stick.*

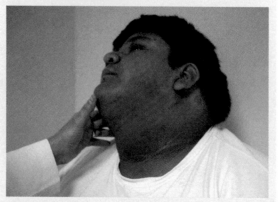

Figure 15-9 *A child with acanthosis nigracans.*

Benedicte Desrus/Alamy Stock Photo

Nursing Care of Type 1 Diabetes

Nursing care for a child with type 1 diabetes is complex. During the early phase of care after a new diagnosis, the nurse should seek to establish a trusting relationship, with this effort then being followed by a great deal of teaching. No matter what the child's age, the family must be included in the teaching sessions so that close family and friends will be prepared to assist the diabetic child as needed. Steps in teaching the newly diagnosed child with type 1 diabetes and the family are summarized in **Box 15-2**. Steps in teaching the newly diagnosed child with type 2 diabetes and the family are summarized in **Box 15-3**.

Hypoglycemia must be avoided. Low blood glucose levels can have severely detrimental effects on the child's brain and organs, leading to lethargy, coma, and death. Periods of hypoglycemia may be associated with too much insulin administered, inadequate food consumption, missed meals or snacks, extra or prolonged rigorous physical activity without a source of nutrition, or consumption of alcohol in adolescence. Children with diabetes must always have a source of glucose that can be rapidly administered orally—for example, juice, dextrose pills, and hard candies for older children. Consumption of 15 to 20 g of carbohydrate is recommended, which equates to two or three 5-g glucose tabs, 2 rolls of Smarties, 15 Skittles candies, ½ cup of apple or orange juice, or 1 teaspoon of brown sugar or honey. The child's blood glucose should be tested again in 15 minutes. If the serum level is still at or less than 70 mg/dL, glucose administration following the preceding

- Signs and symptoms of hypoglycemia (dangerous and associated with the administration of too much insulin), including mild tremors or shakiness, sweating, headaches, palpitations, blurred vision, confusion, poor coordination progressing to seizures, coma, and death. Hypoglycemia is considered a blood glucose level less than 70 mg/dL. Immediate action must be taken to increase the child's blood glucose.
- Signs and symptoms of hyperglycemia (imbalance of insulin, food, and activity; stress; and infections, illnesses, and disease processes), including polyuria (diuresis), polydipsia (tremendous thirst), polyphagia (hunger), fruity odor to the breath, headache, lack of concentration, flushed appearance, spilling of ketones in the urine, and hyperventilation with Kussmaul breathing pattern, progressing to neurologic symptoms of seizures, coma, and death. Hyperglycemia is considered a blood glucose level greater than 250 mg/dL.
- Blood glucose monitoring via a glucometer prescribed to the family for home care.
- Calculation of carbohydrates to be consumed with each meal or snack that contains a significant amount of carbohydrates.
- Calculation of rapid-acting insulin to cover the estimated carbohydrates that the child will consume. Typically, 1 unit of rapid-acting insulin is given for every 15 g of carbohydrates. This ratio will be determined by the pediatric endocrinologist and should be altered accordingly.
- Administration of rapid-acting insulin (lispro [Humalog]) subcutaneously when food is ready to be consumed by the child. Administration sites must be rotated to prevent atrophy or hypertrophy of fat tissue in the subcutaneous skin layer (lipodystrophy).
- Administration of a daily or twice-daily subcutaneous injection of long-acting insulin to stabilize the child's blood glucose over a 24-hour period.
- Appropriate, safe, and rapid responses to periods of dangerous hypoglycemia.
- How to use an insulin pen, if one is ordered.
- How to use an insulin pump, if one is ordered.
- Healthy choices of carbohydrates, such as grains, legumes, milk, and fruits, and limitation of simple sugar carbohydrates, such as candy, refined sugars, and refined grains (white rice). Children should aim to obtain approximately 60% of their daily calories from healthy carbohydrates and 7% from saturated fat, with 1% of these being trans fatty acids (doughnuts and fried foods). Proteins should account for 20% of total calories, and children should be given high-fiber food choices.
- Incorporation of cultural preferences and ethnic foods into a healthy diabetic diet, combined with appropriate carbohydrate counting and insulin administration.
- As the child grows and matures, self-care, blood glucose monitoring, independent carbohydrate counting, and self-insulin administration.
- Purpose, frequency, and meaning of results of HbA_{1c} glycosylated hemoglobin levels.
- Trending patterns in the child's blood glucose, from information that can be electronically downloaded from the glucometer to a computer for graphic display of data.
- When to call the pediatric endocrinology team to adjust the child's insulin doses—illness, infections, participation in a new sport, or rapid growth.

- Healthy eating habits and low carbohydrate consumption
- Encouragement of daily periods of exercise and activity with the entire family
- Encouragement, support, and resources for healthy slow and progressive weight loss
- Monitoring for signs and symptoms of progressing cardiovascular disease such as the development of hypertension
- Long-term complications of diabetes mellitus
- Need for follow-up care, screening, and adherence to oral hypoglycemic medication as ordered

guidelines should be repeated. When stabilized, the child should then consume a protein and carbohydrate snack.

The nutritional needs of a child with diabetes mellitus require a strong foundation of knowledge. The pediatric nurse and the dietician/nutritionist should work together to teach and reinforce the need for diet modification. Because of the many potential health complications associated with diabetes (e.g., kidney failure, heart disease, blindness, dyslipidemia, hypertension, microvascular disease, peripheral neuropathy), a comprehensive educational program with frequent reinforcement must be implemented. Children, especially teenagers, are at risk for struggling with compliance with the medical care required for blood glucose stability, and families struggling to raise a child with diabetes can have adherence issues concerning blood glucose monitoring, insulin dosage calculations (dietary carbohydrate counting), and dietary modification.

Insulin Types, Onset, and Duration

- *Rapid-acting insulins* (lispro [Humalog]; aspart [Novolog]; glulisine [Apidra]): Used before each meal and significant snack with carbohydrate counting (i.e., 1 unit for 15 to 20 carbohydrates). Average onset of action is approximately 15 minutes and peak efficacy is reached in 30 to 90 minutes; duration of action is 3 to 4 hours for lispro and aspart, and approximately 2.5 hours for glulisine.
- *Regular or short-acting insulins* (Humulin R, Novolin R): Onset of action is approximately 30 minutes; peak efficacy occurs in 2 to 3 hours; duration is approximately 3 to 6 hours.
- *Intermediate-acting insulins* (NPH [Humulin N, Novolin N]): Onset of action is approximately 2 to 4 hours; peak efficacy occurs in 4 to 12 hours; duration is 12 to 18 hours.
- *Long-acting insulins* (glargine [Lantus]; detemir [Levemir]): Used for 24-hour basal coverage. Injected once a day, or in some cases twice a day, with onset of action occurring in 1 to 2 hours and peak efficacy in 14 to 24 hours; duration is 26 to 36 hours.

Tips for Administering Insulin in Children

- It is imperative that the correct syringe is used for accurate insulin administration. **Figure 15-10** depicts different syringes with the 0.5 mL (50 units) and 1.0 mL (100 units) syringes being the only ones to use for insulin administration.
- Do not mix rapid-acting and long-acting insulins together in one syringe. The child will require separate injections of each medication.
- Only rapid-acting insulins are used in insulin pumps; refer to the manufacturer's instructions to determine which type of rapid-acting insulin works best in the device.

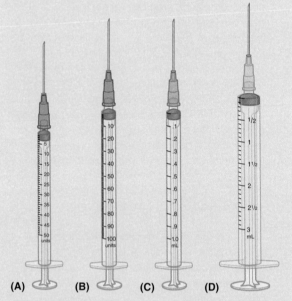

Figure 15-10 *(A) 0.5 mL insulin syringe; (B) 1.0 mL insulin syringe; (C) 1 mL tuberculosis needle; (D) 3 mL syringe for IM injections.*

Case Study

Philip, a 14-month-old child recently diagnosed with type 1 diabetes, presents to the pediatric metabolic/endocrine clinic with severe gastrointestinal distress, fever, dehydration, lethargy, and loss of appetite. His mother is very distressed and appears tired; she is sleep deprived and worried about her child, who she says has had "a stomach bug" for 2 days. Recently divorced, she asks to speak to a social worker concerning her impending loss of living situation and lack of resources to pay for a move. Her 4-year-old child is currently staying with the maternal grandparents, whose own health status is poor.

Upon assessment, the child's vital signs are heart rate of 132 beats/min, respiratory rate of 42 breaths/min, axillary temperature of 101.3°F, oxygen saturation of 91%, blood pressure of 99/42 mm Hg, and significant glucosuria and ketonuria. A finger-stick blood glucose test finds the child's fasting blood glucose to be 372 mg/dL, so intravenous fluids and insulin are initiated to address his dehydration and hyperglycemia. When asked about the child's insulin intake, the mother provides an insulin log but many entries are not filled in.

The pediatric healthcare team gathers in the clinic room with the mother and explains the child needs to be admitted to the pediatric unit for further testing and supportive care. Very distressed, the mother states she is overwhelmed and confused by the child's diabetes regimen and feels as though she lacks the ability to care for the toddler.

Case Study Questions

1. What are the incidence, pathology, clinical presentation, and care required for children with type 1 diabetes mellitus?

(continues)

Case Study *(continued)*

2. What is the most likely reason for this child's symptoms of GI upset, high blood glucose, and ketonuria?
3. How can the pediatric healthcare team support this mother given her feelings of distress and despair?

As the Case Evolves. . .

Philip's mother has agreed to undergo additional education to help her better manage her son's diabetes. The nurse offers her training about signs and symptoms of hypoglycemia.

4. Which of the following signs and symptoms, if stated back to the nurse by the parent, would be considered correct? (Select all that apply.)
   A. Vomiting
   B. Skin flushing
   C. Excessive sweating
   D. Excessive thirst
   E. Fruity odor to the breath
   F. Lethargy

Chapter Summary

- Deviations of the metabolic pathways and biochemical processes in the body are associated with pathological changes and genetic mutations in enzyme function. These pathway pathologies affect carbohydrate, protein, and lipid metabolism.
- Two major groups of metabolic disorders are found in children: (1) inborn errors of metabolism and (2) disorders of metabolic hormones and their production, secretion, and function.
- Metabolic disorders include complications associated with the hypersecretion and hyposecretion of hormones by various endocrine glands. Hormones, which are usually secreted in miniscule quantities, have very specific functions and act only on their target cells.
- The pediatric healthcare team works together to administer state-mandated newborn blood screening tests for many inborn errors of metabolism, confirm positive results, and rapidly initiate therapies (medications, toxic accumulation removal, and diet modification to prevent growth and development complications and lifelong cognitive or neurologic sequelae). If a newborn presents with acidosis, hypoglycemia, or metabolic acidosis, treatment should begin before confirmation of metabolic disorder takes place.
- Hormone-associated metabolic dysfunctions include childhood diagnoses of hypothyroidism, diabetes mellitus, growth disorders, and delayed or premature puberty, among others.
- Care of children with type 1 diabetes mellitus (an insulin-dependent autoimmune disorder) and type 2 diabetes mellitus (resistance or insensitivity to insulin or insufficient production of insulin) requires extensive teaching and support.

- Two major types of insulin are used to treat type 1 diabetes mellitus. A rapid-acting insulin is dosed according to the carbohydrate content of meals; this is coupled with a daily dose of long-acting insulin to provide basal levels as the standard care for stabilizing blood sugars.
- The pediatric nurse has a specific role in accurate screening, early identification of symptoms, implementation of medical management, thorough and safe teaching on care of a child with a metabolic disorder, and ensuring follow-up with surveillance.

Bibliography

Allen, P. J., & Fomenko, S. D. (2011). Congenital hypothyroidism. *Pediatric Nursing, 37*(6), 324–326.

American Diabetes Association. (2015). Facts about type 2. Retrieved from http://www.diabetes.org/diabetes-basics/type-2/facts-about-type-2.html?loc=db-slabnav

American Thyroid Association. (2016). Iodine deficiency. Retrieved from http://www.thyroid.org/iodine-deficiency

Arnold, G. L., & Steiner, R. D. (2014). Phenylketonuria treatment and management: Dietary measures. *Medscape.* Retrieved from http://emedicine.medscape.com/article/947781-treatment#d9

Babey, M., Kopp, P., & Robertson, G. L. (2011). Familial forms of diabetes insipidus: Clinical and molecular characteristics. *Nature Reviews Endocrinology, 7*(12), 701–714.

Bauer, A. J. (2016). Hyperthyroidism. Children's Hospital of Philadelphia. Retrieved from http://www.chop.edu/conditions-diseases/hyperthyroidism-graves-disease

Beaudet, A. L., Scriver, C. R., Sly, W. S., & Valle, D. (2001). Molecular bases of variant human phenotypes. In C. R. Scriver (Ed.), *The metabolic and molecular bases of inherited disease* (8th ed., pp. 3–51). New York, NY: McGraw-Hill.

Dabelea, D., Mayer-Davis, E. J., Saydah, S., Imperatore, G., Linder, B., Divers, J., . . . Hamman, R. (2014). Prevalence of type 1 and type

2 diabetes among children and adolescents from 2001 to 2009. *Journal of the American Medical Association, 311*(17), 1778–1786. doi: 10.1001/jama.2014.3201

Glastras, S. J., Craig, M. E., Verge, C. F., Chan, A. K., Cusumano, J. M., & Donaghue, K. C. (2005). The role of autoimmunity at diagnosis of type 1 diabetes in the development of thyroid and celiac disease and microvascular complications. *Diabetes Care, 28*(9), 2170–2175.

Johnson, S. R., Cooper, M. N., Jones, T. W., & Davis, E. A. (2013). Long-term outcome of insulin pump therapy in children with type 1 diabetes assessed in a large population-based case-control study. *Diabetologia, 56,* 2392–2400.

Knip, M., & Simell, O. (2012). Environmental triggers of type 1 diabetes. *Cold Spring Harbor Perspectives in Medicine, 7,* a007690.

Laffel, L., & Svoren, B. (2011). Epidemiology, presentation and diagnosis of type 2 diabetes mellitus in children and adolescents. *UpToDate.* Retrieved from http://www.uptodate.com/contents/management-of-type-2-diabetes-mellitus-in-children-and-adolescents

Levitsky, L. L. & Sinha, S. (2013). Pediatric Graves disease. *Medscape.* Retrieved from http://emedicine.medscape.com/article/920283-overview

Mayo Clinic. (2014). Diseases and Conditions: Phenylketonuria (PKU). Retrieved from http://www.mayoclinic.org/diseases-conditions/phenylketonuria/basics/symptoms/con-20026275

Mayo Clinic. (2016). Diseases and conditions: Precocious puberty, treatment and drugs. Retrieved from https://www.google.com/webhp?sourceid=chrome-instant&ion=1&espv=2&ie=UTF-8#q=mayo+clinic+precocious+puberty,+treatment+and+drugs

National Center for Chronic Disease Prevention and Health Promotion. (2011). National diabetes fact sheet, 2011. Retrieved from https://www.cdc.gov/diabetes/pubs/pdf/ndfs_2011.pdf

Pearce, E. N. (2015). Is iodine deficiency reemerging in the United States? *AACE Clinical Case Reports, 1*(1), e81–e82.

Phillip, M., Battelino, T., Rodriguez, H., Danne, T., & Kaufman, F. (2007). Use of insulin pump therapy in the pediatric age-group. *Diabetes Care, 30*(6), 1653–1662.

Raghuveer, T. S., Garg, U., & Graf, W. D. (2006). Inborn errors of metabolism in infancy and early childhood: An update. *American Family Physician, 73*(11), 1981–1990.

Saunders, L. M. (2016). Children's health issues: Hereditary metabolic disorders: Disorders of carbohydrate metabolism. *Merck Manual.* Retrieved from http://www.merckmanuals.com/home/children-s-health-issues/hereditary-metabolic-disorders/disorders-of-carbohydrate-metabolism

Sinha, S., & Bauer, A. J. (2014). Pediatric hypothyroidism clinical presentation: History. *Medscape.* Retrieved from http://reference.medscape.com/article/922777-clinical

Szypowska, A., Schwandt, A., Svensson, J., Shalitin, S., Cardona-Hernandez, R., Forsander, G., . . . Madacsy, L.; SWEET Study Group. (2016). Insulin pump therapy in children with type 1 diabetes: Analysis of data from the SWEET registry. *Pediatric Diabetes, 17*(3), 38–45. doi:10.1111/pedi.12416

CHAPTER 16

Gas Exchange and Oxygenation

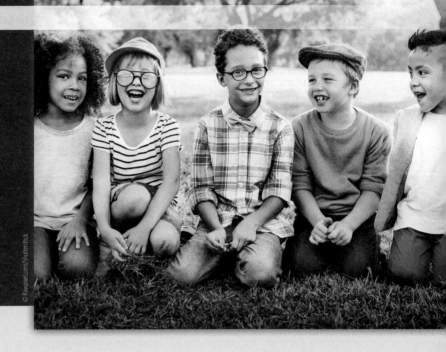

© Rawpixel.com/Shutterstock

LEARNING OBJECTIVES

1. Apply key nursing concepts and the concept of safety across childhood and within each of the developmental stages of childhood (neonate, infant, toddler, preschooler, school age, and adolescent).
2. Incorporate the components of the concept of gas exchange into nursing care for children across the developmental stages.
3. Incorporate the components of the concept of oxygenation into nursing care for children across the developmental stages.
4. Analyze exemplars representing pathology in the concepts of gas exchange and oxygenation—respiratory distress, asthma, cystic fibrosis, and bronchiolitis.
5. Apply pediatric nursing care principles to children experiencing pathology related to respiratory distress, asthma, cystic fibrosis, and bronchiolitis.
6. State the components of essential family education when caring for a child with a respiratory disorder affecting gas exchange and oxygenation.

KEY TERMS

Adventitious breath sounds
Asthma
Atelectasis
Bronchiolitis
Croup
Cyanosis
Cystic fibrosis (CF)
Epiglottitis
Gas exchange
Oxygenation
Rales
Respiratory syncytial virus (RSV)
Retractions
Rhonchi
Stridor
Surfactant
Tonsillitis
Ventilation

Introduction

The pediatric respiratory system is one of the most important systems to understand. Respiratory illnesses, infections, and conditions are common reasons why families seek pediatric health care, and are common causes of illness throughout childhood. Children may present with acute, chronic, or life-threatening respiratory conditions, all of which can affect the stability of the child's well-being and his or her quality of life. Especially vulnerable populations in terms of respiratory disorders are premature infants, immunocompromised children, and children with a chronic illness.

The concepts of gas exchange and oxygenation in the pediatric population begin at the initiation of extra-uterine respiration and continue throughout the entire developmental period of childhood. The most vulnerable period for the newborn is the first 24 hours of life. During this period, the neonate must clear amniotic fluid, initiate a breathing pattern, and maintain effective **gas exchange** with the intake of oxygen (which moves from the lungs into the bloodstream) and the exhalation of carbon dioxide (when moves from the bloodstream into the lungs). Once well established, the infant's respiratory system develops rapidly. The premature newborn has relatively fewer alveoli, reduced quantities of surfactant, and, therefore, more challenges in effective **oxygenation** (the addition of oxygen to the body's systems). **Figure 16-1** illustrates a child's respiratory tract and structures.

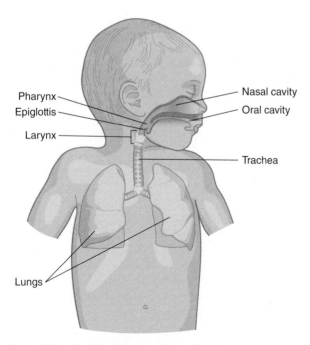

Figure 16-1 *A child's respiratory tract and structures.*

Respiratory System Function

The anatomy and physiology of the respiratory system can be divided into the upper and lower air passageways. The upper airway structures include the nasal cavities, the pharynx, the larynx, and the trachea. The cleansing mechanism of the nasal cilia plays an essential role in maintaining these airways. The lower airway passageways include the main bronchi, bronchioles, and alveoli. Also essential to the respiratory system is the thoracic musculature, which provides for inhalation and exhalation. Red blood cells carry oxygen molecules produced by ventilation and distribute them to the tissues of the body.

Ventilation refers to the process of breathing air into and out of the lungs with the support of the following structures (**Figure 16-2**):

- Intercostal muscles, ribs and diaphragm: Structures that provide support in chest expansion, contraction, and flow of air into the lungs.
- Chemoreceptors: Sensors that respond to a change in the blood oxygen saturation (the percentage of red blood cells with attached oxygen molecules) by sending a chemical message to the brain stem. This process stimulates the child to increase the respiratory rate and depth. High levels of carbon dioxide also stimulate the child's ventilation.
- Respiratory centers in the medulla: In these centers, the child's increased rate or decreased rate of respirations is regulated by nerves that send signals based on oxygenation needs.

A child's respiratory system has several anatomic and physiological differences relative to the respiratory system of an adult. These differences, such as a smaller, narrower airway, can contribute to the development of adverse respiratory conditions. They also affect the assessment and management of an infant or child who presents with a respiratory infection, condition, or compromised state of ventilation.

Respiratory System Differences in Newborns
- Newborns and young infants have a prominent occiput, larger tongue, larger tonsils, shorter and narrower trachea, large and floppy epiglottis, and compliant chest wall, all of which increase the risk of respiratory compromise.
- The newborn has an approximate airway size of 4 to 5 mm, compared to the adult airway size of 18 to 20 mm. The infant's airway is also narrower and shorter than that of an adult at the larynx. The newborn's and infant's airway has the approximate diameter of the child's little finger.
- The newborn's lungs have fewer alveoli than the lungs of an older child. A newborn has approximately 20 to 50 million alveoli, whereas

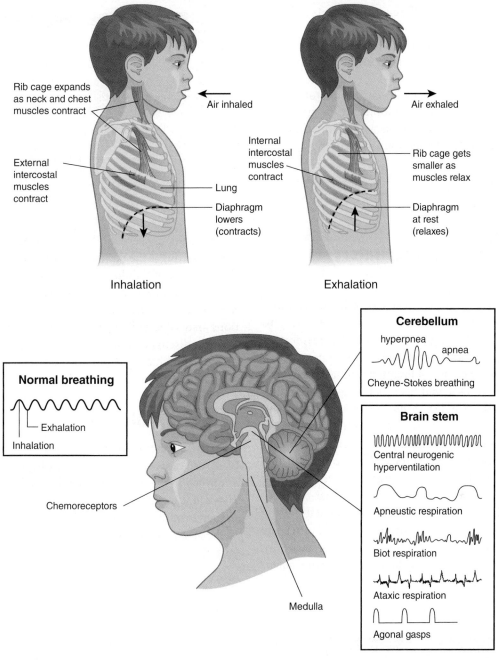

Figure 16-2 *The ventilation process.*

an 8-year-old child has approximately 300 million alveoli. Newborns also have a faster respiratory rate and an uneven respiratory pattern.

- The newborn and the infant rely primarily on their diaphragm and abdominal muscles for breathing. Intercostal muscles are immature and in this developmental stage support only the small chest wall.
- Newborns and young infants have decreased production of mucus, which acts as a cleansing agent to move irritants, particles, and microbes out of the pulmonary system.

- Because of the risk of sudden infant death syndrome (SIDS), newborns and young infants should always be placed on their back to sleep, should never participate in co-sleeping with an adult, and should not have excessive blankets or a body-molding mattress that might trap expired air or compromise air exchange.
- Due to the child's large occiput, the newborn should be placed in a sniffing position for maximal air exchange when the ventilation process is compromised.

Respiratory System Differences in Infants and Children

- A child will experience much louder adventitious breath sounds than an adult in the presence of pathology or distress.
- The infant's and young child's eustachian tubes are at a more horizontal position and are shorter than these structures in adults, leaving the child more prone to fluid retention and middle ear infections.
- The infant is an obligate nose breather and requires suctioning to maintain a patent airway in the presence of copious and thick secretions.

Assessments of the Respiratory System

One of the most important aspects of pediatric nursing across multiple clinical settings is the ability to confidently and thoroughly assess a child's respiratory system. Assessments must include a *visual observation* for air hunger, shortness of breathing, nasal flaring, use of accessory muscles, and head bobbing in the infant. Assessments also include *auscultating* all lung fields—both the upper and lower airways, and the anterior, posterior, and lateral areas—very carefully for adventitious breath sounds (abnormal). **Adventitious breath sounds** include **rales** (popping, bubbling, or high-pitched crackling sounds), **rhonchi** (rattling breath sounds that resemble snoring), wheezing, and **stridor** (high-pitched grating breath sounds). The assessment should include alternate sides of the lung fields for comparison (**Figure 16-3**). Finally, assessments should include *percussion and palpation* and *respiration*.

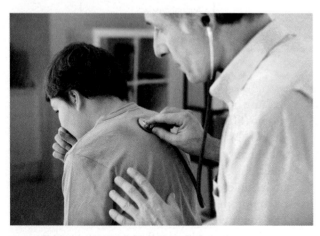

Figure 16-3 *Auscultating a child's lungs.*
© Image Point Fr/Shutterstock

The major concern for the pediatric nurse working in a clinical setting is the rapid identification, assessment, and management of a child with a respiratory pathology. It is not uncommon to encounter children seeking nursing and medical care for treatment of symptoms and complications associated with a variety of pulmonary conditions. We next discuss common oxygenation and gas exchange disorders, including respiratory distress, asthma, cystic fibrosis, and bronchiolitis.

Respiratory Distress

Insufficient intake of oxygen and removal of carbon dioxide (CO_2) can cause a child to experience hypoxemia; low levels of oxygen in the blood can rapidly develop into hypoxia. *Hypoxia* is a general term used to describe low levels of oxygen in body tissue. *Hypoxemia* is a low level of oxygen in the arterial blood, which is assessed by measuring the partial pressure of oxygen (PaO_2).

Risk Factors for Respiratory Distress

Respiratory distress in children, particularly newborns and young children, requires rapid recognition and intervention. Young children, in general, experience rapid decompensation of the respiratory system when acute illness is present. Risk factors associated with respiratory distress include an acute episode of airway obstruction, especially in light of children's narrower airways and their decreased respiratory reserves, and inadequate compensatory mechanisms. Several acute conditions can cause children to have a higher risk for respiratory distress—for example, infant respiratory distress syndrome (previously called hyaline membrane disease), tension pneumothorax, pulmonary embolism or trauma, and viral or bacterial infection causing inflammation. Chronic pulmonary conditions such as cystic fibrosis, asthma, and bronchopulmonary dysplasia also place children at higher risk for rapid respiratory distress when they experience an acute exacerbation of their illness.

Assessments for Respiratory Distress

Assessments for respiratory distress should begin with visual observation of the child's overall appearance and behavior. Work of breathing must be assessed, and the nurse must ensure the child has a patent airway. Level of consciousness, positioning, overall distress, interactive behaviors, and skin color should be determined. The nurse should have access to the child's current weight to prepare for the administration of emergency medications. Oxygen saturations, arterial blood gases, chest radiography, and end-tidal carbon dioxide measurements should all be performed to determine the severity of the child's condition.

Medical Treatment for Respiratory Distress

Mild respiratory distress differs from severe distress in terms of its medical management and treatment. Mild respiratory distress can be managed with positioning, oxygen delivery devices, suctioning, bronchodilators, steroidal anti-inflammatory medications, and fluids. Children with mild distress should not be discharged from a clinic or acute care environment until stable and until the pediatric team deems the child safe enough not to have symptom exacerbation. In contrast, severe respiratory distress requires a team approach to airway management, including rapid-sequence intubation, ventilation, and possibly rapid transport to a higher level of care.

Nursing Care for Respiratory Distress

Nursing care will primarily focus on the early identification and stabilization of the child's compromised airway and gas exchange. The nurse will be a key team member in the rapid response to assist the child with respiratory distress, and should be in a primary position in terms of ensuring communication between team members. This practitioner will assist in the coordination of airway management, oxygen delivery, positioning, specimen collection, and medication management. The nurse should never leave the bedside of the child, but rather assist in coordinating the efforts undertaken during a team response.

Once the child is stable, the nurse works holistically to support the child's emotional state and alleviate the family's anxiety. The family will be very fearful and worried about the child's clinical presentation and status. Knowing that the team is assisting the child will be important, and the nurse can help educate the family on the steps being taken and the rationale for the airway management interventions.

(continues)

PHARMACOLOGY

The influenza vaccine for seasonal infections is now recommended for all children older than 6 months of age. According to the Centers for Disease Control and Prevention (CDC, 2016), the administration of the influenza vaccine to children should be offered to families who seek health care (wellness or illness), whenever they are seen in healthcare environments. Children age 6 months through 8 years who are being vaccinated for influenza for the first time, as well as children who have previously received only one dose of vaccine, should get two doses of vaccine in the current season, with the first dose given as soon as the season's vaccine is available. Children who present with fever of unknown origin, have respiratory symptoms, have had a known exposure, or have recently been hospitalized should be tested for the influenza virus by nasal aspirates and swabs.

Thinking in Concepts to Promote Safety: Respiratory Emergencies

It is imperative that the pediatric nurse have equipment close at hand that will assist the team in securing a patent airway, provide support for ventilation and oxygenation, and control the child's symptoms of respiratory distress. The following essential equipment should be readily available in all clinical settings:

- Emergency ventilation equipment: Masks of various sizes and self-filling resuscitation bags (Ambu bags) (**Figure 16-4**)
- A source of oxygen (wall source or tanks) with the correct "Christmas tree"–style valve that fits the oxygen tubing (**Figure 16-5**)
- Suction equipment, including a variety of suction tip devices such as olive tip, tonsil tip, bulb syringe, and deep sterile suctioning kits (**Figure 16-6**)
- Crash cart (**Figure 16-7**) with intubation equipment; tracheostomy equipment; rescue medications such as racemic epinephrine, epinephrine 1:1000 and 1:10,000, albuterol, sodium

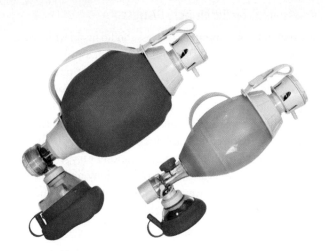

Figure 16-4 *Two sizes (adult and child) of bag-valve mask devices for emergency ventilation.*
© Terayut Janjaranuphab/Shutterstock

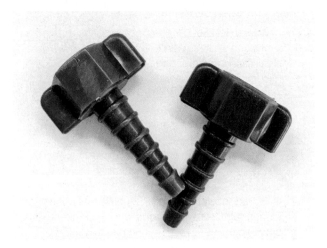

Figure 16-5 *"Christmas tree"–style valve for oxygen tubing.*
© Narumon Numpha/Shutterstock

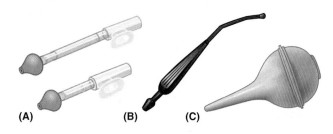

(A)   (B)   (C)

Figure 16-6 *Suction tip devices: (A) olive tip; (B) tonsil tip; (C) bulb syringe.*

bicarbonate, and EpiPen (ACLS Training Center, 2015); and a length-based color-coded resuscitation tape (such as a Broselow tape [**Figure 16-8**]) for rapid determination of emergency medications and equipment for various groupings of weights

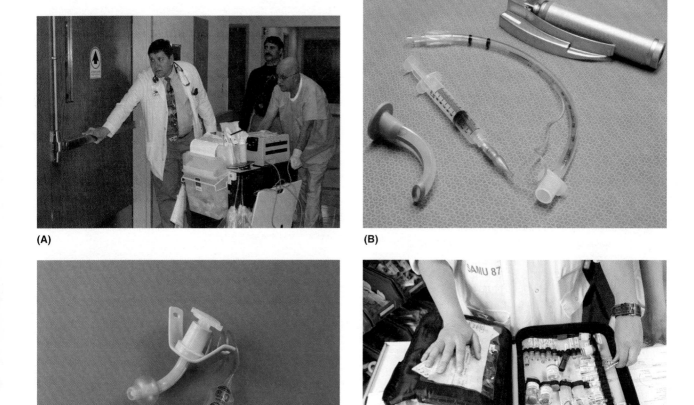

(A)

(B)

(C)

(D)

Figure 16-7 *All clinical settings should have (A) a crash cart readily available with (B) intubation equipment, (C) tracheostomy equipment, and (D) rescue medications.*

(A) © Jones & Bartlett Learning. Courtesy of MIEMSS; (B) © SisterSarah/E+/Getty Images; (D) Phanie/Alamy Stock Photo

RESEARCH EVIDENCE

According to the American Heart Association, children who suffer a complete cardiopulmonary arrest within a hospital setting have a 27% percent chance of survival, whereas the out-of-hospital setting survival rate is 6% for children overall and 3% for infants (Kleinman et al., 2010). Most arrests occur because of respiratory failure, shock, asphyxia arrest (hypoxemia, hypercapnia, acidosis, bradycardia, hypotension, and then cardiac arrest) (Kleinman et al., 2010). It is imperative that the pediatric nurse confidently and rapidly assess a child who presents with respiratory distress, initiate airway support, apply oxygen, and seek team support. A rapid response to respiratory distress can save a child's life.

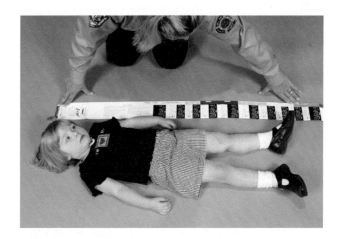

Figure 16-8 *A length-based color-coded resuscitation tape.*

© Jones & Bartlett Learning. Courtesy of MIEMSS.

If a child develops new adventitious breath sounds, the pediatric nurse should report the child's condition immediately:

- Crackles: Popping, bubbling, or high-pitched crackling sounds that occur from air passing through pockets of pulmonary fluids and alveoli (formerly called rales, a term that is falling out of favor).
- Grunting: The sound a child makes when trying to push CO_2 from the lungs on expiration when airways are inflamed, spasming, or narrowed.
- Sibilant rhonchi: Hissing or squeaking sound (wheeze) caused by narrowing of the airways and bronchospasms.
- Sonorous rhonchi: Wheezing caused by secretions in the airways; sounds like a snoring, coarse, deep inspiration or expiration.
- Stridor: Typically found on inspiration; a loud, high-pitched sound that occurs because air is passing a significantly compromised and narrow upper airway. Can be associated with use of fiber-optic bronchoscopy.
- Wheezing: Can be inspiratory, expiratory, or both; whistling sound due to narrowed lower airways.

Data from Bohadana A., Izbicki, G., & Kraman, S. S. (2014). Fundamentals of lung auscultation. *New England Journal of Medicine, 370*, 744–751.

Advanced Airway Management

Airway management is considered an advanced professional skill. National certification as a pediatric advanced life support nurse signifies competency in responding to a child in severe distress or who has suffered a cardiopulmonary arrest. Continued practice through mock codes helps to keep a team of responders ready for a child with advanced needs. Nurses need to be able to confidently respond to a child in distress by taking the following steps:

- Rapidly identifying the symptoms of distress and taking immediate action
- Positioning the child in a high Fowler's position, initiating suctioning, and delivering oxygen therapy
- Requesting team help immediately by calling the rapid response team (RRT) or code team as needed, and supporting the application of the American Heart Association's Neonatal Resuscitation Program (NRP) or Pediatric Advanced Life Support (PALS) program assessment, skills, and algorithms as warranted
- Applying principles of infection control until the source of respiratory distress is identified
- Assembling emergency response equipment and medications
- Providing support and education for the family

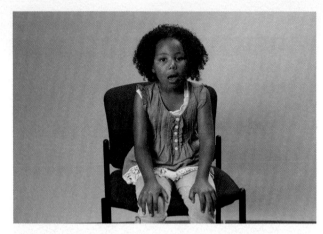

Figure 16-9 *A child tripoding.*
© Jones & Bartlett Learning. Photographed by Glen E. Ellman.

Prevention of Airway Occlusion with Epiglottitis

Epiglottitis is a severe, life-threatening infection of the epiglottis (the small structure that closes the trachea off while swallowing) caused mainly by *Haemophilus influenzae* type B bacteria. The child's epiglottis swells above the vocal cords, causing severe narrowing and potential complete occlusion of the airway. Many children in the United States are vaccinated for *H. influenzae* starting at 2 months of age, but some are not. If a child presents with the abrupt classic "Ds" (drooling, distress, dystonia, dysphagia), is tripoding (**Figure 16-9**), and appears toxic, epiglottitis should be assumed and emergency airway management with possible tracheostomy should be undertaken. Rapid administration of intravenous antibiotics is essential.

Respiratory Distress

A child who presents with respiratory distress needs a team approach to assess, manage, and stabilize the airway. For rapid help, the pediatric nurse should initiate the protocol for the RRT, or if the child is progressing from respiratory distress to respiratory failure, the code team should be called to prevent a full cardiopulmonary arrest.

Asthma

Asthma is considered a chronic inflammatory disease of the lungs that affects the small and large airways. Its pathophysiology is thought to stem from the airways' hyper-responsiveness to specific triggers—which can include anything from allergens to cold air to stress to exercise—to which the child is exposed. Asthma has a strong genetic component and may be associated with atopy; eczema, asthma, and rhinitis often go together. When an infant or young toddler first presents with a hyper-responsive airway leading to wheezing and cough, the primary diagnosis may be reactive airway disease (RAD). A second episode is then considered diagnostic for asthma.

The incidence of asthma is very high. Approximately 9.3% of all children have a confirmed diagnosis of asthma (the total U.S. prevalence is now 6.8 million children) with 50% of new cases occurring in the child's first year of life, followed by 80% occurring by the fifth year of life (CDC, 2015). Asthma deaths are preventable but on the rise: Mortality from this cause is increasing by 6% per year, with 3630 deaths from asthma occurring annually (CDC, 2015). School absences due to asthma are significant, with the number of annual asthma-related school absences of children age 0 to 17 ranging from 9020 to 703,570 depending on the state (Khavjou, Nurmagambetov, Murphy, & Orenstein, 2016). Nationally, children age 5 to 17 collectively missed 10.5 million days of school in 2008 due to asthma exacerbations (CDC, 2013).

The pathology of asthma is typically an inflammatory hypersensitivity response to an external substance or exposure ("trigger") that starts a response cascade. First there is an immediate hypersensitivity in the bronchial mucosa, with immunoglobulin E (IgE) molecules becoming attached to basophils and mast cells. Chemical mediators are then released from these cells, causing a significant series of clinical symptoms:

- Bronchial constriction of the smooth muscles surrounding the outer aspects of the large and small airways
- Copious mucus production by the mucus-producing cells lining the airways
- Inflammation that causes edema and narrowing of the inner luminal tracheobronchial mucosa

Internal stimuli have also been known to cause asthma. For example, extreme emotional responses may produce asthma symptoms.

With continuation of symptoms and the development of severe edema, mucus production, and bronchial constriction, the child may develop serious bronchospasms. If the hyper-responsiveness is not stopped, the child may suffer insufficient oxygenation, CO_2 air trapping, lung hyper-inflammation, severe respiratory distress, and complete obstruction. Asthma deaths can be prevented by rapid responses to a child's early symptoms of an asthma attack.

Diagnosis of Asthma

The diagnostic process for asthma includes a health history, family history of asthma, history of recent viral infections, and identification of symptoms—adventitious breath sounds such as wheezing, coughing, mucus production, and airway hyper-responsiveness. A complete blood cell count may be ordered to assess for infection, and nasal secretions may be assessed for the presence of viruses such as **respiratory syncytial virus (RSV)**, a pathogen that causes mild, flu-like symptoms in most people.

Risk Factors for Asthma

Risk factors associated with asthma include family history of asthma. Risk factors for reactive airway disease include exposure to respiratory infections, cigarette smoke, allergens, and other triggers. Family members must be helped to identify the child's triggers so as to prevent repeated exposures and subsequent episodes of asthma.

Asthma at School: Teachers' and Administrators' Educational Guidelines

Because of the amount of time children spend at school, and their chances of being exposed to triggers there, an asthma exacerbation starting at school is not uncommon. It is imperative that parents disclose their child's diagnosis of asthma to school personnel and provide a list of triggers. It is important to have ready access to rapid-acting bronchodilators in the school environment. Many state laws now encourage children to carry their rapid-acting inhalers with them at all times.

Expeditious identification of asthma symptoms and fast administration of rapid-acting bronchodilator medications can prevent serious asthma attacks at school. Teachers, administrators, and parent volunteers should know what to look for in a child with a confirmed asthma diagnosis who is having an asthma attack:

- Shortness of breath
- Persistent or frequently occurring cough
- Inability to speak in full sentences
- Wanting to sit out of exercise or play activities
- Wheezing
- Tachypnea (any respiratory rate of 60 breaths/min or faster requires immediate transfer to a medical facility from school, without the delay of waiting for a parent to pick a child up)

FAMILY EDUCATION

Asthma Triggers

Avoiding exposure to asthma triggers can prevent asthma attacks and exacerbations. Triggers for asthma include the following factors:

- Animal dander
- Grasses, pine trees, and other vegetation

(continues)

- Cockroach dust (dried remains)
- Dust mites
- Airway irritants such as paint fumes, aerosols, and smoke
- Altitude
- Emotions and stress
- Mold and home allergens
- Fireplace and wood stove smoke
- Cigarette, pipe, e-cigarette, and cigar smoke and fumes
- Food allergies
- Cold air or a change in the weather
- Exercise
- Fragrances
- Gastrointestinal reflux
- Inhaled illegal drugs such as marijuana, cocaine, and methamphetamines

Medical Treatment for Asthma

Prevention is the gold standard for treating asthma. Second to prevention is administration of rapid-acting bronchodilators at the onset of asthma symptoms. (See the **Pharmacology** feature for information on medications used to treat asthma.) A child with moderate to severe asthma will also require daily preventive medications to reduce edema, immunoglobulin reactions, and exacerbations linked to chemical mediators such as leukotrienes, acetylcholine, histamine, and prostaglandins.

PHARMACOLOGY

Because asthma is an inflammatory process, the medications used in this disease address different aspects of the exacerbation process. *Bronchodilators*, usually inhaled beta agonists, are used when symptoms first occur; they "rescue" respiration by opening the bronchi so air can pass through. If the patient's airway is too constricted to allow inhaled bronchodilating medications to enter, IV or injected medications may be needed to interrupt the exacerbation. In clinical settings, rapid-acting anti-inflammatory medications such as *corticosteroids* and *epinephrine* are generally used for this purpose.

Long-acting asthma medications are used as maintenance therapy to reduce systemic inflammation and prevent recurrence of asthma symptoms. Inhaled corticosteroids are favored for use in children, but clinicians should be aware that they may have long-term impacts on growth. These medications may also lead to problematic side effects such as hyperglycemia in children who have or are at risk for diabetes (Egbuonu, Antonio, & Edavalath, 2014).

Short-Acting Asthma Medications

- Short-acting beta-2 agonists (e.g., albuterol)
- Intravenous corticosteroids (e.g., methylprednisolone)*
- Oral corticosteroids (e.g., prednisolone)†
- Anticholinergics (e.g., ipratropium bromide)
- Epinephrine (racemic)*

Long-Acting Asthma Medications

- Inhaled corticosteroids (e.g., fluticasone propionate)
- Long-acting beta-2 agonists (e.g., formoterol fumarate)
- Anti-immunoglobulin E antibodies (anti-IgE) (e.g., omalizumab)
- Mast cell inhibitors (e.g., cromolyn)
- Leukotriene modifiers (LM) (e.g., montelukast sodium)
- Methylxanthines (e.g., theophylline)

* Used primarily in the emergency department setting for treatment of acute exacerbations, not for daily control of symptoms.

† Used primarily after emergency department treatment of an acute exacerbation as prophylaxis against relapse. Courses longer than 5 days provide no additional benefit.

Data from Alangari, 2014; American Lung Association, 2009; Egbuonu et al., 2014; National Heart, Lung, and Blood Institute [NHLBI], 2014a.

Nursing Care for Asthma

The central focus of care for a child of any age experiencing asthma symptoms is airway assessment and management. Pediatric nurses must be confident in assisting a child who is experiencing wheezing, coughing, and asthma symptoms. Rapid assessment of the child's clinical status—including respiratory rate, severity of symptoms, need for transport to a higher level of care, and signs of hypoxemia and hypoxia—is the priority.

After assessment and stabilization, the central focus of nursing care is on educating the child and parents on the avoidance of triggers and care at home and in school, as well as understanding the nature of asthma as a chronic—rather than acute—condition that needs ongoing management. Identifying and correcting mistakes in inhaler technique is important for ensuring medication adherence (Braido et al., 2016). Assessing the caregivers' or child's ability to correctly use a metered-dose inhaler (MDI) or aerochamber, conduct a peak flow evaluation, and follow the personalized asthma action plan can be instrumental not only in reducing the need to seek health care, but also in decreasing the child's chance of a poor outcome, including asthma-related death (**Figure 16-10**). Continuing follow-up to reassess asthma symptoms and update the child's and family's knowledge every 3 to 6 months is an important aspect of care, as the child's asthma symptoms may improve or worsen over time and require a change in regimen.

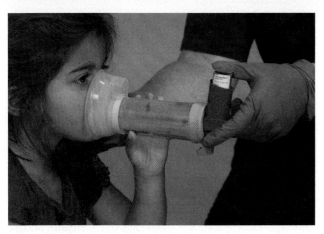

Figure 16-10 *A child using a metered-dose inhaler (MDI) or aerochamber.*

Cystic Fibrosis

Cystic fibrosis (CF) is an autosomal recessive genetic disorder caused by a mutation in the protein cystic fibrosis transmembrane conductance regulator (*CFTR*) gene on chromosome 7, which regulates digestive secretions, sweat, and mucus production. Cystic fibrosis causes cysts and scarring within the pancreas, preventing the normal secretion of digestive enzymes and insulin. In addition, excessive sodium absorption in the lungs causes the normally quite thin respiratory mucus secretions to become thicker, to the point that they obstruct the functioning of exocrine glands.

The potentially fatal combination of blocked exocrine gland secretion and viscous mucus production affects many body systems, including the gastrointestinal, pancreatic, pulmonary, and reproductive system. The problems are caused by the absence of a transmembrane regulator enzyme, which allows the flow of sodium and water into the mucus-producing cells, leading to viscous mucus. Chronic secretion of this thick mucus ("tenacious mucus") blocks the exocrine glands and leads to severe obstruction. The presence of the tenacious mucus also leaves the child vulnerable to chronic pulmonary infections and structural damage.

According to the Cystic Fibrosis Foundation (2015), symptoms that a child might display before being diagnosed with CF include salty-tasting skin; frequent respiratory infections; coughing; wheezing; symptoms of failure to thrive; bulky, greasy stools; and constipation.

Diagnosis of Cystic Fibrosis

The gold standard for CF diagnosis is a sweat chloride test, which will demonstrate elevated levels of chloride in the child's sweat. The noninvasive application of pilocarpine along with a low level of electrical stimulation will cause a child to produce sweat onto a gauze, filter paper, or plastic coil, which is then tested for abnormally high sodium and chloride levels. The test can take as long as 1 hour to complete. Infants from birth to 6 months with sweat test results of greater than or equal to 60 mmol/L are considered positive for this disease (Cystic Fibrosis Foundation, 2015). Children with a level of 40 to 59 mmol/L or more are identified as having a possible positive finding, and those with a level of 60 mmol/L or greater have a positive finding (Cystic Fibrosis Foundation, 2015).

Respiratory infections, bronchitis, atelectasis, pneumonia, and respiratory failure may all indicate a possible diagnosis of CF. Intestinal dysfunctions associated with CF include malabsorption of fat and vitamins A, D, E, and K; gallbladder disease; meconium ileus; diabetes; and nutritional deficiencies.

Median survival for individuals with CF is approximately 37 years for females and 40 years for males (MacKenzie et al., 2014).

Risk Factors for Cystic Fibrosis

Cystic fibrosis occurs in 1 in 2500 Caucasian births and 1 in 17,000 African American births. The only known risk factors associated with CF are race (Caucasian) and having a genetic predisposition to the disease. The probability of having cystic fibrosis is 25% if both parents are carriers of the gene, and 50% that the child will be a carrier. Most children are diagnosed by 2 years of age (Cystic Fibrosis Foundation, 2015).

Medical Treatment for Cystic Fibrosis

Treatment focuses on the removal of tenacious mucus, prevention of pulmonary complications and infections, and the restoration of nutritional balance. Antibiotics; mucolytic agents; mist inhalation; chest physiotherapy; postural drainage; vitamin A, D, E, and K and pancreatic enzyme replacements; and high-calorie diets are mainstays of CF treatment. Use of flutter devices and, in adolescents, high-frequency chest wall oscillation (known as the Vest; **Figure 16-11**) to help dislodge and clear mucus is essential. Intermittent positive-pressure breathing therapy can be effective in improving pulmonary function. In severe cases in which scarring and dysfunction have occurred, lung transplantation or heart–lung transplantation (unilateral or bilateral) may be required for long-term survival.

Nursing Care for Cystic Fibrosis

Family education is the most important aspect of nursing care of a child with cystic fibrosis. The family will be caring for the child and his or her chronic disorder at home. Teaching and reinforcing meticulous care through home chest physiotherapy, secretion drainage, adequate nutrition with a high-calorie and high-fat diet, medication adherence, and knowing when to seek medical assistance for respiratory conditions is paramount.

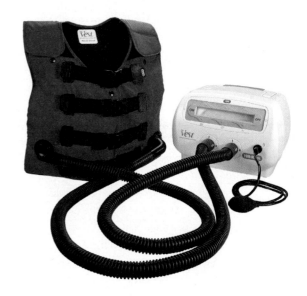

Figure 16-11 *A high-frequency chest wall oscillation device (the Vest).*

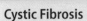

Cystic Fibrosis

Children with cystic fibrosis will need the following drug therapy:

- Annual influenza vaccine
- Antibiotic prophylaxis
- Bronchodilators (e.g., albuterol, salmeterol)
- Anticholinergics (e.g., ipratropium bromide [Atrovent])
- DNase (e.g., dornase alfa)
- Mucolytics
- Hypertonic saline
- Aerosolized aminoglycosides
- Nonsteroidal anti-inflammatory drugs (NSAIDs)
- Vitamin A, D, E, and K supplements
- Mast-cell stabilizers (e.g., cromolyn)
- Corticosteroids
- Digestive enzymes (e.g., Creon, Zenpep, Pancreaze)
- Reflux medications (e.g., ranitidine, lansoprazole, omeprazole)
- Laxatives

A small number of children older than age 6 years with a mutated gene *G55D1* may be able to take ivacaftor (Kalydeco) to target the genetic cause of CF.

Data from National Institutes of Health. (2013). How is cystic fibrosis treated? Retrieved from https://www.nhlbi.nih.gov/health/health -topics/topics/cf/treatment; Cystic Fibrosis Center at Stanford. (2016). Common medications. Retrieved from http://med.stanford.edu /cfcenter/education/english/Meds.html

Bronchiolitis

Bronchiolitis is a viral respiratory infection of the lower airway structures. The infection is caused most frequently by RSV, but can also be caused by an adenovirus, parainfluenza, or rhinovirus (see **Table 16-1** for other respiratory infections and conditions). Bronchiolitis can manifest in any age group throughout the developmental period, but rarely occurs in children older than 2 years. When bronchiolitis is acquired during infancy, the child can be very symptomatic. Infants, with their immature immune systems and lack of immunoglobulins, can develop serious pulmonary infections that require hospitalization. Young infants have anatomic differences that increase their risk for prolonged infection. For example, their relatively few immunoglobulins available to fight infection, coupled with fewer cilia to help remove the infectious material, can cause the infant's infection to take a more serious course.

The pathology of viral bronchiolitis is related to the rapid downward progression of the virus from the upper airways to the lower airways, which leads to significant inflammation, edema, and mucus production. The virus causes the infected cells to fuse with surrounding cells and subsequently destroy cilia in the clumped cells. The mucus and exudates produced cause blockage of the small airways, which can then lead to **atelectasis** (lung collapse). The infant with bronchiolitis frequently needs secretion management, positioning, and oxygen to breathe effectively.

Other symptoms of bronchiolitis include nasal congestion, cough, irritability, fever, wheezing, rhonchi, fine crackles, nasal flaring, retractions, and cough with or without cyanosis. The infant may present with dehydration, tachypnea, tachycardia, fatigue, and copious secretions that lead to shortness of breath and respiratory distress.

Owing to the 2- to 4-day incubation period for bronchiolitis, those caring for the infant with this infection can

TABLE 16-1	Pediatric Respiratory Infections and Conditions: Definitions, Pathology, and Treatment		
Pathology	**Definition**	**Medical Treatment**	**Nursing Care Tips**
Apnea	A 20-second or longer cessation of breathing that is often associated with bradycardia. This condition is associated with prematurity, infection, temperature abnormalities, gastric reflux disease, and immature central nervous system functioning.	Medical treatment is based on identification of the underlying pathology. During an acute episode of apnea, immediate treatment is to stimulate the infant to restore the breathing pattern and reduce bradycardia. Caffeine (orally) may be required in low therapeutic doses to prevent repeated episodes.	Nursing care for a child with apnea is based on careful monitoring with an apnea machine and/or cardiac monitoring. Care must include a rapid response (stimulation) to the child in an acute episode. Careful monitoring of serum levels of caffeine may be ordered. Strict documentation of each episode of apnea with associated activities and behaviors of the child and needed stimulation should be kept for the interdisciplinary team to review.

(continues)

Pathology	Definition	Medical Treatment	Nursing Care Tips
Bronchopulmonary dysplasia (BPD)	Also called chronic lung disease; a respiratory distress condition caused by severe scarring to pulmonary tissues from high levels of prolonged oxygen therapy and mechanical ventilation.	Treatment consists of steroids, bronchodilators, low levels of oxygen, and mechanical ventilation until the infant's lungs mature.	Nursing care for a child with BPD includes promotion of adequate lung function. Care includes meticulous attention to the child's respiratory status, maintaining strict infection reduction techniques, and safety while on ventilation. The family will need support and education while the child is in distress or on a ventilator. Special attention should be given to the infant's growth and development, including nutrition, hygiene, and developmental care. The promotion of safe skin-to-skin contact between the ventilated infant and the parent is essential.
Apparent life-threatening event (ALTE)	A collection of acute symptoms leading the child to display a loss of consciousness, decreased muscle tone, cyanosis, and apnea. Typically occurring in children younger than 1 year of age, this event is frightening to parents, who will often bring their child into the emergency department or call 911 for assistance.	Medical treatment for an ALTE depends on the clinical findings and diagnosis of an underlying pathology. Half of all cases are idiopathic. Male gender, respiratory infections such as RSV and pneumonia, feeding issues, and prematurity are all associated with ALTEs.	Nursing care for a child who has displayed an ALTE focuses on ongoing assessments (apnea monitors, cardiac monitoring, and frequent assessments especially during procedures, blood draws, eating, and crying) and assisting with diagnostics to determine the underlying cause. Parents of a child who has experienced an ALTE should be taught cardiopulmonary resuscitation (CPR).
Epiglottitis	A medical emergency caused by a bacterial infection, *Haemophilus influenzae* type B, that leads to acute inflammation of the epiglottis (the cartilage at the base of the tongue, which prevents aspiration when swallowing), with the potential for extreme respiratory distress and complete upper airway obstruction. Medical history includes a sudden onset of symptoms followed by drooling, dysphagia, dystonia, significant retractions, and stridor. Tripod positioning in young children is common.	Medical management includes rapid identification of the infectious process and immediate administration of antibiotics, steroids, and oxygen. Airway support is essential. Some children in the acute phase will need to have a tracheostomy placed.	A tongue depressor should never be used to assist in visualization of an inflamed epiglottis, as spasm, further inflammation, and complete upper airway obstruction can occur. Primary nursing care includes immediate acquisition and administration of antibiotics and steroids, close monitoring of clinical status, following of arterial blood gases (ABGs), and administration of intravenous fluids.

Pathology	Definition	Medical Treatment	Nursing Care Tips
Respiratory distress syndrome	Associated with a premature infant's immature lungs. A decrease in **surfactant** (a phospholipid that keeps the alveoli open and able to provide adequate gas exchange through a membrane), especially prior to 28 weeks' gestation, causes poor oxygenation and ventilation and damages hyaline membranes. This condition may require mechanical ventilation to reduce acidosis and CO_2 retention, and to promote oxygenation.	This condition is treated with intonation, mechanical ventilation, supplemental oxygenation, and continuous positive airway pressure (CPAP) (NHLBI, 2012). Medications include artificial surfactant replacement, sedation, and medications to maintain safety during mechanical ventilation (NHLBI, 2012).	Nursing care focuses on supporting the infant on a ventilator, administering medications, providing emotional support and teaching for the family. Frequent communication between pediatric team members is crucial to ensure safety of the child with respiratory distress syndrome.
Laryngomalacia or tracheal laryngomalacia	The most common cause of stridor in infancy; a congenital condition caused by immature and soft cartilage in the upper larynx. The condition causes the soft larynx to collapse inward during inhalation (Children's Hospital of Philadelphia, 2017).	Medical treatment consists of surgery if the condition is severe and affects the child's growth and development. Most infants will outgrow this condition by the mid-toddler period.	Nursing care consists of assessing the infant for respiratory distress, apnea and bradycardia, and eating habits. If the infant is displaying respiratory distress, increasing discomfort, or inability to nurse or suck a bottle effectively and has decreased nutritional intake, the primary provider must be notified immediately.
Laryngotracheo-bronchitis (**croup**)	Acute inflammation, edema, and mucus production within the larynx, trachea, and bronchi caused by a virus such as parainfluenza, influenza, enteroviruses, and respiratory syncytial virus. Symptoms include mild fever, a deep "barking" cough, inspiratory stridor and painful breathing, hoarse cry, and, in severe cases, cyanosis. Onset may be sudden and often occurs at night, and is most common in winter or early spring.	Usually lasting 3–5 days, the viral infection takes its course without treatment. Humidified oxygen may help to thin out secretions for more effective clearance and to reduce the inflammation and swelling causing the croupy cough.	Nursing care consists of teaching parents strategies to minimize discomfort and avoid obstruction. Caregivers should encourage quiet, rest, and fluid intake, but avoid cough medicines. Bringing the child into a steamy bathroom for 10 minutes may help alleviate coughing, and holding the child in a sitting position can aid breathing. Parents should be advised to keep close watch on the child's condition and call the healthcare provider immediately in the following circumstances: › The rate of respiration increases or the child has any other difficulty breathing, including retractions. › Exposure to humidity or steam does not improve coughing. › Nostril flaring or a bluish appearance of the skin around the nose or lips develops. › The child begins to drool or is unable to swallow; this may indicate epiglottitis, which is a medical emergency.

(continues)

Pathology	Definition	Medical Treatment	Nursing Care Tips
Nasopharyngitis	The "common cold"; a viral infection that can be caused by more than 200 identified viruses. Symptoms include fatigue, sneezing, coughing, itchy watery eyes, upper and lower airway congestion, and sore throat. The infection is readily transmitted to others through droplets.	Treatment consists of supportive care, rest, secretion control by suctioning (infants), analgesics, humidification, fluids, and antipyretics as needed.	Nursing care is supportive. Provide uninterrupted periods of rest, adequate fluids (the child may need 1.5 times the maintenance volume), and infection control practices.
Otitis media (OM)	A middle ear infection caused by either a virus or a bacterium. It often progresses from an infection that migrated up the young child's shorter, narrower and more linear (straighter) eustachian tube. OM can be directly caused by a respiratory infection, tonsillitis, or adenitis. Signs and symptoms include ear pain or tugging at ears, irritability, fever, decreased appetite, and fluid drainage from the ear.	Antibiotics are administered for OM only if there is clinical evidence of a bacterial infection. A higher white blood cell count, fever, and visualization of pus behind the tympanic membrane are clinical indicators of bacterial OM. For viral OM, the treatment is supportive only, with antipyretics and analgesics. A surgical tympanoplasty with myringotomy (tympanic membrane tube placement) may be required with chronic OM.	Nursing care includes symptom management for ear pain, fever control, fluid intake, and teaching. Parents should be taught not to put their infants to bed with bottles and should be counseled to avoid exposing children to tobacco smoke to reduce risk of OM. Education on the complications of repeated OM includes hearing loss with associated delays in speech development, learning difficulties, and developmental delays.
Pertussis (whooping cough)	A serious bacterial infection of the lungs caused by the infectious agent *Bordetella pertussis*. It is spread by direct contact or droplet. Pertussis presents in three stages: (1) the catarrhal stage, which includes early upper respiratory symptoms (1–2 weeks in length); (2) the paroxysmal stage, which is characterized by frequent cough (a burst of rapid, short coughs followed by a sudden "whooping" inspiration, at times accompanied with cyanosis), mostly at night (4–6 weeks in length); and (3) the convalescent stage, with gradual recovery and less frequent coughing, although occasional paroxysms may recur if a subsequent respiratory infection is contracted.	Treatment consists of antimicrobial therapy with agents such as erythromycin, azithromycin, or clarithromycin.	Parents should be educated about prevention of pertussis via vaccine. Nursing care of the child includes providing antimicrobial therapy, fluids, rest, and oxygen. The infant might need to be admitted to the pediatric intensive care unit if complications occur. Pneumonia, apnea, and atelectasis may occur. Severe cough can cause prolapsed rectum, hernia, rib fractures in teens, and incontinence (American Academy of Pediatrics, Committee on Infectious Diseases, 2009).

Pathology	Definition	Medical Treatment	Nursing Care Tips
Pneumonia	A lower respiratory tract infection that causes inflamed lung parenchyma. The source of infection may be viral, bacterial, fungal, or mycoplasma microbes. Symptoms include cough, tachypnea, fever, and shortness of breath.	Medical treatment for pneumonia will depend on whether the infectious process is viral or bacterial in origin. Antibiotics are required for bacterial pneumonia.	Nursing care for a child with pneumonia will include rest, fluids, antipyretics, analgesics, oxygen, infection control measures, and antibiotics if warranted.
Tuberculosis (TB)	An infection caused by the bacterium *Mycobacterium tuberculosis*. This chronic and highly contagious infection spreads via droplet nuclei. The infection centers on the pulmonary system, but it can also affect the genitourinary and GI systems, bones, joints, and skin. Classic clinical presentations include chronic cough, night sweats, weight loss, sputum production, and fevers. Active TB indicates current infection; latent TB is demonstrated by a positive TB skin test but the bacteria are not active.	Medical treatment for TB in children includes taking up to several anti-TB medicines for several (6–9) months (CDC, 2014).	Nursing care is mainly supportive. The child will be treated at home. Educating the family on adherence to the anti-TB medication is imperative, as resistance may develop. Education on nutrition, rest, home/environment assessment, avoidance of public facilities, hand washing, and screening of relatives to identify latent TB is also important in managing a potential outbreak.
Tonsillitis and adenoiditis	Inflammation of the tonsils, which can be bacterial or viral in origin. Most children present with severe sore throat with pus-covered tonsils and fever.	Treatment for tonsillitis depends on the child's overall clinical presentation. If infection of a bacterial origin is suspected, antibiotics will be ordered. Serial bouts of tonsillitis will lead to surgical or laser removal of the tonsils.	Nursing care for a child with tonsillitis includes preoperative and postoperative care. Symptom management is a high priority prior to surgery. Assessing the child's airway after surgery, especially for continuous swallowing that may indicate bleeding, is a priority.

become ill as well. Itchy eyes, mild sore throat, rhinitis, and fatigue are common adult symptoms. If bacteria are found to be the cause, the pathogen is most likely to be *Chlamydophila pneumoniae* or *Mycoplasma pneumoniae*.

Diagnosis of Bronchiolitis

Diagnosis of bronchiolitis is usually made by rapid enzyme-linked immunosorbent assay (ELISA) of a specimen collected from the infant's or toddler's nasal passageways, looking for RSV, influenza, or other viral causes. In severe cases where pneumonia is also suspected,

a chest X-ray may be ordered. Most young infants with this infection have decreased oxygen saturations. Diagnostics frequently ordered to confirm viral bronchiolitis include the following tests:

- Pulse oximetry
- Arterial blood gases
- Chest radiography to identify over-inflation from mucus plugs, inflammation, and air trapping
- Bacterial cultures
- Rapid ELISA nasal swab for RSV
- Complete blood cell count

Risk Factors for Bronchiolitis

Winter months, attendance of daycare programs, exposure to second-hand smoke, reactive airway disease, and not breastfeeding are risk factors for the development of serious bronchiolitis. Male infants have a higher risk of developing serious infection.

Medical Treatment for Bronchiolitis

Treatment of bronchiolitis is based on the child's clinical presentation. A low oxygen dose with humidification to keep the young child's oxygen saturation greater than 90% is commonly ordered (**Table 16-2** describes oxygen delivery systems). Fluids are often provided either orally, if tolerated, or intravenously, if the child is too short of breath to nurse, suck a bottle, or drink. Some providers may try a dose of rapid-acting bronchodilators such as albuterol to see if the child's symptoms decrease. In severe cases, children will be placed on steroids. Antipyretics and analgesics may be required for fever and symptom management. Premature infants, or those with higher risk factors such as a chronic pulmonary disease or cardiac condition, may receive an

TABLE 16-2 Oxygen Delivery Systems	
Type of System	**Comments**
Nasal cannula	Provides low-to-moderate concentrations of oxygen, 22–40% FiO_2, at lower oxygen flow rates of 0.25–4 L/min.
Simple face mask	Oxygen tubing and mask that fits on the child's head and is secured with an elastic band. May be difficult to secure and maintain on young children who are frightened of the mask. Provides only 35–55% FiO_2 with oxygen delivery at 6–10 L/min. Should be attached to a humidification system for oxygen flows of 4 L/min or greater for comfort and decreased nasal tissue drying.
Oxygen blow-by	Administers very low levels of oxygen mixed with room air. Often larger tubing is placed by the child's face without touching the child. Provides only small amounts of oxygen for children in low-level distress or need.
Oxygen tent	Plastic tent placed over the crib that provides humidified oxygen at up to 50% FiO_2. Requires frequent assessment for moisture and leaks in the setup.
Nonrebreathing mask	Used when a child is in moderate to high levels of respiratory distress. The mask system provides up to 100% FiO_2 by not allowing the child to rebreathe exhaled CO_2. It fits snugly on the child's face and has a reservoir bag that may or may not inflate.
Partial nonrebreathing mask	Provides oxygen at approximately 60–95% FiO_2. The mask does not provide a valve that completely prevents CO_2 from entering back into the child's lungs—hence, its "partial nonrebreathing" name.
Venturi mask	Used when a child needs a specific quantity of oxygen mixed with room air. Color-coded valves provide different mixtures depending on the quantity and percent oxygen required.
Oxygen hood	Large plastic device that fits over the infant's entire head and provides a high concentration of oxygen. It requires frequent assessments for tolerance and skin integrity.
Positive end-expiratory pressure device	Used when the child needs positive end-expiratory pressure to help keep the alveoli open, especially when a child has an acute exacerbation of a chronic pulmonary condition.
Tracheostomy mask	A device that loosely fits over a child's tracheostomy to provide humidified oxygen.
Ventilator	Used for a critically ill intubated child who requires mechanical ventilation. This machine provides support for a child who cannot maintain an independent and effective respiratory rate and depth. It requires several individually set parameters, including inspiratory length, rate, and depth, and oxygen concentration (often titrated). The sophisticated machinery requires precise care provided by a team of physicians, nurses, and respiratory therapists. The goal of use is to wean the child from the ventilator as soon as possible.
Resuscitative bag/mask/valve	A device that should be present at every child's bedside, in all clinic rooms, and on crash carts. It is used to provide emergency resuscitation breathing for a child in extreme distress or who is not breathing. The mask must fit the child's facial structures well to produce an adequate seal.

immunization injection called palivizumab (Synagis), or respiratory syncytial virus immune globulin (RSV-IGIV) monthly during the high-risk late fall and winter seasons to prevent contracting the infection.

Nursing Care for Bronchiolitis

Nursing care is based on the severity of the infant's infection. Frequent assessments for increasing congestion requiring suctioning may be required. Keeping track of intake and output and assessing for dehydration are other important nursing care concerns. The child might have trouble sleeping if he or she has the tight "bronchiolitic" (persistent wet) cough. Keeping the head of the child's bed raised may assist in breathing.

Family education may include infection control measures such as contact isolation, maintaining droplet precautions, and use of a bulb syringe. Providing a low-stimulation environment to promote rest, and comfort measures to reduce crying, will support the child. Overall, this kind of infection is self-limiting, though it may require the nurse to administer analgesics, antipyretics, humidified air, fluids, and antitussives.

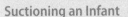

BEST PRACTICES

Suctioning an Infant

Bulb

Pediatric nurses need to teach family members how to use a bulb syringe. The syringe must be compressed prior to placing it in the infant's or young child's nose, and then gently inflated to remove secretions. The mucus should be squirted out immediately and the bulb cleaned with soap and water after each use.

Olive Tip

This device is used by nurses and respiratory therapists to rapidly remove secretions causing a child distress. The olive tip is placed into each nare with the valve open, then rapid on-and-off movements on the valve will pull secretions from the child's nose and pharynx. The device should be cleansed on a regular basis. Keep the tip on the suction tubing ready for use.

Deep Sterile Suctioning

Severe mucus production may require deep sterile suctioning. This procedure is performed by the nurse or respiratory therapist. Sterile kits are used only once and then disposed of. This procedure is considered invasive, with the potential to inflict pulmonary structure damage, and should be performed by professional healthcare team members only with a physician's order.

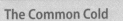

UNIQUE FOR KIDS

The Common Cold

Some viruses that cause the common cold can produce more serious illnesses in infants and toddlers. In these populations, mucus production is increased throughout their smaller airways, inflammation causes edema in the upper airway, fevers can be very high, and irritability ensues with sore throat, persistent cough, and decreased desire to eat and drink. Rest, fluids, secretion management, suctioning if needed with a bulb syringe, and good hand hygiene are all supportive care for the infant or child with the common cold virus.

The U.S. Food and Drug Administration advises against the use of over-the-counter cold and cough medicines in children younger than 2 years. The efficacy of these medications in relieving symptoms is unproven and may be limited, and many parents are unaware of the potential for harm if medications with the same ingredients are given simultaneously, leading to overdose. Some medications are also prone to abuse.

When their children have colds, parents should be advised to encourage intake of fluids, particularly warm, clear beverages such as tea or broth. In older children, honey may be used to soothe an irritated throat and calm coughing, although parents of infants should be advised to avoid the use honey. Topically applied menthol vapor rubs may also provide some symptom relief.

Data from Carr, 2006; "Colds in Children," 2005; Sharfstein, North, & Serweint, 2007.

Case Study

Katy, a 3-year-old child with a history of reactive airway disease, has come to the emergency department for the third time in less than 6 months. Her father brought her in because her work of breathing (WOB) was increasing, she was fatigued, she was not eating or drinking, and the family was out of her albuterol (beta-2 agonist) rapid-acting bronchodilating inhaler. The father indicated that although he did have a prescription refill waiting at the pharmacy, his family was unable to afford the co-payment. The child presents with decreased response time and fatigue, severe retractions, tachypnea, tachycardia, oxygen saturation of 88% on room air, slight circumoral cyanosis after bouts of dry cough, and evidence of dehydration.

Case Study Questions

1. How do this child's symptoms fit with the concepts of oxygenation and gas exchange?
2. What are the immediate assessments and interventions needed to stabilize this child?
3. Which concerns might the pediatric healthcare team have in relation to the family's socioeconomic status?
4. Which other types of medications might be ordered for this child as part of her initial stabilization plan of care?

As the Case Evolves. . .

Katy's family has obtained services to help them pay for Katy's inhaler.

5. Which of the following additional interventions would be appropriate? (Select all that apply.)
   A. Asking Katy and her caregivers to demonstrate how the inhaler is used, so that the correct technique can be taught if necessary
   B. Explaining to the family how to identify and eliminate Katy's asthma triggers
   C. Recommending to Katy's parents that they should bring her to see an allergist or a pulmonologist
   D. Identifying home remedies and over-the-counter medications that can help Katy if they run out of her rescue medication again

Chapter Summary

- Respiratory illness is a common reason why families seek pediatric health care, and is a common cause of illness throughout childhood.
- The concepts of gas exchange and oxygenation in the pediatric population relate to the initial newborn period, when extra-uterine respiration is initiated, and continue to be critical throughout the developmental period of childhood. The most vulnerable period for the newborn in terms of respiration is the first 24 hours of life.
- The anatomy and physiology of the respiratory system can be divided into the upper passageways (nasal cavities, pharynx, larynx, and trachea, plus nasal cilia) and the lower air passageways (main bronchi, bronchioles, and alveoli).
- There are both anatomic and physiological differences in the respiratory systems of children and adults. These differences, such as a smaller, narrower airway, contribute to the development of respiratory conditions in children.
- Insufficient intake of oxygen and removal of carbon dioxide can cause a child with respiratory distress to experience hypoxemia; low levels of oxygen in the blood can rapidly develop into hypoxia.

- Assessments for respiratory distress should begin with visual observation of the child's overall appearance and condition. Work of breathing must be assessed, and level of consciousness, positioning, overall distress, interactive behaviors, and skin color should all be observed.
- The pediatric nurse must have equipment close at hand that will assist the team in securing a patent airway, providing support for ventilation and oxygenation, and controlling the child's symptoms of respiratory distress.
- Reactive airway disease, which may precede a diagnosis of asthma, is associated with risk factors such as exposure to respiratory infections, cigarette smoke, allergens, and other triggers. Family members must be assisted in identifying their child's triggers so that they can prevent repeated exposures and subsequent episodes of asthma.
- Educating the child and family about home care of asthma includes teaching about the individualized asthma action plan, rapid-acting medications, preventive medications, the signs and symptoms of an asthma attack, the child's known triggers, and when to call for immediate help.
- Cystic fibrosis is an autosomal recessive genetic disorder that causes cysts and scarring within the pancreas, preventing the normal secretion of digestive enzymes

and insulin. Excessive sodium absorption in the lungs causes normally thin respiratory mucus secretions to thicken and obstruct exocrine glands.

- Nursing care for a child with a respiratory infection or condition includes educating the family on symptom management, prevention, infectious disease control measures, and adherence to treatment.

Bibliography

ACLS Training Center. (2015). Crash cart supply and equipment checklist. Retrieved from https://www.acls.net/acls-crash-cart .htm

Alangari, A. A. (2014). Corticosteroids in the treatment of acute asthma. *Annals of Thoracic Medicine, 9*, 187–192.

American Academy of Pediatrics, Committee on Infectious Diseases; Pickering, L. (Ed.). (2009). *Red book: 2009 report of the Committee on Infectious Diseases* (28th ed.), Elk Grove Village, IL: Author.

American Lung Association. (2009). Breathe well, live well: Asthma medicines chart. Retrieved from http://www.lung.org/assets /documents/asthma/MedicineChart_Rev09.pdf

Bohadana, A., Izbicki, G., & Kraman, S. S. (2014). Fundamentals of lung auscultation. *New England Journal of Medicine, 370*, 744–751.

Braido, F., Chrystyn, H., Baiardini, I., Bosnic-Anticevich, S., van der Molen, T., Dandurand, R. J., . . . Price, D. (2016). "Trying, but failing": The role of inhaler technique and mode of delivery in respiratory medication adherence. *Journal of Allergy and Clinical Immunology: In Practice, 4*, 823–832.

Carr, B. C. (2006). Efficacy, abuse, and toxicity of over-the-counter cough and cold medicines in the pediatric population. *Current Opinion in Pediatrics, 18*(2), 184–188.

Centers for Disease Control and Prevention (CDC). (2013). *Asthma facts: CDC's National Asthma Control Program grantees*. Atlanta, GA: U.S. Department of Health and Human Services, Centers for Disease Control and Prevention.

Centers for Disease Control and Prevention (CDC). (2014). Tuberculosis (TB): Children. Retrieved from https://www.cdc.gov/tb /topic/populations/tbinchildren

Centers for Disease Control and Prevention (CDC). (2015). Summary health statistics for U.S children: National Health Interview Survey 2012. Retrieved from https://www.cdc.gov/nchs/data /series/sr_10/sr10_258.pdf

Centers for Disease Control and Prevention (CDC). (2016). Children, the flu, and the flu vaccine. Retrieved from https://www.cdc.gov /flu/protect/children.htm

Children's Hospital of Philadelphia. (2017). Laryngomalacia. Retrieved from http://www.chop.edu/conditions-diseases/laryngomalacia

Colds in children. (2005). *Paediatrics and Child Health, 10*(8), 493–495.

Cystic Fibrosis Center at Stanford. (2016). Common medications. Retrieved from http://med.stanford.edu/cfcenter/education /english/Meds.html

Cystic Fibrosis Foundation. (2015). Sweat test. Retrieved from https:// www.cff.org/What-is-CF/Testing/Sweat-Test

Egbuonu, F., Antonio, F. A., & Edavalath, M. (2014). Effect of inhaled corticosteroids on glycemic status. *Open Respiratory Medicine Journal, 8*, 101–105.

Khavjou, O., Nurmagambetov, T., Murphy, L., & Orenstein, D. (2016). *State-level medical and absenteeism costs of asthma among children.* Poster presentation at American Society of Health Economists, June 2016 National Meeting.

Kleinman, M. E., Chameides, L., Schexnayder, S. M., Samson, R. A., Hazinski, M. F., Atkins, D. L., . . . Zaritsky, A. L. (2010). Part 14: Pediatric advanced life support: 2010 American Heart Association guidelines for cardiopulmonary resuscitation and emergency cardiovascular care. *Circulation, 122*(18 suppl 3), S876–S908.

MacKenzie, T., Gifford, A. H., Sabadosa, K. A., Quinton, H. B., Knapp, E. A., Goss, C. H., & Marshall, B. C. (2014). Longevity of patients with cystic fibrosis in 2000 to 2010 and beyond: Survival analysis of the Cystic Fibrosis Foundation patient registry. *Annals of Internal Medicine, 161*(4), 233–241.

National Heart, Lung, and Blood Institute (NHLBI). (2012). How is respiratory distress syndrome treated? Retrieved from https:// www.nhlbi.nih.gov/health/health-topics/topics/rds/treatment

National Heart, Lung, and Blood Institute (NHLBI). (2014a). How is asthma treated and controlled? Retrieved from http://www .nhlbi.nih.gov/health/health-topics/topics/asthma/treatment

National Heart, Lung, and Blood Institute (NHLBI). (2014b). Managing asthma: A guide for schools. Retrieved from http://www.nhlbi.nih .gov/files/docs/resources/lung/NACI_ManagingAsthma-508%20 FINAL.pdf

National Institutes of Health (NIH). (2013). How is cystic fibrosis treated? Retrieved from https://www.nhlbi.nih.gov/health/health -topics/topics/cf/treatment

Rivera, M. L., Kim, T. Y., Steward, G. M., Minasyan, L., & Brown, L. (2006). Albuterol nebulized in heliox in the initial ED treatment of pediatric asthma: A blinded randomized controlled trial. *American Journal of Emergency Medicine, 24*(1), 38–42.

Sharfstein, J. M., North, M., & Serwint, J. R. (2007). Over the counter but no longer under the radar: Pediatric cough and cold medications. *New England Journal of Medicine, 357*, 2321–2324.

Thompson, M., Vodicka, T. A., Blair, P. S., Buckley, D. I., Heneghan, C., & Hay, A. D., for the TARGET Programme Team. (2013). Duration of symptoms of respiratory tract infections in children: Systematic review. *British Journal of Medicine, 347*, f7027.

U.S. Department of Health and Human Services, National Institutes of Health, National Heart, Lung, and Blood Institute. (2015). National Asthma Control Initiative: Keeping airways open—Fact sheet. Retrieved from https://www.nhlbi.nih.gov/health-pro /resources/lung/naci-keeping-airways-open-fact-sheet

Wiebe, K., & Rowe, B. H. (2007). Nebulized racemic epinephrine used in the treatment of severe asthmatic exacerbation: A case report and literature review. *Canadian Journal of Emergency Medicine, 9*(4), 304–308.

CHAPTER 17

Skin Integrity

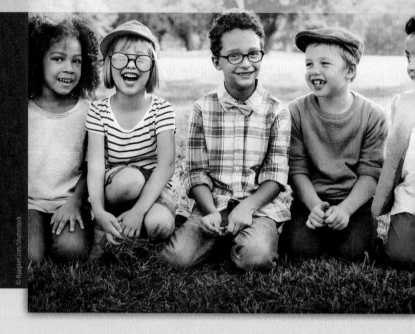

© Rawpixel.com/Shutterstock

LEARNING OBJECTIVES

1. Apply key nursing concepts in caring for a child with a skin integrity condition.
2. Assess the development of the skin in patients from the newborn period through adolescence.
3. Apply appropriate assessment and care for various skin lesions (e.g., macules, papules, plaque, wheals, blisters, nodules, tumors).
4. Analyze exemplars that represent deviations from skin integrity for children: burns, contact dermatitis, pediculosis, and acne.
5. Identify appropriate management methods for common skin conditions in children in relation to etiology, clinical presentation, medical treatments, and nursing education.
6. Apply various nursing care practices to prevent complications with skin integrity conditions.

KEY TERMS

Acne
Burn
Contact dermatitis
Eczema
Lund-Browder chart
Macule
Papule
Primary skin lesion
Pustule
Secondary skin lesion
Urticaria
Vesicle

Introduction

The integumentary system, or skin, is the largest organ in the body. Through its extensive network of blood vessels, human skin receives one-third of the body's total circulating blood. There are two main types of skin: (1) the hairless glabrous skin found on the palms and soles of the feet and (2) hair-bearing skin. The skin has three layers—the epidermis, the dermis, and the subcutaneous layer. Acting as a physical barrier that protects the internal organs and structures, the skin also performs thermoregulation, sense perception, and self-cleaning functions.

The top layer of the skin, the epidermis, consists of dead skin cells that are constantly brushed off and regrow monthly, thereby preventing bacterial colonization. The epidermis contains melanin, which gives the skin its color. Within the epidermis are two distinct sublayers: the stratum layer, which is made up of the corneum, lucidum, granulosum, spinosum, and basale strata layers; and the basal layer. These sublayers contain four types of cells: keratinocytes, melanocytes, Langerhans cells, and Merkel cells. The complex layers of skin are nourished via diffusion of substances from the dermis. In addition, the dermis contains hair follicles with arrector pili muscles, eccrine (sweat) glands, blood vessels, and nerve endings. In the pediatric population, 1 square inch of skin contains approximately 650 eccrine (sweat) glands, 20 blood vessels, 60,000 melanocytes, and 1000 nerve endings.

Across the developmental period, some diseases and genetic anomalies can be diagnosed based on discoloration and lesions of the skin. Many pediatric clinic visits involve skin disorders. Notably, the development of skin loss, blisters, and lesions is very common in children. Infants are especially vulnerable to skin damage, as their epidermis is loosely bound to their dermis, leading to poor adherence of skin layers. Damage to the epidermis and dermis can lead to a secondary infection. The deepest layer of the skin, which consists of subcutaneous fat, provides an anchor for the dermis to the bone and muscle via connective tissue; this fat layer also assists with temperature regulation.

Development of Skin Across Childhood

The outermost layers of the epidermis, or stratum corneum, are not completely developed in preterm infants. As a result, skin barrier function—that is, the ability of skin to protect the body from toxins and pathogenic organisms—is weaker in this vulnerable population. Skin barrier function can be measured by determining the skin's ability to hold on to water and to stay hydrated, which is influenced by the pH (acid–base balance).

The average adult skin has 10 to 20 layers of stratum corneum, whereas the average premature infant has a mere 2 to 3 layers. This section of epidermis develops in the latter part of the third trimester of gestation. A neonate in the neonatal intensive care unit (NICU) may require routine activities such as handling, bathing, exposure to chemicals and cleansers, placement of intravenous catheters, and use of adhesives to attach temperature probes and IV catheters. Unfortunately, all of these activities can break down the integrity of the neonate's skin. Consequently, such infants have a high risk of dehydration through insensible water loss.

The body surface area of neonates and children is relatively larger than the body surface of adults. In addition, neonates' skin is much more permeable, which leads to a greater sensitivity to external irritants and an increased susceptibility to opportunistic infections in these children. Great care must be given to these fragile premature patients. They are kept in humidified isolettes to prevent dehydration for approximately 1 month after birth. The babies are gently handled every 4 hours in the beginning of their NICU stay to allow developmental growth. Their isolettes are covered with dark covers to prevent light from disturbing their premature eyes. The neonates are repositioned using a "hands-on" technique to prevent pressure ulcers and moved gently with their hands crossed over their chest for comfort. Slow movement of very early neonates (less than 28 weeks' gestation) can prevent the fragile blood vessels in the brain from bleeding. Soft blankets, synthetic sheepskin and bendable soft supports are used to create "nests" that keep them in a fetal position with body alignment. Bathing should be limited to sterile saline the first week, followed by minimal use of soap every 4 days.

BEST PRACTICES

Keeping Lesions Moist

In the past, nursing care encouraged the drying out of the base of a wound. Today, best evidence supports the provision of a moist wound base. Epithelial cells fill in the wound and require moisture for their maximum growth and stability. If wet to dry dressing changes are ordered, discuss the appropriateness of the order with the physician. Maintaining sterile wet to wet dressing changes frequently enough to provide wound base moisture will promote healing.

Promotion of Skin Health Across Childhood

Principles of pediatric skin management should be based on early identification and immediate treatment of skin

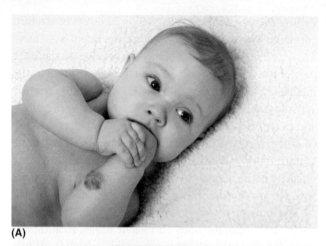

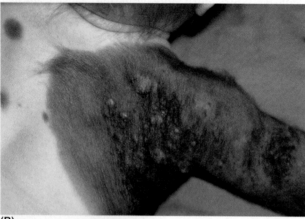

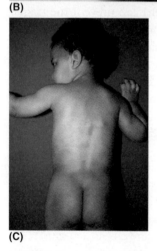

(A)

(B)

(C)

Figure 17-1 *Congenital skin lesions: (A) hemangioma, (B) nevi, and (C) Mongolian spots.*

(A) © gsermek/iStock/Getty Images; (B) © Dr. Ken Greer/Visuals Unlimited, Inc.; (C) © Diomedia/ISM

conditions. Protection against excessive sun exposure and sunburn should be emphasized, as such exposures increase the risk of skin cancers later in life. Common childhood skin conditions include rashes (exanthems), burns, bug bites, cellulitis, scratches, wounds, bruising, acne, eczema, **urticaria** (hives), fungal infections (tinea pedis, tinea capitus, and tinea corporis), impetigo, and parasites such as scabies.

Numerous types of lesions may even be present at birth. The pediatric nurse should assess a newborn's entire skin surface for congenital skin lesions such as hemangiomas, congenital melanocytic nevi, and salmon patches or Mongolian spots (**Figure 17-1**). Although such lesions are usually benign, screening for them at birth offers the nurse an opportunity to educate the parents as to their nature, as well as allows for identification of any more problematic lesions such as skin vesicles, which should prompt evaluation for congenital herpes simplex virus (HSV) infection, or café au lait spots, which might be an early sign of rare disorders such as neurofibromatosis or McCune-Albright syndrome (Lewis, 2014).

FAMILY EDUCATION

Prevention of Sunburns

- Five or more sunburns in childhood can lead to an 80% increased chance of melanoma later in life.
- Babies have the most sensitive skin, which contains little melanin. Sunscreen is not recommended for infants younger than 6 months.
- Stay in the shade: Keep out of the sun from 10 a.m. until 4 p.m.
- Cover up: Wear dry long sleeves of tight-knit cloth. UPF (ultraviolet protection factor) clothing is available.
- Top it off: Wear a wide-brimmed hat that covers the face, ears, and neck.
- Look cool: Sunglasses protect eyes from ultraviolet (UV) rays.
- Sunscreen: Use after babies are 6 months old. Apply a sunscreen with UPF 15 prior to going outside. Remember to apply the sunscreen on the nose, ears, lips, and tops of feet.

The various skin lesions that a pediatric nurse may encounter while caring for children across the developmental period are described in **Table 17-1**. A **primary skin lesion** is the initial change of skin integrity, whereas a **secondary skin lesion** evolves from poor healing due to picking, scratching, or infection of a primary lesion.

A common disorder observed in newborns is erythema toxicum neonatorum (**Figure 17-2**). Referred to as "flea-bite dermatitis," these small papules of white and red color appear on the face and trunk. This is a self-resolving condition, although the presence of the papules causes concern for parents. The pediatric nurse should provide anticipatory guidance and teaching to parents that they should not squeeze or attempt to pop the papules, as they will resolve without intervention.

TABLE 17-1 Skin Lesions	
Macules 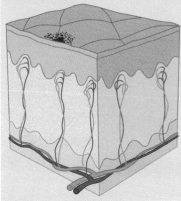	Color change to the skin that is flat, not palpable, and less than 1 cm in diameter Example: petechiae
Patch 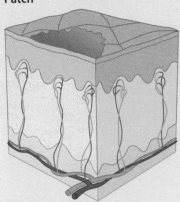	Color change to the skin that is flat, not palpable, and larger than 1 cm in diameter Examples: café au lait spot, vitiligo, white macule
Papules 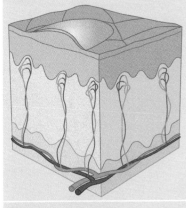	Solid raised lesion with distinct borders that is 1 cm or less in diameter Examples: *Lichen planus*, *Molluscum contagiosum*
Plaque 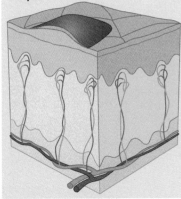	Solid, raised, flat-topped lesion with distinct borders and more than 1 cm in diameter Example: psoriasis

(continues)

TABLE 17-1   Skin Lesions *(continued)*

Nodule

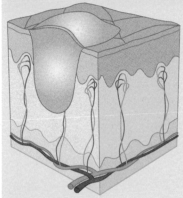

Raised solid lesion with indistinct borders and a deep palpable portion

Examples: rheumatoid nodule, neurofibroma

Wheal

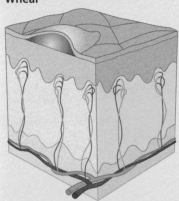

Circumscribed, flat-topped, firm elevation of the skin with a well-demarcated and palpable margin

Example: urticaria from allergic reaction to contactant (an allergic substance)

Vesicle

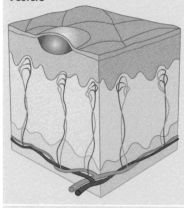

Raised lesion filled with clear fluid that is less than 1 cm in diameter

Examples: varicella, herpes simplex

Bulla

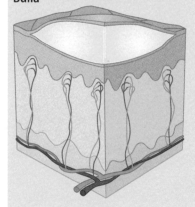

Raised lesion filled with clear fluid that is more than 1 cm in diameter

Example: second-degree burn

TABLE 17-1 Skin Lesions (*continued*)

Cyst

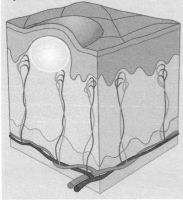

Raised lesion that contains a palpable sac filled with solid material

Examples: epidermal cyst, dermoid cyst

Pustule

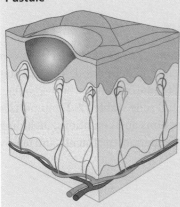

Raised lesion filled with a fluid exudate, giving it a white or yellow appearance

Examples: acne, folliculitis

Atrophy

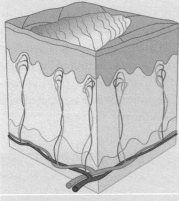

Skin surface is depressed due to thinning or absence of the dermis or subcutaneous fat

Examples: atrophic scar, fat necrosis

Crusting

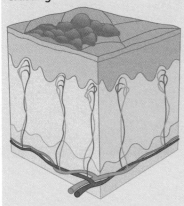

Dried exudates of plasma combined with sloughed skin

Examples: healing varicella lesions after a vesicle opens and drains

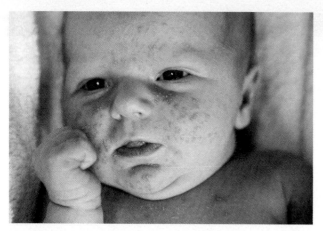

Figure 17-2 *A young infant with erythema toxicum neonatorum.*

David Gee / Alamy Stock Photo

and should not be administered at all (Food and Drug Administration [FDA], 2008, 2016). Older school-age children should not be given such medications unless under the direction of a primary care provider. Part of the reason for these cautions is that the pharmacokinetics of such medications in young children may differ notably from the response in adults. In an early study of the pharmacokinetics of diphenhydramine (Simons, Watson, Martin, Chen, & Simons, 1990), for example, it was found that the drug has a significantly shorter serum half-life in children than in adults, but children's clearance rates are nearly four times as long as the adult rates, offering a greater potential for toxicity when diphenhydramine is dosed repeatedly in young children.

Concept Exemplars

Many potential skin lesions, rashes, and infections can present during the developmental period. This chapter presents four exemplars of these conditions: burns, contact dermatitis, pediculosis, and acne. **Table 17-2** summarizes other common skin infections and conditions, including their etiology, clinical presentation, treatments, and family education needs.

Burns

A **burn** is damage to the skin and other tissues caused by heat, chemicals, electricity, sunlight, or radiation. Burns are the most common household injury for children. In the United States, approximately 300 children visit the emergency department (ED) due to injuries sustained from burns each day (Centers for Disease Control and Prevention [CDC], 2016), for a total of more than 100,000 ED visits for this cause each year. The mortality rate associated with burns is approximately 2 deaths per 300 cases.

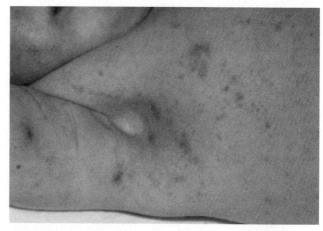

Figure 17-3 *Scabies tracts.*

© CNRI/Science Source

TABLE 17-2 Common Childhood Skin Conditions

Name	Etiology	Assessments	Treatment	Nursing Education
Poison ivy	Urushiols (oils) from poison ivy/oak/sumac lead to a red rash that is extremely itchy. Can cause respiratory distress with asthma-like symptoms if inhaled from the smoke of a burning plant.	Localized streaking red rash from site of exposure within 24–72 hours after exposure. Blisters, pimples, swelling, and severe itching.	Rinse with rubbing alcohol, followed by water. Scrub the child's entire body and scalp, including under fingernails. Calamine lotions, hydrocortisone cream, and cool compresses for comfort and inflammation. Oatmeal baths for itching. Tapered course of steroids if severe.	Advise the patient not to scratch. Keep the skin clean and dry. Teach family members about the ability of the plant oil to spread.
Scabies mite (*Sarcoptes scabiei*)	Pimply rash caused by the parasitic mite *Sarcoptes scabiei* from direct skin contact (**Figure 17-3**). Found in healthcare institutions, schools, and childcare centers.	Red linear rash from burrowing mites, which lay their eggs and leave waste products along tunnels just under the skin. Infection causes white pimples and redness from scratching. Eggs mature in 21 days.	Scabicides topical cream as prescribed by primary care provider. Treatments include 5% permethrin cream (Elimite) administered over the child's entire body. Treatment may need to be repeated in 1 week. Difficult cases of scabies might require a course of oral ivermectin.	Inform the family to wash all linens and towels in hot water. Vacuum car seats, couches, and floors thoroughly. Prevent spread of the mites. Apply the topical cream as prescribed and leave on for the duration as indicated to ensure all mites are killed.
Allergic reactions	Secondary exposure to an agent.	Allergic reaction signs and symptoms vary; typically consist of a rash with pruritus and erythema. Severe reactions can cause anaphylaxis.	Identify triggers and etiology, and then prevent exposure. Provide oral and topical antihistamines. Treat anaphylaxis with intravenous antihistamines, steroids, and epinephrine.	Teach families to avoid triggers. Prevent exposures by communicating with those who care for the child and providing education. Have the child wear a medical bracelet. Carry an epinephrine injectable pen.
Sunburn	Exposure to UVA and UVB rays.	Reddened skin, which can become blistered and peel.	Cool water compresses, aloe vera, topical anesthetic sprays such as Solarcaine, loose cotton clothing. Hydrate the child.	Teach the family to prevent sunburns. Infants should always be covered and wear hats. Sunscreen should be used on children 6 months and older if exposure is inevitable. Educate the family about the connection between sunburns and skin cancer. Keep children covered if outside during the hours of greatest exposure: 10 a.m. to 4 p.m.

(continues)

TABLE 17-2 Common Childhood Skin Conditions (*continued*)

Name	Etiology	Assessments	Treatment	Nursing Education
Atopic dermatitis (**eczema**)	Allergic reaction to an agent, which causes a dry rash from a disruption of the skin barrier. Often associated with the presence of allergies due to an inherited tendency called atopy. Triggers can be food, soap, medications, or contact with plants or animals.	Dry patchy skin, most prominently on the face and inside the elbows and backs of the knees. Can also present as vesicles, papules, or weeping and oozing lesions. In childhood eczema (age of onset: 2–3 years), cluster lesions with lichenification and keratosis pillars may be present.	Apply moisturizers, topical steroid creams, and oral antihistamines such as hydroxyzine, diphenhydramine, loratadine, or fexofenadine.	Educate the family to maintain the skin's barrier function. Lukewarm baths daily for 10–15 minutes. Pat the skin dry—do not rub. Apply medication cream to red rough patches, then gentle moisturizer to face and body soon after the bath. Cool, wet wrap dressings can be used for intense flare-ups.
Candidiasis	Overgrowth of *Candida*, generally in the mucous membranes.	Oral: white patches or plaques in the mouth. Diaper area: beefy red rash developing after diaper dermatitis. Satellite lesions are common.	Nystatin (cream, powder, or ointment), clotrimazole, econazole, miconazole, or amphotericin IV if the case is severe or the child is immunocompromised.	Perform frequent diaper changes; cleanse with cool water. Try to air out the diaper area as much as possible. Apply prescribed medication as directed in a thin layer.
Impetigo	*Staphylococcus aureus* or *Streptococcus pyogenes* infection; highly contagious in the superficial layers of the epidermis. Can occur as a secondary infection after abrasions or chickenpox. Can happen with post-streptococcal glomerulonephritis.	Nonbullous: small vesicles that develop a honey-colored crust, initially in the face. Swollen lymph glands are present. Bullous: less contagious; appears on the face and trunk, and in the buccal areas of the mouth.	Mupirocin has been used, but resistance is occurring. Retapamulin is the first-line topical treatment. Widespread or complicated infections require systemic antibiotics: Augmentin, dicoxacillin, erythromycin, cleocin, Bactrim, Zyvox.	Gently cleanse the honey crusts with water and antibacterial soap with clean washcloths. Teach the family about the application of topical medications, and covering the wounds with clean dressings. Good hygiene is required to prevent spread. Bathing in chlorohexidine is recommended if the infection is spreading.
Cellulitis	Wound in the skin becomes infected with group A beta-hemolytic *Streptococcus*, *Streptococcus pneumoniae*, or *Staphylococcus aureus* that affects the dermis and layers below; can reach the muscle layer. Associated with trauma such as puncture wounds or other infections such as sinusitis or impetigo.	Fever, pain, tenderness, erythema, warmth. Quickly spreads within 24 hours. Glossy tight skin over the affected area, joint stiffness in the area, loss of hair in the area, nausea and vomiting.	Treat with broad-spectrum oral antibiotic therapy for 7–10 days: oxacillin, sulfamethoxazole, or amoxicillin. Severe infections will require IV antibiotics, especially if the infection is invading structures such as the eye socket.	Teach families to cover cellulitis-affected areas with nonocclusive dressings if the infection causes skin tears. Place warm packs on these areas to soothe them.

Assessment

Burns are classified as first-, second-, or third-degree burns, which are equivalent to the terms superficial, partial-thickness, and full-thickness burns. One wound may have several degrees of thickness damage due to the type of agent and the amount of time that the skin was exposed to the irritant. The skin is thinner on the ears, backs of the hands, tops of the feet, and perineum, so burns to these areas tend to cause more serious damage in terms of thickness. For instance, a mild sunburn is a first-degree or superficial burn, appearing red without blisters and pain. The top layer of skin is damaged and will peel away in a few days. By comparison, partial-thickness or second-degree burns can lead to redness and blistering, and parts of the dermis will be damaged. These wounds will appear damp and heal within 10 days. People with more melanocytes (darker skin tones) can lose their pigmentation in these burns.

Deep partial-thickness burns are difficult to differentiate from full-thickness burns and are considered third-degree burns. In this cases, there is more damage to the dermis, and the wounds can appear white and waxy. No capillary refill occurs in the burn tissues, and the nerve endings are destroyed. With deeper burns, there is a high risk for fluid and serum protein loss through weeping. The healing time can be 3 weeks, with scarring and possible contractures occurring. Skin grafts are often required for deep burns and will be performed as a surgical procedure. In the presence of eschar (dead tissues), mechanical debridement may be needed as often as twice each day to allow for epithelization to occur. A child who requires repeated burn wound care

should be prescribed an H_2 antagonist to prevent stress ulcers from forming. Reverse isolation is used to prevent a burn wound from becoming infected.

When assessing a wound, the pediatric nurse should use a marker to outline the wound's perimeter. The date and time of the marking should be visible on the skin or body area. If a wound extends beyond the perimeter of the markings, the wound is expanding and not healing. This expansion could reflect the development of cellulitis, infection, or sinus tracts.

The rule of nines is used in adults and teens to determine total body surface area damaged by burns. In the pediatric patient, a **Lund-Browder chart** is used for this purpose (**Figure 17-4**).

Medical Treatment

With superficial burns, the wound may need cool compresses, application of aloe vera, and symptom management. Partial-thickness burns will require wound care (**Figure 17-5**). Thorough cleaning and the application of a silver sulfadiazine cream may be sufficient.

For full-thickness burns, fluid resuscitation is the primary concern and hypovolemic shock must be prevented. Cardiopulmonary resuscitation (CPR) and airway support may be required if the child's pulmonary system was exposed to heat and smoke. Loss of serum protein via wound weeping may require IV replacement with human albumin or total parenteral nutrition (TPN). The child should be placed on a nothing-by-mouth (NPO) status to prevent paralytic ileus. If the surface area of the burn was large enough to destroy a significant quantity of cells, laboratory

Region	%
Head	
Neck	
Ant. Trunk	
Post. Trunk	
Right arm	
Left arm	
Buttocks	
Genitalia	
Right leg	
Left leg	
Total burn	

Relative percentages of body surface area affected by growth

Age (years)	A ($\frac{1}{2}$ of head)	B ($\frac{1}{2}$ of one thigh)	C ($\frac{1}{2}$ of one leg)
0	$9\frac{1}{2}$	$2\frac{3}{4}$	$2\frac{1}{2}$
1	$8\frac{1}{2}$	$3\frac{1}{4}$	$2\frac{1}{2}$
5	$6\frac{1}{2}$	4	$2\frac{3}{4}$
10	$5\frac{1}{2}$	$4\frac{1}{4}$	3
15	$4\frac{1}{2}$	$4\frac{1}{2}$	$3\frac{1}{4}$
Adult	$3\frac{1}{2}$	$4\frac{3}{4}$	3

Figure 17-4 *The pediatric Lund-Browder chart.*

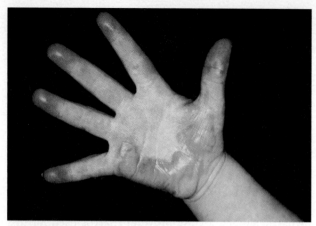

Figure 17-5 *A child with partial-thickness burn.*
© Scott Camazine/Science Source

tests should be monitored to assess the need for packed red blood cell infusions, and to determine whether renal function is declining.

Emergency fluid boluses, fluid maintenance, and fluid resuscitation may all be required for large body surface area burns. To calculate the amount of fluid needed in the first 24 hours to replace fluid lost through the wound, the Parkland formula is generally used. This formula, which was developed by Charles Baxter at Parkland Hospital at Southwestern University Medical Center in the 1960s (Hansen, 2008), states that the volume of fluid required = 4 × body mass (in kg) × percentage of total body surface area encompassed by the burn. Be aware that some sources argue that this formula overestimates the fluids needed for fluid resuscitation (Guilabert et al., 2016).

Nursing Care

Maintaining aseptic technique to prevent a secondary infection in a burn wound is a primary nursing concern. The child's symptoms should be managed carefully by administering the most appropriate pain assessment tool and giving pain management medications. The child will need emotional support and the family will need clear communication concerning all aspects of care. Bringing in the assistance of Child Life specialists to provide distraction, medical play, and education should be a priority in team support for the child.

Contact Dermatitis

Contact dermatitis is a skin rash that can be caused by a variety of irritants. In infants and toddlers, severe diaper rashes are a common form of this condition. Contact dermatitis or diaper dermatitis is often related to the infant's diaper (whether cloth or disposable) or products intended for skin care; urine, soap, detergents, perfumes and baby lotions are just a few possible irritants (Clark-Gruel, Helmes, Lawrence, Odio, & White, 2014; Yu, Treat, Chaney, &

Brod, 2016). In this case, the dermatitis is directly related to the child's perineum being exposed to and aggravated by acidic excrement. Prolonged exposure causes a bright red macular–papular rash with weeping lesions. The infant will present with mild redness that progresses to swelling, blisters, thickening of the skin around the diaper, scaling, crusting, and oozing of fluids. In older children, contact dermatitis can be caused by any number of irritants—for example, poison ivy, harsh soaps or volatile chemicals (e.g., bleach), metals (e.g., nickel, chrome), or allergens such as latex or dyes in beauty products (American Academy of Dermatology, n.d.).

Treatment and Nursing Care

When treating diaper dermatitis, the child's diaper should be removed and the skin cleansed immediately after the child urinates or stools. The skin should be washed completely and gently twice a day, with the removal of all layers of topical treatment and excrements. The skin should be gently cleansed with soft cotton cleansing cloths rather than commercial wipes, which can contain alcohol and other harsh detergents. All folds of the skin should be cleansed well and patted dry. The skin should have a thick layer of vitamin A, vitamin D, and/or zinc oxide protective cream applied. The creams should be left on after diaper changes, except during the twice-daily complete cleansing. Nursing education should include promoting open diaper time to expose the skin to air and not using plastic materials or plastic diaper coverings. The family should be encouraged to reduce the child's stool pH by increasing the consumption of veggies and fruits.

For contact dermatitis in infants beyond the diaper area as well as in older children, the skin should be cleansed well and patted dry; solutions such as Aveeno baths, Burrow's solution, or calamine lotion can then be applied to promote healing. If severe itching occurs, oral antihistamines or hydroxyzine (Atarax) can be used. Emollient lotions may be used if the skin appears dry, but their use should be discontinued if symptoms increase in response to the lotion. If episodes recur, allergy "patch" testing may be needed to determine the cause of the reaction so that it can be avoided (Wentworth et al., 2014). Bacterial overgrowth can occur and may require oral antibiotics.

Pediculosis Humanus Capitus (Head Lice)

Head lice infestations are a common skin infection during childhood. Lice readily pass between children through sharing of common objects such as combs, brushes, hats, over-the-head clothing, and dress-up clothes, and through exposure to infested car upholstery, car seat linings, bedding, and carpets. Lice do not fly; rather, they need an object to pass the mature lice or eggs (nits) between children

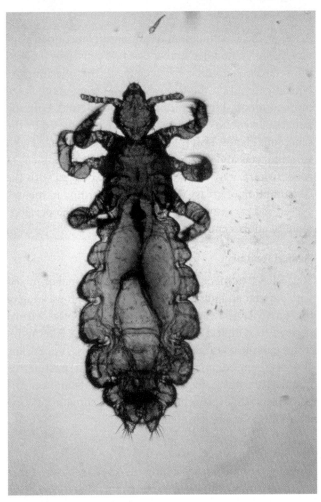

Figure 17-6 *An adult louse.*

Courtesy of Dr. Dennis Juranek/CDC

(CDC, 2015). Classrooms without individual coat racks and children's cubbies for personal item storage are at risk for becoming havens for lice.

The female louse needs a host to provide blood for this species' survival and reproduction. Adult lice cannot live more than 2 days away from a food source. A female louse lives 30 days, lays many hundreds of eggs during her life, and adheres the eggs to the hair shaft using a biological cement as close to the scalp as possible (**Figure 17-6**). The egg sacs then open and the nits hatch in 8 to 9 days (CDC, 2015). The nits (eggs) can stay alive for 10 to 14 days without a host.

Assessment

Children with head lice will complain of a severely itchy scalp, and white nits (eggs) can be found in the hair. The itching is caused by three aspects of the infection: the fast crawling behavior of the six-legged adult parasites, the presence of waste products that irritate the skin, and the parasites' eating behaviors as they drink from a well of blood from scratched skin and open lesions. Children with

head lice can be irritable and unable to sleep soundly. Some develop sores and secondary infections from scratching their scalps. Lice are spread by direct contact from one infected person to another and feed on human blood from areas where intense itching has caused abrasions. The most common age group for infections is 3 to 11 years, and this condition occurs more frequently in girls.

Risk Factors

Sharing of hats, scarves, coats, and hairbrushes carrying lice may spread the infection. Sharing a bed, pillow, couch, or stuffed animal with an infected person allows the parasite to readily pass between children. Contrary to common belief, personal hygiene is not related to lice infestations, as a female louse prefers to lay her eggs on clean hair rather than oily hair (CDC, 2015).

Medical Treatment

Prescription or over-the-counter pediculicides are applied to the child's hair and scalp. Long hair may need two bottles of the treatment. The prescription lotions contain benzyl alcohol, ivermectin, and malathion; spinosad topical suspension is an alternative. The over-the-counter medicines consist of pyrethrins and permethrin 5% shampoos. To rid the hair of lice, the hair should be sectioned off in 1-inch squares, with manual extraction of nits and lice then being performed with a fine-toothed comb (nit comb or dog/cat comb). Careful removal of all egg sacs is imperative to prevent reinfection. Some businesses will perform the extraction of adult lice and nits as a service for a fee.

Nursing Care

Parents and caregivers need to be educated to wash all clothing worn the previous two days, linens, towels, and washable toys in a hot-water washing machine (130°F) and then place the items in a hot dryer (130°F) for at least 5 minutes. All stuffed animals and excess pillows or any item that cannot be washed should be bagged tightly for a minimum of 2 weeks to kill all lice and nits. Hairbrushes and combs should be soaked in hot water (130°F). Parents need to be reminded to vacuum all furniture, floors, and car upholstery thoroughly to remove lice and eggs. Nurses must inform parents and caregivers that fumigants should not be used in the home, because they can be absorbed through the skin, leading to toxicity.

While head lice are the most common form seen in children, body lice and pubic lice might also be found in adolescents in certain circumstances (e.g., homeless children may present with body lice and sexually active youth with pubic lice; Flinders & de Schweinitz, 2004). The latter can be identified by direct observation of the pubic region, and the former by examination of the seams of the clothing, where body lice sometimes can be located. Treatment of these parasites follows a similar course, although further education in hygiene and prevention may also be needed.

If actual lice are not observed, it should be noted that parasitic infestations of scabies or bedbugs may produce similar symptoms (American Academy of Dermatology, 2010). These infestations should be assessed and treated.

PHARMACOLOGY

Stevens-Johnson Syndrome: Toxic Epidermal Necrolysis

- Stevens-Johnson syndrome is a rare and severe reaction to certain medications.
- It starts out as flu-like symptoms: fever, arthralgia, and burning rash on the trunk. The rash begins as macule lesions and then progresses to larger vesicles (bullae), which later rupture.
- The facial and torso skin develop lesions that peel and have the appearance of a full-thickness burn. The lesions can affect the conjunctiva and all mucous membranes.
- Stevens-Johnson syndrome can lead to pneumonia, sepsis, multiple-organ failure, and death (10% morbidity).
- It is treated with corticosteroids, intravenous immunoglobulins, antipyretics, fluid balance and narcotic pain control as needed. Use of a patient-controlled analgesia (PCA) machine is appropriate with painful lesions on the throat, vagina, urethra, and other epidermal surfaces. Severe oral lesions require topical anesthetics and mouthwashes. Debridement of dead tissue may be required; open lesions after debridement can be soothed with Burow's solution on nonadhering dressings.
- Children with lesions throughout the mouth, pharynx, and esophagus will need total parenteral nutrition and intra-lipids.
- Recovery can take weeks.

Data from Foster, C. S. (2015). Stevens-Johnson syndrome. Retrieved from http://emedicine.medscape.com/article/1197450-overview.

Acne

Acne, or the accumulation of pimples (comedones, papules, pustules, nodules, and or cysts), is caused by blocked pilosebaceous glands. For teenagers, these lesions are typically found on the face, chest, and back. Acne is the most common skin condition of the older child. Entering puberty, an excess of sebum (oily fats) is produced by the sebaceous glands. Hair follicles may become plugged with keratinocytes and sebum, leading to the development of acne. Contrary to myth, acne is not associated with the consumption of greasy or oily foods. Hormones, menses cycles, and excessive sweat all contribute to the development of adolescent acne.

Medical Treatment

Suggested treatment for mild acne (comedonal or mixed with papular and pustular) includes thorough washing of the skin twice a day, and the application of a topical benzoyl peroxide and topical antimicrobial medication. Alternative treatments include azelaic or 2% salicylic acids. The first-line choices for moderate acne (mixed papular–pustular or nodular) are oral antibiotics, topical retinoids, and benzoyl peroxides. For severe acne (nodular with conglobate), oral isotretinoins are recommended.

Nursing Care

Nursing care includes teaching the adolescent to cleanse the skin gently with oil-free cleansers. Many teens have success in using cleansers that contain 2% salicylic acid. Adolescents must be encouraged not to pick at their skin or pop pimples, as doing so can force the bacteria around the site of the lesion. The application of very warm clean cloths to a full pustule may help to drain the contents, and is preferred to popping the pustule and spreading the bacteria manually. Although teens should be informed about good nutrition, they need education on how androgen hormones during puberty create more sebum production, causing the lesions.

Case Study

A baby girl was born at 26 weeks' gestation to a mother with pre-eclampsia at a tertiary care hospital. The neonate was stabilized in the delivery room, and then placed on warmed blankets above a preheated, chemically warmed mattress under a radiant warmer. Her pulse oximetry probe was dabbed with cotton prior to placement on her right wrist. After establishing a patent airway via intubation with a 3.0 endotracheal tube, the infant was wrapped in warm blankets with a preheated double newborn hat, shown to her mother, and then brought to the NICU while escorted by her father, the advanced life support nurse, and the neonatologist.

(continues)

Case Study (continued)

In the NICU, the newborn was weighed, measured, and gently cleansed with warmed saline wipes. Deep catheters were placed in her umbilical artery and vein, and intravenous fluids were started at 80 mL/kg, with a bolus of lactated Ringer's and D_{10} IV solution, for hypoglycemia. The NICU nurses transferred the newborn to a preheated isolette with 80% humidity in a swaddle nest with a small roll placed under her shoulders. Footprints were gently taken but no heel sticks were attempted. The nursing staff prioritized the newborn's care, clustered her hands-on care to minimize stimulation, and placed a strip of silicone barrier tape around her feet where her pulse oximetry probe was placed. The silicone barrier tape was changed every 4 hours. The diaper was not fastened to prevent skin tears in the newborn's groin. After 24 hours of midline head positioning, she was placed prone on a surfboard made of synthetic lamb's wool and a warmed infant hat was put on her head. Gentle supportive care with compassionate touch was taught to the parents to avoid overstimulation for this extremely premature, low-birth-weight infant with high risk for skin integrity breakdown.

Case Study Questions

1. What are the preventive skin measures that were provided for this infant?
2. Why was she placed in an isolette with humidity?
3. Why did the NICU nurses use saline wipes and not soap and water to bathe the infant?

As the Case Evolves...

This premature infant has now been in the NICU for 12 weeks and has made good progress. The medical team is discussing when she should go home. This baby is her parents' firstborn, and both parents express nervousness and uncertainty about how to care for her. "We've read a lot of those baby books," explains the father, "but they don't really tell you how fragile a preemie is." He asks the nurse if there is any special information the couple need to know about their premature daughter's skin care.

4. Which of the following teachings provides accurate information for these parents in regard to their daughter's skin care?
   A. The parents should monitor their daughter's skin color and contact their healthcare provider if it appears yellow
   B. This child's skin cannot tolerate oils or sweat, so the parents should bathe their daughter daily in cool, soapy water and towel her dry.
   C. Her prematurity means this child's skin is especially delicate, so the parents should avoid synthetic fibers in her clothes and bedding and be aware that she might develop diaper rash more frequently than non-premature babies would.
   D. Premature babies are prone to eczema, but lotions and ointments should be avoided altogether; baby powder should be used to soothe the itching.

The preemie has been discharged, and her parents ask the nursing staff about whether they should use sunscreen on her face before leaving, given that the summer day is bright and sunny.

5. The pediatric nurse explains that their infant cannot be in the sun unless:
   A. She has reached the age of 6 months, and then only if UPF 15 is applied and a large hat is worn.
   B. She has reached the age of 3 months, and then only during overcast days.
   C. She has reached the age of 3 months, but only between the hours of 10 a.m. and 4 p.m.
   D. She has reached the age of 6 months, but only before the hours of 10 a.m. and after 2 p.m.

Chapter Summary

- The skin is the largest organ of the human body and performs many protective functions.
- Infancy is a time where there is high risk for skin infections, conditions, and lesions. Particularly in premature infants, newborn skin is delicate and susceptible to rashes, eczema, and a variety of outbreaks. Most are self-limiting, and parents should be instructed in how to prevent and care for such episodes.
- Infants and young children are particularly susceptible to skin lesions and damage. Because they are not capable of maintaining good hygiene, they must be prevented from scratching or touching wounds or lesions. Because topical medications are often absorbed systemically, they should be applied in a thin layer under the direction of a healthcare provider.
- Burns are an extremely common cause of injury in children, whether mild (e.g., sunburn) or catastrophic (accidental third-degree burn injuries). Care must be taken to not expose young children to sun. Infants younger than 6 months should not have sunscreen applied nor be exposed to the sun during the hours of 10 a.m. to 4 p.m. Even second-degree burn injuries to children can be extremely serious.
- Other common skin conditions during childhood include eczema, lice, scabies, poison oak or ivy, contact or diaper dermatitis, and acne.

Bibliography

American Academy of Dermatology. (2010). Bedbugs, scabies and head lice—oh my. Retrieved from https://www.aad.org/media/news-releases/bedbugs-scabies-and-head-lice-oh-my

American Academy of Dermatology. (n.d.). Contact dermatitis: Overview. Retrieved from https://www.aad.org/public/diseases/eczema/contact-dermatitis

Centers for Disease Control and Prevention (CDC). (2015). Parasites—lice—head lice: Frequently asked questions. Retrieved from http://www.cdc.gov/parasites/lice/head/gen_info/faqs.html

Centers for Disease Control and Prevention (CDC). (2016). Protect the ones you love: Child injuries are preventable: Burn prevention. Retrieved from https://www.cdc.gov/safechild/burns/index.html

Clark-Greuel, J. N., Helmes, C. T., Lawrence, A., Odio, M., & White, J. C. (2014). Setting the record straight on diaper rash and disposable diapers. *Clinical Pediatrics (Philadelphia), 53*(9 suppl), 23S–26S.

Flinders, D. C., & de Schweinitz, P. (2004). Pediculosis and scabies. *American Family Physician, 69*(2), 341–348.

Food and Drug Administration (FDA). (2008). FDA releases recommendations regarding use of over-the-counter cough and cold products. Retrieved from https://www.fda.gov/ForConsumers/ConsumerUpdates/ucm048682.htm

Food and Drug Administration (FDA). (2016). Use caution when giving cough and cold products to kids. Retrieved from http://www.fda.gov/Drugs/ResourcesForYou/SpecialFeatures/ucm263948.htm

Foster, C. S. (2015). Stevens-Johnson syndrome. Retrieved from http://emedicine.medscape.com/article/1197450-overview

Guilabert, P., Usúa, G., Martín, N., Abarca, L., Barret, J. P., & Colomina, M. J. (2016). Fluid resuscitation management in patients with burns: Update. *British Journal of Anaesthesiology, 117*(3), 284–296. doi:10.1093/bja/aew266

Hansen, S. L. (2008). From cholera to "fluid creep": A historical review of fluid resuscitation of the burn trauma patient. *Wounds, 20*, 9006. Retrieved from http://www.woundsresearch.com/article/9006

Lewis, M. L. (2014). A comprehensive newborn examination: Part II. Skin, trunk, extremities, neurologic. *American Family Physician, 90*(5), 297–302.

Simons, K. J., Watson, W. T. A., Martin, T. J., Chen, X. Y., & Simons, F. E. R. (1990). Diphenhydramine: Pharmacokinetics and pharmacodynamics in elderly adults, young adults, and children. *Journal of Clinical Pharmacology, 30*, 665–671.

Wentworth, A. B., Yiannias, J. A., Keeling, J. H., Hall, M. R., Camilleri, M. J., Drage, L. A., . . . Davis, M. D. (2014). Trends in patch testing. *Journal of the American Academy of Dermatology, 70*, 269–275.

Yu, J., Treat, J., Chaney, K., & Brod, B. (2016). Potential allergens in disposable diaper wipes, topical diaper preparations, and disposable diapers: Under-recognized etiology of pediatric perineal dermatitis. *Dermatitis, 27*(3), 110–118. doi:10.1097/DER.0000000000000177

CHAPTER 18

Cellular Regulation

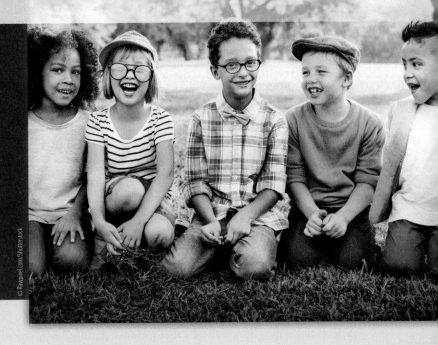

© Rawpixel.com/Shutterstock

LEARNING OBJECTIVES

1. Apply key nursing concepts to care for a child experiencing an oncologic disorder or a hematologic disorder.
2. Analyze the current state of childhood cancer, including incidence, prevalence, and survival rates for various childhood cancers.
3. Evaluate the nursing care needs and medical treatments required for a child with leukemia, lymphoma, or neuroblastoma.
4. Apply guidelines for caring for a child with neutropenia in the hospital or clinic setting, including calculating the absolute neutrophil count and implementing precautions.
5. Formulate effective strategies for symptom control during cancer treatment.
6. Differentiate different types of hematologic disorders found during childhood and identify their etiology, clinical presentation, and treatment.
7. Evaluate the nursing care needs of a child with severe symptomatic anemia requiring blood transfusions, including safe administration, accurate calculation of dose, and care required for an actual or suspected blood transfusion reaction.

KEY TERMS

Anemia
Cryotherapy
Differentiation
Enucleation
Hematopoiesis
Histology
Immunotherapy
Leukemia
Leukocoria
Lymphoma
Malignant
Metastasis
Mitotic index
Nadir
Neuroblastoma
Neutropenia
Radiation
Stem cell
Tumor burden
Vaso-occlusive episode

Introduction

Cellular regulation is a concept used to assess health and identify disorders associated with the cells of the lymphoid and myeloid cell lines, as well as the development of cancerous cells and bleeding disorders. In the science of pediatrics, the concept of cellular regulation opens the door to discussions of hematologic and oncologic pathologies that concern the health, well-being, development, morbidity, and mortality of children from birth through adolescence.

The beginnings of most problems in cellular regulation during childhood derive from genetic aberrations within the cells of the bone marrow (**Figure 18-1**). In the presence of normal physiology, the **stem cells** proliferate to form the various types of new cells that are needed by the body: either the myeloid cell line such as neutrophils, basophils, eosinophils, megakaryocytes (which produce platelets), monocytes (macrophages), or erythrocytes (red blood cells); or the lymphoid cell line, which further differentiates into humoral cells that produce antibodies (B cells) and lymphocyte cells that fight infection (T cells). Lymphocytes are differentiated by their surface proteins (markers); T cells are classified into categories that have specific functions, such as CD3, CD4, CD5, CD7, and CD8.

Stem cells have the capability of developing into many different kinds of cells; the process by which normal stem cell proliferation and differentiation takes place is called **hematopoiesis**. Hematopoiesis is a complex process that occurs in the bone marrow, and it is influenced by a child's health state, nutritional status, exposure to toxic substances, genetic background, and other factors. Children who present with hematologic disorders such as sickle cell anemia, clotting factor disorders, nutritionally based anemia, spherocytosis, congenital neutropenia, or aplastic anemia have a specific problem related to the production, proliferation, circulation, and function of cells originating from the bone marrow. These disorders require long-term management and sometimes frequent blood product or clotting factor transfusions or infusions.

Developmental Issues in Cellular Regulation

Both oncologic and hematologic disorders can be found across the developmental period. Although a newborn is much less likely to present with cancer than, for instance, an adolescent, there are more than 250 types of childhood cancers that can develop at any time during childhood, including the neonatal period (Orbach et al., 2013). The most common forms of neonatal cancer are teratomas, neuroblastomas, soft-tissue sarcomas, **leukemia** (cancer in tissues where blood cell production occurs), renal tumors, and brain tumors (Orbach et al., 2013). Hematologic disorders such as neonatal thrombocytopenia, hemolytic anemia, sickle cell disease, and other blood disorders that are present at or develop at birth arise due to a variety of mechanisms, although many are genetic in nature (Orkin et al., 2009). Hematologic disorders can also arise from cancer treatment, with anemia and neutropenia being common results of chemotherapy. For this reason, the two subjects are often intertwined.

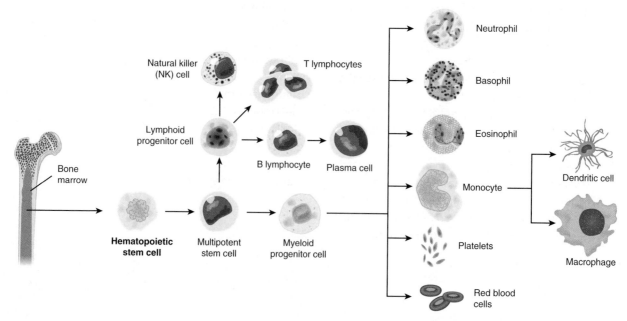

Figure 18-1 *Bone marrow cellular lines from the stem cell.*

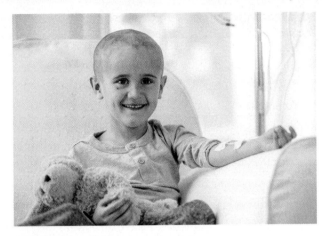

Figure 18-2 *A child receiving chemotherapy.*

© FatCamera/E+/Getty Images.

Childhood Cancer

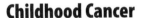

Hematopoiesis begins during fetal development, with production of these cell lines taking place in the fetus's spleen and liver. After birth, the hematopoietic stem cell produces new cell lines in the cavities of the child's bone marrow. While adult cancers are often related to aging and exposure to environmental factors that promote mutations (e.g., radiation, pollutants), in children most cancers tend to be related to a congenital gene mutation, sometimes inherited, that leads to the proliferation of cancer cells. For instance, children with Down syndrome (trisomy 21) are at higher risk of developing acute lymphocytic leukemia (ALL) (National Cancer Institute, 2016b), and children with certain forms of leukemia who present with the Philadelphia chromosome are at higher risk for poor outcomes and shorter survival rates. Children who have retinoblastoma have an inherited gene mutation called *RB1*. Children with documented exposure to ionizing radiation have a much higher chance of developing cancer due to mutations to their genetic material that lead to uncontrolled abnormal cell growth.

Management of the various types of cancer proceeds according to specific and unique treatment plans called protocols. Treatment protocols may follow guidelines provided by organizations such as the Children's Oncology Group (COG), an international consortium of pediatric oncologists and clinics that pool data for assessment of treatment regimens and data collection and analysis of outcomes. The most common types of cancer in children, representing approximately 75% of all pediatric cancer

diagnoses, are leukemias, **lymphomas** (cancers that develop from lymphocytes), nephroblastomas (Wilms' tumor), and central nervous system (CNS) tumors, including brain tumors and neuroblastomas. Leukemias account for approximately 30% of all childhood cancers, and CNS tumors for approximately 32% (American Cancer Society, 2016).

Children have a different experience with cancer than adults do. During periods of rapid growth, such as during the first year of life (birth to 1 year of age) and during the adolescent period, children have a higher risk of complications and cancer progression and decreased response to treatment (**Figure 18-2**). Children often need to take multiple antineoplastic (chemotherapy) drugs over an extended period of time to achieve remission.

Although childhood cancer across the developmental period is rare, the number of new cases (incidence) is rising. With research-based treatments, however, survival rates are steadily improving (National Cancer Institute, 2015a). In 1975, a simple majority of childhood cancer victims had a 5-year survival rate (50%), but as of 2010, that percentage had increased to 80% (National Cancer Institute, 2015a). Survival rates depend on the age of the child at diagnosis, the administration of multidrug treatments, and the type of cancer. Survival rates for acute leukemia have skyrocketed and now exceed 90%. Unfortunately, other, less common childhood cancers continue to have low survival rates. Overall, mortality rates are declining due to the effectiveness of the cancer treatment protocols for children.

Because of the use of multiple drugs and/or radiation therapy delivered at high doses relative to their body surface area (BSA) to treat their cancer, children who have had a childhood cancer diagnosis are at risk for the development of "late effects" such as chronic illness or even a secondary cancer in later childhood or in adulthood (National Cancer Institute, 2016a). Lifelong surveillance is required, to include blood analysis, diagnostics, and regular medical check-ups.

TABLE 18-1 Staging of Childhood Cancer

Staging a child's cancer gives information about treatment plans. Typically, TNM (tumor size, lymph node involvement, and presence of **metastasis**) staging is used for solid childhood tumors. Staging may also include specifics on the location of the tumor, the cell type, and the structures involved.

T: Tumor Size

At diagnosis, the child may have one or several small or large tumors present. The size of the tumor(s) helps to determine how extensive the cancer diagnosis is. For some larger tumors, surgical debulking may be required to reduce the tumor burden before other therapies are initiated.

Tx = The tumor cannot accurately be sized.

T0 = The tumor cannot be found.

T1–T4 = The tumor size is determined; it may be further distinguished by size and surrounding tissue involvement.

N: Lymph Node Involvement

Nx = Positive lymph nodes cannot be accurately measured.

N0 = The adjacent or close-by lymph nodes have no cancer cells detectable within them.

N1–N3 = Nodes surrounding the tumor are positive; denotes the number of lymph nodes involved.

M: Presence or Absence of Metastasis

Mx = The presence of metastasis cannot be measured.

M0 = There is no evidence of local, regional, or widespread metastasis of the original tumor cells.

M1 = Metastasis (distant growth of tumor cells) has been detected.

Medical Treatments for Childhood Cancer

After determining the cancer diagnosis and the staging (**Table 18-1**), if appropriate, childhood cancers are treated with well-established standard therapies and in clinical trials. Guidelines produced by consortia such as the Children's Oncology Group and the National Comprehensive Cancer Network (NCCN) offer the interdisciplinary oncology healthcare team a roadmap specifically created for the treatment of a certain cancer—one that is sometimes tailored to specific patient populations.

For instance, the COG guideline for ALL provides a plan of care for girls that lasts 2 years, while the plan of care for boys lasts 3 years. The guideline identifies the minimally acceptable complete blood count (CBC) laboratory findings representing bone health (e.g., the number of platelets must be equal to or more than 75,000, and the absolute neutrophil count must be equal to or more than 750, prior to giving chemotherapy that causes further decreases in bone marrow hematopoietic cell production). Approximately 7 to 10 days after a child receives a course of chemotherapy, the antineoplastic drugs suppress the production of all three cell lines (red blood cells [RBCs], neutrophils, and thrombocytes) to their lowest level (**nadir**). This leaves the child at risk for severe anemia, bleeding, and infection risk.

Children's responses to medical treatment of their cancer depends on four principles. The extent of disease at diagnosis highly influences their ability to fight progression of the disease. Understanding the tumor **histology**, or the types of cells in the tumor tissue, allows the pathologist to identify the type of cancer and predict factors such as rapid division of the cancer cells and responsiveness to chemotherapeutic agents. The tumor cells' **mitotic index** is the percentage of tumor cells currently in the process of division: The more that are dividing, the better they will respond to chemotherapy. Their **differentiation** indicates how closely the tumor cell resembles its mother cell: The more the tumor cell looks like the original cell, the better. A highly differentiated cell is very similar to its sister cell; in other words, the more differentiated it is, the more similar the cancer cell is to the other cancer cells. In general, more-similar cancer cells grow and spread more slowly and are more responsive to treatment. Lastly, the **tumor burden** (i.e., the number of cancer cells, the tumor size, or the amount of cancer in the body) is important. If the child's tumor is large, and is spread throughout the child's body, the more difficult the tumor is to treat.

Chemotherapy treatment typically proceeds through four phases. Nevertheless, each oncology diagnosis will have a unique treatment plan and may or may not include these four phases:

- *Induction:* The first phase of chemotherapy given to a child after initial diagnosis to "induce" a remission. The goal is to have "minimal residual disease" or no disease at the end of induction.

- *Consolidation:* The second phase of cancer treatment. This is defined as the treatment phase implemented after induction therapy to consolidate the gains obtained; or further reduce the residual cancer cells remaining.
- *Intensification:* An additional phase of cancer treatment, administered as needed for positive minimal residual disease or a continued presence of tumor.
- *Maintenance:* The long final phase of childhood cancer treatment that includes chemotherapy to maintain a remission or zero minimal residual disease. For instance, in treatment of childhood leukemia, the maintenance phase can last one or two years and includes weekly IV push therapy with vincristine and oral chemotherapy.

Chemotherapy is considered the gold standard of cancer treatment. Very few childhood cancer diagnoses are treated with radiation or surgery alone. Cancer chemotherapy uses highly cytotoxic drugs that inhibit the process of cell division; some of them specifically target cells that divide rapidly, which is a characteristic of many (but not all) cancer cells (Mitchison, 2012). Because the medication cannot distinguish between normal and cancerous cells, it also affects normal cells that reproduce rapidly, including blood cells/bone marrow, hair, and gut mucosal cells. For this reason, patients on cancer chemotherapy often experience short-term toxicities and side effects such as nausea, alopecia (hair loss), mucositis, pancytopenia, and other problems associated with cell damage. In addition, long-term consequences from chemotherapy may include learning disabilities and cognitive effects.

Each neoplastic drug is considered either cell cycle specific or cell cycle nonspecific (i.e., specific or not specific for the mitosis cycle). The cell cycle is the multiple-step process that a cell goes through to divide (**Figure 18-3**). The first stage of mitosis is interphase, when the cell is not dividing but is preparing to divide. During this phase of the cell cycle, the cell is identified as being in either G_1 (centriole replication), S (DNA replication of all 46 chromosomes), or G_2 (growth). In the next phase, known as the M phase, the cell divides in five distinct steps: prophase, metaphase, anaphase, telophase, and cytokinesis. In cytokinesis, two identical cells are produced. Chemotherapy may either disrupt cellular division during the cell cycle, or disrupt the cell regardless of which mitotic phase it is in.

Cell-cycle-specific agents include the following therapies:

- Plant alkaloids (inhibit mitosis)
  - Etoposide (G_2)
  - Vincristine (M)
  - Vinblastine (M)
  - Paclitaxel (G_2 and M)
- Antimetabolites (inhibit protein synthesis)
  - Hydroxyurea (S)
  - Methotrexate (S)
  - 6-Mercaptopurine (6MP) (S)
  - 6-Thioguanine (6TG) (S)
  - Cytarabine (S)

Cell-cycle-nonspecific agents include the following therapies:

- Antitumor antibiotics such as daunomycin and dactinomycin
- Alkylating agents such as thiotepa and cyclophosphamide
- Asparaginase such as L-asparaginase and PEG-L-asparaginase
- Nitrosoureas such as carmustine
- Topoisomerase-1 inhibitors such as irinotecan
- Heavy metals such as carboplatin and cisplatin

All types of chemotherapy agents cause bone marrow toxicity and a subsequent nadir, requiring specialized protective nursing care.

RESEARCH EVIDENCE

Types of Childhood Cancer Treatments

Eight types of treatments are used for childhood cancer:

- *Chemotherapy:* Antineoplastic drugs administered intravenously, intrathecally, intramuscularly, and intra-cavitary that work by inhibiting cellular growth and division.
- *Surgery:* Surgical debulking or tumor removal. Surgery can also be used to diagnose, determine the location, or palliate cancer.
- **Radiation**: High-energy X-rays that take the form of either external radiation beams directed at the tumor(s) or internal radiation via implantation of radioactive seeds, wires, catheters, or injection. Radiation disrupts the electrons orbiting around the tumor cell nucleus by the process of ionization.
- *Hormone therapy:* Use of certain hormones, such as corticosteroids, to inhibit cancer cell growth or block cancer cell action. Receptor-positive cancer cells are responsive to hormonal therapy.
- *Biologic therapy:* Use of the child's own immune properties to fight cancer directly. Interferon-beta is a type of biologic cancer therapy.
- **Immunotherapy**: Immune cells are used to stimulate cancer-fighting properties, such as cytotoxic T lymphocytes to treat Epstein Barr virus.

(continues)

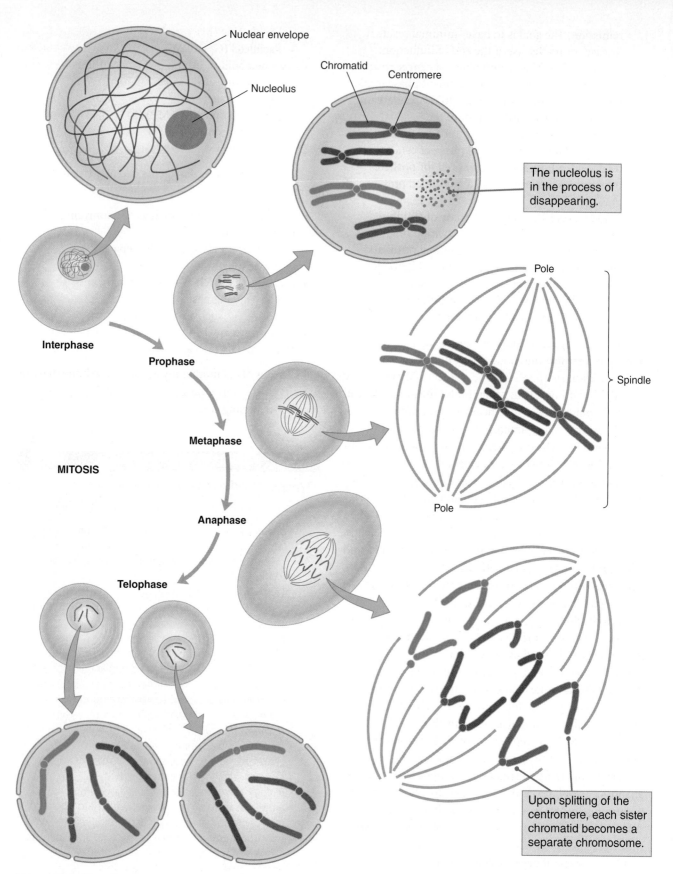

Figure 18-3 *The cell cycle.*

- *Targeted therapy:* Drugs or other substances that target specific cancer cells and produce minimal damage to surrounding or associative cells . Vascular endothelial growth factor (VEGF) and tyrosine kinase inhibitor (TKI) are two examples of targeted therapy. VEGF works by inhibiting the growth of new blood vessels that would normally feed tumor cells.
- *Watchful waiting:* Careful monitoring of the child, the child's condition, and the suspected or confirmed tumor. This option is used when the tumor's growth or malignant properties are questionable. Some rare cancers can disappear without external treatment through the work of the child's own immune system; others may be so slow growing that immediate treatment is not warranted.

Data from National Cancer Institute. (2015b). Unusual cancers of childhood treatment (PDQ)—Patient version: Treatment option overview. Retrieved from https://www.cancer.gov/types/childhood-cancers/patient/unusual-cancers-childhood-pdq#section/_11

BEST PRACTICES

Cancer Therapy Blood Analysis to Determine the Nadir

Pediatric nurses caring for children who are receiving cancer therapy need to be astute in obtaining laboratory specimens from central lines. Children with cancer typically are treated over an extensive period of time and will have an implanted port (**Figure 18-4**) or a tunneled central line catheter (**Figure 18-5**). The assessment for nadir includes an evaluation of the child's hemoglobin, hematocrit, platelet count, and absolute neutrophil count (ANC).

Understanding how to interpret a complete blood count (CBC) with manual differentiation so as to determine the level of protection and safety required for the child is an imperative in nursing. Children receiving cancer treatment often need blood transfusions for symptomatic hemoglobin levels less than 8 g/dL and platelet infusions for frank bleeds or counts of less than 10,000 (providers must follow their roadmap protocols).

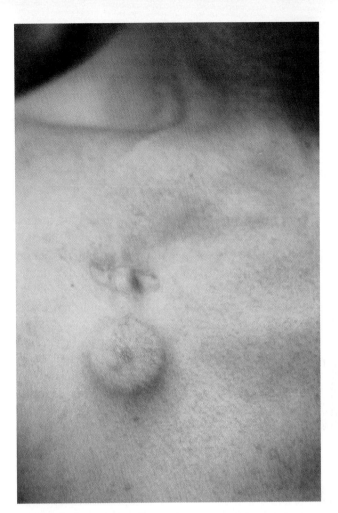

Figure 18-4 *An implanted port.*
© Glasshouse Images/Corbis/Getty Images.

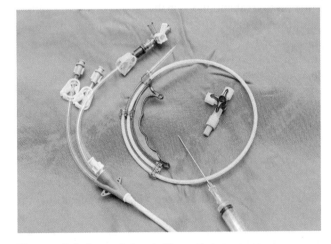

Figure 18-5 *A tunneled central line catheter.*
© pirke/Shutterstock.

Although childhood cancer is generally rare, some forms occur more commonly than others. The remainder of this section gives an overview of the diagnosis and treatment for more commonly seen pediatric cancers.

Hematologic Cancers

Acute Lymphoblastic Leukemia

Cancer that begins in the bone marrow and is found throughout the child's blood is called acute lymphoid leukemia or acute lymphocytic leukemia (ALL); it is the most common of all childhood cancers (National Cancer Institute, 2016b). The overall 5-year survival rate for ALL is more than 90% (National Cancer Institute, 2016b).

In this disease, tiny blasts (i.e., immature cancerous white blood cells) infiltrate and fill the child's bone marrow in great numbers. This infiltration prevents the bone marrow from producing normal cells. With time, blast cells will also infiltrate the child's ovaries, testes, lymph nodes, and spinal fluid, and then move to organs such as the spleen, liver, and skin. A child who presents as quite ill with positive blasts in the CBC blood smear should undergo further evaluation, including immunophenotyping to determine which proteins are expressed on the tumor cell membrane. This information about the cancer cell's genetics allows the oncologist to determine the expected response to treatment, and determine whether the child is considered a low risk, medium risk, or high risk. Many more factors influence this picture, but early determination of the ALL blast properties can help the oncologist determine the best course of action (Pui, Mullighan, Evans, & Relling, 2012).

Treatment of ALL consists of inserting a central line for safe drug therapy and rapidly initiating chemotherapy drugs. Chemotherapy guidelines for ALL may include the administration of the medications into both the blood and the intrathecal space to maximize killing of ALL cancer cells dwelling in the child's cerebral spinal fluid. Some children with ALL are eligible for a stem cell and/or bone marrow transplantation (Saletta, Seng, & Lau, 2014).

Acute Myeloid Leukemia

Compared to ALL, acute myeloid leukemia (AML; also called acute nonlymphocytic leukemia or acute myelogenous leukemia) is a less common type of leukemia that is more difficult to treat and more challenging to achieve a remission (Saletta et al., 2014). As in ALL, blasts fill the bone marrow spaces and then build up in significant numbers within the blood circulation in children with AML. When the AML cells enter into organs and form solid tumors, the resulting groupings of cells are called chloroma. Children who demonstrate AML cellular genetic material that places them at high risk are considered candidates for bone marrow transplantation. In some high-risk children with AML, stem cell transplantation may be warranted to either provide new bone marrow stem cells or assist in a more rapid recovery after multidrug high-dose chemotherapy treatment (Leung et al., 2012).

Hodgkin Lymphoma

The body's lymphatic system is made up of tiny thin tubes where clear lymphatic fluid carries lymphocytes. Hodgkin lymphoma is a cancer of the lymphatic system in which abnormal lymphatic cells proliferate and form tumors. Two main types of Hodgkin lymphoma are distinguished: nodular and classical. Most of the tumors associated with this disease present in the child's upper body, such as in the chest, in the neck, or behind the breastbone. After staging the tumor, a pediatric oncologist will treat the tumor(s) with chemotherapy, or with radiation for more advanced disease.

Central Nervous System Tumors

Starting in the brain or spinal cord, central nervous system (CNS) tumors can be either benign (noncancerous) or **malignant** (cancerous). Unfortunately, even a benign CNS tumor is still potentially extremely harmful: Even though it does not metastasize, it can have highly detrimental effects on the local brain and nerve tissue. Depending on its location, a benign tumor can affect a child's vital functions, memory, thoughts, emotions, and sensory experiences; thus, children with these types of tumors can have significant disabilities (**Figure 18-6**).

During the developmental period, children generally present with one of five types of CNS tumors: astrocytoma, germ cell tumor, medulloblastoma, brain stem glioma, or ependymoma. Treatment can include surgery, radiation, chemotherapy, or a combination of these treatments. Most children with tumors in the brain will need care from a team consisting of specialists in both pediatric oncology and pediatric neurology, as both the disease and its treatment present many challenges for the family and the child's long-term functioning. Many families consider entering their children into clinical trials when making their treatment decisions.

Neuroblastoma

Neuroblastoma is a CNS cancer that arises from the branches of nerves that run out of or exit from the spinal cord. Most young children with neuroblastoma present with tumors in their abdominal cavities. Classic signs of this childhood tumor include a large, bloated abdomen,

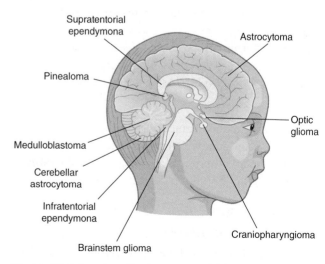

Figure 18-6 *Location of brain tumors in children.*

bone pain, refusal to walk, skin tumors, loss of appetite, and, if tumors are present in the local area, bowel or bladder abnormalities. Most neuroblastomas are found in children younger than age 5; in rare cases, an infant may be born with this type of tumor.

Surgery to remove the tumor or reduce its bulk, chemotherapy, radiation, and retinoic acid (Retin-A) are all used to treat neuroblastomas. Retinoic acid, a form of vitamin A, has been shown to be effective in reducing the chance that the child's tumor will return (relapse) and is administered after standard treatment is complete (Park, Eggert, & Caron, 2010; Peinemann, van Dalen, Kahangire, & Berthold, 2015).

Soft-Tissue and Bone Cancers

Ewing Sarcoma

One type of cancer that affects both bones and nearby soft tissues is the so-called Ewing tumors. Three types of Ewing tumors are distinguished: (1) undifferentiated Ewing sarcoma, which occurs most often; (2) peripheral primitive neuroectodermal (PNET); and (3) extraosseous Ewing sarcoma. Ewing tumors occur most commonly in adolescence (Saletta et al., 2014). Treatment of this type of neoplasm is determined by the location and size of the tumor, and by whether the tumor has metastasized to distant sites. Surgery, chemotherapy, radiation, and bone marrow transplantation are all used to treat Ewing sarcoma in children.

Wilms' Tumor (Nephroblastoma)

Cancer of the kidneys accounts for approximately 7% of all childhood cancers, and in children younger than age 15, most of these cases involve Wilms' tumors. The mean age of diagnosis with these nephroblastomas is 3 to 4 years. Approximately 10% of the children who develop this cancer have congenital deformities. In addition, numerous specific genetic mutations have been identified for Wilms' tumor, leading to the recommendation that a referral for genetic counseling be offered under certain circumstances when Wilms' tumor is diagnosed (National Cancer Institute, 2016c). Conditions that should raise suspicion of a genetic anomaly include aniridia, developmental delay, hypospadias, cryptorchidism, pseudohermaphrodism, overgrowth, and hemihyperplasia. A child who is diagnosed with Wilms' tumor and who has one or more of these conditions should be assessed for genetic abnormalities. In most children, only one kidney is affected, but bilateral tumors are sometimes found, albeit more often in girls than in boys.

Children presenting with Wilms' tumor may by asymptomatic, or they may have symptoms such as abdominal

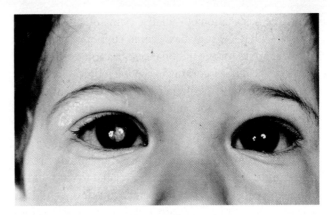

Figure 18-7 *A child with leukocoria.*
Courtesy of National Cancer Institute (http://www.cancer.gov)

pain (present in 40%), a lump or swelling in the abdomen, fever, hematuria, hypertension, and hypercalcemia (National Cancer Institute, 2016c). Nursing care for these patients should address their symptoms as well as assist caregivers in obtaining the necessary treatment. Because this form of cancer is relatively rare, referral to pediatric oncology specialists with experience in treating Wilms' tumor and/ or a clinical trial is recommended by the National Cancer Institute (2016c).

Retinoblastoma

Typically first identified by a child's parents, a retinoblastoma is a tumor located on or within the retina of the eye. Commonly, a parent or caregiver will notice an abnormal whitish glow on the child's retina when light falls on the eye in a particular angle—a phenomenon called **leukocoria** (**Figure 18-7**). Retinoblastomas are rare in children, but more than 40% of all cases have a genetic link. If the tumor is localized without metastasis, there is currently a 90% cure rate.

Treatment for retinoblastoma includes **enucleation** (removal) of the affected eye, followed by the introduction of a custom-made prosthesis. **Cryotherapy** (use of liquid nitrogen), radiation, and laser therapy may be required to eliminate remaining cells. The goal of therapy is medical treatment of the cancer and the prevention of visual impairment or blindness.

Nursing Care of the Pediatric Patient with Cancer

Pediatric oncology nursing is a specialized field of nursing science. Cancer treatments must be administered by a chemotherapy- or biotherapy-certified RN who has shown not only a commitment to this vulnerable population, but also mastery of the necessary knowledge, theory, and safe skills. The Association of Pediatric Hematology/Oncology Nurses (APHON) provides written support materials to prepare nurses for the national certification exam.

Pediatric nurses working in schools, clinics, and emergency rooms must be prepared to identify a child with cancer who is in trouble; one with the potential for serious side effects such as anemia, dehydration, and neutropenia with fevers (sepsis is a life-threatening complication); and one who needs care of a central line or implanted port. All nurses must have basic knowledge related to caring for a child with cancer and should be able to assess a child for severe symptoms such as pain and nausea using developmentally appropriate subjective and objective assessment tools, symptoms of stomatitis (mouth sores) or mucositis (mucous membrane sores anywhere in the body), anemia, evidence of bleeding and petechiae, neutropenia, and pending sepsis (**Figure 18-8**). In addition, all nurses should be able to assess a central line for complications or a port site for subtle evidence of infection.

Evidence of Infection in Children Undergoing Cancer Therapy

In children receiving cancer therapy that causes pancytopenia, classic evidence of infection may be absent. Owing to their depressed bone marrow function and subsequent reduced production of granulocytes (both mature, segmented neutrophils that can fight infection and immature new granulocytes known as bands), these children may not have any of the cells that would normally cause a cell-mediated reaction at the infection site. For instance, in a child with cancer who is receiving chemotherapy and is now in nadir, and who has a central line insertion site infection, there may not be any redness, swelling, pain, or pus at the line insertion site because there are no neutrophils to respond to the infection. Lymphocytes may be severely reduced to the point of not being able to launch a T-cell killer infection-fighting presence. The ANC can be very low, critically low, or actually zero in children with cancer, in which case the child may be highly vulnerable to infection yet not produce clear symptoms by which to identify an infection. *The only clinical sign of infection that children with cancer display may be a fever* (defined as a temperature of 38°C [100.4°F] or greater taken orally). Report fevers immediately in children on cancer treatment, as antibiotics must be initiated immediately to be lifesaving. Time from identification of the fever to reporting the fever to the medical staff to start of antibiotics should be *less than 1 hour.*

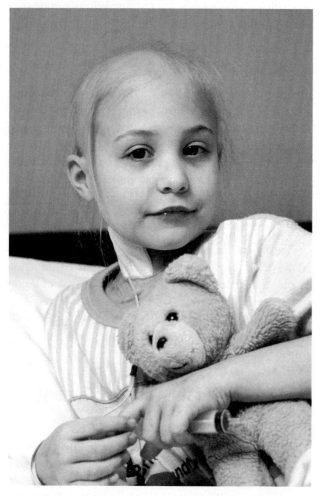

Figure 18-8 *A child with alopecia from cancer treatment.*
Courtesy of Bill Branson/National Cancer Institute.

Educating families during cancer treatment is an ongoing responsibility of the pediatric nurse. Teaching and then reinforcing emotionally difficult and complex topics to families who have diversity in language, culture, health literacy, and desire to learn is quite challenging. From diagnosis of childhood cancer, through the phases of induction, consolidation, intensification, and maintenance through long-term follow-up (surveillance), there is much that the family needs to understand and decision making in which they need to participate. Communication is key in keeping a child with cancer safe. Families must feel as if they can readily contact the pediatric oncology care team to report clinical changes, concerns about the child's condition, fevers, symptoms, and side effects. Cancer is highly disruptive to the flow of family life, and stress, financial strain, marital problems, and sibling rivalry are just a few of the challenges that families may face. Mobilizing support systems to assist the family is a powerfully important role of the pediatric nurse. Child Life specialists, social workers, child psychologists, school administrators and teachers, neighbors, and extended family all need to help provide for the family enduring the crisis of long-term childhood cancer treatment.

The pediatric nurse must also teach a family how to care for a child with side effects of chemotherapy. Understanding the cells of the bone marrow, knowing how to calculate an ANC, and knowing how to implement and maintain neutropenic precautions at home and in the hospital are essential education components. Having all adults in the child's circle know precautions to take when the child has **neutropenia** (a low number of neutrophils in the blood) can save lives. Neutropenic precautions include the following measures:

- Post neutropenic precaution signage on the child's hospital room door.
- Post hand washing signage on the child's hospital room door.
- Place the child in double-door isolation when possible.
- Place the child in a positive-pressure room when possible.
- Screen all visitors for infectious diseases, including taking a child visitor's temporal temperature.
- Refrain from including fresh fruits or fresh vegetables on food trays due to the potential for microbial contamination.
- Refrain from placing fresh flowers in the room due to the potential for *Aspergillus* contamination.
- Decontaminate the child's full skin surface daily with a skin cleanser (e.g., Hibiclens), or at least

thoroughly bathe the child daily and assess for skin infections, bruising, and petechiae.
- Designate all equipment used to only the child, including vital signs equipment, stethoscope, and oxygen saturation. Monitor equipment and any other supplies that would normally be shared between patients. Clean designated equipment frequently to prevent spread of infection.
- Do not administer pain medications that contain acetaminophen (Tylenol) or ibuprofen (Motrin) and that could mask a fever unless specifically instructed to do so by the pediatric oncologist.
- Measure daily weights and calculate a daily ANC to help guide the level of isolation that the child requires for protection from infection.
- If the child is neutropenic, then the child is likely to be pancytopenic: Do not take rectal temperatures, administer injections, perform rectal digital exams, use tampons, or trigger any cause of bleeding due to thrombocytopenia. Assess for anemia with daily lab values.
- Take special care of the child's mucous membranes, especially in the mouth. Because chemotherapy prevents cells from dividing, the mucous membranes, which are constantly dividing and replenishing, are particularly susceptible to these drugs' effects. Inflammation and infection of mouth sores is not just painful, but also dangerous because of the potential for introduction of bacteria. The child should brush with a soft toothbrush at least twice daily; rinse the mouth with salt and soda, Peridex (to decrease bacterial load), or "magic mouthwash"; should not floss; and should eat foods that are neither too hot nor too spicy.

The nurse should teach the family how to interpret their child's daily lab tests and how to calculate an absolute neutrophil count so they can understand the need for neutropenic precautions and help keep their child safe in the hospital, in the clinic, and at home. The child's ANC will also help determine whether the child should stay home from school for a period of time. For a child receiving chemotherapy and in the nadir, the ANC is calculated by multiplying the total white blood cell count (WBC) by the percentage of neutrophils (segmented or mature) and bands (immature baby neutrophils) found in the CBC with manual (not automated) differential.

Example 1

Total WBC = 3000
Segmented neutrophils = 19%
Bands = 4%
$$ANC = (3000)(0.19 + 0.04)$$
$$= 690$$

This child is considered mildly neutropenic.

Example 2

Total WBC = 1400
Segmented neutrophils = 11%
Bands = zero
ANC = (1400) (0.11)
     = 154

This child is considered severely neutropenic and needs strict precautions to prevent infection, sepsis, and life-threatening consequences.

Hematologic Disorders

Disorders related to the hematologic system include genetic disorders, acquired disorders, nutrition-related disorders, and situational conditions such as hemorrhage. Genetic disorders include congenital anemias and red blood cell dysfunctions such as sickle cell anemia. Acquired disorders are associated with changes in the RBCs that occur with some infectious diseases, such as parvovirus infection causing aplastic disorders or malaria.

Anemia

Defined as a condition or disease that significantly reduces either the total measurable circulating RBC count or the amount of hemoglobin, **anemia** strains the child's body by reducing the availability of oxygen. Healthy hemoglobin provides all cells with the needed amounts of oxygen. The processes of growth, tissue repair, mental capacity, and energy production all require adequate oxygen. Anemia interrupts the delivery of oxygen in one of five ways:

- Impaired production of RBCs or impaired production of hemoglobin
- Disturbances in the metabolic pathways, such as nutritional disorders, conditions, or deficiencies
- Decreased production or efficacy of erythropoietin, the renal hormone
- Small prolonged bleeds, occult GI bleeds, or frank hemorrhage leading to a reduced level of hematocrit
- Conditions of hemolysis or destruction in which either antibodies destroy RBCs or toxins, chemicals, parasites, and microbes destroy circulating RBCs

Nutrition-related anemia is the most common anemia in the infant, toddler, and preschool stage, and often is associated with over-consumption of milk (Lundblad, Rosenberg, Mangurten, & Angst, 2016; Ziegler, 2011). A young child who consistently consumes more than 24 ounces of milk per day is at risk for not consuming foods rich in iron and complete proteins, which in turn increases the child's risk of developing anemia. An infant who is given cow's milk before the first birthday may experience irritation of the GI mucosa leading to occult bleeds, which can further deplete iron stores.

Children with anemia will present with classic symptoms including fatigue, irritability, pallor, dizziness, and dyspnea. If the child is experiencing active bleeding, the nurse may observe vomiting, diarrhea, and melena (blood in the stools). If the child is actively bleeding in the genitourinary system, hematuria may be present. In severe cases, the child's symptoms can progress to severe syncope, poor concentration, decreased level of consciousness, seizures, and death. Any child who presents with symptoms of anemia should have an immediate CBC and reticulocyte analysis performed, along with a diet history and physical examination. In young children, the family should be questioned about the child's average consumption of cow's milk (Lundblad et al., 2016).

In older children, especially adolescent girls, anemia may accompany lifestyle choices such as vegan, vegetarian, or "fad" diets, if iron-rich foods are not included in the diet (e.g., spinach) or if B vitamins are not obtained through supplementation (Grooms, Walsh, & Monnat, 2013). If a school-age child or teen claims to follow a vegetarian/vegan or "special" diet, whether the rationale is for weight loss or moral justifications, the child and caregivers should be given appropriate feedback on the need for supporting intake of iron and B vitamins to avoid both iron-deficiency and pernicious anemia (Grooms et al., 2013). Anemia may occur secondary to eating disorders, but in a child with normal weight who claims a standard diet but nonetheless presents with pernicious anemia, the possibility of a malabsorption syndrome (e.g., celiac disease) should be considered (Hoffman et al., 2013).

Medical Treatment for Anemia

The pediatric healthcare team will determine the severity of the child's presenting anemia. A long course of oral iron supplementation may be sufficient if the parents make dietary changes to stop the progression of the child's state of anemia. In more severe cases, the child may be hospitalized for intravenous iron dextrose solutions and possibly packed red blood cells (PRBC) transfusion.

Additional laboratory evaluations may include a direct Coombs test (which assesses for the presence of antibodies causing the child to experience hemolysis), serum iron, transferrin, osmotic fragility for spherocytosis, lead levels, and hemoglobin electrophoresis to allow the determination of which type of hemoglobinopathy is present.

Anemia Therapy: Transfusion

Children who have a hematologic condition that requires an immediate intervention for anemia will be given a PRBC transfusion, in which the vast majority of serum and white blood cells are removed, leaving RBCs behind. Minute quantities of donor serum and white blood cells are the source of most transfusion reactions. Other transfused blood products are listed in **Table 18-2**.

Nursing Care of a Child Receiving a Transfusion

Children receiving transfusions require specialized care. The pediatric nurse must provide developmentally appropriate nursing care to such a child. Eliciting the support and engagement of the Child Life team will assist the child in understanding why the transfusion is needed and what the child can expect.

Safety must be maintained during the transfusion. A large-gauge angiocatheter should be used that is stabilized for

TABLE 18-2	Transfused Blood Products and Their Indications

Whole Blood

Given only in extreme emergencies where large volumes of blood are required as lifesaving hemorrhage treatments. ABO and Rh compatibility must be matched.

Packed Red Blood Cells (PRBC)

Given when a child's hemoglobin or hematocrit is low (typically 8 g/dL or less) and the child is symptomatic. For children, PRBC transfusions are given in a dose of 10–15 mL/kg from one donor if possible. A single unit of donor PRBCs can be divided into alloquots (4 packs) so the blood can be preserved for future transfusions. Limiting a child's exposure to transfused foreign proteins is essential to prevent alloimmunization (i.e., the production of antibodies against transfused cells). One transfusion dose of PRBCs typically raises a child's hemoglobin by 1 g/dL and the hematocrit by 3%.

Platelets

Small particles of the cell walls from the thrombocytes, which are essential for the production of clots. Many children who experience pancytopenia from cancer treatment will require lifesaving platelet transfusions. If a child's count is 20,000 or fewer cells and there is evidence of bleeding, the child will need a platelet transfusion. A cross-match is typically performed between the donor and the recipient, but is not required. ABO and Rh compatibility between the donor and the recipient is preferred to reduce alloimmunization.

Fresh-Frozen Plasma

Administered to a child to increase coagulation factors: factor IX (stable) or factor V and factor IX (unstable). Fresh-frozen plasma may be given to patients with traumatic injuries and children with significant burns.

Granulocyte Infusions

Associated with a very high risk of severe incompatibility reactions. The administration of granulocytes is rarely performed, and is viewed as a last effort to combat infections in children with severe and prolonged immunocompromised states.

the administration of the blood product. Transfusions should be given over no longer than 4 hours, and bags should be hung on blood "Y" tubing with 0.9% normal saline (NS) only. Dextrose solutions will cause hemolysis of the transfused cells. The child should have designated vital signs equipment set up next to the bed so that rapid measurements can be taken as needed and per protocol. All blood products must be double-checked by two registered nurses at the bedside, with the child's identification also being verified. Documentation of the double-checking safety procedures is imperative.

Blood product transfusions are not without risks. Children who will receive transfusion therapy must have all risks and benefits described to the family, and written consent must be obtained unless the child is being transfused after a life-threatening injury within emergency services. Transfusion reactions, if they are going to occur, typically become evident within the first 5 to 15 minutes after the transfusion being administered (see also **Box 18-1** for examples of painful transfusions). Medications to treat transfusion reactions should be made available, but not necessarily drawn up. These medications include antipyretics, antihistamines, epinephrine, corticosteroids, and bags of 0.9% NS for rapid fluid resuscitation if the child's blood pressure falls.

BOX 18-1 When Transfusions Hurt

The following conditions may lead to pain during a transfusion:

- Iron overload, which requires chelation therapy (hemochromatosis) to reduce the risk of liver, heart, and tissue damage.
- Graft-versus-host disease, in which transfused blood products attack bone marrow cells, leading to fevers, rash, diarrhea, abdominal pain, and increased liver function tests. Leukocyte-depleted and irradiated blood products must be administered to kill the remaining WBCs that cause this condition.
- Acquisition of infectious diseases from blood product transfusion (rare but still possible). These infections include cytomegalovirus (CMV), human immunodeficiency virus (HIV), and hepatitis B.

Febrile Reactions

- Oral temperature of 38°C (100.4°F) or higher.
- Report the fever but do not stop the transfusion unless instructed to do so. Administer oral acetaminophen at 10 to 15 mg/kg per dose as ordered. Acetaminophen may also be administered intravenously.

- Febrile reactions are frequently caused by the presence of a small quantity of donor serum in the infused product. Children who have this reaction should be premedicated for fevers for all subsequent transfusions.

Severe Urticaria

- Itching anywhere on the body; may also cause areas of redness and swelling on the skin, or look patchy.
- Report the reaction immediately to the ordering primary care provider or the hospitalist, and follow that professional's orders. The transfusion may or may not be stopped.
- Administer diphenhydramine orally or intravenously, typically 1 mg/kg per dose. Follow the institutional protocol for safe administration. Do not rapidly push intravenous antihistamines.

Hemolytic Reactions or Acute Immune Reactions

- Symptoms vary. Children may experience headache, dizziness, fever, skin flushing, general back pain, flank pain, body aches, chills, and increasingly bloody or darker urine. Late effects may include jaundice from the bilirubin liberated from the lysed RBCs.
- Turn off the transfusion immediately, as the donor cells that were transfused are being hemolyzed by antibodies (most likely due to ABO or Rh incompatibility). Call the primary physician who ordered the blood immediately (hematologist, oncologist, or hospitalist). Do not leave the child. Start a 0.9% NS line with all new tubing down to the IV hub or central line access point.
- Run the line at a to-keep-open (TKO) rate until orders are received for IV rate or boluses. Carefully send the transfusion tubing, blood bag, and any other transfusion equipment used to the blood bank. Be prepared for orders for lab draws (CBC, Coombs test, urinalysis, bilirubin, blood cultures, urinalysis, and others as ordered).

Chills and Rigors

- Children will demonstrate mild to severe shaking and uncontrolled trembling. Feelings of body chills such as one gets with a rapid fever may occur.
- Stop the transfusion and run 0.95% NS. Report the reaction immediately. In the type of reaction, children are reacting to the small amount of donor serum in the transfused blood product. Prepare for the administration of a small amount of a narcotic given IV to stop the shaking and rigors. Children may also need acetaminophen.

Sepsis

- Children will demonstrate fever, tachycardia, and possibly tachypnea if acidosis develops; hypotension is often a late sign. Children may also exhibit lethargy or a change in level of consciousness.
- Sepsis is a medical emergency. Do not leave the child, but call for help immediately if sepsis is suspected. The transfused product may be contaminated with cold storage organisms called halophiles—this can be a lethal blood transfusion reaction. Stop the transfusion and start 0.95% NS on new tubing. Prepare for the administration of several 0.9% NS boluses. Have the team bring the crash cart to the child's room. The child may need immediate transfer to a higher level of care (PICU) or IV vasopressors. Be prepared to draw labs, blood cultures, and arterial blood gases (ABGs). Carefully have someone take the transfused product, tubing, and all transfusion equipment used to the blood bank for analysis of the presence of bacteria.

Severe Respiratory Conditions

- Transfusion-related acute lung injury (TRALI) can present either as acute or with a slow onset. The reaction can start within 1 to 6 hours. Children will show shortness of breath, decreasing oxygen saturation readings, tachypnea, and overall distress.
- Due to the accumulation of antibodies against the transfused unit, the child may be third-spacing fluids and having a severe immune reaction that presents in the lungs. If the transfusion is still being administered, stop the transfusion and start 0.9% NS in new tubing. Report the child's reaction and symptoms immediately.

Alloimmunization

- Children will show evidence of hemolysis and demonstrate a poor response to the transfused blood product.
- Alloimmunization is caused by an immune response that generates antibodies to the foreign proteins of the transfused product. Children may demonstrate either an immediate reaction or a delayed reaction related to hemolysis.
- Report the symptoms to the ordering physician. If the blood product is still infusing, stop the transfusion and start a 0.9% NS line on new tubing. Save all transfusion equipment and the transfused blood bag for laboratory analysis.
- Future transfusions of blood products will require premedication of the child, consisting of

dihydramine and corticosteroids. A child who has this kind of reaction will need to have subsequent transfusions of HLA-matched blood to lower the quantity of antibodies transfused.

Anaphylaxis

- A severe and rapid reaction to the transfused product, which leads to an overwhelming immune response.
- Call the rapid response team immediately, and bring the crash cart to the room. Stop the transfusion and start a 0.9% NS line on new tubing. Begin NS IV boluses. Prepare lifesaving medications such as epinephrine, antihistamines, steroids, and vasopressors. Save all transfusion equipment and the transfused blood bag for laboratory analysis. Be prepared to draw blood for laboratory analysis as ordered. Transfer the child to a higher level of care (PICU).

Sickle Cell Anemia

Children with an autosomal recessive congenital (genetic) disorder of hemoglobin leading to rigid sickle-shaped RBCs are diagnosed with sickle cell disease (SCD). Fetuses and young infants have highly efficient hemoglobin F (fetal), which is subsequently replaced with hemoglobin A (adult). Through newborn screening for inborn errors of metabolism, infants may be identified early with the life-changing condition of hemoglobin S (sickle), and prevention of complications can start early.

Sickle cell disease is predominately found in the African American community and has an incidence rate of approximately 1 case per 500 live births. Most children with SCD are symptomatic by middle infancy. Early diagnosis is made through hemoglobin electrophoresis, which determines the types of hemoglobin present. Children with SCD are monitored by their sickle cell index (sickled solubility), a measure of the percentage of circulating sickled cells. An increasing percentage indicates that the affected cells are becoming grouped together in the small vasculature, which can lead to tissue hypoxia and eventually ischemia. The presence of abnormal sickle S hemoglobin (HgbS) in SCD leads to vaso-occlusive states described as **vaso-occlusive episodes**. In these events, the child experiences both chronic pain and acute peaks of pain, requiring drug therapy. Significant hemolytic anemia occurs due to the fragility of the sickled cells. Cellular waste products build up in the spleen, and the child is at risk for needing a splenectomy before rupture occurs.

A vaso-occlusive episode begins with a trigger. For example, a state of hypoxia, hypoxemia, infection, fatigue, dehydration, or emotional distress can trigger the production of larger quantities of sickle cells from the bone marrow. The vaso-occlusive episode (formerly known as a vaso-occlusive crisis) produces increased viscosity of the circulating blood and can lead to obstruction and stroke. One or more of the following sickle cell anemia–associated crises or episodes can occur:

- *Vaso-occlusive crisis:* Associated sickled clots form in small vascular areas such as the joints, lungs, tissues of the abdomen, fingers, and feet.
- *Hyperhemolytic crisis:* A rapid increase in sickled RBC destruction leads to hemolyzed cellular debris and bilirubin buildup in the tissues (jaundice) and kidneys.
- *Aplastic crisis:* The child's bone marrow decreases production of both normal-shaped RBCs and sickle cells.
- *Sequestration crisis:* Large numbers of hemolyzed sickled RBCs are transported to the spleen. The child may develop signs of shock including tachycardia, hypotension, syncope, dizziness, and overall reduced circulatory volume.

The final concerning complication with sickle cell anemia is the development of acute chest syndrome. In this condition, the fine pulmonary vasculature in the child's lungs becomes clogged with sickle cells and clots, leading to symptoms of pneumonia, reduced ventilation, reduced gas exchange, and a severe state requiring intensive care and possibly intubation with ventilation.

Medical Management of Sickle Cell Anemia

Medical management of sickle cell anemia requires an interdisciplinary team approach. In children and adolescents with SCD, their disorder impacts all aspects of their lives. Preventing acute vaso-occlusive episodes, reducing the risk of severe life-threatening complications of the disease, decreasing the complications associated with multiple blood transfusions (if required), increasing the presence of hemoglobin F, and effective symptom management are mainstays of medical management. Commonly used medications and medical interventions for sickle cell disease are listed in **Table 18-3**.

Nursing Care for Sickle Cell Disease

Although a pediatric nurse can encounter a child or adolescent with SCD in any clinical setting, pediatric hematology nurses provide specialized care to this vulnerable population. Children and teens with SCD need tremendous emotional help, support, compassion, honesty, and active listening skills. Having a lifelong chronic disease that is marked by

TABLE 18-3 Medications and Other Interventions for Sickle Cell Disease

Medications

› Prophylaxis for infection prevention: daily oral penicillin or amoxicillin

› Pulmonary inhalers such as albuterol to dilate the bronchus and bronchioles and improve lung function

› Vitamin D and calcium for reduced serum levels

› Hydroxyurea to increase hemoglobin F production

› Gabapentin for inflammation associated with sickled clots and pain

› Aspirin, if indicated, for coagulation prevention

› Folic acid to increase the mean corpuscular volume (MCV) of the RBCs

› Antibiotic therapy if the presenting trigger is infection

› Deferoximine (Desferal) or deferasirox (Jadenu) to remove increased levels of iron from transfusion therapy and hemolysis

› Pain medications: Motrin, Tylenol with Codeine, Vicodin, Norco, and morphine as needed

› Patient-controlled analgesia (PCA) if the child is hospitalized for a pain crisis or vaso-occlusive episode and needs intravenous fluids and intravenous pain management: usually morphine or Dilaudid

› Intranasal Fentanyl for rapid pain management in emergency room settings

Other Interventions

› Oxygen therapy if the child presents with abnormal arterial or capillary blood gases or low oxygen saturations

› Intravenous fluid resuscitation if the child presents with dehydration, increased percentage of sickle cells, and vaso-occlusion

› Warm packs on areas of vaso-occlusion for pain and increased circulation to the affected areas

› Blood transfusion therapy if the child is severely anemic and in hemolysis

› Rest to improve healing

› Nutrition for tissue repair and cell production

› Counseling for stress reduction and improved coping

---

painful exacerbations and vaso-occlusive episodes renders these special children vulnerable to emotional distress.

Children with SCD face the prospect of recurring acute episodes of pain. This pain is directly related to the occlusion of small vessels, which become clogged with sickled (banana-shaped) red blood cells. The clogged vessels then become inflamed, which draws neutrophils to the area, and blood flow in the area becomes static. This process leads to tissue hypoxia, acidosis, and eventually ischemia. Inflammation also damages the vascular endothelium. Pain can be found in a variety of areas of the body (**Table 18-4**). During these painful episodes, the nurse must perform accurate subjective and objective pain assessments, to be followed with effective pain management.

The pediatric nurse working with this population must understand the pathology of SCD, know how to identify it, and prevent exposure to and reduce triggers in the child's life. Education is paramount for the child and family. Providing rapid interventions for vaso-occlusive episodes and understanding how to effectively assess and manage pain provides safety for the child, prevents complications, and

TABLE 18-4 Areas of Sickle Cell Disease–Related Pain: Vaso-occlusion, Hypoxia, and Ischemia of Tissues

Dactylitis: acute pain and swelling of the fingers

Osteomyelitis: inflammation of bone tissue

Arthritis: inflammation of the joints

Priapism: prolonged and painful erections due to the presence of viscous blood/clots in the penis; these clots may require extraction or vasodilation via medications

Pneumonia: inflammation and infection of the pulmonary system, which can precede acute chest syndrome

Splenic sequestration: pooling of RBCs and hemolyzed RBC components

Cholecystitis: inflammation and infection of the gallbladder, necessitating removal of this organ

Acute chest syndrome: a severe life-threatening condition in which microscopic clots form in the pulmonary vasculature, affecting ventilation and gas exchange

builds trust. Working closely with the interdisciplinary team to implement management of the child's care may mean that the pediatric nurse takes the primary role in ensuring effective communication between the family and the healthcare team. All children with SCD need a case management approach to care and continued education throughout the developmental period.

Complications of SCD are associated with the various types of the disease. When children are diagnosed with HbSS (i.e., with two copies of the sickle gene), they have a greater chance of experiencing acute complications such as pain crises, bacteremia, aplastic crisis, and acute chest syndrome. Early identification of signs and symptoms of these complications can reduce the need for prolonged hospitalization, severe injury, and death. Monitoring for signs of complications includes observing verbal indications of increasing pain, tachycardia, tachypnea, hypertension, and inconsolability in young children. Pain may or may not be associated with a vaso-occlusive episode.

QUALITY AND SAFETY

Children who are hospitalized with sickle cell anemia and require a surgical intervention should not be given a prolonged course of preoperative or postoperative oxygen therapy. When this therapy is given, the child's bone marrow will stop or reduce production of reticulocytes. Oxygen therapy should be used judiciously and should be discontinued as soon as safe.

Factor Deficiencies

Some children may present with an X-linked recessive bleeding disorder requiring factor replacement. Hemophilia is one such disorder; in fact, it is the most common severe inherited coagulation disorder. Hemophilia A (factor VIII deficiency; occurs more often in boys) and hemophilia B (factor IX deficiency) are the most common forms of hemophilia. Patients with hemophilia are cared for the pediatric hematology oncology team. In such children, the pediatric nurse must be able to provide rapid assessments for evidence of bleeding, both frank and occult, and be skilled at the administration of and education about intravenous factor replacement.

Infants may be first diagnosed with hemophilia when they display bleeding episodes during or after a circumcision, venipuncture, or a surgical intervention. The severity of the disorder (mild, moderate, severe) is graded based on the percentage of factor produced by the child. Absence of either factor VIII or factor IX leads to severe impairment of thrombin and fibrin generation. Classic clinical presentations are bruising (ecchymotic areas on the skin), bleeding gums, hematuria, epistaxis (nosebleeds), joint pain from bleeds into joints (synovitis and hemiarthrosis), bleeding with rigorous play leading to injuries, and significant bleeds with trauma.

Active bleeding requires immediate venous access for IV factor replacement. Children may require administration of 1-deamino-8-D-arginine vasopressin (DDAVP) to increase their factor VIII level prior to a surgical procedure such as wisdom teeth extraction.

Case Study

Marisol, a 16-year-old Hispanic girl, has been in the PICU for severe pancreatitis for over a week. She originally presented to the pediatric emergency department with severe abdominal pain, elevated temperature, nausea, and dyspepsia. Her initial diagnosis was based on her elevated pancreatic enzymes and clinical presentation. Her family speaks only Spanish and has been present at her bedside continuously.

As her condition progressed, Marisol developed pancytopenia and received a consultation from the pediatric oncologist. After both serum laboratory analysis and a subsequent biopsy of a large lymph node on her neck, Marisol was diagnosed with lymphoma. She was very distressed about the diagnosis and immediately displayed signs of

withdrawal, was very concerned about the future and her schooling, and appeared depressed. Because Marisol is the family's "interpreter," her parents are not sure what is happening and seem very confused and alarmed by their daughter's behavior.

Case Study Questions

1. Now that a diagnosis of lymphoma has been verified, what are the appropriate first steps in a family-centered model of care for this teen and her family?
2. How is lymphoma treated?
3. Which special care needs arise for a teenager facing lengthy treatments with multiple inpatient admissions?
4. Which resources can a nurse mobilize for this patient?

(continues)

Case Study *(continued)*

As the Case Evolves. . .

After the initial diagnosis of lymphoma is made, the nurse sits down with Marisol and her family. A medical interpreter is brought in so that Marisol does not have to interpret for her parents. The nurse answers the parents' initial question—"What is wrong with our daughter?"—by explaining that Marisol has lymphoma and describing what that means. The interpreter then tells the nurse that Marisol's father is asking, "What do we do next to treat this disease?"

5. Which of the following responses is appropriate to explain the next step of treatment?
   A. "Your daughter will likely need a combination of drug therapy and radiation, and the treatment regimen will probably last a number of weeks, maybe months, depending on her response."
   B. "We will work with you to find an appropriate clinical trial for your daughter to participate in."
   C. "We will run some tests to identify the kind of lymphoma she has and which stage it is at. That information will help determine the right treatment regimen when you go see a pediatric oncology specialist."
   D. "For most lymphomas, we usually take a 'watch and wait' approach until we see whether the disease is undergoing rapid change. So not much will happen for a few months, although your daughter will need frequent checkups."

Marisol has begun her treatment protocol. At the end of the third week of chemotherapy, Marisol's mother approaches a bilingual nurse and expresses concern about how sick the treatment makes her daughter. She says, "After this is over, I'm not sure I will ever bring my daughter to see a doctor again!" The nurse recognizes that a key responsibility is to reinforce the family's understanding and compliance with cancer surveillance.

6. Which of these follow-up measures will Marisol's mother need to have explained to her?
   A. Twice-yearly computed tomography (CT) scans
   B. A full body assessment by the pediatric oncology team
   C. The national recommendations for childhood immunization
   D. Regularly scheduled appointments to check for signs of relapse

During her first course of chemotherapy, Marisol complains to her mother that she is nauseous, fatigued, breathless, dizzy, and chilled, and says her heart keeps racing. Her mother brings her in for an evaluation, and Marisol is found to have iron-deficiency anemia.

7. Which of the following is an appropriate therapeutic response?
   A. Encourage Marisol to eat more iron-rich foods
   B. Prescribe an iron supplement and consider use of a colony-stimulating factor medication
   C. Prescribe a B-vitamin supplement
   D. Initiate a RBC transfusion

Chapter Summary

- Cellular regulation is a concept used in understanding health and disorders associated with the lymphoid and myeloid cell lines, as well as the development of cancerous cells and bleeding disorders.
- Cancer in children is rare, and requires a specialized team approach and care at institutions that specialize in the treatment of childhood cancers.
- Children have a different experience with cancer than adults do. During periods of rapid growth, such as during the first year of life and during the adolescent period, children are at higher risk for cancer and exhibit decreased responses to treatment. Children with cancer often need to receive multiple antineoplastic (chemotherapy) drugs over an extended period of time to achieve remission.
- The cause of childhood cancer is often difficult to pinpoint because a child has not had a lifetime of toxic exposures (e.g., smoking, drinking, radiation,

sun exposure, asbestos). Genetic mutations—a known cause of cancer—are often the triggers for cancer in children.
- Children with Down syndrome (trisomy 21) are at higher risk for developing acute lymphocytic leukemia (ALL). Children with certain forms of leukemia who present with the Philadelphia chromosome are at higher risk for poor outcomes and shorter survival rates.
- A child's response to medical treatment depends on four principles: tumor histology, mitotic index, differentiation, and tumor burden.
- Medical care for childhood cancer involves complex chemotherapy treatment plans that incorporate radiation, surgery, biotherapy, and immunotherapy. Multiple side effects can occur, including both short-term and delayed effects.
- Other cellular regulation disorders include anemias related to nutritional disorders, genetic disorders such as sickle cell anemia, hemolytic conditions, and factor deficiencies such as hemophilia.

- ◆ Care is provided to children with cellular regulation disorders by a specialized interdisciplinary team of pediatric oncology hematology professionals. Nevertheless, any pediatric nurse can encounter a child with past or current history of a disorder of cellular regulation.

Bibliography

American Cancer Society. (2016). Cancers that develop in children. Retrieved from http://www.cancer.org/cancer/cancerinchildren/detailedguide/cancer-in-children-types-of-childhood-cancers

Grooms, L. P., Walsh, M., & Monnat, L. E. (2013). Treatment of anemia in the adolescent female. *Pediatric Annals, 42*, 36–39.

Hoffman, R., Benz, E. J., Jr., Silberstein, L. E., Heslop, H., Weitz, J., & Anastasi, J. (2013). *Hematology: Basic principles and practice* (6th ed.). Philadelphia, PA: Elsevier Saunders.

Leukemia and Lymphoma Society. (2013). Long-term and late effects of treatment for childhood leukemia or lymphoma facts. No. 15. Retrieved from https://www.lls.org/sites/default/files/file_assets/longtermlateeffectschildhood.pdf

Leung, W., Pui, C.-H., Coustan-Smith, E., Yang, J., Pei, D., Gan, K., . . . Campana, D. (2012). Detectable minimal residual disease before hematopoietic cell transplantation is prognostic but does not preclude cure for children with very-high-risk leukemia. *Blood, 120*, 468–472.

Lundblad, K., Rosenberg, J., Mangurten, H., & Angst, D. B. (2016). Severe iron deficiency in infants and young children, requiring hospital admission. *Global Pediatric Health, 3*. doi:10.1177/2333794X15623244

Mitchison, T. J. (2012). The proliferation rate paradox in antimitotic chemotherapy. *Molecular Biology of the Cell, 23*(1), 1–6.

National Cancer Institute. (2015a). Childhood cancers. Retrieved from http://www.cancer.gov/types/childhood-cancers

National Cancer Institute. (2015b). Unusual cancers of childhood treatment (PDQ)—Patient version: Treatment option overview. Retrieved from https://www.cancer.gov/types/childhood-cancers/patient/unusual-cancers-childhood-pdq#section/_11

National Cancer Institute. (2016a). Late effects of treatment for childhood cancer (PDQ). Retrieved from https://www.cancer.gov/types/childhood-cancers/late-effects-hp-pdq

National Cancer Institute. (2016b). Childhood acute lymphoblastic leukemia treatment. Retrieved from https://www.cancer.gov/types/leukemia/hp/child-all-treatment-pdq

National Cancer Institute. (2016c). Wilms tumor and other childhood kidney tumors treatment (PDQ). Retrieved from https://www.ncbi.nlm.nih.gov/books/NBK65842/

Orbach, D., Sarnacki, S., Brisse, H. J., Gauthier-Villars, M., Jarreau, P.-H., Tsatsaris, V., . . . Doz, F. (2013). Neonatal cancer. *Lancet Oncology, 14*, e609–e620.

Orkin, S. H., Nathan, D. G., Ginsburg, D., Look, A. T., Fisher, D. E., & Lux, S. E. (Eds.). (2009). *Hematology in infancy and childhood* (7th ed.). Philadelphia, PA: Saunders Elsevier.

Park, J. R., Eggert, A., & Caron, H. (2010). Neuroblastoma: Biology, prognosis, and treatment. *Hematology/Oncology Clinics of North America, 24*, 65–86.

Peinemann, F., van Dalen, E. C., Kahangire, D. A., & Berthold, F. (2015). Retinoic acid post consolidation therapy for high-risk neuroblastoma patients treated with autologous hematopoietic stem cell transplantation. *Cochrane Database of Systematic Reviews, 1*, CD010685.

Pizzo, P. A., & Poplack, D. G. (Eds.). (2016). *Principles and practice of pediatric oncology* (7th ed.). Philadelphia, PA: Wolters Kluwer.

Pui, C.-H., Mulligan, C. G., Evans, W. E., & Relling, M. V. (2012). Pediatric acute lymphoblastic leukemia: Where are we going and how do we get there? *Blood, 120*, 1165–1174.

Saletta, F., Seng, M. S., & Lau, L. M. S. (2014). Advances in paediatric cancer treatment. *Translational Pediatrics, 3*(2), 156–182.

Withycombe, J. S., Andam-Mejia, R., Dwyer, A., Slaven, A., Windt, K., & Landier, W. (2016). A comprehensive survey of institutional patient/family educational practices for newly diagnosed pediatric oncology patients. *Journal of Pediatric Oncology Nursing, 33*(6), 414–421. doi: 10.1177/104354216652857

Ziegler, E. E. (2011). Consumption of cow's milk as a cause of iron deficiency in infants and toddlers. *Nutrition Reviews, 69*(suppl 1), S37–S42. doi:10.1111/j.1753-4887.2011.00431.x

CHAPTER 19

Cardiovascular: Perfusion

Guest Author: Lu Sweeney, RNC-NIC, MS, CNS, CHSE

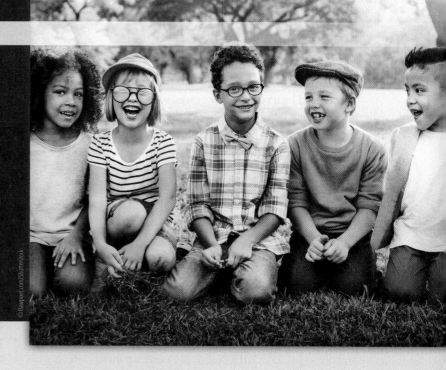

LEARNING OBJECTIVES

1. Evaluate the function of the three fetal cardiac shunts in utero and during the postnatal transition.
2. Critically analyze congenital cardiac anomalies and associated pathophysiology.
3. Assess whether heart defects are cyanotic (right-to-left cardiac blood flow) or acyanotic (left-to-right cardiac blood flow), and incorporate those findings into nursing care.
4. Evaluate acquired cardiac dysfunction related to infectious or other processes.
5. Apply developmentally appropriate nursing assessments to care for children who have cardiovascular disorders.
6. Incorporate care practices needed for health promotion and avoidance of disease exacerbation in a child with a cardiac defect or dysfunction.
7. Evaluate safety challenges for the child with a cardiovascular disease with tissue perfusion and oxygenation.
8. Apply concepts of nursing care, health promotion, and complications prevention to a care plan for a child with congestive heart failure.
9. Apply nursing concepts regarding safe administration of cardiac medications to a child, including evaluation of medication effects and appropriate patient/parent teaching.

KEY TERMS

Acquired heart disease
Acyanotic
Congenital heart defect
Congenital heart disease
Congestive heart failure
Cyanotic
Fetal circulation
Hypoxemia
Oxygenation
Perfusion

Introduction

Cardiovascular (CV) disease in children occurs either due to a **congenital heart defect** (born with the malformation) or **acquired heart disease** (acquired sometime after birth). Such defects involve the physical structures in the heart and can alter heart function, circulatory function, or both. Congenital heart defects (CHDs) are the most frequent kind of birth defect and are the largest cause of birth defect-related fatalities in the first year of life, affecting nearly 1% (approximately 40,000) of babies born in the United States each year (Centers for Disease Control and Prevention [CDC], 2015). Of the 1% born with CHDs, 25% have a critical congenital heart defect (CCHD) requiring at least one invasive intervention before the infant reaches his or her first birthday. In 2004, hospitalization costs for infants with congenital heart conditions amounted to $1.4 billion (CDC, 2015). Higher risk of congenital heart defects can be related to maternal conditions such as diabetes, smoking, and obesity (CDC, 2015; National Center on Birth Defects and Developmental Disabilities, 2016).

This chapter explores broad categories of **congenital heart disease** and acquired cardiac disease (ACD), along with the nursing care that children with these conditions require. Congenital conditions predominantly involve structural issues that affect blood flow and, therefore, perfusion. Acquired heart conditions can result from a multitude of etiologies, such as maternal diseases (diabetes), infectious processes (rheumatic fever), or a combination of factors, or as a secondary result from another illness.

Cardiopulmonary System Functioning from Infancy to Childhood

Cardiopulmonary development begins very early in pregnancy. Functioning atria, ventricles, valves, and vessels are in place at eight weeks into the pregnancy; therefore, congenital malformations occur early in fetal development as well (Blackburn, 2003). The fetal circulation supports the fetus's overall growth but directs the majority of the blood supply away from the developing lungs. These shunts, or blood flow pathways, persist because of pressure changes inside the cardiopulmonary system that force pathways to stay propped open or reverse the blood flow, similar to water flowing upstream or pooling behind a dam.

After birth, the circulatory system transitions to the normal, familiar function: circulation of oxygen-carrying blood flowing in from the lungs and out to the body, and return of the deoxygenated blood to the lungs for reoxygenation. The myocardium contracts in response to electrical impulses from inherent pacemakers in the heart, sending blood with oxygen-carrying red blood cells (RBCs) out through the circulatory and pulmonary vascular system.

Core principles of cardiac function are as follows:

- **Fetal circulation**: The right ventricle and atrium circulate deoxygenated blood to the lungs, and then the oxygenated blood returns to the left atrium and ventricle to be pumped to the rest of the body (**Figure 19-1**).
- **Oxygenation**: Adequate RBCs must be present in the blood to carry oxygen. Adverse effects of anemia—most often related to iron deficiency—not only impact oxygen delivery to tissues, but can also have negative effects on development of cognition and academic and verbal skills in children ranging from infancy to adolescence (Halterman, Kaczorowski, Aligne, Auinger, & Szilagyi, 2001). Transfusion may be needed in case of inadequate oxygenation.
- Precision: Precisely timed cardiac cycles of contraction and refilling phases are managed by an innate system of electrical conduction, pacemaking nodes, and cardiac muscle fibers located throughout the heart. Disruption of conduction can result in arrhythmias, which negatively affect perfusion and oxygenation (**Figure 19-2**).
- **Perfusion**: Episodes of low blood pressure can lead to poor tissue perfusion (delivery of blood to the body's cells) and shock. Hypotension can be a late sign of compromise in children, so care and treatment should be initiated before it occurs. The opposite condition, hypertension, can also lead to poor health outcomes in children, similar to those noted in adults, and is thought to be under-diagnosed. Priority goals for the healthcare team related to blood pressure are to prevent hypotension and hypertension.
- Protection: When critical illness or fluid loss occurs, a child's body will recognize this state and protectively reduce blood flow to noncritical areas, reserving the bulk of the oxygen delivery for the heart and brain. Prompt corrective treatment is essential because the child will not be able to compensate indefinitely; cardiovascular collapse and death will eventually result from such a condition.
- Homeostasis: Critical to adequate blood pressures and perfusion is optimized fluid and electrolyte status for the child's specific needs. Fluid overload, which is sometimes worsened by low urine output, can lead to heart failure. Lack of adequate intravascular fluid volume can lead to hypotension and, possibly, shock. Sodium, chloride, and potassium levels, along with other blood chemistries, are vital to monitor and correct as needed.
- Elimination: Renal function is critical to maintaining fluid and electrolyte balance, which supports

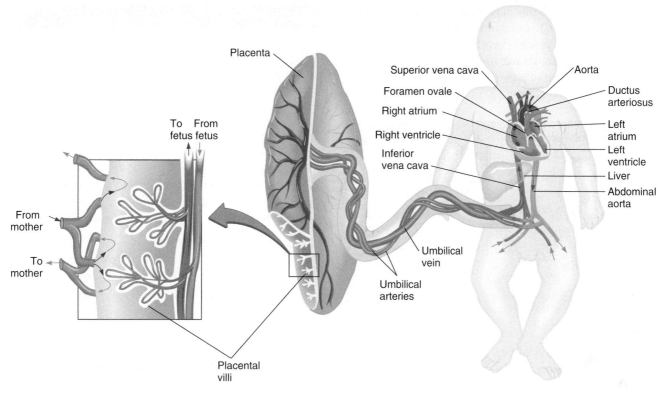

Figure 19-1 *Fetal circulation.*

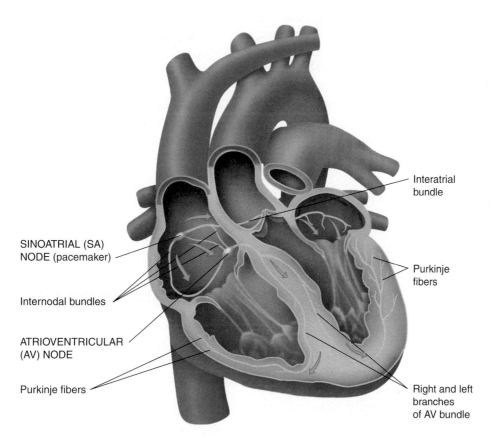

Figure 19-2 *The cardiac electrical conduction system.*

CV function. Urine output can be a strong indicator of the effectiveness of vital organs' perfusion owing to the kidneys' sensitivity to poor blood flow. Oliguria or anuria due to poor kidney perfusion can be a result of poor cardiac function.

In the developing child, the CV features evolve with progression through developmental stages. Gradual shifts in baseline values of vital signs is a normal part of growth and development. Progression from a more rapid heart rate to a less rapid one with increasing age as well as higher-trending blood pressure measurements are considered part of this evolution and, when they are within the expected ranges, considered normal. The heart grows in size at the same rate as body weight increases. Blood volume capacity increases from 40 mL in the infant to 600 to 800 mL in the adult. Just as in adults, heart health can greatly influence how successful the child is at living a healthy lifestyle regarding food choices and daily activity. Genetic and environmental factors also play key roles.

Healthcare providers should be familiar with the changes in the functional cardiovascular system expected at each developmental level:

- *Newborns (birth to 28 days):* The newborn phase is the most rapidly adaptive, featuring the transition to air-breathing from maternal/placental oxygenation. Corresponding changes in the newborn's circulatory system occur that support perfusion through the new non-fetal blood flow pathways—specifically, through the closure of the three fetal shunts owing to shifts in pulmonary and systemic pressures (**Table 19-1**).

The newborn and infant myocardium or cardiac muscle is relatively stiff. As a consequence, the heart cannot expand the volume of blood that fills the chambers to be subsequently pumped and distributed, if such expansion is needed to meet increased perfusion demands owing to illness, dehydration, or other volume loss such as bleeding. Instead, the only way to improve cardiac output is by

TABLE 19-1 Three Fetal Shunts and Anticipated Closure
Foramen ovale (flap-like opening between the atria): Directs the majority of blood away from the lungs. This intracardiac shunt should close after birth, when blood pressure in the lungs decreases (pulmonary vasodilatation) and left-sided heart pressure increases.
Ductus arteriosus (connects the descending aorta and left pulmonary artery): Diverts the majority of blood away from the fetus's lungs in utero. If this extracardiac shunt persists beyond the neonatal period, it can produce left-to-right (increased blood flow to the lungs) shunt-related symptoms. May become bidirectional in blood flow for a few hours after birth.
Ductus venosus (connects the umbilical vein to the fetal inferior vena cava): Allows for fetal mixed blood to bypass the liver. This shunt, which is outside the heart, is permanently closed with clamping of the umbilical cord after birth.

increasing the heart rate. Tachycardia in the newborn or young child can be compensatory and signal impending cardiovascular collapse. Tachycardia of the newborn must be assessed to rule out other causes and then treated.

- *Infants (1 month to 1 year):* Total blood volume doubles from the newborn's 20 mL/kg to 40 mL/kg by age 6 months. An infant's hematocrit tends to be approximately 30% at 2 months of age, but subsequently increases to 38% to 42% for late adolescent girls (non-anemic) and 40% to 45% for late adolescent boys. Sex differences in hematocrit become significant at puberty.
- *Toddlers and preschoolers (1–5 years):* Blood volume quadruples to 160 mL by 2 years of age.
- *School age and adolescence (6–18 years):* By the school-age developmental period, children have heart rates and blood pressure near the adult range. Adolescents experience a doubling in heart weight. Systolic blood pressure increases in boys and plateaus in girls. Lung size increases, and both respiratory rate and vital capacity decrease (Rudolph, Rudolph, Lister, First, & Gershon, 2011).

Causes of Congenital Heart Defects

Some inherited syndromes can include a CHD, including the following conditions, all of which have strong genetic components (Oster et al., 2016):

- Chromosomal syndromes: Down syndrome (trisomy 21), Edwards syndrome (trisomy 18), Patau syndrome (trisomy 13), and Turner syndrome
- Genetic associations: CHARGE syndrome and VATER/VACTERL association
- Chromosomal deletion/microdeletions: DiGeorge syndrome (22q11 deletion) and Williams syndrome

Positive family history of CHD, particularly in siblings, increases concern for CHD recurrence. Several maternal–fetal factors can increase risk (Oster et al., 2016):

- Prematurity: less than 37 weeks' gestation
- Multiple-gestation pregnancy
- Preeclampsia
- Advanced maternal age: 40 years or older
- Maternal infections such as rubella and influenza
- Infertility treatment
- Maternal activities: alcohol or substance abuse, first-trimester smoking
- Maternal use of medications: angiotensin-converting enzyme (ACE) inhibitors, thalidomide, retinoic acid, NSAIDs, phenytoin, and lithium
- Maternal conditions: phenylketonuria (PKU), diabetes, hypertension, obesity, and thyroid disorders

RESEARCH EVIDENCE

Challenges in Identification of Pediatric Hypertension

Hypertension in children can be over-diagnosed (temporary blood pressure increase due to stress or fear of going to the doctor) or under-diagnosed due to difficulty in remembering the complex variations in normal values for different age, sex, and height groups. A consensus guideline defines hypertension as blood pressure measurements on three visits that measure at or higher than the 95th percentile for age, height, and sex (Hansen, Gunn, & Kaelber, 2007).

Not all pediatric CV disease is present at birth, however. Due to increasing trends of pediatric obesity and associated hypertensive changes, evidence of damage to the heart and blood vessels is now being seen earlier in the life span. These vascular changes are usually seen in adults who do not follow heart-healthy lifestyles or diets, but are increasingly being observed in children with comorbid hypertension, elevated cholesterol and triglycerides, and type 2 diabetes.

QUALITY AND SAFETY

In addition to using written tables for normal and abnormal blood pressure ranges, pediatric nurses can access a wide range of healthcare applications for mobile devices. An example is the color-coded BP Centiles app developed by the SMART Platforms project through Boston Children's Hospital (https://apps.smarthealthit.org/app/4). This government-funded group creates modular information technology that is usable by different healthcare IT systems.

Assessments of the Cardiovascular System

Assessment of the CV system in children begins with a health history of pertinent family history, and then progresses to questions related to CV illnesses, surgeries, injuries, or accidents. An ideal circumstance of a quiet, alert child for physical assessment of this system is important to obtain the best baseline data. This is especially true for the initial assessment so as to better detect changes in condition.

UNIQUE FOR KIDS

Measuring Blood Pressure in Pediatric Patients

The following are nationally accepted National Institutes of Health (NIH) guidelines for measuring blood pressure (BP) in pediatric patients:

1. Routine BP measurements should be started at 3 years of age.
2. Select the correct cuff size based on the child's arm size. A good rule of thumb is that the correct cuff size is the largest cuff that fits on the upper arm with space below for the stethoscope head.
3. Measurement of BP should be performed on the right arm of a seated, relaxed child.
4. The "gold standard" BP technique is measurement by auscultation.
5. Practical advantages of using an automated BP device (which correlates "reasonably well" with auscultation technique) are quick results at a slight distance from the child and reduction of technique error by health care personnel.
6. In the event of an elevated BP as measured by an automated device, repeat the measurement by auscultation.

Modified from U.S. Department of Health and Human Services, National Institutes of Health, National Heart, Lung, and Blood Institute. (2007). A pocket guide to blood pressure measurement in children. Retrieved from http://www.nhlbi.nih.gov/health/resources/heart/hbp-child-pocket-guide-html.

The nurse begins with a visual assessment of the child's chest, noting whether there appear to be visible vibrations related to the heartbeat. General appearance of small or thin stature from poor weight gain, signs of chronic **hypoxemia** (low level of oxygen in the blood) such as clubbed fingers, and dysmorphic features are also noted. Physical assessment includes systematic auscultation of heart sounds for murmurs (noting extra sounds S_3 or S_4, location, pitch, timing, intensity, quality, duration, and radiation), lung sounds, height, weight, vital signs including blood pressure (BP) measurements in all four extremities (if BP readings demonstrate different pressures between upper and lower extremities, report immediately), and presence and quality of the child's peripheral pulses. The nurse should also assess for evidence of chronic hypoxemia such as cyanosis, poor weight gain, tachypnea, dyspnea, polycythemia, and clubbing. The nurse must assess hydration status, including mucous membranes moisture and turgor; skin temperature of extremities; mottling; capillary refill time; diaphoresis; urine output; and level of the liver border. An abnormally located liver border can indicate fluid overload due to congestive heart disease; in such cases, peripheral edema, presence of cyanosis or pallor, and signs of fatigue may be observed.

Diagnostics

The pediatric healthcare team has access to an array of diagnostics and tools for assessing children for cardiac abnormalities. These tools include chest X-ray to determine heart size and position, 12- or 15-lead electrocardiography (ECG) to detect arrhythmias, echocardiogram to delineate anatomy, and ventricular function test to detect abnormal flow. An echocardiogram is a noninvasive tool that can diagnose cardiac disease with nearly the same accuracy as the invasive, definitively diagnostic cardiac catheterization. Such catheterization is associated with significant risks of injury, bleeding, and infection as well as procedural and postoperative nursing care. This procedure includes cannulation of a large vein, usually in the femoral area, to directly view structures, obtain myocardial biopsies, assess conduction, and measure cardiac flow and pressures. It is also associated with some potential benefits—namely, some defects can be repaired or mitigated using the less invasive, interventional catheterization versus an open chest procedure.

BEST PRACTICES

The pediatric care team can best support the child with CV using a patient- and family-centered care approach. The care team consists of parents, doctors, nurses, social workers, Child Life specialists, counselors, dieticians, pharmacologists, case managers, and community partners.

Successful collaboration relies on the following key principles:

- Listening, respecting, and incorporating family culture and preferences into the plan of care
- Optimizing organizational flexibility to facilitate patient and family choice for healthcare approaches
- Ensuring unbiased, clear, and complete ongoing information at the level and language to optimize patient and family participation in decision making
- Ensuring formal and informal (peer-to-peer) support in each developmental stage as appropriate while maintaining confidentiality under the provisions of the Health Insurance Portability and Accountability Act (HIPAA)
- At a systems level, active involvement of patients and families in policy making, program development, family advisory councils and task forces, and quality improvement projects
- Identifying and enhancing strengths of the children themselves, empowering them to actively participate in their own healthcare decision making

Data from American Academy of Pediatrics. (2012). Patient- and family-centered care and the pediatrician's role. *Pediatrics, 129*(2), 394–404.

Other assessments include serum chemistry, blood calcium, hematocrit, hemoglobin, antistreptolysin-O (ASO) titer and throat culture if streptococcal infection is suspected, C-reactive protein, arterial blood gases, liver function panels, renal panels, serum lactate, erythrocyte sedimentation rate, blood urea nitrogen, creatinine, complete blood count (CBC), platelet and differential, and blood culture for specific pathogens. In patients with congestive heart failure (CHF), the brain natriuretic peptide (BNP) level can be elevated. Cardiac troponin may be elevated with cardiomyopathy, myocarditis, and sepsis, all of which ultimately result in decreased perfusion.

QUALITY AND SAFETY

Assessments That May Indicate Impending Heart Failure

The following findings require immediate intervention and communication to the healthcare provider:

- Increased respiratory rate and, although less common than in adults, presence of crackles
- Lethargy
- Decreased perfusion—prolonged capillary refill time and/or decreased or absent pulses
- Pallor, mottling, and cool extremities
- Oliguria
- Unanticipated weight gain
- Noncompliance with ordered medications

Assessment of a Newborn with Cyanosis: Acrocyanosis Versus Central Cyanosis

When assessing a newborn with cyanosis, respiratory status, activity, and location of the dusky blue color are important to note (**Figure 19-3**). If cyanosis is confined to extremities, leaving the face and trunk pink, it is likely the temporary benign finding of acrocyanosis as the baby transitions to extrauterine life. Cyanosis (central) resulting from pathological processes leaves the infant's entire skin surface—particularly nail beds, circumoral area, and mucous membranes—with a dusky color.

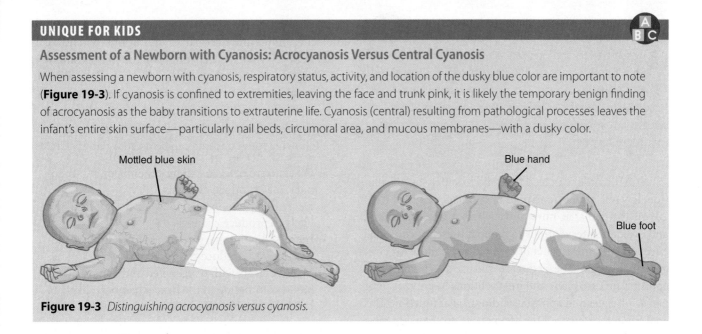

Figure 19-3 *Distinguishing acrocyanosis versus cyanosis.*

A valuable tool put in place across the United States by the Department of Health and Human Services is the Newborn Screening for Critical Congenital Heart Defects program. Twelve critical defects needing repair in the first year can be detected with this screening, even in an asymptomatic baby (Oster et al., 2016). The simple screening maneuver consists of placing a pulse oximetry probe on the right extremity (the only extremity with preductal blood flow) and a second pulse oximeter probe on either of the infant's feet—they both receive postductal blood flow—and comparing the two values. If the difference in the two simultaneous readings is greater than 3%, further diagnostic testing for a CCHD is needed.

Pain Effects on Perfusion

Children rarely experience the same type of chest pain as adults do from ischemia. More commonly, pain in the pediatric thorax is related to pulmonary processes such as pleural pain, musculoskeletal issues, dermatologic conditions, and inflammatory processes. Myocardial infarction, however, may be a complication of Kawasaki disease (a severe and acute condition of panvasculitis, which is treated with intravenous immunoglobulin [IVIG] and aspirin), which is a form of acquired heart disease. Given this risk, the pediatric nurse must assess all chest pain thoroughly and critically.

Pain increases the demands on the CV system if it is severe or undertreated. Most healthy children can tolerate the resulting tachycardia, tachypnea, and correlated blood pressure changes, but children with CV disease may decompensate further. To evaluate a child's pain, the nurse should conduct a thorough health history, specifically describing the chief complaint including timing, influencing factors, triggers, and severity. Developmentally appropriate pain tools should be used in this evaluation. Results from objective pain tools, subjective pain tools, and physiological measurements of vital signs should be combined to assess a child's complaint of pain. Prompt interventions with appropriate and adequate pharmacologic and nonpharmacologic strategies are critical.

Care Management of a Child with a CV System Disorder

Several CV conditions affecting perfusion have lengthy and complex management. Some disorders require several surgeries and long-term medical management if the child is to attain normal or near-normal cardiovascular function. Congenital defects affecting critical blood flow pathways demand immediate corrective surgery. The timing of the closure of the patent ductus arteriosus (PDA) fetal shunt can mean that an infant with an undetected CCHD is sent home and then suffers the risk of acute decompensation or dies when the PDA closes. Some CV disorders that significantly affect perfusion can cause complications in the cardiopulmonary system, such as congestive heart failure, as well as in all organs that are sensitive to reduced perfusion. A child with an acute or chronic CV condition that becomes incompatible with life may be a candidate for heart or heart/lung transplantation.

A CV disorder can lead the child to suffer social isolation, low self-esteem, and poor body image (Luyckx et al., 2014). The pediatric nurse must assess, plan, implement, and evaluate interventions to combat these psychosocial effects. The primary goal of care for any child with congenital or acquired heart disease is to use developmentally appropriate care plans and interventions to prevent poor perfusion states and optimize cardiovascular function. This goal applies throughout the life span, as survivorship rates are improving and more children with CHD/CCHD are surviving into late adolescence and adulthood.

The following approach to nursing care will optimize support for the child with a CV condition:

- Develop a holistic nursing plan of care that includes multidisciplinary participation.
- Offer empathetic care by being sensitive to the privacy needs of the parents and child, providing care breaks to the parents, and facilitating a calm and healing environment.
- Monitor vital signs, lab tests, and diagnostic procedures to detect developing or subclinical complications.
- Provide efficient care to reduce discomfort and fatigue; encourage robust nutrition; and provide frequent rest breaks, hygiene, and comfort to prevent crying, particularly when the child is cyanotic.
- Encourage safe recommended physical activity, which can improve physical status and quality of life.
- Monitor precise daily weights, as well as intake and output, to determine nutritional, fluid, and electrolyte status.
- Adhere to the medication regimen, while monitoring for intended effects and unwanted reactions.
- Monitor for effective or poor coping by the child and family. Use anticipatory guidance and coordinate care team resources, including social services and Child Life specialists.

Congenital Heart Defects

There are several approaches to categorizing CHDs. A very generalized organization is to group the defects into **acyanotic** (left-to-right cardiac blood flow) and **cyanotic** (right-to-left cardiac blood flow) types, but each child's defect is unique and the cardiac "shunt" or blood flow can change or reverse itself, depending on the child's condition, leading to symptoms that seem contrary to the acyanotic or cyanotic categories. This can complicate assessment and clinical decision making. To better understand the underlying processes that impact blood flow with different defects, the following four concepts can be used to classify CHDs:

- Obstructive defects: can be systemic or, if pulmonary, may produce cyanosis
- Decreased pulmonary flow: right-to-left flow and likely to produce cyanosis
- Increased pulmonary flow: left-to-right flow and less likely to produce cyanosis
- Mixed defects with oxygenated and deoxygenated blood comingling in the heart chambers: likely to result in cyanosis (Rudd & Kocisko, 2014)

Some patients with CHDs/CCHDs will be "ductal dependent" temporarily. In other words, they depend on the ductus arteriosus staying open longer than usual to allow necessary blood flow to the lungs if the defects prevent any other flow to the lungs once the ductus closes naturally. Oxygen and lack of maternal prostaglandins are two key factors that cause the closure of the ductus—which is the rationale for intentionally using medications (prostaglandin E_1 [PGE-1]) and accepting lower oxygen saturation ranges to keep this pathway open in children who would cease to perfuse and oxygenate, until immediate surgical intervention can be accomplished. **Table 19-2** and **Table 19-3** identify some CHDs that are representative of numerous malformation variations.

A simple bedside test that can help distinguish between cardiac or respiratory causes in children who are hypoxemic is a hyperoxygenation test. In this test, the infant is put on 100% oxygen for 20 minutes and a blood gas sample is drawn. Infants with cyanotic CHD will not have significantly increased Po_2.

Congestive Heart Failure

Congestive heart failure is typically a secondary pathology to a CHD or acquired CV dysfunction. It results from

TABLE 19-2   Selected Acyanotic Disorders

Ventricular Septal Defect (VSD)

Diagnosis: Opening in the ventricular septal wall, which allows mixing of blood from the oxygenated left ventricle to the deoxygenated right ventricle. This results in increased pulmonary flow and decreased pulmonary compliance, causing stiffer lungs and less effective ventilation (**Figure 19-4**).

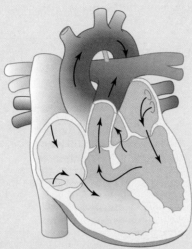

Figure 19-4 *Ventricular septal defect.*

Assessment: Most common CHD; left-to-right shunt. The child may be asymptomatic or present with a murmur. A late harsh murmur may sometimes be heard after pulmonary pressures decrease at 4 to 8 weeks of age. Shortness of breath, failure to thrive (FTT), feeding difficulties, and a lower left sternal border systolic thrill can be present.

Treatment: Echocardiogram will show an enlarged left atrium. Chest X-ray may show an enlarged heart and increased lung vascularity. Large defects must be surgically closed. Small defects may be repaired via cardiac catheterization with a patch. Postoperative care and observation should continue for cyanosis, respiratory distress, and bleeding at the catheter insertion site. The child may need several months of treatment with blood thinners and dental antibiotic prophylaxis, with corresponding nursing care and education. Annual check-ups with the child's cardiologist are encouraged.

Atrial Septal Defect (ASD)

Diagnosis: An opening in the septum between the left and right atria. It can be due to persistence of a fetal shunt, involving the foramen ovale. Flow is left to right; flow may be increased to the lungs.

Assessment: May have a harsh, loud murmur or be asymptomatic. The size of the right atrium may potentially be increased, and the child may have mild CHF.

Treatment: Large defects must be surgically closed. Small defects may be repaired via cardiac catheterization with a patch. The child may need several months of treatment with blood thinners and dental antibiotic prophylaxis, with corresponding nursing care and education. Annual check-ups with the cardiologist are encouraged.

Aortic Stenosis (AS)

Diagnosis: Stenosis (narrowing) of the aortic valve and adjacent vessel wall that obstructs flow from the left ventricle to the aorta. May have aortic valve regurgitation. The increased workload on the left ventricle leads to hypertrophy (enlargement) of the left ventricular wall. The child will be ductal dependent if the AS is severe.

Assessment: Risk factors include group A *Streptococcus* infections. Findings include a lower systolic BP and narrow pulse pressure (difference between the systolic and diastolic values), fatigue, activity intolerance (can lead to sudden death), syncope, shortness of breath, systolic murmur, and chest pain.

(continues)

TABLE 19-2   Selected Acyanotic Disorders (*continued*)

Treatment: Diagnostics such as echocardiogram, chest X-ray, cardiac catheterization with balloon valvuloplasty (widening the opening by pulling a small balloon through it) if possible, or open-heart aortic valve replacement. PGE-1 infusion may potentially be implemented prior to surgery. The nurse should prepare for treating arrhythmias, CHF, and pain, and should provide preoperative and postoperative teaching. Provide discharge instructions and teaching including dental/preprocedural antibiotic prophylaxis, as valve replacement increases the risk of bacterial endocarditis.

Coarctation of the Aorta (CoA)

Diagnosis: Constriction of the aorta that spares upper-body perfusion but decreases flow to the lower extremities, distal to the left subclavian artery. Usually distal to the carotid arteries, sparing blood flow to the head. Ventricular septal defect (VSD) is common.

Assessment: Associated with Noonan syndrome. Systolic murmur. BP is higher in the right (preductal) arm than in the lower extremities (postductal). Weaker femoral and lower-extremity pulses. Cardiomegaly and right-sided heart failure due to constriction of aortic outflow. Headache, shortness of breath, and poor feeding, growth, and development. Can present as hypertension in teens.

Treatment: Cardiac catheterization with balloon dilation of the stenotic area and stent placement. Monitor for restenosis. Periodic follow-up with the cardiologist.

Patent Ductus Arteriosus (PDA)

Diagnosis: Persistent fetal circulation pathway between the aorta and the pulmonary arteries, resulting in left-to-right flow and risk of CHF (**Figure 19-5**). In utero, this condition allows blood oxygenated by the placenta to flow away from the lungs and into the systemic circulation. Most ducts close within 48 hours in term infants; the risk of delayed closing increases with increasing prematurity.

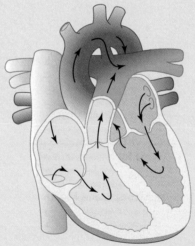

Figure 19-5 *Patent ductus arteriosus.*

Assessment: Murmur is best heard at the upper left sternal border. Pulmonary congestion and enlarged heart on chest X-ray. Active precordium, bounding peripheral pulses, and increased capillary refill time. Tachypnea, apnea or labored respirations, and poor feeding. Diaphoresis with feeding. Weight increase from retained fluid. Wide pulse pressures with low diastolic BP. Labile oxygen saturations.

Treatment: Pharmacologic closure of symptomatic babies with PDA can be attempted by using courses of indomethacin or ibuprofen. Adverse side effects include bleeding, pulmonary hemorrhage, and compromised perfusion to the gut and kidneys, so infants are monitored closely and may be placed on NPO (nothing by mouth) status for therapy. If drug therapy does not result in duct closure, then surgical ligation is performed.

TABLE 19-3   Selected Cyanotic Disorders: Right-to-Left Flow

Tetralogy of Fallot (TOF)

Diagnosis: Four malformations that result in mixed blood and restricted blood flow to the lungs, usually resulting in a right-to-left shunt: pulmonary stenosis (PS), overriding aorta, right ventricular hypertrophy, and ventricular septal defect (VSD).

Assessment: Third most common heart defect. Associated with DiGeorge syndrome and Down syndrome. Occurs more often in males. Right-to-left shunt. Murmur, dyspnea when active, and polycythemia. As the PDA closes, cyanosis increases. Clubbed digits can be found. A "boot-shaped" cardiac silhouette may be observed on X-ray (**Figure 19-6**).

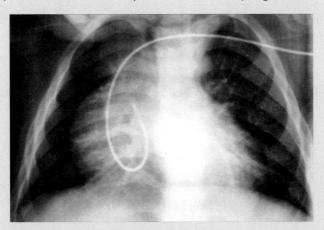

Figure 19-6 *X-ray of "boot-shaped" heart in tetralogy of Fallot.*
© Diomedia / ISM / SOVEREIGN

Treatment: The most common method of treating TOF is complete intracardiac repair in infancy. With infants who are too small or weak to tolerate the surgery, the healthcare team may opt for a previously common strategy—performing a procedure to temporarily improve blood flow to the lungs so that complete repair of the defect can be performed when the child is older and stronger (National Heart, Lung, and Blood Institute, 2011). Priorities are to manage CHF symptoms, minimize hypoxia, and provide enough nutrition to support growth and development. The nurse and family should prevent crying, dehydration, constipation, fever, and pain, which can provoke hypercyanosis "tet" spells (acute profound decreases in pulmonary flow) and lead to hypoxic brain injury. Immediate interventions include putting the child in a knee-to-chest position to increase systemic vascular resistance and pulmonary flow. This position should be coupled with oxygen administration, anticipation and prevention of provoking conditions, and calming of the child. In severe cases, the pediatric nurse may need to give morphine to decrease pain and dilate the child's pulmonary vasculature, thereby stopping the tet spell.

Dextro-Transposition of the Great Arteries (d-TGA)

Diagnosis: Defect in which the two great vessels—the pulmonary artery and aorta—are reversed. Oxygenated blood cycles to and from the lungs without going to the systemic circulation. Deoxygenated blood does not circulate to the lungs. This severe disorder is ductal dependent. An "egg on a string" cardiac silhouette can be observed on X-ray.

Assessment: Profound cyanosis, tachypnea, and negative hyperoxygenation test.

Treatment: Prompt intravenous access and administration of PGE-1 to stabilize the child prior to an immediate surgical intervention, which consists of an initial balloon atrial septostomy and a later arterial switch procedure (Jatene switch). Nursing care includes maintaining oxygen saturation, giving PGE-1 and ACE inhibitors to promote coronary perfusion, and providing postoperative care.

Tricuspid Atresia (TA)

Diagnosis: Rare. *Atresia* means completely blocked or missing. The malformed tricuspid valve blocks blood flow from the right atrium to the right ventricle, radically decreasing blood flow to the lungs. If no VSD is present, then the TA is ductal dependent and the PDA must be maintained for survival.

(continues)

TABLE 19-3   Selected Cyanotic Disorders: Right-to-Left Flow (*continued*)

Assessment: Cyanosis, murmur, dyspnea, clubbing, and poor growth. Echocardiogram, ECG, chest X-ray, and cardiac catheterization are all indicated. This condition requires three-stage surgical repair and possibly heart transplant.

Treatment: Maintain PGE-1 infusion. Prepare the child and parents for surgery. Anticipatory guidance and counseling are required for the adjustment to a lifelong cardiac care plan and for the possibility of heart transplant. Monitor for CHF, tachycardia, and chronic diarrhea.

Hypoplastic Left Heart Syndrome (HLHS)

Diagnosis: Second most common CHD; ductal dependent. Severe underdevelopment of the left side of the heart, aortic valve, aorta, left ventricle, and mitral valve results in pulmonary congestion and edema.

Assessment: The child will be asymptomatic until the ductus arteriosus closes, at which point the child becomes tachypneic, dyspneic, and cyanotic and demonstrates ashen skin color coupled with poor perfusion and a murmur with gallop. Immediate three-stage surgical repair must be initiated, and the family must anticipate the need for heart transplant.

Treatment: Parents are given the option of supportive care only, which usually leads quickly to death; staged reconstructive surgery; or heart transplant. The risks and benefits of the two therapeutic options are approximately equivalent, as the difficulty and risk of the staged surgery is balanced by the difficulty of obtaining a suitable heart for transplantation (Si, Ohye, Bove, & Hirsch-Romano, 2014). Echocardiogram, chest X-ray, preparation for surgery, and provision of postoperative care are included in the child's treatment plan. The initial surgery in the staged reconstruction is undertaken as soon as possible (ideally less than 1 month) after birth, and subsequent surgeries complete the reconstruction. Lifelong medications and follow-up with cardiology team will be required. The nurse should prepare the caregivers for their child having a severe condition and provide support. The child will have an increased risk for bacterial endocarditis, so an infection prevention protocol will be needed.

a chronic or acute decrease in the ability of the heart to pump adequate amounts of blood to the body, which causes congestion or backup of fluid into the systemic vascular and/or pulmonary vasculature, negatively impacting perfusion. CHF is directly related to a malfunctioning ventricular muscle.

In addition to assessing for the four main signs of CHF (tachycardia, tachypnea, enlarged heart, and enlarged liver), the pediatric nurse should note the following symptoms of a child experiencing CHF: (1) generalized pallor; (2) diaphoresis; (3) murmurs including S_3 and S_4; (4) cool extremities with weak pulses and slow capillary refill; (5) poor appetite and growth failure; (6) fatigue and activity intolerance; and (7) oliguria.

Signs of systemic (peripheral) venous congestion include peripheral edema, jugular vein distention (not seen in infants), liver and spleen enlargement, and ascites. Pulmonary congestion linked to heart failure can be manifested as tachypnea, dyspnea, grunting, stridor, retractions, exercise intolerance, and recurring respiratory infections.

The main goals of treatment to improve the cardiac output for patients with CHF are the following: (1) reduce cardiac workload; (2) maximize contractility; (3) improve perfusion and oxygenation; (4) minimize fluid overload; and (5) provide optimal nutritional support.

Digoxin Therapy

One of the medication mainstays of treatment of CHF is digitalis glycoside (digoxin) therapy, which can improve the contractility of the heart without increasing heart rate, improve cardiac output, and improve perfusion and oxygenation. Digoxin is available as an oral elixir with a 0.05 mg/mL concentration. Infant doses are calculated in micrograms (1000 mcg = 1 mg). An initial digitizing dose is given; then, depending on its effects, a maintenance dose is determined. Two nurses must double-check the dosing and the amount drawn up. Digoxin has a very narrow therapeutic window with a high potential for overdose and toxicity. Signs of digoxin toxicity include nausea, vomiting, anorexia, abdominal pain, visual disturbances, bradycardia, and arrhythmias.

RESEARCH EVIDENCE

Assessment of Capillary Refill Time

Current research has resulted in a recommendation for a standardized method to assess capillary refill time (CRT) in patients. Moderate pressure on the fingertip for 5 seconds with an ambient temperature between 20 and 25°C (68°F–77°F) results in the most reliable measurement (Fleming et al., 2015).

Medications Used for Diuresis for CHF

Diuretics used to treat CHF disease are given in the morning to allow maximum rest at night.

- *Furosemide (Lasix):* Loop diuretic. Monitor electrolyte levels, especially potassium. Watch for ototoxicity and development of renal calculi with long-term use. Encourage consumption of foods with high potassium content, and watch for signs of dehydration and allergic response.
- *Bumetanide (Bumex):* Loop diuretic. Monitor electrolyte levels, especially potassium. May worsen ototoxicity with aminoglycoside use. Encourage consumption of high-potassium foods; avoid sun exposure. Watch for signs of dehydration or nausea/vomiting.
- *Spironolactone (Aldactone):* Potassium sparing. Give missed doses when discovered, but do not double-dose. Maintain strict intake and output (I & O) records. Monitor potassium levels.
- *Hydrochlorothiazide (Diuril):* Potassium sparing. Give missed doses when discovered, but do not double-dose. Take with food. Avoid sun exposure. NSAIDs decrease effectiveness. Call the physician if dehydration, nausea, or diarrhea occurs.

The following guidelines should be followed when administering digoxin:

- Take the child's apical pulse for a full minute prior to giving the dose. If available in the healthcare setting, an ECG strip can be saved for confirmation of an accurate heart rate and documentation.
- Do not give digoxin if the heart rate is less than 90 beats/min for infants or less than 70 beats/min for older children. The adult threshold is less than 60 beats/min. Written drug orders should specify the heart rate required for dosing.
- Oral dosing is twice daily, usually at 8 a.m. and 8 p.m.
- Do not mix digoxin with food; give water after the dose to prevent tooth decay due to the sweetened elixir.
- If a dose is missed, do not make it up. Instead, give the next dose on schedule.
- Do not redose the medication if the child vomits.
- If more than two consecutive doses are missed, contact the physician or practitioner.
- Closely monitor the child for signs of toxicity.
- Provide effective caregiver teaching for safe home administration of digoxin.
- Store digoxin in a safe location, preferably one that is locked.

- Have Poison Control Center contact information readily available, and notify the healthcare team immediately in the event of an unintentional overdose.

Acquired Cardiac Disorders

Although much more common in adults, acquired heart disease can occur in children throughout the age spectrum and developmental period. Common acquired cardiac disorders in children are explored in this section.

Rheumatic Heart Disease

Diagnosis

Rheumatic fever is an inflammatory disease affecting the connective tissues that occurs after the child experiences a group A beta-hemolytic *Streptococcus* (GABHS) infection such as strep throat or scarlet fever. These infections can cause heart valve damage, which then contributes to the development of rheumatic heart disease (RHD). Antibodies produced cause lesions to develop in joints and heart connective tissues. Untreated RHD can cause clusters of bacterial or fungal organisms that can embolize to the brain, kidneys, and lungs.

Risk Factors

Children at risk have untreated streptococcal infections, with symptoms appearing approximately two weeks after the infection's onset. Rheumatic fever primarily affects children between ages 5 and 15 years. RHD has familial tendencies.

Treatment

If rheumatic fever or rheumatic heart disease is suspected, then a throat culture may be taken to confirm the presence of a streptococcal infection. ECG and echocardiogram may be performed, looking for cardiomegaly and carditis. Assessments for symptoms of rheumatic heart disease include (1) fever; (2) a very painful, swollen, red joint (usually a knee, elbow, shoulder, or ankle, in which the swelling and inflammation recede and move to another joint); (3) nosebleeds; (4) brief periods of skin rashes (less common); (5) shortness of breath; (6) chest pain, abnormal heart rhythm, or murmur; and (7) abdominal pain.

Nursing care includes care and monitoring of CHF, administration of antibiotics, and anti-inflammatory medications. Patient and family teaching focus on screening school-age children for sore throat. Provide education about antibiotic dental prophylaxis. If heart valve damage is significant, valve replacement will be necessary.

Kawasaki Disease

Diagnosis

Kawasaki disease (KD) is the leading cause of acquired heart disease in children. This inflammatory process affects the skin, blood vessels (when blood vessels are affected throughout the body, the condition is called panvasculitis), mucous membranes, and the lymph system. Although its cause is unknown, KD has been documented to follow viral infections and toxic exposures. The condition is not contagious, but it can mimic other infectious diseases such as scarlet fever or measles.

Symptoms of KD include high fever, conjunctivitis, enlarged lymph nodes, red lips, and a "strawberry" tongue (**Figure 19-7**). The child may demonstrate edematous and erythematous hands and feet, extreme irritability, groin rash, and signs of cardiac involvement on echocardiogram and X-ray. Initially, the child will show increased white blood cells (WBCs), lymphocytes, and platelet counts.

Although complete cure is possible, KD causes scarring of the coronary arteries and can lead to coronary aneurysm to the point that 73% of patients have a myocardial infarction within the first year after diagnosis (Brogan et al., 2002). Close monitoring for progression of the vascular inflammatory process is needed.

Risk Factors

Risk factors include Asian descent and age younger than 6 years. Nevertheless, KD can strike persons of all races and any age group.

Treatment

Immediate administration of intravenous immunoglobulin (IVIG) is required, with significant improvement usually noted within 24 hours. High-dose aspirin therapy is used for 6 to 8 weeks, which can be lifesaving despite the risk of Reye syndrome associated with this medication. Monitoring is needed for CHF, myocarditis, leaky heart valves, and pericardial effusions.

Sub-bacterial Endocarditis

Diagnosis

When the cardiac endocardium becomes inflamed by infection with a streptococcal or staphylococcal organism, the resulting sub-bacterial endocarditis (SBE) can be life threatening.

Risk Factors

Risk factors associated with SBE include a past history of heart valve damage, and replacement of or damage to the endocardium. Organisms entering the body via dental work, tooth brushing, cuts, catheters, or respiratory infections may cause the initial infection. Symptoms include fever, chills, shortness of breath, cough, murmur, joint pain, petechiae, flank pain, weight loss, and fatigue. Skin and nail signs may be present. Retinal Roth spots are seen early.

Treatment

Blood cultures, CBC, and echocardiogram are all required for confirmation of SBE. Intensive antibiotic therapy is necessary. The nurse will monitor for stroke, poor cardiac output and CHF, and antibiotic-induced nausea, vomiting, and diarrhea. The nurse should prepare the child and family for valve replacement surgery.

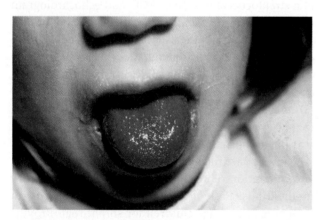

Figure 19-7 *Symptoms of Kawasaki disease include "strawberry" tongue.*

© Dr. Ken Greer/Visual Unlimited, Inc.

Pediatric Care Team: Focus on Child Life Specialists

Play is the essential work of the child. Play can be therapeutic and very soothing for children with healthcare issues. Without an opportunity to play, children cannot achieve their optimal developmental goals. Thus, play must be preserved and play opportunities planned for hospitalized children.

Child Life specialists (CLS) are bachelor's- or master's-prepared professionals with expertise in helping children and families deal with life's challenging events. They provide emotional support for families, deliver education, and encourage optimal development of children facing challenges, particularly those related to health care and hospitalization.

CLS promote effective coping through play, preparation, education, and self-expression activities. Some hospitals have designated play rooms, which are protected areas where no medical care can interrupt play, and programs designed and managed by CLS.

Case Study

Chang Hung, a 14-month-old child with trisomy 21 and a ventricular septal defect, was admitted to the pediatric unit with tachypnea, tachycardia, poor appetite, and decreased activity. His concerned parents were at his bedside continuously. Initial vital signs were temperature of 98.2°F, heart rate of 144 beats/min, respiration rate of 56 breaths/min, BP of 92/68 mm Hg, and oxygen saturation of 93% on room air. The toddler had mild edema to distal extremities; was pale, mottled, and thin; and appeared fatigued. He had subcostal retractions, clear lung fields, soft systolic heart murmur, hypoactive bowel sounds, and a palpable liver border 2 cm below the costal margin. He was tachypneic and diaphoretic when eating or drinking. Urine output was 1 mL/kg/hr, and he had slightly cool extremities with weak peripheral pulses. Capillary refill time was delayed, at 4 to 5 seconds. His chest X-ray revealed cardiomegaly and mild pulmonary edema.

This patient was ultimately diagnosed with congestive heart failure (CHF). Orders were to start digoxin, diuretics, and ACE inhibitors. A 23-guage peripheral intravenous saline lock was started. Oxygen was immediately delivered at 2 L/min via nasal cannula, and efforts were made to keep the child comforted. His parents were encouraged to participate in his care.

Case Study Questions

1. What will the pediatric healthcare team, including the nurse, evaluate to determine whether the plan of care and medications are having the desired effect?

2. Are there any nursing concerns or special administration guidelines for digoxin?

3. Which concerns for nutritional support will the healthcare team have for this child? Which interventions are warranted?

As the Case Evolves. . .

Chang Hung is experiencing a number of cardiovascular conditions at the time of his admission. A new nurse arrives on the unit and reviews the child's chart.

4. Which of the following conditions will the nurse identify as a direct outcome of an error of fetal development?
    A. Congestive heart disease
    B. Tachycardia
    C. Ventricular septal defect
    D. Cardiomegaly

5. Chang Hung has now been stabilized and is to be discharged to home care. The nurse knows that more teaching is necessary when the mother, who has received discharge teaching in caring for her infant, makes which of the following statements?
    A. The heartbeat must be more than 90 beats per minute so our son can have his digoxin.
    B. It is okay for our son to get his digoxin a few hours early even if he is nauseated, has diarrhea, or is dizzy.
    C. We should give our son exactly the amount that the doctor ordered.
    D. The doctor will order blood tests to check how much digoxin is in our son's blood.

Chapter Summary

- Congenital heart disease has roots early in the fetal development of the heart. Complex malformations can occur that often require invasive interventions and lifelong management.
- Congenital heart defects can be loosely grouped into acyanotic (left-to-right shunt) and cyanotic (right-to-left shunt) lesions.
- Acquired heart disease occurs after birth; examples include rheumatic heart disease, Kawasaki disease, and sub-bacterial endocarditis. Untreated streptococcal infections are associated with many of these disorders.
- Congestive heart failure can result from congenital heart disease or an acquired heart disease as a major complication. Four core symptoms of CHF are tachypnea, tachycardia, hepatomegaly, and cardiomegaly.
- To promote safety and positively impact quality of life, a holistic multidisciplinary approach to management of pediatric patients with CV disease is optimal. Robust teaching regarding signs and symptoms, medication administration, long-term prognosis, and care after discharge will have a positive effect.
- Increased survivorship of children with CHD into the teen and adult years necessitates adaptation of medical management and nursing plans of care that meet the developmental needs of the children as they grow and mature.

Bibliography

American Academy of Pediatrics. (2012). Patient- and family-centered care and the pediatrician's role. Committee on Hospital and Institute for Patient- and Family-Centered Care. *Pediatrics, 129*(2), 394–404.

Antonucci, R., Zaffanello, M., Puxeddu, E., Porcella, A., Cuzzolin, L., Pilloni, M. D., & Fanos, V. (2012). Use of non-steroidal anti-inflammatory drugs in pregnancy: Impact on the fetus and newborn. *Current Drug Metabolism, 13*(4), 474–490.

Behrman, R. E., Kliegman, R. M., & Jenson, H. B. (Eds.). (2011). *Nelson textbook of pediatrics* (19th ed.). Philadelphia, PA: W. B. Saunders.

Blackburn, S. T. (2003) *Maternal, fetal and neonatal physiology: A clinical perspective* (2nd ed.). St. Louis, MO: Saunders/Elsevier.

Boyle, L., Kelly, M., Reynolds, K., Conlan, M., & Taylor, F. (2015). The school-age child with congenital heart disease. *American Journal of Maternal Child Nursing, 40*(1), 16–23.

Brogan, P. A., Bose, A., Burgner, D., Hingradia, D., Tulloh, R., & Michie, C. (2002). Kawasaki disease: An evidence based approach to diagnosis, treatment and proposals for future research. *Archives for Disease in Childhood, 86*, 286–290.

Centers for Disease Control and Prevention (CDC). (2015) Congenital Heart Defects (CHDs): Data & statistics. Retrieved from http://www.cdc.gov/ncbddd/heartdefects/data.html

Centers for Disease Control and Prevention (CDC). (2016). Congenital heart defects (CHDs): Data & statistics. Retrieved from https://www.cdc.gov/ncbddd/heartdefects/data.html

Donoghue, A., Berg, R. A., Hazinski, M. F., Praestgaard, A. H., Roberts, K., & Nadkarni, V. M. (2009). Cardiopulmonary resuscitation for bradycardia with poor perfusion versus pulseless cardiac arrest. *Pediatrics, 124*(6), 1541-1542.

Fleming, S., Gill, P., Jones, C., Taylor, J. A., Van den Bruel, A., Heneghn, C., & Thompson, M. (2015). Validity and reliability of measurement of capillary refill time in children: A systematic review. *Archives of Disease in Childhood, 100*, 239-249.

Fulton, D. R., & Saleeb, S. (2016). Management of isolated ventricular septal defects in infants and children. *UpToDate*. Retrieved from https://www.uptodate.com/contents/management-of-isolated-ventricular-septal-defects-in-infants-and-children

Go, A. S., Mozaffarian, D., Roger, V. L., Benjamin, E. J., Berry, J. D., Borden, W. B., . . . Turner, M. B. On behalf of the American Heart Association Statistics Committee and Stroke Statistics Subcommittee. (2013). Heart disease and stroke statistics—2013 update: A report from the American Heart Association. *Circulation, 127*, e6-e45.

Halterman, J. S., Kaczorowski, C., Aligne, A., Auinger, P., & Szilagyi, P. G. (2001). Iron deficiency and cognitive achievement among school-aged children and adolescents in the United States. *Pediatrics, 107*, 1381-1386.

Hansen, M. L., Gunn, P. W., & Kaelber, D. C. (2007). Under diagnosis of hypertension in children and adolescents. *Journal of the American Medical Association, 298*, 8.

Luyckx, K., Goossens, E., Rassart, J., Apers, S., Vanhalst, J., & Moons, P. (2014). Parental support, internalizing symptoms, perceived health status, and quality of life in adolescents with congenital heart disease: Influences and reciprocal effects. *Journal of Behavioral Medicine, 37*, 145.

Mahle, W. T., Newburger, J. W., Matherne, G. P., Smith, F. C., Hoke, T. R., Koppel, R., . . . Grosse, S. D. On behalf of the American Heart Association Congenital Heart Defects Committee of the Council on Cardiovascular Disease in the Young, Council on Cardiovascular Nursing and Interdisciplinary Council on Quality of Care and Outcomes Research; and the American Academy of Pediatrics Section on Cardiology and Cardiac Surgery, and Committee on Fetus and Newborn. (2009). Role of pulse oximetry in examining newborns for congenital heart disease: A scientific statement from the American Heart Association and American Academy of Pediatrics. *Circulation, 120*, 447–458.

National Center on Birth Defects and Developmental Disabilities. Center for Disease Control and Prevention. (2016). Facts about birth defects. Retrieved from https://www.cdc.gov/ncbddd/birthdefects/facts.html

National Heart, Lung, and Blood Institute. (2011). How is tetralogy of Fallot treated? Available at: https://www.nhlbi.nih.gov/health/health-topics/topics/tof/treatment

Oster, M. E., Aucott, S. W., Glidewell, J., Hackell, J., Kochilas, L., Martin, G. R., . . . Kemper, A. R. (2016). Lessons learned from newborn screening for critical congenital heart defects. *Pediatrics, 137*(5), e20154573. doi: 10.1542/peds.2015-4573

Papp, L. A. (2007, July 16). Heart sounds: Lub dub and so much more: Making sense of the rhythmic beating of the adult heart. *Advance for Nurses: Northern California and Northern Nevada.*

Rudd, K., & Kocisko, D. (2014). *Pediatric nursing: The critical components of nursing care.* Philadelphia, PA: F. A. Davis.

Rudolph, C. D., Rudolph, A. M., Lister, G. E., First, L. R., & Gershon, A. A. (Eds.). (2011). *Rudolph's pediatrics* (22nd ed.). New York, NY: McGraw-Hill.

Sadler, T. W. (2004). *Langman's medical embryology* (9th ed.). Philadelphia, PA: Lippincott Williams & Wilkins.

Satau, G. M. (2015). Pediatric congestive heart failure workup. Retrieved from http://emedicine.medscape.com/article/2069746-workup

Si, M.-S., Ohye, R. G., Bove, E. L., & Hirsch-Romano, J. C. (2014). Surgical treatment of pediatric hypoplastic left heart syndrome. *Medscape.* Retrieved from http://emedicine.medscape.com/article/904137-treatment#d10

U.S. Department of Health and Human Services, National Institutes of Health, National Heart, Lung, and Blood Institute. (2007). A pocket guide to blood pressure measurement in children. Retrieved from http://www.nhlbi.nih.gov/health/resources/heart/hbp-child-pocket-guide-html

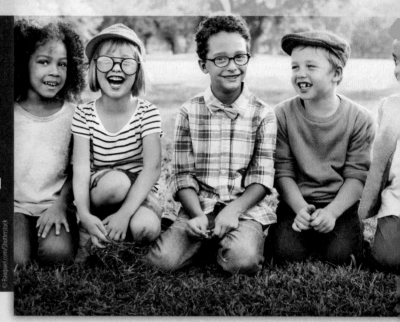

CHAPTER 20

Sensory Perceptions: Impairments and Disorders

Guest Author: Madelene Yee-Kopperdahl, RNC-NIC, BSN, RN

LEARNING OBJECTIVES

1. Assess the level of sensory maturation during fetal and neonatal development.
2. Apply knowledge of decibel levels of common sounds in the environment in offering advice to patient caregivers on an acceptable decibel level that will not cause hearing loss.
3. Differentiate between conductive and sensorineural hearing loss.
4. Apply pharmacologic knowledge of medications that are ototoxic to children.
5. Analyze visual stimulation that is age appropriate for each developmental group: infant, toddler, preschooler, school age, and adolescent.
6. Assess for pathophysiology of retinopathy of prematurity (ROP), and identify precautions that the bedside nurse should implement to prevent ROP.
7. Evaluate strategies of play therapy for patients with vision impairment and hearing loss.
8. Apply nursing concepts regarding the pathology and care practices for a child with sensory integration disorder.
9. Assess patients with autism spectrum disorders according to their diagnosis, and implement appropriate medical management, nursing care, and family education.

KEY TERMS

Autism spectrum disorders
Decibel
Early intervention
Hearing loss
Otitis media
Retinoblastoma
Retinopathy of prematurity
Sensory integration
Sensory perception
Sensory processing

Introduction

Sensory perception is a concept that describes the use and experience of the sensory organs across the developmental period. This concept includes normal development of the sensory organs as well as the deviations that can occur. Deviations in sensory perception can be primary (existing from birth) or secondary, where the child suffers a disease, injury, or traumatic event. The pediatric nurse works with the healthcare team to ensure that patients enjoy a healthy state of being that promotes sensory development. Focusing on safety allows the child to have an expected sequential development of sensory organ maturation. Anticipatory guidance for parents includes promoting a complete immunization schedule, as childhood infectious diseases can cause injury to the sensory organs. When children experience trauma, disease, or injury that affects the sensory organs, the nurse works with the family and interdisciplinary team to prevent the development of sensory deprivation.

The concept of sensory perception includes various sensory organs and sensory experiences. The seven sensory experiences include the olfactory (smell), gustatory (taste), visual, auditory, proprioceptive (sense of body awareness), vestibular (sense of movement and balance), and tactile senses. A child's cognition, neurologic health, level of consciousness, orientation, health, and well-being all highly influence sensory perception (**Figure 20-1**). Children with neurologic conditions that affect level of consciousness or the ability to process sensory input may have a severe reduction in their sensory perception.

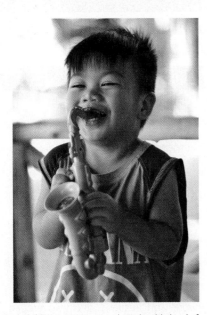

Figure 20-1 *A child's cognition, neurologic health, level of consciousness, orientation, health, and well-being all highly influence sensory perception.*
© Wasu Watcharadachaphong/Shutterstock.

Brain injuries from anoxia, cerebral palsy, hypoxic ischemic encephalopathy, brain tumors, and Guillain-Barré syndrome are examples of such neurologic conditions.

Sensory Development

Maturation of the sensory system occurs in a specific sequence during fetal development. This process begins with development of tactile sense, vestibular sense, proprioception, and gustatory taste buds (differentiating sweet, salty, bitter, and sour). The most abundant number of taste buds (7000) are developed by birth. Development of the olfactory sense follows, then hearing, and finally vision (Kenner & McGrath, 2010). Most of these senses are functional between 24 and 32 weeks' gestation, except for vision. By the time the infant reaches six months of age, depth perception, color, acuity, and eye movements (tracking) have developed, but it takes up to a year for vision to fully develop (Kenner & McGrath, 2010).

Maternal health, environment, maternal recreational and prescribed medication use, and prematurity are just a few of the conditions that can alter the fetus's brain development during the critical time of sensory maturation. If a fetus is subjected to any of these conditions, the connections (synapses) that build the framework for brain development may be changed or altered. For example, if a baby is born prematurely, typical sources of stimulation (e.g., noise, lights, pain from heel sticks) can alter normal brain development. Although prematurity will not alter the sequence in which the senses mature, it will alter the foundation of the sensory system as a whole compared to that of the term-gestation baby.

Immediate skin-to-skin contact, also known as kangaroo care, has been adopted as a standard in many delivery rooms, including for women who have undergone cesarean sections. This tactile contact provides the sensations that the term newborn needs. The feel of the mother's warmth, her smell, her voice, and even the taste of her skin typically draw the baby into a natural position for breastfeeding (Bergman & Bergman, 2010). Studies have shown that skin-to-skin contact after delivery can stabilize neonatal breathing, temperature, and blood sugar; reduce crying; and produce a much calmer newborn. This exposure to the external environment is the first step in which the newborn begins to establish a sense of trust with the immediate surroundings.

Nurses need to include the co-parent in the skin-to-skin contact. The inclusion of the co-parent not only builds a bond, but also creates a safe environment for the neonate. Safety is one of the foundational principles of the first stage of development according to Erik Erikson's stages of psychosocial development.

Hearing Disorders

The sensation of hearing is a complex process. Sound waves traveling through the external and internal structures of the ear stimulate the auditory nerve, which then sends signals to the brain. The brain interprets these electrical signals as sounds. This form of communication allows us to understand our environment, with the stimulation influencing our behaviors and actions.

Hearing begins when sound travels through the canal from the outer ear, hitting the eardrum (tympanic membrane). As the eardrum vibrates from these sound waves, the bones of the middle ear—malleus, incus, and stapes—connect with the cochlear of the inner ear, which is filled with fluid, and transmit the sound forward. A membrane in the cochlea is separated into two parts: an upper segment and a lower segment. Sensory hair cells situated on top of this membrane move in tandem with the vibrations of the sounds coming into the cochlea. This vibration allows chemoreceptors to rush in, creating a signal that the auditory nerve carries to the brain and interprets as a specific sound with meaning (National Institutes of Health [NIH], National Institute on Deaf and Other Communication Disorders [NIDCD], 2014).

Hearing loss is categorized as conductive, sensorineural, or mixed. Conductive hearing loss involves problems with the ear canal, eardrum, or middle ear structures. Common causes of conductive hearing loss are malformation of the outer ear structures, repeated ear infections, foreign body, and perforation of the eardrum.

Sensorineural hearing loss (SNHL) involves damage to the auditory nerve or the inner ear structures. Causes of SNHL include exposure to loud noise, head trauma, family history, illness, or ototoxic drugs. Ototoxic medications include antibiotics such as aminoglycosides, antifungals, nonsteroidal anti-inflammatory drugs (NSAIDs), chemotherapy, loop diuretics, and salicylate medications (Bisht & Bist, 2011). In some cases (e.g., with NSAIDs or aspirin), the toxicity depends on the dose and is reversible; in others, the damage may be permanent (e.g., with neomycin, a highly ototoxic antibiotic) (Taneja, Varshney, Taneja, & Varshney, 2015). It is the bedside nurse's role to administer these ototoxic drugs according to the recommendations. The nurse must be aware of potential side effects and drug compatibility.

Mixed hearing loss is a combination of conductive hearing loss and SNHL, which may involve all ear structures: outer, middle, inner ear and the auditory nerve.

Warning signs of possible hearing loss include, but are not limited to, tinnitus, buzzing noise, slight muffling of sounds, difficulty understanding speech despite hearing sound, and the perception of being unsure of the direction sound is coming from. Sound is measured in **decibels** (dB), a unit

of measurement of the intensity of sound (**Table 20-1**). Ear protection is recommended when an individual is exposed to sounds of 85 dB for greater than 8 continuous hours. Children exposed to sounds registered at 70 dB continuously for

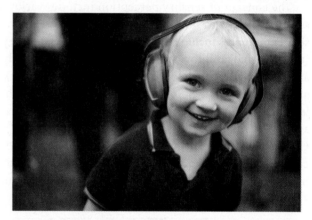

Figure 20-2 *Ear muffs can provide protection from hearing loss.*
© PeopleImages/DigitalVision/Getty Images

TABLE 20-1 Decibel Levels of Everyday Sounds
45 dB: Refrigerator motor
50 dB: Rainfall
60 dB: Typical speech
75 dB: Washing machine
85 dB: Busy city traffic
90 dB: Gas mower, hair dryer
100 dB: iPod
110 dB: Leaf blower, rock concert
120 dB: Ambulance, jack hammer
140 dB: Fireworks and jet airliner directly overhead

Data from Hearing Loss Association of America. (2017). Prevention of hearing loss. Retrieved from http://www.hearingloss.org/content/prevention-hearing-loss

24 hours are considered at risk for hearing loss, according to the National Institute of Health's National Institute on Deafness and Other Communication Disorders (NIDCD, 2017).

Children are more sensitive to sounds than adults are, and the same sounds can register up to 20 dB greater in a child than in the average adult. According to the NIH's NIDCD (2017), 17% of teens age 12 to 19 have some degree of hearing loss—a phenomenon that is believed to be related to use of MP3 players and other mobile auditory music devices at high volume levels.

The state of California, as well as many other states, has established a newborn hearing screening program (NHSP) that is available to all families prior to discharge from the hospital. This screening seeks to identify hearing loss early and link families to resources by the time the infant reaches six months of age. Infants born at home, at birthing centers, or at other alternative birthing sites should have follow-up care that includes assessment by the screening program. For further information on this required or offered screening, contact the National Center for Hearing Assessment and Management (http://www.infanthearing.org/screening/).

Acute Otitis Media

Otitis media—ear infection—may have either a viral or a bacterial origin. Acute otitis media (AOM) is defined as an inflammation of the middle ear space with a rapid onset of signs and symptoms of an acute infection such as fever and ear pain. It occurs most frequently in children younger than 24 months, and is usually preceded by an upper respiratory infection (URI). AOM is usually diagnosed by otoscopic visualization of the tympanic membrane for pus, bulging, purulent drainage, or redness. Depending on whether URI symptoms are present, waiting 72 hours for clinical improvement has been recommended, rather than immediately starting antibiotic treatment. However, antibiotic treatment is recommended for children younger than 6 months due to their immature immune systems. Myringotomy—the placement of eardrum tubes via a procedure involving a surgical incision of the eardrum (tympanoplasty)—may be indicated if the pain is severe (Hockenberry & Wilson, 2009).

PHARMACOLOGY

Current practice guidelines state that healthcare providers should not immediately prescribe oral antibiotic therapy for otitis media in childhood. Although otitis media is the most common childhood infection for which antibiotics are prescribed, and there has been a decrease in the complication of mastoiditis, antibacterial medications are not encouraged unless the child does not demonstrate clinical improvement.

Visual Disorders

During fetal development, the eye develops at 16 weeks' gestation. Blood vessels begin to form at the optic nerve, providing oxygen and nutrients to the developing retina. The retina grows rapidly, especially during the last 12 weeks of pregnancy, and its development continues up to 1 month after birth.

According to the National Eye Institute (NIH/NEI, 2011), 4% of preschoolers have myopia (nearsightedness) and 21% have hyperopia (farsightedness). Another childhood visual disorder—astigmatism (irregular curvature of the eye)—is found in 10% of preschoolers. These three disorders represent the most common visual disorders in children and are collectively classified as refractive errors, or errors associated with abnormalities of the eye shape that alter the conversion of light into signals for brain interpretation. Refractive errors are correctable. The preschooler developmental stage is an important time to conduct visual screening and treatment prior to the child engaging in elementary school academics.

Two other visual conditions that are less common but not rare, affecting approximately 3% of children (Friedman et al., 2009), are strabismus (crossed eyes) and amblyopia (lazy eye). These misalignments of the eyes affect vision by disrupting the brain's ability to merge left- and right-eye images appropriately. Ultimately, the brain suppresses signals from one eye or the other, leading to an effect of functional blindness in one eye. Both conditions can be corrected via vision training, orthoptics, surgery, botulinum toxin injection, or a combination of approaches. Most authorities agree that obtaining early treatment for either condition (e.g., before age 5) produces the best results (Bradfield, 2013; Wright & Spiegel, 2013).

Box 20-1 lists the various visual disturbances found in children.

BOX 20-1 Visual Disturbances in Childhood

- Albinism-related visual disturbances
- Amblyopia
- Aniridia
- Astigmatism
- Cataract
- Cortical visual impairment
- Diabetic retinopathy
- Glaucoma
- Hyperopia
- Myopia
- Nystigmatism
- Optic nerve atrophy
- Retinoblastoma
- Retinopathy of prematurity
- Strabismus

Retinopathy of Prematurity

Retinopathy of prematurity (ROP) is a disorder in which the blood vessels in the retina develop abnormally, potentially leading to blindness. A variety of factors may contribute to ROP, including prematurity, low birth weight, and hypoxia. Premature infants born at less than 31 weeks' gestation and weighing less than 1250 g are at highest risk. Oxygen is considered a contributing factor in the development of ROP, which explains why it is important to monitor oxygen saturation levels for all infants who receive oxygen and adjust the Fio$_2$ according to the specified institutional parameters (NIH/NEI, 2016a).

ROP occurs in two phases. Phase 1 occurs between 30 and 32 weeks of life. In this phase, blood vessel growth halts due to hyperoxia from the supplemental oxygen that many premature babies receive to support their immature respiratory system. Phase 2 begins later, during weeks 32 to 34 of life. This phase is marked by abnormal blood vessel growth, which can potentially cause retinal detachment (Friddle, 2013).

Severity of ROP is classified based on the zone, extent, stage, and presence of disease (**Figure 20-3**). There are five stages (I–V), ranging from mild to complete retinal detachment. Approximately 90% of infants with ROP have a mild case and do not require any treatment. In contrast, those with the most severe form of ROP may have impaired vision and possibly blindness from retinal detachment. On an annual basis, approximately 1100 to 1500 premature infants develop severe ROP, requiring treatment; 400 to 600 infants are classified as legally blind from ROP each year (NIH/NEI, 2016a).

Treatment modalities for ROP include laser therapy and cryotherapy. The goal of treatment is to slow or reverse the abnormal blood vessel growth in the retina, but both of these therapies are known to affect peripheral vision. Their long-term side effects are not known.

Light reduction in the neonatal intensive care unit (NICU) has not been shown to decrease the incidence of ROP in low-birth-weight infants based on studies supported by the National Eye Institute. Instead, prevention of ROP focuses on preventing preterm births, early screening and detection for infants born at less than 28 weeks' gestation and weighing less than 1500 g, and

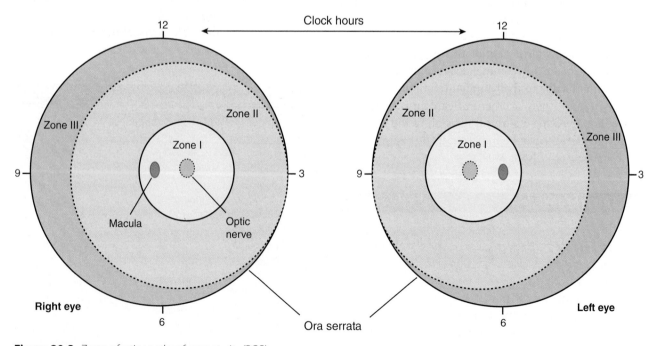

Figure 20-3 *Zones of retinopathy of prematurity (ROP).*

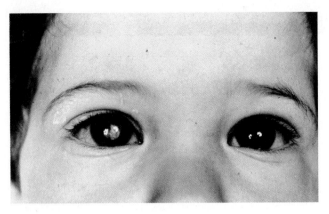

Figure 20-4 *Leukocoria or cat's eye.*

Courtesy of National Cancer Institute (http://www.cancer.gov)

decreasing exposure to bright light (even though there is no direct correlation between increased ROP incidence and lighting). Use of supplemental oxygen must be monitored and maintained according to saturation limits to help prevent fluctuations in blood oxygen levels. ROP should be treated once diagnosis is confirmed by eye exam (NIH/NEI, 2016a).

Retinoblastoma

Retinoblastoma is a rare tumor of the retina that typically affects children younger than 5 years of age. This congenital ocular tumor is usually unilateral, although 30% of tumors may be bilateral. Approximately 40% of retinoblastomas are inherited via a mutated gene that may predispose them to other cancers later in life, such as melanoma, osteosarcoma, lung cancer, or breast cancer, particularly if radiation therapy was part of their treatment (American Cancer Society, 2015; NIH/NEI, 2016b). Parents may seek medical treatment for their child after discovering a whitish glow in their young child's eye. The term often used to describe this phenomenon is "cat's eye"; the medical term for this finding is leukocoria (**Figure 20-4**).

Retinoblastoma typically manifests with two initial signs: white eye reflex and strabismus. Redness and pain, which are often seen associated with glaucoma, are also potential symptoms. Definitive diagnosis is made through parent interview, ophthalmic exam, ultrasound, and computed tomography. Prognosis is positive, with a 90% success rate after treatment. Treatment includes radiation, laser therapy, cryotherapy, and chemotherapy. If required for containment or structural damage, the child's eye may be removed (enucleation) and a prosthesis provided (Hockenberry & Wilson, 2009). Blindness is a late sign of this disorder.

Concepts in Communication Development for Visually Impaired or Hearing-Impaired Children

For infants who are born with a hearing or visual impairment, it is very important to feel secure and safe in their familiar environment. This is the first step toward building trust in the first year of life. Bonding with the primary caregiver forms one of the most important relationships for the child; it acts as a foundation for trust to be created with the outside world. Parents need to form that trusting bond, read their children's cues as they learn to communicate, interpret their needs, and act promptly to provide what is needed.

Every child's reaction to sensory stimulation is different. It is up to the caregivers to read these cues, interpret them, and engage the child to communicate with family members and others. To be successful, caregivers must provide a safe environment for the child, build trust, include the child in the activity from beginning to end, and develop their own language for activities such as saying hello or goodbye, diaper changes, play, thirst, hunger, or boredom. Parents and caregivers also need to pause and watch the child's reactions, as it may take some time for the child to respond to cues that a non-impaired child would react to immediately. The child may become frightened, confused, or even angry if someone unexpectedly touches him or her without warning.

In hearing-impaired children as well as in children with other neurologic impairments such as apraxia (Tierney, Pitterle, Kurtz, Nakhla, & Todorow, 2016), use of sign language has been known to start young, as early as infancy. Helping children identify a language with which they can communicate with others helps them to understand the outside world (Napoli et al., 2015). While learning, it is important to observe for signs of overstimulation. The child should be encouraged to explore the surroundings together with the caregiver, with each guiding the other. Children benefit from having choices, having some degree of control over their own environment so they will not feel alone, and interacting with others. Their environment should be adjusted as needed so that children have their space for activities and play; routines are very important to them. The nurse should encourage the use of all the senses, including tactile, olfactory, and gustatory senses, if appropriate, to understand their outside world (Gleason, 2008). **Table 20-2** offers ideas for play activities involving visual stimulation.

Sensory Processing Disorders

In **sensory processing** disorder (SPD), also known as sensory integration disorder or dysfunction, the process of translating all incoming sensory stimulation in a meaningful

TABLE 20-2 Play Activities for Visual Stimulation of Different Age Groups

Infant

› Infants are able to distinguish color differences beginning at 2–3 months of age.

› Caregivers should provide objects with high contrast such as black-and-white patterns, checkerboards, circles, and yellow-and-black patterns.

› Caregivers should bring their face to within 6–10 inches in front of the infant; play with the infant in this visual range and show various facial expressions.

› With infants between 4 and 7 months, shades of reds, blues, and yellow are most beneficial, along with complex patterns and shapes.

› Provide infants with large picture books, music boxes, mobiles hung over the crib, push–pull toys, jack-in-the-boxes, and strings of big colorful beads.

› Play peek-a-boo with infants to increase object permanence.

Toddler

› Physical growth and motor skills slow during the toddler period, but intellectual, social, and emotional development increases. The toddler benefits from activities that promote interaction through visual play.

› Toddlers enjoy parallel play, imitation, language learning, dressing up, drawing, finger painting, sorting objects by shape and color, and playing with balls, trucks, and building blocks.

› Provide toddlers with a large cement surface and give them colored chalk to scribble designs or color in shapes.

Preschool

› Young children benefit from three- to four-piece puzzles, objects that can be sorted and are colorful, matching objects to a picture book, water play, jumping, running, associative play, hand puppets, clay modeling, and medical kits.

› Play ideas include drawing with large crayons of various bright colors on large sheets of paper. Activities can include copying shapes and then coloring them in, or providing an outline of a body and having the child color in hair, eyes, and body parts.

School Age

› School-age children benefit from discovering aspects of space (e.g., planets, constellations), table games, checkers, simple card games, music, and sports lessons.

› Many visually stimulating arts and crafts projects specifically designed for this age group are available. Provide opportunities to play with colored yarn, colored string, and colored art supplies.

Adolescent

› The teenage period is marked by puberty, mood swings, identity, sexuality, dating, peers, body image, bullying, being self-centered, and developing self-esteem. Being prompted to draw, paint, and color their emotions and life experiences is beneficial.

› Teens benefit from higher-level visually stimulating projects, such as stencils, advanced coloring projects, ceramics, free drawing, and painting.

---

way is affected. In the 1970s, Jane Ayers, an occupational therapist, identified **sensory integration** dysfunction as problems in managing and translating sensory inputs obtained through the vestibular, proprioception, tactile, auditory, and visual senses. Ayers developed two assessment tools—the Southern California Sensory Integration Tool (SCSIT) and the Sensory Integration Praxis Tool (SIPT)—to aid occupational therapists in their evaluation of children having difficulty in school, whether behavioral or academic. Ayers also developed child-directed, play-based tools to

assist in SPD treatment that helped the child handle normal activities such as eating with utensils, dressing, and play (www.thespiralfoundation.org).

Children with SPD have difficulty interpreting sensations in a meaningful way. They struggle to cope with everyday life activities such as dressing, eating, and playing. Use of gross and fine motor skills, attention and behavior, self-esteem, eating, and sleeping are all influenced by how the brain interprets these incoming sensory signals. The senses help children interpret the world and adapt that understanding

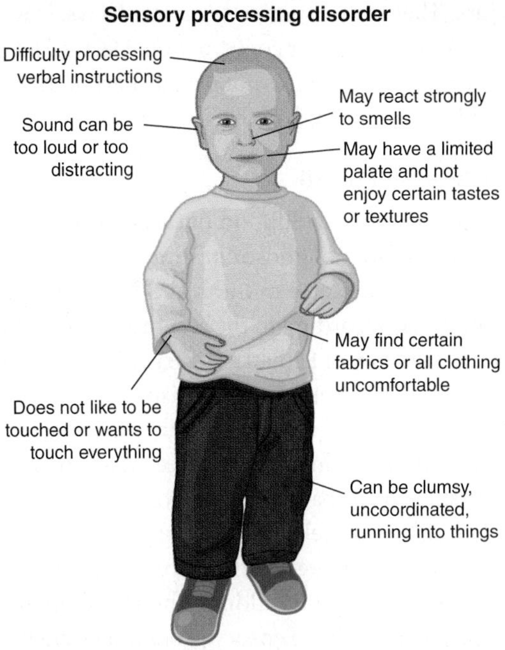

Sensory processing disorder

Difficulty processing
verbal instructions

Sound can be
too loud or too
distracting

May react strongly
to smells

May have a limited
palate and not
enjoy certain tastes
or textures

May find certain
fabrics or all clothing
uncomfortable

Does not like to be
touched or wants to
touch everything

Can be clumsy,
uncoordinated,
running into things

Figure 20-5 *Features of sensory processing disorder.*

based on their environment. Successful sensory interpretation then increases self-esteem, confidence, and sense of identity (**Figure 20-5**).

In contrast, poor integration of sensory input may distract, confuse, and frustrate children with SPD, prompting them to act out with inappropriate behavior in the classroom and be labeled a "problem child." This labeling and categorization can further alienate these children from their peers. Children with SPD may have difficulty academically and socially, leading to feelings of isolation; they may be disruptive, confused, angry, and prone to behavioral outbursts; and they may have a lack of physical coordination that makes them reluctant to participate in sports. Such children may also underreact to sensory stimulation (e.g., tactile, vestibular, proprioception, hearing, vision, smell, and taste stimuli). As caregivers, teachers, and advocates, nurses need to provide a safe, nurturing, and stimulating environment to support every child's developing brain and build each child's trust in the world.

Three major categories of sensory processing disorders are distinguished (Spiral Foundation, 2015):

- Sensory modulation dysfunction: Under- or over-response to stimulation, such as hypersensitivity to sounds, a tendency to be easily distracted by movements, or overreaction to certain textures.
- Sensory discrimination disorder: Difficulty in recognizing and processing sensations such as touch. The child may have difficulty with balance and coordination, enjoy spinning around, chew on nonfood items, or grab items too tightly.

- Praxis disorders: Problems with motor planning. A child with a praxis disorder may not track with eyes or make eye contact, or may have difficulty speaking. He or she may not enjoy sports or may have difficulty reading.

Because there is no universally accepted diagnostic tool for SPD, other behavioral or developmental disorders must be considered during the diagnostic process. Sensory integration difficulties may be a factor in autism spectrum disorders, attention-deficit/hyperactivity disorder (ADHD), anxiety/behavioral disorders, and developmental dis-coordination (American Academy of Pediatrics [AAP], 2012).

Symptoms of SPD must be thoroughly evaluated to rule out behavioral, developmental, and medical disorders. In addition, nurses should educate families that sensory integration therapies have insufficient data to support their use as interventions, set time limits and specific goals and parameters when monitoring for effect of sensory integration therapies, and recognize that occupational therapy may be time limited depending on resources and insurance, so that the plan of treatment must include clear priorities (AAP, 2012).

Autism Spectrum Disorders

Autism spectrum disorders (ASD) is a group of disorders that affects brain development. As of 2013, the fifth edition of *Diagnostic and Statistical Manual of Mental Disorders* (*DSM-5*) grouped subtypes of autism into ASD, including "classic autism disorder," childhood disintegration disorder, pervasive developmental disorder—not otherwise specified (PDD-NOS), and Asperger syndrome (Lai, Lombardo, Chakrabarti, & Baron-Cohen, 2013).

The incidence of ASD is approximately 1 in 68 children, and 1 in 42 males; that is, boys are 5 times more likely to be diagnosed with ASD than girls. Almost half of children currently diagnosed with ASD demonstrate average or above-average intelligence, compared to one third of those diagnosed a decade ago. Risk factors for ASD include low birth weight, prematurity, having a sibling with ASD, and genetic disorders such as fragile X syndrome, Rett syndrome, and tuberous sclerosis (Christensen et al., 2016; National Institute of Mental Health, 2016).

In 2000, the CDC established the Autism and Developmental Disabilities Monitoring (ADDM) Network. The primary goals were to accurately track the number of children with ASD, provide characteristics of ASD (including gender, race/ethnicity, age at evaluation and diagnosis, and intellectual ability), determine whether ASD is common in a particular group of children, and understand the impact of ASD on the child, family, and community (CDC, 2016a).

Children with ASD may have varied characteristics in different degrees that affect verbal and nonverbal communication, social interactions, and repetitive behaviors. ASD is associated with problems in motor coordination, attention, physical health, and intellectual abilities. The wide and varied range of signs and symptoms of ASD include not showing eye contact, crying outbursts, delayed language, repetitive words or phrases, rocking, preoccupation with lining up objects in a certain way, gastrointestinal symptoms (constipation or diarrhea), seizure disorders, altered sleep patterns, sensory processing problems, and eating nonfood items. Children and adults with ASD may be of above-average intelligence, very detailed oriented, and able to retain information over a long period of time; be strong visual and auditory learners; and excel in math, science, music, or art (CDC, 2016b). Children with ASD also have challenges with social interactions. They may avert their gaze and not look at a person speaking to them. Language development may be delayed, and they may interpret social or verbal cues incorrectly. Children with ASD take language very literally and may not understand the intent behind another person's use of language, such as with jokes or sarcasm. They may respond to stimuli by physically hurting themselves through repetitive behaviors such as head banging or rocking to help them cope with situations they do not understand (CDC, 2016b).

Asperger syndrome falls under the broad category of ASD. Children with Asperger syndrome are considered to have a high-functioning form of autism, as their difficulties usually involve social interactions and repetitive behaviors. They may experience motor delays, leading to clumsiness or poor motor coordination. Delayed language or cognitive development is not usually part of the clinical picture of Asperger syndrome.

Treatment Goals for ASD

ASD begins in early childhood but lasts throughout the lifetime. Therefore, diagnostic testing of developmental delays should begin at 9 months and be repeated at 18 and 24 months, according to the recommendations of the American Academy of Pediatrics. There is no single means of medical detection or cure for autism.

Children with ASD are often prone to associated medical conditions, including seizures, sleep disturbances, and gastrointestinal disturbances such as constipation, diarrhea, and inflammatory bowel disease (Coury et al., 2012). These disorders must be treated with appropriate medical care in addition to therapy to address the child's neurologic and social dysfunctions. Sensory processing difficulties in children with ASD may cause them to be overly sensitive to textures or sounds, or not sensitive enough to lighting or temperature. **Early interventions** (i.e., support for children and families that begins soon after birth, so as to minimize the extent of the problem experienced by the young child) will benefit these children over the long term, as they learn and build coping skills to deal with behavior and personal relationships. Therapies will aid in decreasing symptoms and increase capabilities in handling their environment. Treatment plans must be individualized, as not every child has the same set of symptoms or reactions to their surroundings.

Case Study

Baby JR is an ex-30 weeks' gestation male with multiple medical issues during his 15-month hospitalization. JR's mother has type 1 diabetes, requiring multiple daily insulin injections that continued during this pregnancy. Because of his prematurity and immature lungs, this infant required a tracheostomy at 1 month of age, as well as diuretics, aerosol treatments, and aminophylline to treat his chronic lung disease. A MIC-KEY button (gastrostomy tube) was surgically placed prior to discharge, as he had difficulty taking his required daily nutrition orally.

JR had several bouts of pneumonia during his hospital stay and developed septic shock and endocarditis from severe sepsis. He had clonus in his lower extremities and was later, after discharge, diagnosed with cerebral palsy. He developed some degree of sensorineural hearing loss from ototoxic medications he was given. His family and caregivers in the hospital learned sign language so as to communicate with him.

This infant's family consists of a young married couple in their mid-20s with intact family support; those family members reside approximately 30 minutes from the hospital.

Case Study Questions

1. Which anticipatory guidance for discharge needs would this family require? Include multidisciplinary support: general health, medications, speech, physical therapy, and occupational.

(continues)

Case Study (continued)

2. Which ongoing education support needs will this family have?
3. Which type of respite support should be coordinated for the family?

As the Case Evolves...

The pediatric nurse is working with JR's parents to help them learn how to care for their son. Both are young, first-time parents, and the nurse finds that they have a few misconceptions about concerns that will arise during their son's infancy and early childhood.

4. Which of the following statements, if made by one of the participating parents, would require more teaching?
   A. "If my child has an ear infection, I need to make sure he completes the entire course of antibiotics."
   B. "Ear infections can be directly related to other viral infections, such as those in the sinuses and throat."
   C. "Immunizations through the infant period are important to prevent ear infections."
   D. "Tugging on the ear may be a clue that my son has an ear infection."

Chapter Summary

- Building a foundation of trust during the first year of life is vital to brain development as the child learns to cope with the outside world on an emotional, social, and intellectual level.
- Pediatric nurses, caregivers, and parents must allow children to explore their environment and learn about themselves in their own way.
- The concept of sensory perception includes normal development of the sensory organs as well as the various deviations that can occur. Deviations in sensory perception can be primary or secondary.
- Maternal health, environment, maternal recreational and prescribed medication use, and prematurity are just a few of the conditions that can alter the fetus's brain development during the critical time of sensory maturation. If these conditions persist, the connections that build the framework for brain development may be changed or altered.
- Hearing loss is categorized as conductive, sensorineural, or mixed.
- Retinopathy of prematurity (ROP) is a disorder in which the blood vessels in the retina develop abnormally, potentially leading to blindness. A variety of factors may lead to ROP, including prematurity and low birth weight.
- Retinoblastoma is a rare congenital ocular tumor that is usually unilateral. Parents may seek medical treatment for their child after discovering a whitish glow in their young child's eye, known as "cat's eye" or leukocoria.
- Almost half of children currently diagnosed with autism spectrum disorder demonstrate average or above-average intelligence, compared to one third of those diagnosed a decade ago. Risk factors for ASD include low birth weight, prematurity, sibling with ASD, and genetic disorders such as fragile X syndrome, Rett syndrome, and tuberous sclerosis.
- Children with ASD may have varied characteristics in different degrees that affect their verbal and nonverbal communication, social interactions, and repetitive behaviors. ASD is associated with problems in motor coordination, attention, physical health, and intellectual abilities.

Bibliography

American Academy of Pediatrics (AAP). (2012). AAP policy statement: Sensory integration therapies for children with developmental and behavioral disorders. *Pediatrics, 129,* 1186.

American Academy of Pediatrics (AAP). (2014). AAP policy: Screening examination of premature infants for ROP. *Pediatrics, 131,* 189-195.

American Cancer Society. (2015). Retinoblastoma: Fact sheet. Retrieved from http://www.cancer.org/acs/groups/cid/documents/webcontent/003135-pdf.pdf

Bergman, J., & Bergman, N. (2010). *Hold your premie: A work book on skin-to-skin contact for parents of premature babies* (2nd ed. revised). Cape Town, South Africa: New Voices Publishing, 1–130.

Bisht, M., & Bist, S. S. (2011). Ototoxicity: The hidden menace. *Indian Journal of Otolaryngology Head and Neck Surgery, 63*(3), 255–259.

Bradfield, Y. S. (2013). Identification and treatment of amblyopia. *American Family Physician, 87*(5), 348-352.

Centers for Disease Control and Prevention (CDC). (2016a). Autism and Developmental Disabilities Monitoring (ADDM) Network. Retrieved from http://www.cdc.gov/ncbddd/autism/addm.html

Centers for Disease Control and Prevention (CDC). (2016b). Facts about ASD. Retrieved from http://www.cdc.gov/ncbddd/autism/facts.html

Christensen, D. L., Baio, J., Braun, K. V., Bilder, D., Charles, J., Constantino, J. N., . . . Yeargin-Allsopp, M. (2016). Prevalence and characteristics of autism spectrum disorder among children aged 8 years: Autism and Developmental Disabilities Monitoring Network, 11 sites, United States, 2012. *MMWR Surveillance Summary, 65*(SS-3), 1–23.

Coury, D. L., Ashwood, P., Fasano, A., Fuchs, G., Geraghty, M., Kaul, A., . . . Jones, N. E. (2012). Gastrointestinal conditions in children with autism spectrum disorder: Developing a research agenda. *Pediatrics, 130*(suppl 2), S160–S168.

Daniel, E. (2007), Noise and hearing loss: A review. *Journal of School Health, 77*, 225–231.

Friedman, D. S., Repka, M. X., Katz, J., Giordano, L., Ibironke, J., Hawse, P., & Tielsch, J. M. (2009). Prevalence of amblyopia and strabismus in white and African-American children aged 6 through 71 months: The Baltimore Pediatric Eye Disease Study. *Ophthalmology, 116*(11), 2128–34.e1-2.

Friddle, K. (2013). Pathogenesis of retinopathy of prematurity: Does inflammation play a role? *Newborn and Infant Nursing Reviews, 13*, 161–165.

Gleason, D. (2008). Early interactions with children who are deaf-blind. Retrieved from http://files.eric.ed.gov/fulltext/ED531843.pdf

Graven, S., & Browne, J. (2008). Sensory development in the fetus, neonate, and infant: Introduction and overview. *Newborn and Infant Nursing Reviews, 10*, 7.

Hockenberrry, M. J., & Wilson, D. (2009). *Wong's essentials of pediatric nursing* (8th ed.). St. Louis, MO: Elsevier.

Kenner, D., & McGrath, J. (2010). *Development care of newborns and infants* (2nd ed.). Chicago, IL: National Association of Neonatal Nurses.

Lai, M. C., Lombardo, M. V., Chakrabarti, B., & Baron-Cohen, S. (2013). Subgrouping the autism "spectrum": Reflections on DSM-5. *PLoS Biology, 11*(4), e1001544.

Napoli, D. J., Mellon, N. K., Niparko, J. K., Rathmann, C., Mathur, G., Humphries, T., . . . Lantos, J. D. (2015). Should all deaf children learn sign language? *Pediatrics, 136*(1), 170–176.

National Institutes of Health (NIH). (2016). Genetics home reference: Retinoblastoma. Retrieved from https://ghr.nlm.nih.gov/condition/retinoblastoma

National Institutes of Health (NIH), National Eye Institute (NEI). (2011). National Institutes of Health release data from largest pediatric eye study. Retrieved from https://nei.nih.gov/news/statements/pediatric

National Institutes of Health (NIH), National Eye Institute (NEI). (2016a). Facts about retinopathy of prematurity. Retrieved from https://nei.nih.gov/health/rop/rop

National Institutes of Health (NIH), National Eye Institute (NEI). (2016b). Retinoblastoma. Retrieved from https://nei.nih.gov/health/retinoblastoma

National Institutes of Health (NIH), National Eye Institute (NEI). (n.d.). Astigmatism. Retrieved from https://nei.nih.gov/healthy eyes/astigmatism

National Institutes of Health (NIH), National Institute on Deaf and Other Communication Disorders (NIDCD). (2014). NIDCD Fact Sheet. Hearing and balance: Noise induced hearing loss. Pub No. 99-4233. Retrieved from https://www.nidcd.nih.gov/sites/default/files/Documents/health/hearing/NIDCD-Noise-Induced-Hearing-Loss.pdf

National Institutes of Health (NIH), National Institute on Deafness and Other Communication Disorders (NIDCD). (2017). Noise-induced hearing loss. Retrieved from https://www.nidcd.nih.gov/health/noise-induced-hearing-loss

National Institute of Mental Health. (2016). Autism spectrum disorder. Retrieved from https://www.nimh.nih.gov/health/topics/autism-spectrum-disorders-asd/index.shtml

Spiral Foundation. (2015). What is sensory integration? Retrieved from http://www.thespiralfoundation.org/aboutspd.html

Taneja, M. K., Varshney, H., Taneja, V., & Varshney, J. (2015). Ototoxicity, drugs, chemicals, mobile phones and deafness. *Indian Journal of Otology, 21*, 161-164.

Tierney, C. D., Pitterle, K., Kurtz, M., Nakhla, M., & Todorow, C. (2016). Bridging the gap between speech and language: Using multimodal treatment in a child with apraxia. *Pediatrics, 138*(3). [Epub ahead of print]. pii: e20160007. doi: 10.1542/peds.2016-0007

Wright, K. W., & Spiegel, P. H. (eds.). (2013). *Pediatric ophthalmology and strabismus* (2nd ed.). New York, NY: Springer Science+Business.

CHAPTER 21

Intracranial Regulation

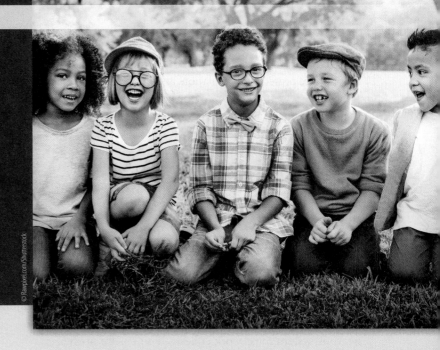

© Rawpixel.com/Shutterstock

LEARNING OBJECTIVES

1. Define key words and phrases related to the concept of intracranial regulation and neurologic disorders during childhood.
2. Understand the anatomy and physiology of the central and peripheral nervous systems, including how these structures grow, mature, and change during childhood.
3. Apply principles of homeostasis to children with head injury, structural defects, or space-occupying lesions producing increased intracranial pressure.
4. Differentiate the assessment, diagnosis, medical treatment, and nursing care for commonly seen neurologic disorders found across the developmental levels.
5. Contrast the various infection control practices used when children present with infectious processes within the neurologic system, including viral and bacterial meningitis.
6. Create a teaching plan for a family whose child was recently diagnosed with a seizure disorder.
7. Evaluate the impact of childhood trauma affecting intracranial regulation—such as shaken baby syndrome—on the victim, family, and healthcare providers.
8. Analyze the differences in types, assessments, treatments, and care for children with cerebral bleeds.

KEY TERMS

Absence seizure
Abusive head trauma
Brudzinski's sign
Cerebrospinal fluid
Concussion
Epidural hematoma
Febrile seizure
Grand mal seizure
Increased intracranial pressure
Kernig's sign
Meningitis
Seizure disorder
Subdural hematoma

Introduction

The concept of intracranial regulation is complex. The bony cranium houses a variety of neurologic structures that require protection, regulation, and integration so that they can provide the systems of the body with messages to maintain homeostasis and functional status. Intracranial regulation requires that the central nervous system (the command center) and the peripheral nervous system (the response center) work together to support the child's maturation, growth and development, cognitive development, and safety through appropriate responses to harmful stimuli.

Neurologic System Function

Understanding the anatomy and physiology of the central and peripheral nervous system is the foundation for connecting symptoms with disorders or injuries. The entire nervous system must work cohesively to ensure normal function, sensory experiences, and involuntary and voluntary motor responses. The three core components of the child's nervous system are the central nervous system (CNS), the peripheral nervous system (PNS), and the autonomic (involuntary) nervous system (ANS). All three of these components must communicate, coordinate, and interact appropriately to provide the child with full physical, emotional, and intellectual properties and activities. The central nervous system serves as the command center for the entire nervous system, constantly interpreting and integrating stimuli and initiating both voluntary and involuntary movements. The nervous system not only controls the functions of the body, but allows for adaptation to the environment, both consciously and unconsciously.

Developmental Factors

Neurologic development begins in the fifth week of fetal development, with neurons (impulse conductor cells) eventually being produced during weeks 15 to 30 of gestation. With healthy and consistent development, the newborn begins life with neurologic stability and predictable growth and maturity. The identification of lags in developmental milestones is a key indicator that the child is experiencing a neurologic disorder.

Central Nervous System

The central nervous system includes the brain and the spinal cord, which are housed in and protected by the bony cranium and the vertebral column, respectively. To provide room for expansion of the brain, the newborn presents with open anterior and posterior fontanels (**Figure 21-1**).

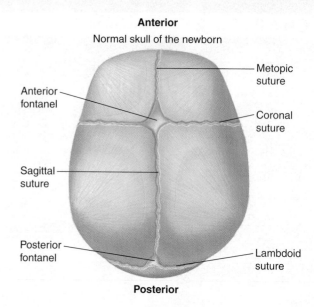

Figure 21-1 *Anterior and posterior fontanels on a newborn's skull.*

The posterior fontanel closes first, by age 2 months; the larger anterior fontanel closes by 12 to 18 months of age.

The brain consists of three main structures: the cerebrum, cerebellum, and brain stem. Within the brain structures are neurons with myelin sheaths (not fully present until late adolescence), **cerebrospinal fluid** (CSF), meninges, and the ventricles where the CSF is produced and reabsorbed by the choroid plexus lining the four ventricles of the brain (**Figure 21-2**).

The outer layer of the brain, the cerebrum, is the largest brain structure and is in control of motor, sensory, and intellectual functioning. The outermost layer is the cerebral cortex (gray matter), which is made up of neuron cell bodies. In contrast, the inner layer of the cerebrum consists of the basal ganglia and the axons (white matter). The cerebrum is divided into two hemispheres connected by the corpus callosum, a fibrous band of nerves that share information between the hemispheres. The right side of the brain controls the left side of the body, and vice versa. Directly below the corpus callosum is the thalamus. Considered an information relay center, this tissue is responsible for transporting information via nerves to the areas of the cerebrum. The cerebrum is also divided into four specific lobes, each with its own function: the temporal lobe (taste, hearing, and smell), the parietal lobe (sensory coordination), the occipital lobe (visual stimuli interpretation), and the frontal lobe (voluntary motor movements). Directly under the thalamus is the hypothalamus, which provides autonomic brain regulation of sleep, appetite, blood pressure, core body temperature control, breathing patterns and depth, and peripheral nerve transmissions in response to emotions and behaviors.

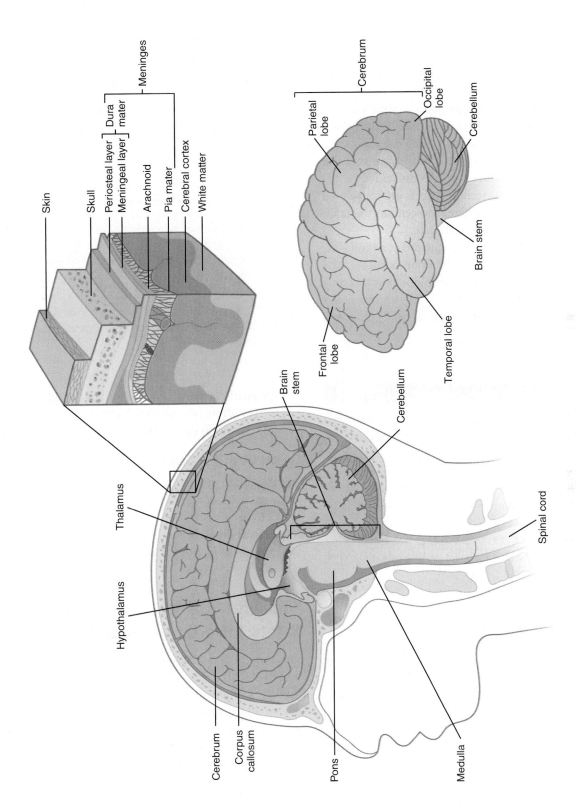

Figure 21-2 *The structures of the brain, protective coating, and the spinal cord.*

Skin

Skull

Periosteal layer
Meningeal layer — Dura mater

Arachnoid

Pia mater

Cerebral cortex

White matter

Meninges

Thalamus

Hypothalamus

Cerebrum

Corpus callosum

Pons

Brain stem

Cerebellum

Medulla

Spinal cord

Cerebrum

Parietal lobe

Occipital lobe

Cerebellum

Brain stem

Frontal lobe

Temporal lobe

Below the hypothalamus is the base of the brain, called the cerebellum. The cerebellum regulates equilibrium, smooth-muscle movements, sensory impulse coordination with muscle activity, and muscle tone.

The most posterior segment of the brain is the brain stem. Here, information about the basic functions of the respiratory, cardiac, and vasomotor systems are transmitted between the higher levels of the brain and the body.

The most central anatomic components of the brain are the neurons. Numbering in the hundreds of billions, these cells are considered conductor cells for nerve impulses.

The spinal cord, which is bathed in CSF, consists of a central band of tissue, with 31 pairs of spinal nerves extending from this cord. Ascending tracts are considered sensory (toward the brain), whereas descending tracts are reserved for motor responses to stimuli.

In summary, one can think of the head as a vault containing many vital structures. The brain occupies 80% of the space in the cranium, cerebral blood flow accounts for 10% of the cranial volume, and CSF fills the remaining 10%. **Box 21-1** provides information on head circumference in children.

RESEARCH EVIDENCE

The pediatric nurse should understand the principles underlying the Monro-Kellie doctrine. Specifically, research has shown that the brain's physiology is governed by a rule concerning space and pressure, which must remain consistent and stable. If any of the three elements of fixed space—brain tissue, blood circulation, or CSF—is altered, the fixed bony cranium must activate compensatory mechanisms by altering one of these three components to maintain normal and expected levels of intracranial pressure (Dunn, 2002; Kukreti, Mohseni-Bod, & Drake, 2014).

Peripheral Nervous System

Structures of the peripheral nervous system include those neurologic structures that are outside of the brain and spinal cord. Thirty-one pairs of spinal nerves and 12 cranial nerves make up the PNS (**Table 21-1**; **Figure 21-3**). Both the autonomic nervous system and the somatic (voluntary) nervous system are a part of the PNS. The somatic nervous system regulates higher brain processing, reflexes, shivering, and all conscious thought. The autonomic nervous system regulates two antagonistic systems:

- Parasympathetic nervous system (rest and digest): Releases the cholinergic neurohormone acetylcholine to conserve energy

---

BOX 21-1 Head Circumference Measurements

Head circumference measurements are essential for monitoring brain growth and should continue from birth to at least the second birthday. Normal patterns of growth are as follows:

- At birth, the average head circumference is 34 to 35 cm.
- From birth to 1 year of age, the head circumference grows by 2 cm per month for the first 3 months, by 1 cm per month for the next 3 months, and by 3 cm total over the last 6 months. Thus, head circumference increases, on average, by 12 cm during the first year of life.
- From 1 year to 3 years of age, head circumference growth slows, averaging only 1 to 3 cm per year.
- The average head circumference for 12-month-olds is approximately 45 to 47 cm.
- By age 3, the head circumference measurement averages 48.5 cm.
- More than 50% of brain growth occurs during the first 12 months of life.

Data from Centers for Disease Control and Prevention, National Center for Health Statistics. (2001). Data table of infant head circumference-for-age charts. Retrieved from http://www.cdc.gov/growthcharts/html_charts/hcageinf.htm

---

- Sympathetic nervous system (fight or flight): Releases adrenergic catecholamines to provide energy to respond to stressful stimuli

Cerebrospinal Fluid Regulation

Both acquired and congenital disorders can lead to the dysregulation of CSF. The overproduction of CSF, or the decreased absorption of CSF, can lead to **increased intracranial pressure** (i.e., increased pressure inside the skull) in children whose fontanels and suture lines are closed.

Thinking in Concepts to Promote Safety: Intracranial Regulation

The concept of intracranial regulation refers to the process of stabilization and homeostasis of the tissues and fluid present in the child's bony cranium. During insults due to injury, trauma, infection, or space-occupying lesions, the process of regulation will include stabilizing pressure within the bony cranium. Many disorders and injuries during childhood can lead to the dysregulation of, or increase in, intracranial pressure (ICP). Three compensatory mechanisms serve to regulate the intracranial space:

- The ability to decrease the production and increase the absorption of CSF

TABLE 21-1   Cranial Nerves Mnemonic

Cranial Nerves	Mnemonic: "On old Olympic towering tops, a Finn and German viewed some hops."
I Olfactory: Sense of smell	On
II Optic: Visual sensory	Old
III Oculomotor: Extraocular eye movements, upper eyelid elevation, papillary construction	Olympic
IV Trochlear: Extraocular eye movement, inferior	Towering
V Trigeminal: Jaw movements including chewing, biting	Tops
VI Abducens: Extraocular eye movements, lateral	A
VII Facial: Sense of taste in anterior area of the tongue, muscle movement of expressions, forehead muscle movement	Finn
VIII Acoustic: Auditory sensory	And
IX Glossopharyngeal: Swallowing ability and coordination, throat sensations and taste in the posterior portion of the tongue	German
X Vagus: Gag reflex, swallowing, abdominal and thoracic visceral movements	Viewed
XI Spinal accessory: Ability to move head and shoulders, rotation of the head	Some
XII Hypoglossal: Tongue movements	Hops

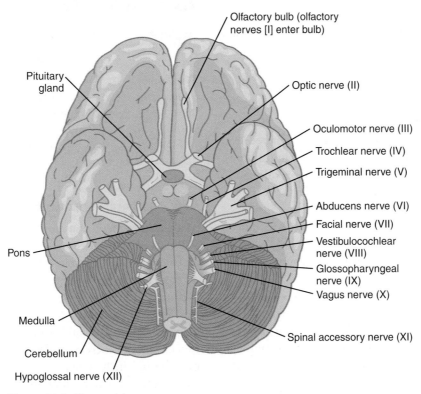

Figure 21-3 *The cranial nerves.*

- The ability to vasoconstrict blood vessels within the brain and surrounding tissues of the head
- The ability to secrete hormones that reduce fluids within the cells and tissue of the brain (aldosterone)

Increased Intracranial Pressure

Increased ICP is not uncommon in children. Indeed, traumatic brain injury (TBI) associated with childhood injuries and trauma is a significant cause of morbidity and mortality in children both in the United States and around the world. The three principal causes of TBI in children are motor vehicle accidents, falls, and intentional injury by assault (child abuse); the last type of trauma is associated with more severe injuries (Deans, Minneci, Lowell, & Groner, 2013).

When a child presents with increasing head circumference measurements, bulging fontanels, misshapen skull bones, irritability, vomiting, increased muscle tone, decreased or altered consciousness, or the setting-sun eyes sign, the pediatric medical team should assess for the presence of increased ICP. Increased ICP can be caused by a rise in the pressure of the ventricles where CSF is produced and absorbed, or it can stem from the presence of a lesion such as a tumor, infectious mass, bleed, clot, or brain tissue swelling. Medical diagnoses such as meningitis, stroke, hydrocephalus, encephalitis, and aneurysm rupture can increase ICP as well. Rapid assessment, confirmation, and medical treatment are warranted in children who present with symptoms of increased ICP.

Increased ICP is directly related to decreased brain tissue perfusion and brain tissue anoxia. In many cases, it represents a secondary brain injury after a child has suffered a traumatic brain injury via a significant head trauma.

Assessments for Increased ICP

Symptoms of increased ICP in infants include altered level of consciousness; separation of the bony cranium sutures; nonpulsating, bulging fontanels; and projectile vomiting and irritability with inconsolability and a shrill, high-pitched cry. In older children, vomiting, headache, lethargy, weakness, diplopia, and seizures can denote increased ICP. Infants may display Macewen sign, also known as cracked pot sign, in which an obvious enlarged venous system appears on the top of the head (**Figure 21-4**).

To assess this condition, the medical team will order a lumbar puncture, magnetic resonance imaging (MRI) or computed tomography (CT), or placement of an intraventricular catheter, which is inserted into the ventricle through a small hole drilled in the skull for pressure readings. If a child's Glasgow Coma Scale score (discussed in detail later in this chapter) is between 3 and 8, the child must undergo

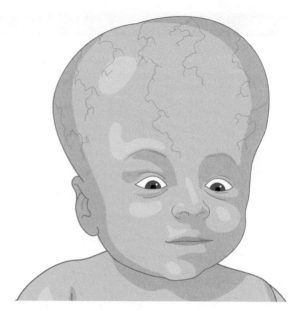

Figure 21-4 *Macewen sign.*

immediate ICP monitoring in an intensive care unit, and will require intubation for respiratory support. Pressure monitoring is done by cannulation of the ventricles or by placement of microtransducer-tipped ICP monitors, which are inserted through a skull bolt into the subdural space or the brain parenchyma (tissues).

UNIQUE FOR KIDS

Normal values for ICP vary depending on the child's age. For infants, ICP should be between 1.5 and 6 mm Hg; young children should have ICP between 3 and 7 mm Hg; and older children and young adults should have ICP readings between 10 and 15 mm Hg. When a child experiences increased ICP with pressure readings exceeding 20 mm Hg for more than 5 minutes, the child will need to be treated to prevent morbidity (Kukreti et al., 2014).

Medical Treatments for Increased ICP

Medical treatment of a child with suspected increased ICP starts with the identification of the associated trauma and stabilization of the injury. If rapid reduction of ICP is required, the pediatric team should administer medications to sedate and/or intubate the child, perform procedures to drain cerebrospinal fluid, and administer osmotherapy to pull fluids from the child's body. Intubation criteria for increased ICP in the setting of traumatic brain injury include hypoxia, hypocapnia, hypercarbia, chest wall dysfunction, and a drop in Glasgow Coma Scale score (Kukreti et al., 2014).

Some institutions have established policies on hyperventilation as a rapid means to reduce ICP. Hyperventilation is reserved for cases in which acute brain herniation is a risk, as this procedure can reduce brain oxygenation (Brasher & Tasker, 2013). Because P_{CO_2} acts as a vasoconstrictor when hyperemia is present, hyperventilation is undertaken to reduce P_{CO_2} and increase blood flow in the child's brain.

The goal of medication therapy for increased ICP is to maintain the child's osmolality to 360 mOsm/L. The following medications are indicated for this purpose:

- Mannitol 5% to 20% IV, to reduce vascular volume (net reduction of brain water) (0.25 to 1 g/kg IV bolus)
- Pentobarbital (nembutal sodium), as barbiturates reduce intracranial hypertension and decrease cerebral metabolic rates
- Osmitrol 5% intravenously, to provide the maximal vascular osmolality
- Hypertonic saline, to shift fluids out of brain tissue without inducing profound osmotic diuresis

BEST PRACTICES

Hypotonic solutions should not be used in patients who have experienced a traumatic brain injury resulting in increased ICP, as extracellular fluid (ECF) shifts to intracellular fluid (ICF) compartments will occur, leading to greater brain tissue edema.

Other procedures used to rapidly reduce ICP include placing the child in a barbiturate coma, implementing a decompressive craniectomy (skull bone removal to provide room for brain swelling), and use of hypothermia to 32–33°C (which provides neuroprotection by reducing cerebral metabolism). After stabilization associated with a traumatic brain injury or a documented increase in production of or lack of absorption of CSF, the child's condition may require surgical placement of a shunt to remove CSF from the ventricles of the brain.

Ventricular-Peritoneal Shunts

Shunt placement consists of the surgical implantation of a drainage system that extends from the inner cavity of one of the larger brain ventricles, down to the child's peritoneal cavity (**Figure 21-5**). The shunt provides for gravity-induced drainage of excessive CSF causing increased intracranial pressure. Nursing care includes daily measurement of head circumference, protection from postoperative infection, and early identification of shunt failure by monitoring for signs of increased ICP.

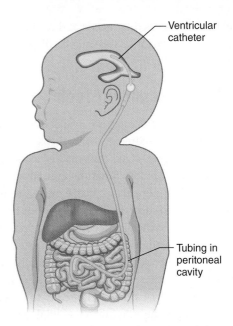

Ventricular catheter

Tubing in peritoneal cavity

Figure 21-5 *Placement of a ventricular-peritoneal shunt.*

QUALITY AND SAFETY

When a child with a ventricular-peritoneal (VP) shunt experiences a sudden onset of symptoms associated with increasing ICP (e.g., projectile vomiting, headaches, fussiness, inconsolable crying), the nurse should suspect a shunt complication. Such complications can include kinking of the tubing leading to obstruction, clogging of the shunt tubing by infection or cellular debris, and disconnection of the tubing or migration of the tips of the tubing as the child grows.

Nursing Care of the Child with Increased ICP

Caring for a child who has experienced a traumatic brain injury or a pathological condition where the production or absorption of CSF is dysfunctional requires specialized training. The pediatric nurse will provide protection from harm, protection from infection during ICP monitoring, and care of the intubated child. The height of bed is raised to 30 degrees, the child's head is maintained in a midline position, and the child's airway is maintained. The child's pain and anxiety levels (if the child is not sedated) should be a priority, as both of these factors can increase cerebral metabolic demand. Maintaining a calm environment, reducing coughing, and reducing discomfort and sensory stimuli will assist the pediatric patient in maintaining a lower ICP.

Parents of a child with increased ICP will be in distress and need supportive nursing care. A social worker should be brought in to assess their needs and resources. Parent education on the various assessments, diagnostics, and treatments is also required.

Neurologic Assessment Tools

A variety of assessment tools are available to determine neurologic health in children. A comprehensive assessment should include a mental status exam as well as assessments of motor function, sensory function, cranial nerve function, and reflexes. The pediatric nurse must assemble the equipment needed to successfully assess a child's neurologic status. Depending on the practice setting, various supplies should be readily available for the healthcare team to use.

In practice, neurologic assessments usually focus on the problem or concern presented by the child. It is more typical for the pediatric nurse to be ready to check pupil reaction with a pen light, a full set of vital signs, motor function assessment, sensory function assessment, and level of consciousness assessment.

Pediatric Glasgow Coma Scale

A frequently used rapid test of a child's neurologic status is the Pediatric Glasgow Coma Scale (**Figure 21-6**). The nurse, or other members of the pediatric healthcare team, can use this scale to test the child's best response to motor movement, verbal response, and eye opening. Unique to pediatrics, this scale does not require that the child be able to verbalize his or her response; that is, the adult version of the Glasgow Coma Scale was modified to allow even preverbal children to be tested with this tool.

Scores on the Pediatric Glasgow Coma Scale range from 3 to 15. Often, if a child's score is 8 or less, the child will require rapid transport to a higher level of care and intubation. Remember: "If it's 8, intubate." A score of 7 typically indicates the child is in a coma. A score of 3 may indicate brain death.

Reflexes

Children's reflexes can be organized into two larger categories: those associated with the newborn and young infant, and those associated with older children. Primitive reflexes can be found in the newborn through the first several months of life, but most of them disappear by the sixth to eighth months of life. Deep tendon reflexes are present in older children and persist throughout the life span.

Pediatric Glasgow Coma Scale (GCS)

Activity	Score	Infant	Score	Child
Eye opening	4	Open spontaneously	4	Open spontaneously
	3	Open to speech or sound	3	Open to speech
	2	Open to painful stimuli	2	Open to painful stimuli
	1	No response	1	No response
Verbal	5	Coos, babbles	5	Oriented conversation
	4	Irritable cry	4	Confused conversation
	3	Cries to pain	3	Cries
	2	Moans to pain	2	Inappropriate words
	1	No response	1	Moans
				Incomprehensible words/sounds
				No response
Motor	6	Normal spontaneous movement	6	Obeys verbal commands
	5	Localizes pain	5	Localizes pain
	4	Withdraws to pain	4	Withdraws to pain
	3	Abnormal flexion (decorticate)	3	Abnormal flexion (decorticate)
	2	Abnormal extension (decerebrate)	2	Abnormal extension (decerebrate)
	1	No response (flaccid)	1	No response (flaccid)

Figure 21-6 *The Pediatric Glasgow Coma Scale.*

Data from Pediatric Advanced Life Support, 2012, the American Heart Association.

Primitive Reflexes

- Babinski reflex: Assesses for pyramidal tract dysfunction, with the infant dorsiflexing the great toe and then quickly fanning out the toes. This reflex may be present up to 1 year of age.
- Moro reflex: Change in equilibrium when the head falls back slightly (no more than 3 to 5 cm); the infant will open the hands, extend and abduct the arms, and then bring them back together. This reflex disappears by 6 months of age.
- Tonic neck reflex/fencer's stance: With a slight movement of the infant's head to either side while lying supine, the child will extend the arm and leg out on the side where the head was turned, mimicking a fencer's pose. This reflex disappears by 6 to 7 months of age.
- Dancing reflex: Placing supportive hands on the newborn's chest wall, and then holding the infant with feet just touching a surface, causes the child to display small dancing movements.
- Crawling reflex: When the newborn is placed prone, the infant makes slight crawling movements.
- Startle reflex: When a newborn or young infant hears a sudden sound, the child will display the same signs as noted with the Moro reflex.
- Sucking reflex: Assesses afferent fibers of cranial nerves V and IX, and efferent fibers of cranial nerves VII, IX, and XII.

Deep Tendon Reflexes

Deep tendon reflexes test the efferent neurons in the anterior horn of the spinal cord. Hyperreflexia may indicate a lesion above the level of the spinal reflex pathway, whereas hyporeflexia is a diminished response to the tapping of the area and can also indicate disease. The following deep tendon reflexes are typically tested:

- Biceps reflex (C5–6)
- Brachioradialis reflex (C5–6)
- Knee jerk reflex or patellar (L2–4)
- Ankle jerk reflex (S1–2)

Reflexes are never used by themselves as a diagnostic tool for neurologic health or disease, but rather are considered part of a more extensive assessment for neurologic health or problems. Deep tendon reflexes are graded using a 0 to 4+ scale, where 0 is an absence of reflex response and 4+ indicates a clonus type of reaction with repeating reflex demonstration. A score of 2+ is considered a normal and expected reflex response.

Motor Function

The assessment of motor function is considered an overall gross examination of the child's central or peripheral

UNIQUE FOR KIDS

Distraction has been shown to enhance the chance of obtaining a deep tendon reflex response. One often-successful method is to have the child grasp the hands together and then, just before eliciting the reflex, ask the child to quickly pull apart the grasped hands.

nervous system health. Motor function testing in children includes gait, presence of ataxia, motor strength, and bilateral abilities. Simple play that includes retrieving a ball, playing catch, or skipping down a hallway can assist in the assessment of motor function.

Levels of Consciousness

Expected levels of consciousness for a child may be described as awake, wakefulness, alert, oriented, playful, and in a state of expected interaction, as appropriate for the child's developmental level. Determining a child's level of consciousness on the following continuum helps to determine whether a child has recently experienced or is currently experiencing a neurologic disorder:

- Alert
- Drowsiness
- Confusion
- Stupor
- Obtunded
- Coma

Neurologic Diagnostic Exams

A child who presents with neurologic symptoms may need to undergo invasive and noninvasive diagnostic exams and laboratory analysis to detect the cause and form a diagnosis. The following tests are often used in children to determine pathology.

- *Electroencephalogram (EEG):* EEG is a measurement of electrical activity within the brain to assess the location and severity of seizure activity. It is usually conducted over a 24-hour period and uses a video to capture activity.
- *Lumbar puncture:* Sterile placement of a needle into the subarachnoid space of the lumbar spinal column (L3-4 or L4-5) may be performed to obtain specimens, assess level of pressure, and administer medications such as intrathecal chemotherapy.
- *MRI of the head:* MRI, a noninvasive diagnostic procedure without ionizing radiation, is used to evaluate the brain, CNS, and bones, and to look for masses, tumors, and lesions.

- *Positron emission tomography (PET) scan:* PET scan is used to detect tumors, lesions, and trauma. Radioactive chemicals are administered and then tracked to detect abnormalities.
- *Electromyography:* This technology, which records electrical activity during muscle rest and activity, is used to diagnose nerve and muscle disorders.
- *Nerve conduction velocity:* This test measures the ability of a nerve to send an electrical conduction via flat electrodes; one electrode sends a signal to the nerve, and the other detects the muscle response.
- *Ventricular tap:* Needle placement into an infant's bulging fontanel is directed at the subdural space or the ventricle via the anterior fontanel. This method is used to find an etiology for excessive head growth and increased ICP.
- *ICP monitoring:* This process allows for the assessment of pressure readings (20 mm Hg or higher) within the ventricles through subarachnoid bolts or intraventricular catheter placement.
- *Laboratory analysis:* Lab tests may assess for spinal infections, inflammation (C-reactive protein [CRP] or erythrocyte sedimentation rate [ESR]), infection (blood cultures), urinalysis, serum levels of anticonvulsants, toxins and illicit drugs, complete blood cell count (CBC) with differentiation of the white blood cell (WBC) count, viral cultures for meningitis, metabolic testing for protein disorders, and genetic testing for neurologic disorders.

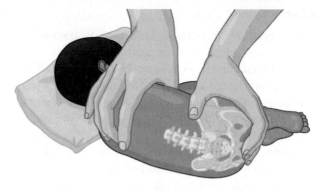

Figure 21-7 *An infant in a fetal position, held tightly in a curl, for optimal positioning during a lumbar puncture.*

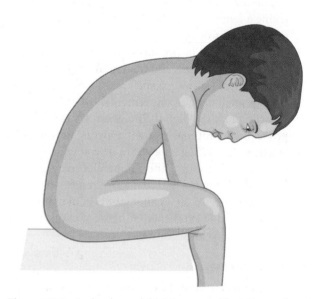

Figure 21-8 *A school-age child sitting up and flexed forward, ready for a lumbar puncture.*

Definitions of Neurologic Impairments or Disorders

Under the concept of intracranial regulation, a variety of disorders may be encountered in childhood, ranging from the newborn period through adolescence. This section describes neurologic disorders that can be either acquired or considered congenital.

Abusive Head Trauma (Shaken Baby Syndrome)

The form of child abuse previously referred to as "shaken baby syndrome" and now more commonly called **abusive head trauma** is a severe form of nonaccidental cerebral trauma leading to encephalopathy (American Academy of Pediatrics [AAP], 2015; Parks, Annest, Hill, & Karch, 2012). Abusive head trauma is associated with high morbidity and mortality. Leaving few external signs, the injury is multifactorial and includes retinopathy (diagnostic marker), shearing of the brain vasculature, subdural hemorrhages (diagnostic marker), diffuse brain tissue injury, respiratory distress, and increased ICP. Children may present with paralysis, coma, and multiple fractures. A single vigorous shaking episode of an infant or young child can lead to long-term consequences or death (AAP, 2015).

The injury associated with abusive head trauma is described as being a whiplash type of injury. During the shaking episode, the child's brain experiences an abrupt and uncontrolled coup-contrecoup injury through an accelerated, then decelerated movement of the brain in the cranium, with or without a rotator component. These injuries are also described as translational forces producing linear movement of the brain (Frasier & Coats, 2015). Impact injuries may be noted as well. If impact injuries are present, the severity of the consequences of abusive head trauma increases. Central apnea associated with extension of the medulla oblongata, mostly associated with severe shaking, can be fatal. Death is reported in as many as 36% of severe abusive head trauma cases (Matschke et al., 2009).

Diagnosis

Radiographic and ophthalmologic findings are used to confirm a diagnosis of abusive head trauma (Frasier & Coats, 2015). "Flame-like" hemorrhages of the retina (**Figure 21-9**), bleeding in the optic nerve, and swelling of the eye structures are confirmatory findings (AAP, 2015). Subdural hematoma (SDH) is not exclusively seen in abuse cases, but the presence of SDH is strongly associated with cases of abuse (AAP, 2015), but not with accidental injury. Thus, if SDH is present, the possibility of abuse should be considered. Children who present with respiratory distress with no obvious adventitious breath sounds should also be considered for abusive head trauma.

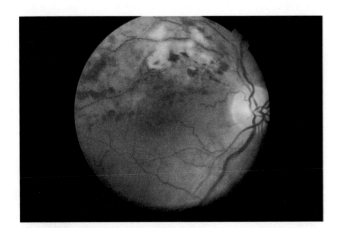

Figure 21-9 *"Flame-like" retinal hemorrhages indicative of abusive head trauma.*

© Michael Abbey/Science Source

Risk Factors

Occurring in all social, ethnic, and economic strata, abusive head trauma is associated with parental stressors including alcohol use, drug abuse, disability of the child, teenage parenting, and violent tendencies of the caregiver (Matschke et al., 2009). Unrealistic expectations, single parenthood, instability of the home life, parental depression, and maltreatment history of the parent are other risk factors (Paul & Adamo, 2014).

Medical Treatment

Treatment for abusive head trauma is supportive. Children may need to be intubated and monitored for increased ICP in the pediatric intensive care unit (PICU). The sequence of medical management is to initiate vital life support, suspect that the child has been shaken, investigate for retinal bleeds, conduct diagnostic imaging (MRI or CT), and involve social services and law enforcement agencies (Christian, 2016).

Understanding the long-term consequences of abusive head trauma, which may include blindness, cognitive impairment, learning disabilities, seizure disorders, motor dysfunction, cerebral palsy, and hydrocephalus, can assist the medical team in providing supportive care.

Nursing Care

The most important aspect of nursing care is prevention of abusive head trauma. Nurses are in the ideal position to offer preventive education to families being discharged from maternity units, nurseries, neonatal intensive care units (NICUs), and pediatric clinics. Understanding that children younger than 3 to 4 years are at highest risk for child abuse, nurses must develop educational programs that address the prevention and consequences of child abuse. Physical vulnerabilities of children must be communicated, such as their disproportionally larger heads, weak neck muscles, and inability to communicate needs. Inconsolable crying, male sex, colic, increased medical needs, and prematurity are all factors that put a child at risk for abusive head trauma (Walls, 2006).

RESEARCH EVIDENCE

In a clinical trial, educational materials were deemed effective in improving parental understanding of general crying, unsoothable crying, dangers of shaking, and behaviors of walking away when frustrated and caregiver self-talk (Barr et al., 2008). The findings supported the contention that abusive head trauma prevention materials are effective in promoting education concerning risk factors.

Meningitis

Three primary layers of connective tissue surround and protect the brain. The dura mater, the thickest protective layer, lines the skull bones and folds into the brain fissures to provide protection and stability. The arachnoid membrane, the middle protective layer, is much thinner and more fragile. The final layer, closest to the brain tissue, is the pia mater; this layer is extremely thin and very vascular. Collectively, these layers are referred to as the meninges. Inflammation or infection of these layers, called **meningitis**, can be viral, bacterial, or aseptic in nature.

Diagnosis

Prior to administering antibiotic therapy to a pediatric patient, it is important for the healthcare team to collect blood cultures and cerebrospinal fluid via a lumbar puncture (Bonadio, 2014). Bacterial meningitis can be caused by a variety of microbes, but the two most commonly isolated in children are *Streptococcus pneumoniae* and *Neisseria meningitidis*. In the past, *Escherichia coli*, *Haemophilus influenzae* type B (Hib), and beta-hemolytic *Streptococcus* also were common culprits. *E. coli* infection has until fairly recently been easily managed with beta-lactam antibiotics, so *E. coli* meningitis has become unusual (although growing antibiotic resistance may change that status), while effective vaccines have reduced the incidence of HiB- and beta-hemolytic *Streptococcus*–related cases (Brouwer, Tunkel, & van de Beek, 2010; Peña et al., 2008).

Risk Factors

Children may be exposed to bacteria that reach the meninges via bloodstream infections. When a child has bacterial otitis media, sinusitis, mastoiditis, or pharyngitis, the bacteria can enter the bloodstream and directly infect the meninges. Bacterial meningitis can progress into the CSF, which includes few WBCs, and flourish to the point that it becomes a very significant and potentially lethal infection. Children who are on long-term corticosteroids or who are immunosuppressed are particularly vulnerable to complicated meningitis. Meningitis is associated with the following signs and symptoms:

- Vomiting
- Fever
- Irritability, exacerbated by cuddling and close holding or rocking
- Nuchal rigidity (pain and resistance to neck flexion)
- Change in eating or feeding patterns
- Headache
- Lethargy
- Seizures

- Change in level of consciousness
- **Kernig's sign**: severe hamstring stiffness, such that the child cannot straighten the leg when the hip is flexed to 90 degrees (**Figure 21-10**)
- **Brudzinski's sign**: severe neck stiffness, which causes the child's hips and knees to flex when the neck is flexed (**Figure 21-11**)
- Photophobia

Medical Treatments

Medical treatments for bacterial meningitis consist of the rapid initiation of antibiotic therapy. Medication classes used for this purpose include ampicillins, cephalosporins, aminoglycosides, and penicillins. Intravenous or oral corticosteroids may be used on a trial basis to reduce inflammation and prevent complications such as hearing loss. If the meningitis is determined to have a viral etiology, the treatment is supportive, including bed rest, fluids, analgesics, and infection precautions.

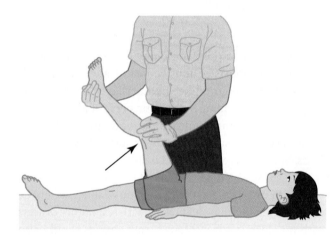

Figure 21-10 *Kernig's sign.*

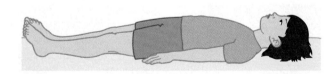

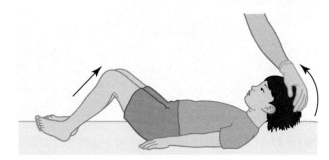

Figure 21-11 *Brudzinski's sign.*

Nursing Care

Children who present with symptoms of meningitis should be immediately placed on droplet and contact precautions. Isolation precautions should be maintained for no less than 24 hours of intravenous antibiotic therapy. All specimens should be collected before the administration of antibiotics. The child should be kept at rest, with lower stimulation; specifically, lights should be kept low and noise should be minimized.

Brain Tumors

As the most common solid tumors found across childhood, brain tumors have the highest rates of mortality of any of the childhood malignancies (Ward, DeSantis, Robbins, Kohler, & Jemal, 2014). The vast majority of brain tumors are located in the supratentorial region (above the cerebellum). The etiology of most childhood brain tumors remains unknown. Fourteen types of brain tumors are distinguished, based on the tumor histology (tissue type). The most common brain tumors in children are medulloblastoma, ependymoma, and astrocytoma (American Brain Tumor Association, 2014). There are no known risk factors for development of childhood brain tumors.

Diagnosis

The diagnosis of brain tumors includes recent medical history, neurologic examination, and diagnostic procedures. Children may report vomiting and nausea, especially upon rising in the morning and resolving after vomiting, and headaches. Neurologic symptoms may include tingling, weakness, abnormal paresthesia, trouble walking or balance issues, and vision, hearing, and speech problems. Brain MRI with gadolinium injection, CT, and PET scans are most frequently ordered to assess for brain tumors. A lumbar puncture is performed to determine whether the disease has spread to the CSF or surrounding cord tissues. If the child presents with back pain or pain that extends from the back out the arms or down the legs, spinal metastasis is suspected.

Medical Treatment

Treatment for brain tumors is complicated. The child might initially undergo a tumor biopsy so definitive histology can be determined. The child typically will have a tumor resection if able, or a tumor reduction if the tumor is not resectable. If the tissue type is radiosensitive, radiation treatment is administered over the course of several weeks. The total radiation dose is determined and then divided based the desired treatment length. Chemotherapy may be included with treatment. Treatment protocols may follow guidelines provided by organizations such as the Children's Oncology Group (COG), an international consortium of pediatric oncologists and clinics that pool their data to support assessment of treatment regimens and data collection and analysis of outcomes.

Nursing Care

Nursing care includes assessment for and immediate reporting of complications associated with the presence of the tumor and the treatment of the tumor. A space-occupying lesion can lead to increased ICP, neurologic symptoms, and discomfort. The nurse should monitor for pain, nausea and vomiting (especially on rising in the morning), changes in visual acuity, diminishing productivity at school (e.g., due to tumor-induced strabismus and nystagmus), personality changes, increasing head circumference, ataxia, and clumsiness. Children with brain tumors should be placed on seizure precautions and assisted with ambulation until independence is fully assessed. Safety is key for a child with a neurologic tumor.

If a child has undergone a surgical biopsy or resection of the tumor, immediate postoperative needs include bed rest with the head of the bed elevated by 10 to 20 degrees for several hours. Postoperative pain assessments, neurologic status, vital signs, mental status, and emotional status should all be evaluated.

QUALITY AND SAFETY

In the immediate postoperative period for a child undergoing surgical manipulation of a brain tumor, the nurse must be cautious not to contribute to increased ICP. The nurse should treat pain immediately, never place the child in a Trendelenburg position, monitor for hyperthermia associated with brain edema, and keep the child comfortable and calm.

Children with brain tumors and their families need very special and empathetic nursing care. These children may undergo many months or years of treatments, surgeries, and diagnostics. Support and hope are needed to assist the family in tolerating the multiple healthcare interactions and facing the unknowns associated with whether their child can be cured.

Seizure Disorders

Seizure disorders occur when a wave of abnormal and excessive electrical activity in a child's brain causes changes in motor movements, levels of awareness, and behavior. The term *epilepsy* is used to denote a tendency to have recurrent seizures. The term *convulsion* is sometimes used to describe a grand mal, tonic-clonic seizure. Severe seizure activity can be very frightening to parents, as the child may lose consciousness, experience uncontrollable jerking movements, froth at the mouth with excessive saliva, and bite the tongue.

Numerous etiologies are associated with childhood seizure activity, but the majority of children who have an epileptic disorder have no identifiable cause. Eighty-percent of seizures that occur in the first year of life have no etiology that can be isolated in diagnostic exams or laboratory analysis. Across childhood, seizures can be associated with overall or diffuse brain dysfunction such as occurs with rapid-onset high fevers, exposure to toxins, exposure to drugs, neoplasms or tumors, space-occupying lesions, hypertension, or bleeds.

Diagnosis

A 24-hour EEG with video is the cornerstone of diagnosing seizures not associated with fevers in children. Either an MRI or a CT may also be performed in an attempt to detect the presence of brain abnormalities predisposing the child to the erratic electrical currency generated in the brain that leads to seizure activity. **Table 21-2** identifies the international classifications used for childhood epileptic seizures.

Risk Factors

Risk factors for children presenting with seizures include a variety of pathologies, trauma, injuries, and bleeds. Periods of anoxia to the brain are associated with the development of seizure activity.

Medical Treatment

Current medications administered to children include single-medication regimens as well as multidrug regimens for nonresponsive patients or in case of continued seizure activity. **Box 21-2** summarizes the medications used for treating pediatric seizures.

TABLE 21-2	International Classification of Seizures
Partial Seizures	
› Simple partial seizures	
› Complex partial seizures	
Generalized Seizures	
› **Absence seizures**: Most often noted in a child's classroom, when the child "checks out" and is nonresponsive for a brief period	
› Atonic seizures: Noted as an abrupt loss of the child's muscle tone	
› Myoclonic seizures: Brief, symmetrical, repetitive movements	
› Clonic seizures: Jerking, rhythmic muscle movements, such as flexion of the child's extremities	
› Tonic seizures: Sustained muscular contraction	
› Tonic-clonic seizures (**grand mal seizure**): Combination of abnormal muscular activity including tonic (sustained contraction) and clonic (jerking movements) features	
› **Febrile seizures**: Seizure that occurs in children ranging from 3 months to 6 years of age, which is not classified as an epileptic seizure disorder. Fevers that have rapid onset, but are not always high, can cause a child to have a generalized grand mal seizure lasting 1–2 minutes. Febrile seizures have familial tendencies and lower the threshold for subsequent fever-induced seizure activity. Anticonvulsants are rarely ordered for children who experience such seizures; treatment is preventive, through the administration of antipyretics at the onset of a suspected febrile illness and on an around-the-clock basis until the illness ends.	

BOX 21-2   Medications for Treatment of Seizures in Children

- Carbamazepine (Tegretol or Carbatrol)
- Clonazepam (Klonopin)
- Ethosuximide (Zarontin)
- Lamotrigine (Lamictal)
- Levetiracetam (Keppra)
- Oxcarbazepine (Trileptal)
- Phenobarbital (Luminal)
- Phenytoin (Dilantin)
- Tiagabine (Gabitril)
- Topiramate (Topamax)
- Valproic acid (Depakote or Depakene)

Data from Goldenberg, M. M. (2010). Overview of drugs used for epilepsy and seizures: Etiology, diagnosis, and treatment. *Pharmacy and Therapeutics, 35*(7), 392–415.

PHARMACOLOGY

Children who test positive for the HLA-B*1502 allele should not take the common antiseizure medication carbamazepine due to their increased risk of developing Stevens-Johnson syndrome. HLA testing may be suggested for children in higher-risk ethnic groups (Schachter, 2016).

FAMILY EDUCATION

Families of children who are prescribed phenytoin need education on the side effects of gingival hypertrophy, rash, folic acid depletion, and increased body hair (Schachter, 2016).

Nursing Care

Besides promoting safety in all aspects of the child's home, recreational, and academic life, the second most important aspect of nursing care of a child with a seizure disorder is to support the child and family with medical adherence, demonstrated by adequate and safe ranges of serum anticonvulsant therapy. Education is paramount so that families will understand the importance of ensuring consistent anticonvulsant medication administration, at the same time each day, so dips in serum concentrations of the medications do not occur. Many children with complicated seizure disorders have a low seizure threshold and need their medications taken on time and with great consistency. Families need to be taught to document any seizure activity, including precipitating factors, seizure activity witnessed, and length of each seizure.

When interacting with families whose child is suspected of having a seizure, the pediatric nurse should ask the following questions:

- In which setting did the seizure activity occur? At which time of day?
- Which activity was the child participating in just before the seizure began?
- What were the precipitating factors occurring just prior to the seizure?
- Did the child describe a sensory experience (aura) prior to the seizure?
- What did the seizure behavior look like? Was it general or focal? What were the limb movements like?
- What was the duration of the seizure activity?
- What the child's postseizure behavior? Was there a postictal state (i.e., somnolence, confusion, sleepiness, fatigue)?
- What is the child's medical history, current state, and overall state of health?

Other Neurologic Disorders

Muscular Dystrophy

Muscular dystrophy comprises a group of inherited progressively degenerative diseases that cause muscle weakness, atrophy, and degeneration. When the disease has a childhood onset, it tends to be Duchenne muscular dystrophy, which mostly affects males.

The pathology of muscular dystrophy is linked to a genetically induced reduction or absence of dystrophin, a muscle protein. As muscle fibers degenerate, the body fills the vacated space with connective tissue layers and adipose tissue. Key signs of muscular dystrophy are waddling gait, weakened pelvic floor, wide stance when standing, and Gower's sign (difficulty with rising from a sitting or lying position). Progression of the disease is rapid, with most

RESEARCH EVIDENCE

Ketogenic Diets and Neuroprotection Properties

Previous research has shown that a ketogenic diet—which consists of significant carbohydrate restriction and high fat intake (80% to 90% of calories)—can reduce seizures in children with medication-resistant or hard-to-control disorders. A strict ketogenic diet appears to promote certain chemical neuroprotective properties. For example, ketone bodies such as β-hydroxybutyrate may protect nerves against cellular injury by increasing anti-inflammatory and antioxidant effects, as well as increasing energy reserves for neurons affected by injury (Martin, Jackson, Levy, & Cooper, 2016). Activation of adenosine triphosphate (ATP)–sensitive potassium channels and inhibition of glutamatergic excitatory synaptic transmission are other mechanisms that have been suggested as being protective (Danial, Hartman, Stastrom, & Thio, 2013).

affected children no longer being able to ambulate by 12 years of age. Diagnosis is confirmed by muscle biopsy, electromyography, and increased serum creatine kinase levels due to muscle breakdown.

There is no known cure for muscular dystrophy, so treatment is supportive. Nursing care focuses on providing a safe environment, promoting an emotional support system for the child and family, encouraging good nutrition, and supporting the respiratory system.

Cerebral Palsy

Cerebral palsy (CP) is a nonprogressive, neuromuscular disorder that is most commonly associated with pathology induced by a hypoxic or anoxic birth incident affecting the segment of the brain that controls motor function. Many maternal influences have been known to contribute to CP, including infections (especially rubella), drug ingestions, periods of anoxia, isoimmunization, toxemia, and diabetes. Perinatal influences include prolapsed cord, placenta abruptio, and delay in delivery of the newborn's head. The three types of CP are spastic (affecting the cortex), ataxic (cerebellum), and athetoid (basal ganglia).

Many children with CP have poor control of motor movements, and some experience paralysis. In some cases, cognitive function and intelligence may not be affected at all, but different forms of cognitive and other neurologic impairments (e.g., speech, vision) occur to varying degrees (Odding, Roebroeck, & Stam, 2006). Typical clinical symptoms include abnormal motor performance, delayed gross motor development, thin extremities, abnormal gait (e.g., scissors gait), hypertonia, flexion, contractures, sensory defects, and feeding difficulty.

Treatments for CP are not curative. Medications used for such patients include baclofen to relieve spasticity and muscle relaxants. Nursing care involves family support and education to prevent injury, reduce contraction of muscles through range of motion (ROM) exercises, and assessments for nutrition risks and skin breakdown.

Guillain-Barré Syndrome

Guillain-Barré syndrome is a progressive ascending polyneuritis leading to paralysis. Without resolution, this progressive condition can be fatal if severe respiratory distress leads to complete respiratory failure. The pathology stems from the body's autoimmune attack on the myelin (phospholipid protein) sheath of peripheral nerve cells. In children, the etiology of Guillain-Barré syndrome is often associated with a resolving gastrointestinal viral infection or some other immune system stimulus.

There is no treatment for this syndrome. Medical support to maintain adequate ventilation may be required while the condition takes its course. Most children recover from Guillain-Barré syndrome; few have lasting neurologic sequelae.

Neural Tube Defects

Neural tube defects, which include spina bifida, are structural defects of the central nervous system due to inadequate closure of the neural tube during fetal development. This state may produce any of several defects, all with variable severity. Research has shown that inadequate maternal consumption of folic acid at conception and in the first trimester of pregnancy increases the risk of neural tube defects in the fetus.

Spina bifida (**Figure 21-12**) is divided into two main classifications:

- Meningocele, where the bony spinal column is open, allowing for a sac to protrude that contains CSF and the meninges
- Myelomeningocele, where the protrusion includes the CSF, the meninges, and a segment of the child's spinal cord

Medical treatment for spina bifida consists of surgical repair. Nursing care includes immediate care of the sac after delivery, preoperative and postoperative care of the incision, and education for the family on the complications associated with the varying severity of the defect. Children may have motor limitations and weakness, decreased bladder function and increased risks for urinary tract infection, inadequacy of bowel control, increased risk for hydrocephalus, increased ICP, meningitis, and paralysis. Complications depend on the severity of the spinal cord involvement. Children with spina bifida are also at increased risk for latex allergies.

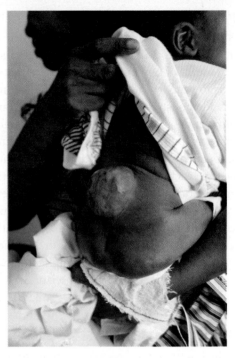

Figure 21-12 *A child with spina bifida.*
© Diomedia/BSIP

Hypoxic Ischemic Encephalopathy

Hypoxic ischemic encephalopathy (HIE) is often the pathological consequence of a near-drowning experience, but may be present in newborns who are asphyxiated at birth (Fatemi, Wilson, & Johnston, 2009) and can sometimes be seen in children who have suffered intentional injuries, such as choking or abusive head trauma (AAP, 2015). In neonates, the injury can lead to cerebral palsy and multiple disabilities.

The child who has suffered a nonfatal drowning may have irreversible multisystem injuries, including multi-organ hypoxia from prolonged hypoxemia. The lungs, brain, and kidneys are most likely to be affected with HIE. Within the brain, the tissues most susceptible to injury are the hippocampus, insular cortex, and basal ganglia. Long-term consequences related to submersion accidents depend on the duration of submersion and the success of aggressive resuscitation efforts in the field (Suominen & Vahatalo, 2012).

Concussions

Concussions in childhood are mainly associated with sports injuries or head injuries during recreational activities. As many as 53% of child athletes have reported experiencing a concussion by the time they enter high school. The majority of concussions occur in children age 10 to 19. Considered a mild TBI, the impact of a direct hit to the head causes the child's brain to develop neuropathy such as micro-bleeds and axonal injury.

Single concussions are considered to produce a transient brain injury; subsequent concussions can increase the risk for greater neurodegenerative impairment, including memory loss, traumatic encephalopathy, post-traumatic stress disorder, and cognitive defects. Due to the potential short- and long-term effects of a repeat concussion (particularly if the first one is incompletely healed), children who suffer from a concussion should be protected from a recurrence until a doctor's examination pronounces the first incident completely resolved (Harmon et al., 2013).

Concussion symptoms are organized into four categories: thinking/remembering, physical, emotional/mood, and sleep (Centers for Disease Control and Prevention [CDC], 2016a). The first category includes difficulty concentrating, thinking clearly, or remembering new information, and can be expressed as "feeling slow." Physical symptoms include dizziness, poor balance, nausea, vomiting, headache, fatigue, photophobia, and poor coordination. Emotional or mood symptoms include anxiety, irritability, and depression. Sleep disturbances may range from insomnia to hypersomnia, or involve difficulty falling asleep. Loss of consciousness is not needed to make a diagnosis of a concussion. Symptoms can start immediately following impact, or they can be progressive or be delayed (Semple et al., 2015).

Severe Lead Poisoning

Despite national efforts to reduce exposure, children continue to be exposed to significant levels of lead in more than 4 million homes in the United States. *Healthy People 2020* and the Centers for Disease Control and Prevention have undertaken initiatives designed to reduce childhood lead blood levels that are more than 10 mcg/dL. The CDC uses a blood serum level of 5 mcg/dL to identify children who have been exposed to lead and need case management. Medical management with chelation therapy is needed when levels reach 45 mcg/dL; prior to that point, it is more effective to remove lead sources from the child's environment than to rely on chelation therapy (Lowry, 2010). Serum blood levels of lead that reach 90 mcg/dL have been associated with neurologic consequences, including cerebral edema (CDC, 2016b).

Cerebral Bleeds

Cerebral vascular accidents in childhood are rare, but are associated primarily with prematurity, trauma, anatomic malformations such as Chiari malformation or arteriovenous malformation, or aneurysm. Children who experience cerebral bleeds require rapid identification and treatment. Symptoms include severe sudden headaches; vomiting; dizziness; trouble with movement, speech, or vision; and seizures.

Two types of cerebral bleeds are distinguished:

- **Subdural hematoma**: Caused by an injury or accident, it is considered a slower venous bleed leading to a clot below the dura mater but outside of brain tissue. Veins tear and bleed often from skull fractures.
- **Epidural hematoma**: Caused by an injury to the head, it is considered a rapid arterial bleed where a clot forms above the dura mater. This cerebral arterial bleed is also associated with skull fractures.

Childhood Migraines

Migraine headaches are not uncommon in children, and the average age of symptom onset is 7. There is a link between childhood migraines and hereditary factors. Symptoms of childhood migraines include unilateral or bilateral pain often described as pounding or throbbing, nausea, vertigo, vomiting, body paresthesias, and photosensitivity. Migraines can be exacerbated by menses in adolescent females.

Treatment for migraines should be holistic and include rest, stress management, diet, removal of known environmental triggers (e.g., lights, weather changes, altitude changes, odors, screen time) and stress-related triggers, adequate sleep, and exercise. Some children are very sensitive to nitrates in food, so their consumption should be avoided.

Medical management requires one or more of the following pharmacologic categories: abortive medications that work on blood vessel receptors, preventive medications to influence the onset of a migraine episode, and rescue analgesic medications for immediate pain relief (Johns Hopkins Medicine, 2015). Specific medications for childhood migraines include the following agents:

- Beta blockers
- Antiseizure medications
- Tricyclic antidepressants
- Naproxen
- Acetaminophen
- Ibuprofen
- Triptans

PHARMACOLOGY

Preventive Therapies Used in Childhood Migraine Headaches

- Antidepressant: amitriptyline
- Antihistamines: cyproheptadine
- Antiepileptics: levetiracetam, divalproex sodium, or topiramate
- Calcium-channel blockers: flunarizine

Case Study

Martin, a 17-year-old adolescent, has just begun summer training for his third and final year on the high school football team. Currently in great physical shape, he has been gearing up throughout the summer for a vigorous physical team sport by working out and running. Playing as the linebacker, Martin experienced a moderate concussion with a brief loss of consciousness during a preseason practice game with his own team members. The game was put on hold while 911 was called. Paramedics responded by driving onto the playing field and picking Martin up for rapid transport to the nearest emergency department (ED). In the ED, the healthcare team conducted a physical exam, followed by a health history. Knowing the circumstances surrounding the injury, the pediatric team prepared for diagnostics.

Case Study Questions

1. How is a concussion diagnosed?
2. What are the clinical signs and symptoms of a concussion?
3. What are the components of a nurse-led developmentally appropriate teaching session for young athletes at risk for concussions?
4. What are the risks of continuing to participate in a football game after a child has experienced a concussion?

As the Case Evolves. . .

Martin has been diagnosed with a concussion. This is the first concussion he has experienced, and his parents ask the nurse which symptoms they might expect.

5. Which of the following answers are correct? (Select all that apply.)
   A. Headache, blurry vision, and dizziness
   B. Excessive hunger or thirst
   C. Hyperactivity and high energy
   D. Anxiety, nervousness, and depression
   E. Insomnia, difficulty falling asleep, or excessive sleepiness

Martin has been recovering from his concussion at home. He has experienced a few symptoms of headache, dizziness, poor coordination, forgetfulness, and anxiety. Four days after the initial injury, he decides to "clear his head" by going for a bike ride. Unfortunately, he forgets to put his helmet on. While turning onto the street, Martin loses control of his bike and falls, hitting his head against a signpost on the sidewalk. A nurse who works at the local hospital and who helped treat Martin during his visit 4 days ago is walking nearby. Recognizing him, the nurse comes to Martin's aid, only to find that he is unconscious, with dilated pupils.

6. What is the correct next action to take?
   A. Stay with Martin until he returns to consciousness and tell him to walk (not ride) back to his house and explain what happened to his parents.
   B. Assist Martin in returning home once he wakes up and advise his parents to follow up with his pediatrician as soon as possible.
   C. Call Martin's parents to come get him and advise them to bring him to a rapid-care clinic.
   D. Call 911 for immediate emergency transport and care.

Chapter Summary

- The bony cranium houses a variety of neurologic structures that require protection, regulation, and integration to provide the systems of the body with messages needed to maintain homeostasis and functional status.
- Intracranial regulation requires that the central nervous system (the command center) and the peripheral nervous system (the response center) work together to support the child's maturation, growth and development, cognitive development, and safety through appropriate responses to harmful stimuli.
- Neurologic development begins in the fifth week of fetal development, with neurons (impulse conductor cells) being produced in weeks 15 through 30 of fetal development.
- With healthy and consistent development, the newborn begins life with neurologic stability and predictable growth and maturity.
- Acquired and congenital disorders can lead to the dysregulation of cerebrospinal fluid (CSF). The overproduction or decreased absorption of CSF can lead to increased intracranial pressure in children whose fontanels and suture lines are closed.
- Traumatic brain injuries associated with childhood injuries and trauma are a significant cause of morbidity and mortality in children both in the United States and around the world.
- When a child presents with increasing head circumference measurements, bulging fontanels, misshapen skull bones, irritability, vomiting, increased muscle tone, and/

or the setting-sun eyes sign, the pediatric medical team should assess the child for increased ICP.

- A comprehensive neurologic assessment includes a mental status exam, as well as assessments of motor function, sensory function, cranial nerve function, and reflexes.
- A child who presents with neurologic symptoms should undergo invasive and noninvasive diagnostic exams and laboratory analysis to identify the cause and form a diagnosis.
- Abusive head trauma, formerly known as shaken baby syndrome, is a severe form of non-accidental cerebral trauma that leads to encephalopathy and is associated with high morbidity and mortality. Leaving few external signs, such an injury is multifactorial in nature and produces retinopathy, shearing of brain vasculature, subdural hemorrhages, diffuse brain tissue injury, respiratory distress, and increased ICP.
- Other neurologic conditions noted in children include muscular dystrophy, cerebral palsy, Gullain-Barré syndrome, neural tube defects, hypoxic ischemic encephalopathy, concussions, and migraines.

Bibliography

American Academy of Pediatrics. (2015). Understanding abusive head trauma in infants and children: Answers from America's pediatricians. Retrieved from http://www.ncsl.org/Portals/1/Documents/fsl/Understanding_AHT_Infants_Children_AAP_FINAL_6-15.pdf

American Brain Tumor Association (ABTA). (2014). Brain tumors in children. Retrieved from http://www.abta.org/adolescent-pediatric/brain-tumors-in-children.html

Barr, R. G., Rivara, F. P., Barr, M., Cummings, P., Taylor, J., Lengua, L., & Meredith-Benitz, B.A. (2008). Effectiveness of educational materials designed to change knowledge and behaviors regarding crying and shaken-baby syndrome in mothers of newborns: A randomized clinical trial. *Pediatrics, 123*(3), 972–980.

Bonadio, W. (2014). Pediatric lumbar puncture and cerebrospinal fluid analysis. *Journal of Emergency Medicine, 46*(1), 141-150.

Brasher, R. C., & Tasker. R. C. (2013). Elevated intracranial pressure (ICP) in children. *UpToDate,* Topic 6077, Version 8.0. Retrieved from http://www.uptodate.com/contents/elevated-intracranial-pressure-icp-in-children

Brouwer, M. C., Tunkel, A. R., & van de Beek, D. (2010). Epidemiology, diagnosis, and antimicrobial treatment of acute bacterial meningitis. *Clinical Microbiology Reviews, 23*, 467–492.

Centers for Disease Control and Prevention (CDC). (2001). Growth charts: Data table of infant head circumference-for-age charts. Retrieved from http://www.cdc.gov/growthcharts/html_charts/hcageinf.htm

Centers for Disease Control and Prevention (CDC). (2016a). What are the signs and symptoms of concussion? Retrieved from http://www.cdc.gov/traumaticbraininjury/symptoms.html

Centers for Disease Control and Prevention (CDC). (2016b). Lead: What do parents need to know to protect their children? Retrieved from https://www.cdc.gov/nceh/lead/acclpp/blood_lead_levels.htm

Christian, C. (2016). Child abuse: Evaluation and diagnosis of abusive head trauma in infants and children. *UpToDate.* Retrieved from http://www.uptodate.com/contents/child-abuse-evaluation-and-diagnosis-of-abusive-head-trauma-in-infants-and-children

Covassin, T., Elbin, R. J., Stiller-Ostrowski, J. L., & Kontos, A. P. (2009). Immediate Post-Concussion Assessment and Cognitive Testing (ImPACT) practices of sports medicine professionals. *Journal of Athletic Training, 44*(6), 639–644.

Danial, N. N., Hartman, A. L., Stastrom, C. E., & Thio, L. L. (2013). How does the ketogenic diet work? Four potential mechanisms. *Journal of Child Neurology, 28*, 1027–1033.

Deans, K. J., Minneci, P. C., Lowell, W., & Groner, J. I. (2013). Increased morbidity and mortality of traumatic brain injury in victims of nonaccidental trauma. *Journal of Trauma and Acute Care Surgery, 75*(1), 157–160.

Dunn, L. T. (2002). Raised intracranial pressure. *Journal of Neurology, Neurosurgery, and Psychiatry, 73*(suppl 1), i23–i27.

Fatemi, A., Wilson, M. A., & Johnston, M. V. (2009). Hypoxic-ischemic encephalopathy in the term infant. *Clinics in Perinatology, 36*, 835–858.

Frasier, L. D., & Coats, B. (2015). Abusive head trauma: Clinical, biomechanical, and imaging considerations. In P. K. Kleinman (Ed.), *Diagnostic imaging of child abuse* (pp. 343–344). Cambridge, UK: Cambridge University Press.

Goldenberg, M. M. (2010). Overview of drugs used for epilepsy and seizures: Etiology, diagnosis, and treatment. *Pharmacy and Therapeutics, 35*, 392–415.

Harmon, K. G., Drezner, J. A., Gammons, M., Guskiewicz, K. M., Halstead, M., Herring, S. A., . . . Roberts, W. O. (2013) American Medical Society for Sports Medicine position statement: Concussion in sport. *British Journal of Sports Medicine, 47*(1), 15–26.

Johns Hopkins Medicine. (2015). Headaches in children. Retrieved from http://www.hopkinsmedicine.org/healthlibrary/conditions/pediatrics/headaches_in_children_90,P02603/

Kukreti, V., Mohseni-Bod, H., & Drake, J. (2014). Management of raised intracranial pressure in children with traumatic brain injury. *Journal of Pediatric Neurosciences, 9*(3), 207–215.

Lowry, J. (2010). Oral chelation therapy for patients with lead poisoning. Retrieved from http://www.who.int/selection_medicines/committees/expert/18/applications/4_2_Lead OralChelators.pdf

Martin, K., Jackson, C. F., Levy, R. G., & Cooper, P. N. (2016). Ketogenic diet and other dietary treatments for epilepsy. *Cochrane Database of Systematic Reviews, 2*, CD001903.

Matschke, J., Herrmann, B., Sperhake, J., Korber, F., Bajanoswki, T., & Glatzel, M. (2009). Shaken baby syndrome: A common variant of non-accidental head injury in infants. *Deutsches Arzteblatt International, 106*(130), 211–217.

Odding, E., Roebroeck, M. E., & Stam, H. J. (2006). The epidemiology of cerebral palsy: Incidence, impairment and risk factors. *Disability and Rehabilitation, 28,* 183–191.

Parks, S. E., Annest, J. L., Hill, H. A., & Karch, D. L. (2012). *Pediatric abusive head trauma: Recommended definitions for public health surveillance and research.* Atlanta, GA: Centers for Disease Control and Prevention.

Paul, A. R., & Adamo, M. A. (2014). Non-accidental trauma in pediatric patients: A review of epidemiology, pathophysiology, diagnosis and treatment. *Translational Pediatrics, 3*(3), 195–207.

Peña, C., Gudiol, C., Calatayud, L., Tubau, F., Domínguez, M. A., Pujol, M., . . . Gudiol, F. (2008). Infections due to *Escherichia coli* producing extended-spectrum beta-lactamase among hospitalised patients: Factors influencing mortality. *Journal of Hospital Infection, 68*(2), 116–122.

Sanger, T. D., Delgado, M. R., Gaebler-Spira, D., Hallet, M., & Mink, J. W. (2003). Classification and definition of disorders causing hypertonia in childhood. *Pediatrics, 111*, e89.

Schachter, S. C. (2016). Antiseizure drugs: Mechanism of action, pharmacology, and adverse effects. *UpToDate.* Retrieved from http://www.uptodate.com/contents/antiseizure-drugs-mechanism-of-action-pharmacology-and-adverse-effects?source=search_result&search=antiseizure+drugs+mechanism+of+action+pharmacology&selectedTitle=1%7E150

Semple, B. D., Lee, S., Sadjadi, R., Fritz, N., Carlson, J., Griep, C., . . . Noble-Haeusslein, L. J. (2015). Repetitive concussions in adolescent athletes: Translating clinical and experimental research into perspectives on rehabilitation strategies. *Frontiers in Neurology, 6*, 69.

Suominen, P. L., & Vahatalo, R. (2012). Neurologic long term outcome after drowning in children. *Scandinavian Journal of Trauma, Resuscitation and Emergency Medicine, 2012*, 20–55.

Walls, C. (2006). Shaken baby syndrome: A role for nurse practitioners working with families of small children. *Journal of Pediatric Health Care, 20*(5), 304–310.

Ward, E., DeSantis, C., Robbins, A., Kohler, B., & Jemal, A. (2014). Childhood and adolescent cancer statistics, 2014. *CA: A Cancer Journal for Clinicians, 64*, 83–103.

CHAPTER 22

Genitourinary Elimination

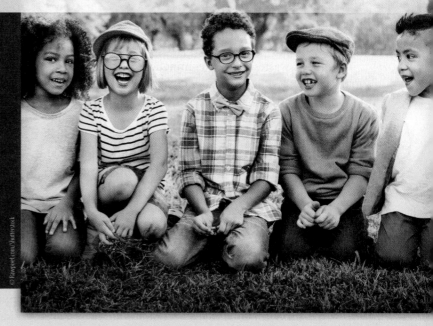

LEARNING OBJECTIVES

1. Apply key nursing concepts in caring for a child with a genitourinary tract disorder.
2. Incorporate understanding of the child's genitourinary and renal development into care plans for genitourinary and renal disorders.
3. Apply understanding of the relationship between the genitourinary system and the essential electrolytes—sodium, potassium, magnesium, phosphorus, and calcium—to treatment plans for children with genitourinary and renal disorders.
4. Evaluate the clinical presentation of dehydration across childhood, including assessment findings.
5. Assess the clinical presentation of childhood genitourinary/elimination conditions, including those related to infectious processes and those associated with anatomic anomalies.
6. Analyze nursing care concerns for a child presenting with a urinary tract infection, and describe the nursing care and medical treatments for urinary tract infections across the developmental period.
7. Differentiate between glomerulonephritis and nephrotic syndrome, including differences in their pathology, laboratory values, clinical presentations, and nursing care.

8. Assess the pathology of other childhood genitourinary conditions, including enuresis, testicular torsion, undescended testes, ambiguous genitalia, and others.
9. Evaluate a family teaching plan for a child with enuresis.

KEY TERMS

Acidosis
Alkalosis
Ascites
Diurnal enuresis
Enuresis
Epispadias
Glomerulonephritis
Hemolytic uremic syndrome (HUS)
Hypospadias
Nephrotic syndrome
Uremia

Introduction

Genitourinary elimination involves multiple systems, but most prominently the renal system. The production of the body's wastes and the elimination of urine involves the processes of nutrient and fluid consumption, absorption, distribution, and excretion of the end products of metabolism. The renal system has ultimate responsibility for body fluid regulation and balance. The field of urology encompasses the study and functions of the kidney, renal, pelvis, ureters, bladder, urethra, and reproductive organs (**Figure 22-1**).

Pediatric Renal Function

The kidneys perform six functions:

- *Elimination of liquid waste products* from the blood within a process of detoxification in the form of urine.
- *Production of the hormone erythropoietin*, which stimulates the bone marrow to produce red blood cells.
- *Production of the chemical renin*, which stimulates the production of first angiotensin I, then

angiotensin II, leading to vasoconstriction in response to a lower total vascular fluid volume.
- *Stimulation of the hormone aldosterone through the presence of the chemical angiotensin II.* Aldosterone's function is to elicit the reabsorption of sodium and water, thereby returning blood pressure to normal after it falls.
- *Regulation of fluids and electrolytes* by absorption or excretion of sodium and other electrolytes.
- *Regulation of acid–base balance* through the action of bicarbonate molecules.

Developmental Influences to Genitourinary Elimination

Developmental aspects of the genitourinary system and urinary elimination include fluid regulation, electrolyte balance, and waste elimination. A young child has an immature renal system, and this immaturity affects the kidneys' function and efficiency. Developmental differences in children influence not only fluid and electrolyte balance, but also the process of waste elimination. In the infant, the kidneys are unable to concentrate waste products into the form of urine for excretion. Consequently, infants' urine has a lower specific gravity (typically 1.010 or less) than the urine of older children or adults. Infants and young children need a higher rate of metabolism to support their rapid growth and energy production. On average, this rate is 2 to 3 times higher than the metabolic rate in adults, which also means that infants and young children require greater amounts of body water. Furthermore, insensible water loss is greater for infants and young children due to their overall increased heart rates, respiration rates, gastrointestinal peristaltic rates, and fever heights (**Box 22-1**).

Newborns and young infants are highly susceptible to defects that occur during fetal development. Neonates who present in the first days of life with a single umbilical artery, congenital malformation, abdominal mass, or chromosomal abnormality may be more susceptible to the development of a pediatric genitourinary disorder or disease. Also, a specific set of diagnoses in the mother

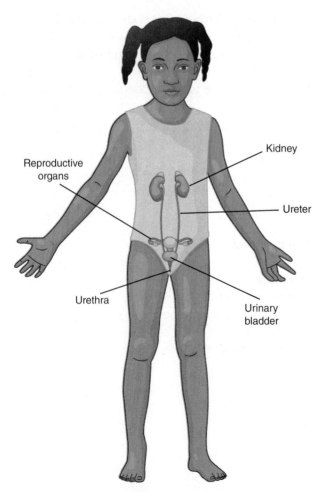

Reproductive organs

Kidney

Ureter

Urethra

Urinary bladder

Figure 22-1 *The genitourinary system.*

BOX 22-1 Body Water

The percentage of total body weight that is accounted for by water is far different in premature infants, newborns, and young infants than during later phases of life:

- Premature infants have approximately 90% of their total weight as body water.
- Infants have approximately 70% to 80% of their total weight as body water.
- Adolescents have 55% to 65% of their total weight as body water.

during pregnancy should put the pediatric healthcare team on alert to look for the development of renal disease or disorder in a newborn. These maternal conditions include the following diagnoses:

- Oligohydramnios
- Polyhydramnios
- New-onset or preexisting diabetes
- Alcohol or cocaine ingestion
- Hypertension

During the newborn period and early infancy, children demonstrate less efficacy in the regulation of fluids, waste products, concentration of urine, and overall balance of the electrolytes. Metabolism is much higher during early life compared to the rest of the life span, and the total kilocalories required for growth are the highest of any time in life. Nevertheless, the newborn's renal system remains immature and is not able to function with the same efficiency as an older child's renal system. As a result, any disorders in the renal system leave the newborn and infant vulnerable to dehydration, poor pH regulation, fluid retention, hypertension, and **uremia** (buildup of urea and other waste products in the body).

An infant has less body water reserves within the intracellular space for conservation during disorders or conditions that lead to fluid loss. With an overall body water turnover rate of 50%, infants are at greater risk for dehydration and fluid imbalances. Owing to their relatively large body surface area, they are also at greater risk for evaporation of fluids with skin exposure, fevers, and heat loss.

One of the most important skills unique to the care of pediatric patients is performing accurate intake and output (I&O) measurements. Children produce approximately 1 to 2 quarts of urine each day, with the kidneys filtering 120 to 150 quarts of blood to produce this output. Because of young children's renal maturity challenges and their susceptibility to fluid imbalances, the pediatric nurse must keep meticulous records of all output in relation to the child's intake. As children grow and mature, and become better able to concentrate their waste products, the number of times they urinate begins to decline.

Daily body weights and weighing of all diapers is the most effective means to determine a child's fluid status. Diapers are first weighed when dry, and this value is then subtracted from the weight of the soiled diaper. One gram of urine weight is considered equivalent to 1 mL of urine volume. Average urine production for hydrated children across the developmental period is as follows:

- Newborn: 10 mL/hr
- Infant: 5-10 mL/hr
- Toddler and preschooler:15-20 mL/hr
- School-age child: 10-25 mL/hr
- Adolescent: more than 30 mL/hr

Genitourinary Disorders in Children

Disorders of the genitourinary elimination system are common during childhood, with approximately 1.2 million children presenting with a urinary tract infection each year. According to the American Society of Pediatric Nephrology (2015), 300,000 children develop conditions in which blood and protein are present in urine. This clinical presentation is consistent with conditions such as glomerulonephritis, nephrotic syndrome, and hemolytic uremic syndrome.

Assessment of the genitourinary system should be conducted both during visits where the child is ill or during well-child visits. Fluid status, skin turgor, weight for height and age, vital signs, peripheral pulses, and general appearance should all be assessed. Three common clinical presentations—febrile illness, diarrhea, and vomiting—contribute to the need for meticulous assessments and screening of fluid status. Because the genitourinary system is a part of the body's acid-base balance, children with moderate to high fluid losses should be assessed for acid-base imbalances, particularly metabolic **acidosis** (increased acidity of the blood) and metabolic **alkalosis** (abnormally low hydrogen ion concentration in the blood). Metabolic acidosis is associated with excessive vomiting, whereas metabolic alkalosis is associated with excessive and prolonged diarrhea. During periods of acidosis, the child will compensate by blowing off excess carbon dioxide (CO_2) via the respiratory system or, alternatively, the renal system will retain bicarbonate (HCO_3) to correct metabolic acidosis or release HCO_3 to correct metabolic alkalosis.

BEST PRACTICES

Common Diagnostic Exams Performed in Pediatric Patients to Identify Disorders of Urinary Elimination

- Urinalysis
- Urine culture and sensitivity (**Figure 22-2**)
- Specific gravity
- Creatinine clearance
- Voiding cystourethrogram
- Renal angiogram
- Glomerular filtration rate
- Blood urea nitrogen
- Blood creatinine
- Intravenous pyelogram

Nursing Care for Children with Genitourinary Disorders

Children who will need nursing care for their genitourinary disorder may present with a variety of concerns. Infection, inflammation, obstruction, and complications associated

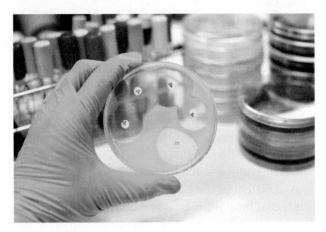

Figure 22-2 *A urine culture and sensitivity laboratory study.*

© Jarun Ontakrai/Shutterstock

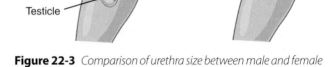

Figure 22-3 *Comparison of urethra size between male and female infants.*

with congenital anomalies in the genitourinary or reproductive system are commonly seen. Using the nursing process, the pediatric nurse formulates an appropriate focused assessment, decides on priority nursing diagnoses, and then formulates goals and interventions that will best suit the child's physiological, physical, developmental, and emotional needs. Young children, in particular, need comprehensive nursing care focused on developmental influences. For instance, infants and young children who are acutely ill typically do not take in oral fluids at the rate and quantity required for balance and healing. Children who present with continued fever, acute gastrointestinal infections with diarrhea and vomiting, and complications associated with common urinary tract infections (UTIs) will have extra fluid losses and, in turn, higher fluid needs. The daily calculation of a child's fluid maintenance requirements is essential to ensure these needs are being met.

Infectious Processes

Children of any age or sex may present with a genitourinary system infection. Their relatively short urethras (**Figure 22-3**), urinary reflux, anatomic anomalies, and sitting in a soiled diaper with stool make children more susceptible to genitourinary infectious processes. Rapid diagnosis and prompt treatment of such infectious processes can help prevent strictures, scarring, or issues with infertility in adolescence or adulthood. Kidney infections are called pyelonephritis, urethra infections are called urethritis, and bladder infections are called cystitis.

Urinary Tract Infections

Compared to adults, young children have shorter urethras that leave them more susceptible to urinary tract infections. Girls have very short urethras (3 to 5 cm in length), which allows bacteria to readily migrate up to the bladder and

cause infection. It is imperative that girls learn to wipe from front to back after defecating to avoid this risk. Infant boys who are not circumcised have a slightly increased risk for the development of a UTI (*MedlinePlus*, 2014).

A UTI is formally defined as more than 5×10^4 colonies of bacteria per milliliters of urine. Common microbial culprits in pediatric UTIs are gram-negative aerobic bacteria, with gram-positive bacteria being encountered less often. Pediatric nurses should be aware that there is a developmental pattern to the microbes that cause UTIs in children (Imam, 2013; Qureshi, 2005):

- Infants are most susceptible to *Escherichia coli* infections due to sitting in diapers soiled with stool.
- Toddlers are most susceptible to *E. coli* and *Klebsiella* infections.
- Preschoolers are most susceptible to *E. coli*, *Klebsiella*, and *Pseudomonas* infections.
- School-age children are most susceptible to *Klebsiella*, *Pseudomonas*, and *Proteus mirabilis* infections.
- Adolescents are most susceptible to *E. coli*, *Klebsiella*, *Pseudomonas*, *Staphylococcus saprophyticus*, and groups B and D streptococcal infections.

PHARMACOLOGY

In female pediatric clients, the use of antibiotics profoundly disrupts the homeostatic presence of normal microflora in the vaginal area, which can lead to persistent *E. coli* colonization. Genital flora, including lactobacilli and staphylococci, provide a natural resistance to urinary pathogens until antibiotic therapy disrupts their presence (Finer & Landau, 2004).

Recurrent UTIs in children are often associated with voiding dysfunctions, incomplete bladder emptying, incontinence with inadequate cleansing, chronic constipation affecting the function of the detrusor muscle, and high-grade vesicoureteral reflux. As many as 50% of infants and 30% of children who present with UTIs have genitourinary structural anomalies (Weinberg, 2015). Children who present with abnormal or infrequently found bacteria, severe flank pain, high fever, nausea and vomiting, and chills require an immediate workup for possible retrograde infection (bacteria that have moved from the bladder into the kidneys). Presence of heme, white blood cells (WBCs), casts, leukocyte esterase, and foul smell are common in urine associated with UTI.

Nursing Care for a Child with UTI

Nursing care of a child with a suspected or confirmed UTI includes patient teaching, family education, symptom management, and medical treatment initiation. The pediatric nurse should assess a child for the following indicators:

- Frequency, urgency, and pain (dysuria) associated with urination
- Presence of a foul odor of urine
- Color of urine: pink or red denotes presence of blood
- Clarity of the urine: WBCs make the urine cloudy
- Specific gravity and pH of the urine
- Presence of associated symptoms such as fever, dehydration, poor sucking or feeding behaviors, or nausea
- Abdominal pain, pelvic pain, or flank pain

Care should include the following measures:

- Providing large quantities of the child's favorite oral fluids at the desired temperature
- For hospitalized patients, starting and maintaining a patent IV for fluid replacement and antibiotics
- Encouraging fluid consumption of more than 100 mL/kg/day
- Treating the child's fever and discomfort

At discharge or in outpatient settings, parents of infants and toddlers should be taught how to clean female genitalia after stooling to ensure all feces is removed from the child's outer and inner labia and to reinforce wiping from front to back in potty-training girls. Dietary strategies for UTI prevention include encouraging children to maintain an adequate fluid intake (Lotan et al., 2013) and consume plain yogurt containing *Lactobacillus* and *Bifidobacterium*

cultures, as there is some indication that probiotics in combination with antibiotic therapy may offer protection against UTI recurrence (Tewari & Narchi, 2015).

Rates of UTI in boys who are uncircumcised have been found to show only a 2.2% increase throughout childhood, but are 8-fold higher during the male infant's first year of life (Hinfey & Steele, 2015). These data do not support the supposition that circumcision in male children is a medical necessity. Proper hygiene after stooling is the most important step in preventing the development of UTIs.

Frequently prescribed antimicrobials for urinary tract infections in pediatric patients include the following agents (Herbert & Roth, 2015; Iman, 2013):

- Ampicillin (Omnipen)
- Amoxicillin (Amoxil)
- Cephalexin (Keflex)
- Gentamicin (Garamycin)
- Co-trimoxazole (Bactrim, Septra)
- Nitrofurantoin
- Trimethoprim/sulfamethoxazole (TMP/SMX)

Oral or IV fluids should be administered during treatment. Fluids in amounts up to 100 mL/kg/day may be ordered.

Research demonstrates that consuming cranberry juice capsules after having genitourinary or reproductive surgery in which a urinary catheter is placed can reduce the risk of developing a UTI. (Foxman, Cronenwett, Spino, Berger, & Morgan, 2015).

Pyelonephritis

Pyelonephritis is often observed in infants and young children who present with an acute febrile UTI where bacteria have ascended. Considered an upper genitourinary tract infection, pyelonephritis is an infection of the structures of the kidneys. Approximately one out of every 30 UTIs (lower genitourinary tract) will develop into pyelonephritis (Urology Care Foundation, 2015). Common bacterial culprits include *Escherichia coli* (90% of cases), *Klebsiella*, *Enterococcus faecalis*, and *Streptococcus* and *Staphylococcus* (both gram-positive bacteria and both rare etiologies) (Hinfey & Steele, 2015).

If a child with a UTI has a fever, the child's condition should prompt suspicion of pyelonephritis and be treated promptly with appropriate antibiotics. Adolescents who present with symptoms of UTI accompanied with chills, fever, and flank pain should be assessed for pyelonephritis. Young children may also demonstrate nausea, vomiting, and diarrhea when this type of infection is present. Complications of this condition may include dehydration, hypertension, renal scarring, and renal failure. Treatment consists of oral fluids and oral antibiotics for children with mild infection, and IV fluids and IV antibiotics for children who are experiencing associated gastrointestinal distress or gastrointestinal fluid losses and/or who appear quite ill from the infection.

Sexually Transmitted Infections

Sexually transmitted infections (STIs) during childhood occur mostly in the adolescent developmental period. When younger children present with STIs, it is imperative that the pediatric healthcare team assess for child sexual abuse.

Sexually transmitted infections are, by nature, infections that are passed during either sexual intercourse or during some form of genital contact. Thus, while testing for STIs, the team frequently tests females for pregnancy.

Children at highest risk for STIs are those between the ages of 15 and 19 (Child Trends Databank, 2015), those with a recent history of sexual intercourse or intimate genital contact without condom use, and those who are intravenous drug users. According to the Centers for Disease Control and Prevention (CDC, 2011), STIs are a critical health challenge, with at least 19 million new cases per year, costing more than $17 billion to treat. The three top treatable STIs found in high-risk children are syphilis, chlamydia, and gonorrhea (CDC, 2011; Child Trends Databank, 2015) (**Table 22-1**). Untreated STIs and delayed treatment of STIs are associated with infertility.

Children, particularly young teenagers, must be offered health screening for STIs if infection is suspected. Some pediatric healthcare settings offer STI testing whether or not children state they are or have been sexually active. Determining whether a child is sexually active is not as important as offering screening. Young teens, especially,

TABLE 22-1 Common Sexually Transmitted Infections in Adolescents			
Infection	Microbe	Symptoms	Treatment
Chlamydia	*Chlamydia trachomatis*	Dysuria	Oral azithromycin (often only a single dose is administered)
Gonorrhea	*Neisseria gonorrhoeae*	Dysuria Vaginal discharge Penile discharge	Ceftriaxone (often only a single dose is administered)
Genital herpes (**Figure 22-4**)	Herpes simplex type 1 Herpes simplex type 2	Itching Burning Tingling Pain Blisters	No treatment is available; no cure is obtainable
Genital warts (condyloma acuminatum) (**Figure 22-5**)	Human papillomavirus	Warts (small growths) on the anus, penis, labia, and cervix	No treatment is available; no cure is obtainable
Syphilis (**Figure 22-6**)	*Treponema pallidum*	Primary stage: single chancre or multiple chancres (lesions) Secondary stage: skin rashes on different areas of the body Latent stage: hidden symptoms at first progressing to internal organ infection and damage	Penicillin
Trichomoniasis	*Trichomoniasis protozoa* (parasite)	Malodorous discharge, either clear, white, yellow, or green in color Intense itching	Metronidazole or tinidazole

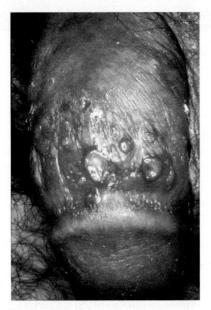

Figure 22-4 *Genital herpes.*

Courtesy of CDC/Dr. N.J. Flumara.; Dr. Gavin Hart

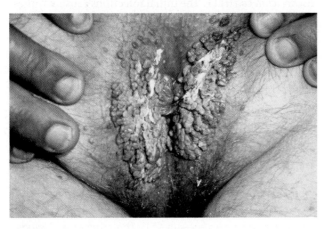

Figure 22-5 *Genital warts.*

© Dr. Ken Greer/Visuals Unlimited, Inc.

may not be honest about their sexual activity, number of partners, or type of sexual activity in which they have participated. Additionally, adolescents may not perceive themselves to be at risk (Schneider, FitzGerald, Byczkowski, & Reed, 2016). Nurses who identify children at risk or suspect children to be at risk should offer testing immediately, especially in cases of actual or suspected child sexual abuse or rape.

If symptomatic, children and teens with STIs may present with genital discharge with or without odor, genital pain, dysuria, and lesions. Nevertheless, the majority of males and females with chlamydia are asymptomatic (Committee on Adolescence & Society for Adolescent Health and Medicine, 2014). Keeping privacy paramount, the pediatric nurse will assist with physical assessment and specimen collection.

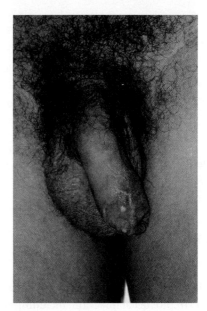

Figure 22-6 *Syphilis chancre.*

© Dr. Ken Greer/Visuals Unlimited, Inc.

Many states now allow young teenagers to seek medical care for STI diagnosis, STI treatment, and birth control without parental or guardian consent. Even so, adolescents may have questions about confidentiality, which the nurse should be prepared to answer.

Treatment for STIs includes oral antibiotics, oral antivirals (for herpes), and follow-up for assessment of adherence to the medications.

Acute Glomerulonephritis

Glomerulonephritis is a kidney condition that develops following an infectious process—typically 1 week to 10 days after a streptococcal infection. The kidney's small collection tubules, which are attached to blood vessels and which are where urine is filtered from the blood, are called the glomeruli and nephrons (**Figure 22-7**). When a child experiences a significant streptococcal infection, the antigen-antibody complexes that result from the body's immune response, which seeks to destroy and remove the streptococcal bacteria's cellular wastes, become deposited in the glomeruli and clog the final filtration system. The clogged nephrons become inflamed, impairing the kidney's ability to filter liquid waste. Aside from streptococcal infections, inflammatory diseases of the arteries and genetic dispositions are the most common causes of acute glomerulonephritis (AGN).

Nursing Care for a Child with Acute Glomerulonephritis

The child with AGN will present with dark brown urine whose appearance mimics that of strongly brewed tea. The child's total urine output will decline as the child progresses

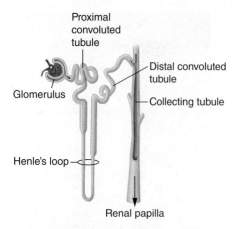

Figure 22-7 *Kidney glomeruli and nephrons.*

to renal failure. In many cases, the child will have a recent history of a streptococcal infection, including sore throat, tooth abscesses, UTIs, skin infections, or other strep-related symptoms. Often, the child with AGN feels fatigued and experiences dyspnea, headache, joint pain, rash, elevated blood pressure, and edema. The edema associated with AGN appears in the early morning as puffy eyes and then progresses to the rest of the body. The clinical presentation is aligned with the changes happening in the body, which lead toward acute renal failure.

Laboratory findings will include positive strep throat cultures, blood cultures, and/or urine cultures. The medical team will order chest X-rays to identify the cause of pulmonary congestion, as well as a renal ultrasound and renal biopsy. The following laboratory analyses can also be used to demonstrate the presence of the AGN pathology:

- Elevated erythrocyte sedimentation rate (ESR)
- Depressed complement C3 and C4 levels
- Mild to moderate elevated blood urea nitrogen (BUN) and creatinine
- Elevated anti-DNase B titer
- Elevated antistreptolysin-O titer

Medical treatment for AGN focuses on the immediate treatment of any remaining streptococcal infections, restoration of fluid balance, reduction of urea buildup, and restoration of kidney function. Potential interventions include antibiotics, diuretics, antihypertensives, and phosphate binders to reduce buildup of phosphates in the blood.

Nursing care focuses on the acuity of the situation at hand. A child with AGN can present as very sick and, therefore, requires astute assessments and care. Daily weights on the same scale to accurately determine the response of fluid and waste-product removal and edema reduction are imperative. Symptom management becomes important, as the child will suffer headaches, body aches, malaise, arthralgia, gastrointestinal distress, and hypertension.

Hemolytic Uremic Syndrome

Hemolytic uremic syndrome (HUS) is a rare and potentially lethal form of kidney failure in children who develop an infection caused by either *Escherichia coli* 0157.H7 or *Escherichia coli* 0111. The initial infections caused by these agents may be acquired from eating contaminated foods or raw meat. Outbreaks of HUS are more common in the summer and are closely associated with the consumption of inadequately cooked meats, intake of unpasteurized dairy products or juices, and contaminated swimming pools, water parks, daycare facilities, and fast-food restaurants. HUS can also be associated with certain medications.

The presence of bacteria in the blood damages red blood cells and causes massive lysis of the cells. This pathology of HUS leads to acute nephropathy, microangiopathic hemolytic anemia, and thrombocytopenia. If a child has seizures associated with HUS, his or her prognosis is considered guarded.

HUS is most commonly seen in young children between 4 months and 4 years of age. Common early presentations include complaints of severe abdominal pain, followed by vomiting and bloody, watery diarrhea. Upon assessment, the team will find dehydration and small bruises on the lining of the mouth. The kidneys become overwhelmed as the number of damaged and lysed red blood cells (RBCs) increases, and their passageways become clogged to the point that the child experiences renal failure with subsequent uremia and fluid retention. The child with HUS will need rapid transport to a higher level of care (intensive care unit [ICU]) for fluid management, edema reduction, dialysis, and management of any bleeding, anemia, and electrolyte disturbances that may be present.

Other Pediatric Disorders of the Genitourinary System

Many childhood genitourinary disorders can be classified into one of four general categories: obstructive disorders, disorders related to nerve or structural damage, and disorders that pertain to specific sexes. **Table 22-2** introduces several of these pediatric genitourinary disorders.

Nephrotic Syndrome

Nephrotic syndrome, also called minimal change nephrotic syndrome, is a complex set of symptoms, considered idiopathic in nature, that occurs more often in male children than female children. Associated with the development of large pores on the final filtration membrane of the child's kidney, it is characterized by a significant loss of serum protein into the urine (**Table 22-3**). There are four cardinal symptoms of nephrotic syndrome:

- Severe proteinuria
- Severe hypoproteinemia
- Hyperlipidemia
- Generalized edema, especially noted in the abdomen (**ascites**)

TABLE 22-2 Other Pediatric Genitourinary Disorders

Genitourinary Obstructive Disorders

› Kidney stone: A solid material that evolves when urine components become highly concentrated and form a small stone. The stone can become lodged in the ureter. This condition is associated with severe pain and blood in the urine.

› Polycystic kidney disease: A hereditary condition in which clusters of fluid-filled cysts are found anywhere throughout the kidney structure, and possibly other organs such as the liver. These cysts can grow large and lead to kidney function failure.

› Hydronephrosis: An obstruction of urinary outflow of the kidney by any means, which causes urine to build up, typically within the renal pelvis. Several types of obstruction may block the bladder outlet, or the presence of kidney stones may lead to hydronephrosis.

Genitourinary Disorders Associated with Nerve Damage or Structural Damage

› Neurogenic bladder: Nerve damage resulting in abnormal retention of urine or leaking of urine from the bladder, typically caused by a spinal cord injury.

› Ureterocele: A congenital condition marked by abnormality in the ureter. Often having a cyst-like nature, the affected area is usually located near the distal end of the ureter where it opens into the urinary bladder. The segment of tissue balloons outward, forming a sac-like pouch.

› Vesicoureteral reflux: Reflux of urine up into the ureters before or after urination.

Male Genitourinary Disorders

› **Hypospadias**: An abnormally positioned opening of the urinary meatus, which may be located in various areas of the penis or base of the penis—most commonly on the underside of the penis.

› **Epispadias**: Abnormal positioning of the urinary meatus on the upper side (dorsum) of the penis (**Figure 22-8**).

› Undescended testicle (cryptorchidism): Testicles typically descend by 9 months of age; cryptorchidism is marked by one or both of the testes remaining in the abdomen. The scrotal sac keeps the testicles 2–3°F cooler than the body temperature. The longer the testicles remain in the warmer environment of the abdomen, the greater change of dysfunction and infertility.

› Priapism: The inability of an erect penis to return to the flaccid state. Surgery, clot evacuation, or medications such as pseudoephedrine, amphetamine, or phenylephrine may be required to reduce the erection and prevent hypoxia and tissue damage. High-flow priapism (less common) requires interventions and is associated with nerve dysfunction in conditions such as spinal cord injury. Low-flow priapism (80–90% of pediatric cases) is caused by blood not returning to the body. A sickle cell anemia vaso-occlusive episode can cause a child or teen to experience priapism.

› Testicular torsion: The rotation and twisting of the spermatic cord, which causes extreme pain, swelling, and reduced blood flow to the scrotum. This condition requires surgical intervention.

(continues)

TABLE 22-2   Other Pediatric Genitourinary Disorders (*continued*)

Female Genitourinary Disorders

› Female genital mutilation (**Figure 22-9**): The intentional removal or alteration of the female genital organs for nonmedical reasons associated with culture or religion; also called female genital cutting or female circumcision. Mostly performed in African and Middle Eastern regions, the procedure is conducted on females ranging in age from infants to adolescents. It is illegal in many parts of the world and is classified as a violation of the human rights of female children and adults (World Health Organization, 2016).

› Labia cyst (Bartholin gland cyst): The blockage of flow from and development of cysts in the Bartholin glands, which are located on either side of the vaginal opening and secrete substances to lubricate the vaginal lips. Typically painless, the cysts are not treated unless they are very painful or become infected.

TABLE 22-3   Distinction Between Glomerulonephritis and Nephrotic Syndrome

Manifestations	Glomerulonephritis	Nephrotic Syndrome
Streptococcal antibody titers	Present	Absent
Edema	Puffiness of face and eyes, especially in morning; edema spreads during day to extremities and abdomen	Generalized
Skin	Child may appear pale; skin is warm to the touch	Extreme skin pallor; skin is warm to the touch and appears shiny
Weight	Increased in acute stage	Increased from retention of sodium and water
Gastrointestinal symptoms	Anorexia, vomiting	Anorexia, diarrhea, and malabsorption
Urine analysis and output	Urine is smoky brown, cloudy, and severely reduced in volume. Specific gravity is elevated. Proteinuria and hematuria are present. Microscopic examination reveals red blood cells and leukocytes.	Urine appears darkly opalescent and frothy. Specific gravity is extremely elevated. Massive proteinuria is present. Microscopic examination reveals hyaline casts and oval fat bodies. Output may be reduced.
Vital signs	Mild to moderately elevated blood pressure	Usually within normal limits; blood pressure may be low or normal
Malnutrition	Absent	Present due to loss of protein and anorexia
Blood examination	Serum electrolytes are normal unless the child is in renal failure. Azotemia may occur as a result of decreased glomerular filtration; it is reflected in elevated blood urea nitrogen and creatinine levels in approximately 50% of children. Hematocrit may be decreased because of hemodilution. Hypoproteinemia and hyperlipidemia may occur.	Serum electrolytes are usually normal. Serum sodium level is usually low. Serum protein and albumin levels are greatly reduced. Hematocrit may be normal or elevated because of hemoconcentration. Hyperlipidemia and elevated triglycerides occur as a result of alterations in the lipid metabolism pathway (Kim & Trachtman, 2014).

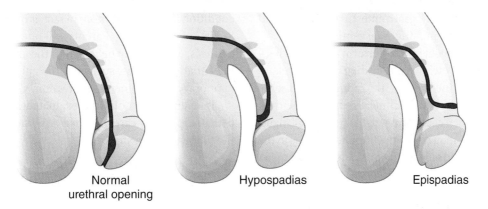

Figure 22-8 *Abnormal positioning of the urinary meatus on the penis: hypospadias and epispadias.*

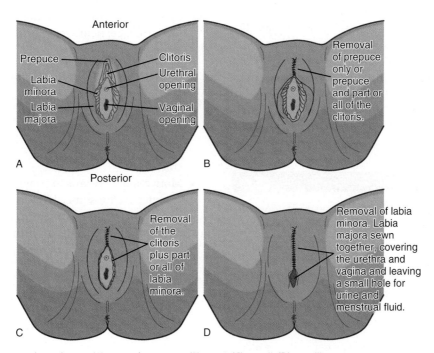

Figure 22-9 *Female genital mutilation: (A) normal anatomy, (B) type I, (C) type II, (D) type III.*

Assessments for the diagnosis of nephrotic syndrome in a child include the following indicators:

- Fluid accumulation (edema)
- Weight gain with abdominal swelling
- Golden yellow, foamy urine
- Fatigue
- Decreased appetite
- Nausea and anorexia

Medical treatment of nephrotic syndrome is generally supportive. Diuretics, sometimes in combination with albumin (Duffy, Jain, Harrell, Kothari, & Reddi, 2015), may be required to restore fluid balance. In addition, antihypertensive agents may be ordered as needed.

Nursing Care for a Child with Nephrotic Syndrome

Corticosteroids are the mainstay of medical treatment of nephrotic syndrome, and may be required for an extensive length of time. In turn, nurses should monitor for significant steroidal side effects, including hyperglycemia, hypertension, poor growth, and adrenal suppression (Madani et al., 2011). Dietary support and education will be required to reinforce the need for adhering to a high-protein, low-salt diet.

The child with nephrotic syndrome will need to have frequent vital signs monitoring to assess for potential fluid overload, daily weights, and frequent assessment of skin integrity due to the marked edema associated with this condition. Poor nutrition, gastrointestinal distress, and fatigue should prompt nursing interventions.

Families must be taught how to perform a dipstick check for the presence of proteinuria. A finding of +1 correlates with 30 mg/dL of urine protein. The family must also be educated to assess the child for clinical signs of protein release, including sudden changes in weight, increasing fatigue, shortness of breath, changes in appetite, and changes in the appearance of the child's urine (frothy, golden and viscous).

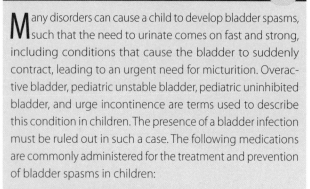

PHARMACOLOGY

Steroidal anti-inflammatory medications are the primary medical treatment for pediatric nephrotic syndrome. A lengthy course of treatment is often required to decrease the pore size on the final glomerular membrane. Unfortunately, these lengthy treatment regimens put children at risk for side effects, which include hyperglycemia, excessive hunger, emotional lability, hypertension, immunosuppression, and poor wound healing.

PHARMACOLOGY

Many disorders can cause a child to develop bladder spasms, such that the need to urinate comes on fast and strong, including conditions that cause the bladder to suddenly contract, leading to an urgent need for micturition. Overactive bladder, pediatric unstable bladder, pediatric uninhibited bladder, and urge incontinence are terms used to describe this condition in children. The presence of a bladder infection must be ruled out in such a case. The following medications are commonly administered for the treatment and prevention of bladder spasms in children:

- Anticholinergics (oxybutynin, bromide, or propantheline)
- Belladonna
- Opium suppositories
- Antibiotics in the presence of infection

Enuresis

Enuresis is a term used to describe a type of a voiding dysfunction that occurs after a child has mastered urinary toilet training. In the most common form of enuresis, the child experiences involuntary urination during the night. Daytime urinary incontinence is called **diurnal enuresis**. The

condition is not uncommon; in fact, it may affect as many as 20% of all children. Parents will often delay reporting enuresis, as they may believe that the child is experiencing situational stress, such that the episode represents a temporary developmental regression.

True enuresis should be evaluated by a professional pediatric primary care provider. Assessments can include the following indicators:

- Length of time of the incontinence
- Time of day of the incontinence (diurnal or nighttime)
- Presence of trauma
- Stressors in the child's life
- Conscious holding of urine during the day
- Associated medical conditions such as overflow incontinence, neurogenic bladder, cystitis, or sphincter dysfunction

Ideas for interventions include the following:

- Restriction of oral fluids after evening meal
- Toileting directly before climbing into bed
- Emotional support; never scolding, belittling, judging or demonstrating frustration toward the child
- Motivational rewards for staying dry (controversial, but effective for some children)
- Bed alarms that signal wetness from urination
- Desmopressin acetate, a synthetic form of antidiuretic hormone, to reduce the production of urine
- Anticholinergic therapy (oxybutynin chloride), for diurnal enuresis

QUALITY AND SAFETY

The pediatric nurse caring for a child with a genitourinary disorder must keep in mind several aspects of safety and support:

- Monitor for fluid imbalance and assess for changes in vital signs, especially the development of hypertension.
- Be aware of the complexity of acid–base imbalances, and monitor for increasing metabolic acidosis.
- Remember that obstructive disorders can lead to permanent scarring and renal dysfunction.
- Provide privacy to children during genitourinary assessments; even young children are sensitive to physical exams, touching of genitalia, and exposure of private areas.

Case Study

A pediatric nurse recognizes a family approaching the nursing desk in the hallway of the hospital unit. This is the third admission within 6 months for this young boy and his family. The child has an existing diagnosis of nephrotic syndrome. Even as the family is approaching, the nurse notes that the child is very edematous, with eyes puffy enough to cause the child to look as though his eyes are closed.

Case Study Questions

1. What are the cardinal signs of nephrotic syndrome that the nurse would recognize during visual and physical assessment?
2. The grandfather joins the family later in the evening. He asks the nurse to explain what the pathology of nephrotic syndrome is, in nontechnical terms. What would the nurse say?
3. The nurse anticipates medical treatments and plans for which medications and intravenous administrations?
4. Which dietary needs does this child have that the nurse will need to specify during his stay?

As the Case Evolves. . .

This family sits down with the nurse to discuss their son's recent visit to the hospital. The nurse reviews with them the dietary restrictions for a child with idiopathic nephrotic syndrome.

5. Which of the following statements, if made by the parents, would indicate a need for additional teaching?
   A. "We make sure we don't add any salt to his food, and we buy low-sodium products."
   B. "He eats only a limited amount of very lean meat, and we don't give him any eggs or dairy products at all."
   C. "We make sure he drinks plenty of water—at least 32 ounces per day, so he stays well hydrated."
   D. "We focus his diet around whole grains, vegetables, and nuts."

Chapter Summary

◆ Genitourinary elimination most prominently involves the renal system, which has the ultimate responsibility for body fluid regulation and balance.
◆ Developmental differences in children influence fluid and electrolyte balance as well as waste elimination. These differences, in turn, influence nursing care.
◆ More than 1 million children present with urinary tract infections each year.
◆ Children of any age or sex may present with a genitourinary system infection. Their relatively short urethras, urinary reflux, anatomic anomalies, and sitting in a soiled diaper with stool make children more susceptible to genitourinary infectious processes.
◆ Genitourinary disorders include pyelonephritis, sexually transmitted infections, acute glomerulonephritis, and hemolytic uremic syndrome.
◆ Many childhood genitourinary disorders can be classified into one of four general categories: obstructive disorders, disorders related to nerve or structural damage, and disorders that pertain to specific sexes. Examples include kidney stones, ureterocele, hypospadias, and labia cyst, respectively.
◆ Enuresis affects as many as 20% of all children. True enuresis should be evaluated by a professional pediatric care provider.

Bibliography

American Society of Pediatric Nephrology. (2015). Online resources: Genitourinary and kidney disorders. Retrieved from http://www.bmsch.org/health-library/greystone---pediatric-library-categorized-v1/article/topic-index---genitourinary-and-kidney-disorders/

Ayoob, R. M., & Schwaderer, A. L. (2016). Acute kidney injury and atypical features during pediatric poststreptococcal glomerulonephritis. *International Journal of Nephrology, 2016*, 5163065.

Centers for Disease Control and Prevention (CDC). (2011). STD trends in the United States: 2010 national data for gonorrhea, chlamydia, and syphilis. Retrieved from http://www.cdc.gov/std/stats10/trends.htm

Child Trends Databank. (2015, January). Sexually transmitted infections (STIs). Retrieved from http://www.childtrends.org/?indicators=sexually-transmitted-infections-stis

Committee on Adolescence & Society for Adolescent Health and Medicine. (2014). Policy statement from the American Academy of Pediatrics: Screening for nonviral sexually transmitted infections in adolescents and young adults. *Pediatrics, 134*(1), 302–311.

Duffy, M., Jain, S., Harrell, N., Kothari, N., & Reddi, A. S. (2015). Albumin and furosemide combination for management of edema in nephrotic syndrome: A review of clinical studies. *Cells, 4*(4), 622–630.

Finer, G., & Landau, D. (2004). Pathogenesis of urinary tract infections with normal female anatomy. *Lancet Infectious Diseases, 4.* Retrieved from http://middleeast.thelancet.com/journals/laninf/article/PIIS1473-3099(04)01147-8/fulltext

Foxman, B., Cronenwett, A., Spino, C., Berger, M., & Morgan, D. (2015). Cranberry juice capsules and urinary tract infection after surgery: Results of a randomized trial. *American Journal of Obstetrics and Gynecology.* Retrieved from http://dx.doi.org/10.1016/j.ajog.2015.04.003

Herbert, K. L., & Roth, C. C. (2015). Pediatric urinary tract infection organism-specific therapy. *Medscape.* Retrieved from http://emedicine.medscape.com/article/1976563-overview

Hinfey, P. B. & Steele, R. W. (2015). Pediatric pyelonephritis. *Medscape.* Retrieved from http://emedicine.medscape.com/article/968028-overview#a7

Imam, T. H. (2013). Bacterial urinary tract infections. *Merck Manual: Professional Version.* Retrieved from http://www.merckmanuals.com/professional/genitourinary-disorders/urinary-tract-infections-(uti)/bacterial-urinary-tract-infections

Kim, M., & Trachtman, H. (2014). Dyslipidemia in nephrotic syndrome. In A. Covic, M. Kanbay, & E. V. Lerma (Eds.), *Dyslipidemias in kidney disease* (pp. 213–239). New York, NY: Springer Science + Business.

Lotan, Y., Daudon, M., Bruyère, F., Talaska, G., Strippoli, G., Johnson, R. J., & Tack, I. (2013). Impact of fluid intake in the prevention of urinary system diseases: A brief review. *Current Opinion in Nephrology & Hypertension, 22*, S1–S10.

Madani, A., Umar, S., Taghaodi, R., Hajizadeh, N., Rabbani, A., & Z-Mehrjardi, H. (2011). The effect of long-term steroid therapy on linear growth of nephrotic children. *Iranian Journal of Pediatrics, 21*(1), 21–27.

MedlinePlus, U. S. National Library of Medicine. (2014). Urinary traction infection: Children. Retrieved from https://medlineplus.gov/urinarytractinfections/children.html

Mills, M., White, S. C., Kershaw, D., Flynn, J. T., Brophy, P. D., Thomas, S. E., & Smoyer, W. (2005). Developing clinical protocols for nursing practice: Improving nephrology care for children and their families. *Nephrology Nursing Journal, 32*(6), 599–607.

National Institute of Diabetes and Digestive and Kidney Disorders. (2011). Urinary tract infections in children. Retrieved from https://www.niddk.nih.gov/-/media/E3EC257A60164794AA9FB27CB4278902.ashx

Qureshi, A. M. (2005). Organisms causing urinary tract infections in pediatric patients at Ayub Teaching Hospital Abbottabad. *Journal of Ayub Medical College Abbottabad, 17*(1), 72-74.

Schneider, K., FitzGerald, M., Byczkowski, T., & Reed, J. (2016). Screening for asymptomatic gonorrhea and chlamydia in the pediatric emergency department. *Sexually Transmitted Diseases, 43*(4), 209–215.

Tewari, K., & Narchi, H. (2015). Recurrent urinary tract infections in children: Preventive interventions other than prophylactic antibiotics. *World Journal of Methodology, 5*(2), 13–19.

Urology Care Foundation. (2015). Kidney (renal) infection-pyelonephritis. Retrieved from http://www.urologyhealth.org/urologic-conditions/kidney-(renal)-infection-pyelonephritis

Weinberg, G. (2015). Urinary tract infection in children (UTI). Retrieved from https://www.merckmanuals.com/professional/pediatrics/miscellaneous-bacterial-infections-in-infants-and-children/urinary-tract-infection-uti-in-children

World Health Organization. (2016). Female genital mutilation. Retrieved from http://www.who.int/mediacentre/factsheets/fs241/en/

CHAPTER 23

Mobility

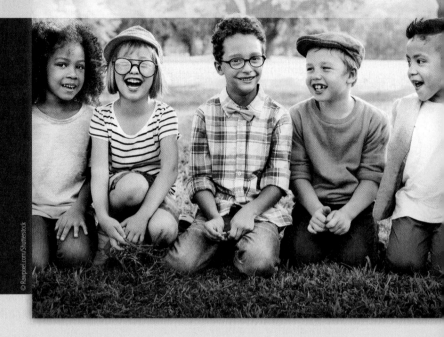

© Rawpixel.com/Shutterstock

LEARNING OBJECTIVES

1. Apply key nursing concepts for care associated with issues of mobility in children across the developmental period.
2. Evaluate the anatomy and physiology of the musculoskeletal system as it pertains to early growth and development.
3. Analyze alterations in normal fetal development, and in growth and development for children, that lead to alterations in expected mobility.
4. Assess congenital mobility issues during childhood.
5. Incorporate into nursing practice an understanding of the incidence, pathophysiology, clinical presentation, and management of acquired disorders of mobility during childhood.
6. Analyze components of nursing care required to provide education and support for childhood mobility issues.

KEY TERMS

Barlow's sign
Club foot
Congenital hip dysplasia
Dislocation
Duchenne muscular dystrophy
Epiphyseal plate
Legg-Calvé-Perthes disease
Limb-length discrepancies
Ortolani's sign
Ossification
Scoliosis
Slipped capital femoral epiphysis
Spina bifida

Introduction

Mobility—a functional feature of anatomic development that helps children explore and manipulate the environment—is a key factor in growth and development. After the newborn period, an infant develops the musculoskeletal system by increasing strength, agility, and movement. While the young infant's musculoskeletal system contains a complete set of 206 bones, and all muscles in place, myelination of central and peripheral nerves must occur for the infant to transition from having reflex responses only to slowly exhibiting purposeful movement, coordination, and locomotion. Within the first year of life, a child moves from a state of dependence and immobility, to learning to raise the head, roll over, sit up, and rapidly crawl, and then to walking.

The musculoskeletal system structures should be intact at birth. Through the process of maturation, cartilage (embryonic connective tissue) is replaced with osteoblasts via **ossification** within bony structures. Progressing outwardly from the diaphysis (hard shaft portion), ossification is required for bone strength. This process continues until the child is in late adolescence, when skeletal maturation reaches completion.

A young child's bones are more porous and less dense than those of adults and, therefore, are more prone to fractures. Bones become strong and less pliable as the young child grows. After ossification, the bones grow via the **epiphyseal plate**, or the growth plate. Muscles, as they mature through hypertrophy, provide greater stamina, coordination, and strength to the growing child.

Disorders affecting a child's musculoskeletal system can have a major impact on how the child learns to engage in mobility, independence, and play. Pediatric nurses who interact with children and their families should keenly assess how each child's musculoskeletal system matches up with the achievements expected for the child's developmental stage. Early identification of motor delays, or early identification of congenital or acquired disorders, can initiate the management or treatments of many musculoskeletal conditions.

Assessments for Issues in Mobility

Assessment for congenital conditions starts with a newborn's first evaluation. The interdisciplinary team works to identify disorders as early as possible. The initial assessment of a newborn should include an examination to identify birth trauma, such as fracture of the collarbones, and congenital disorders such as club foot, congenital hip dysplasia, and **limb-length discrepancies** (i.e., differences in the lengths of the arms or the legs). A complete health history of the pregnancy and birth, followed by a thorough physical exam of the newborn, allows for early identification of congenital conditions. Later assessments will evaluate whether the child is experiencing intrinsic factors affecting mobility, such as developmental motor delays, abnormal bone structures and gait, or scoliosis, as well as extrinsic factors that may affect mobility, such as child abuse. If the pediatric team suspects a disorder, further evaluation is warranted, including the following steps:

- Radiographic assessment
- Bone scans
- Computed tomography (CT) scans
- Magnetic resonance imaging (MRI)
- Positron emission tomography (PET) scans
- Diffusion tensor imaging (DTI)
- Swallowing studies

Developmental Perspectives on Mobility-Related Issues

Since each child is unique and develops on his or her own timeline and sequence, the pediatric nurse must be able to identify deviations in what would normally be expected during each developmental state. For instance, a toddler who is not walking by age 16 months should be referred for further evaluation. It may be that the parents are overly protective and not allowing or challenging the child to progressively gain more locomotion, or it may be that muscle biopsies are needed to check for muscular dystrophy. A child with an awkward gait may need to be further assessed for a neurologic disorder affecting the child's musculoskeletal system. A young teen with uneven shoulders and a rib hump should be evaluated for scoliosis. The pediatric team must incorporate the assessment of developmental milestones, and normal or expected growth and development, into each well-child or sick-child encounter.

Congenital and Idiopathic Disorders

Congenital disorders of the musculoskeletal system are conditions that affect mobility and have been present since birth. These disorders may develop while in utero, or they may occur during the birthing process. This section outlines four exemplars of congenital and idiopathic disorders with the potential to affect mobility during childhood: congenital hip dysplasia, spina bifida, club foot, and scoliosis.

Congenital Hip Dysplasia (Developmental Dysplasia of the Hip)

Identified as early as hours after birth, **congenital hip dysplasia** (CHD) affects the hip joint. Either the hip joint is shallow enough to allow the head of the femur to slip slightly (preluxation) from the acetabulum, or it is so shallow that the femoral head can move around the hip socket (subluxation). In the most extreme cases, the femoral head is found out of the socket completely (**dislocation**). The development of CHD is influenced by family history, in-utero positioning (frank breech), presentation of twins, newborn's overall size, and oligohydramnios (Noordin, Umer, Hafeez, & Nawaz, 2010). Culturally, families who wrap and carry their newborns in a consistent abducted position (legs together, straight) can also influence the extent of the condition after birth.

During a newborn assessment, two techniques are typically performed to assess for this condition. To assess for **Ortolani's sign**, the child is placed in a supine position with the knees flexed 90 degrees (**Figure 23-1**). The provider then places the pads of his or her fingers over the greater trochanter, with the thumb placed internally at the upper thigh. While abducting the hip outward, a positive Ortolani's sign would be found if a clicking sound is heard while the femoral head is slipping back into the acetabulum. A positive **Barlow's sign** is identified when, using the same technique but adducting the child's hip joint, the femoral head slips back out of the socket to a state of dislocation (**Figure 23-2**). Other possible positive findings are the Allis sign, where the nurse identifies unequal knee height in the newborn while lying in the supine position, flexing the thighs in a 90-degree position toward the trunk, or the presence of unequal thigh skin folds while the newborn is supine and the thighs are flexed. The nurse who identifies any positive sign should report the findings immediately so treatment can be initiated. In an older child, the pediatric nurse may identify a slight limb-length discrepancy, history of delayed walking, waddling gait, or presence of a limp.

Treatment for CHD should be initiated within two months to attain the best outcomes. For young infants

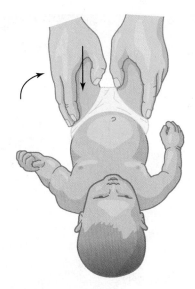

Figure 23-2 *Barlow's sign.*

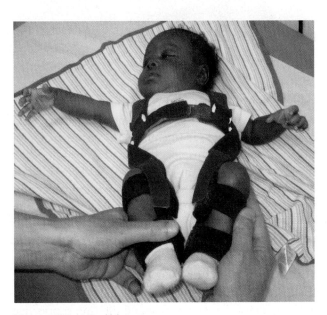

Figure 23-3 *A Pavlik harness.*
Courtesy of International Hip Dysplasia Institute

(less than 3 months of age), the pediatric team will place a Pavlik harness to maintain a flexed and abducted position that holds the femoral head into the acetabulum, so as to deepen the socket contour as the child grows (**Figure 23-3**). This device includes an adjustable strap system to allow for rapid infant growth. Older infants and young children will require skin traction, followed by the placement of a spica cast to hold the femoral head and acetabulum in the desired abducted position (**Figure 23-4**).

Spina Bifida

Commonly associated with the neurologic system, **spina bifida** presents as a weakened area or gap in the bony

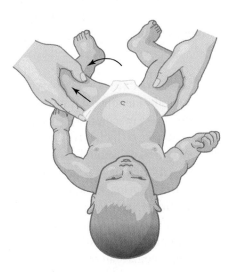

Figure 23-1 *Ortolani's sign.*

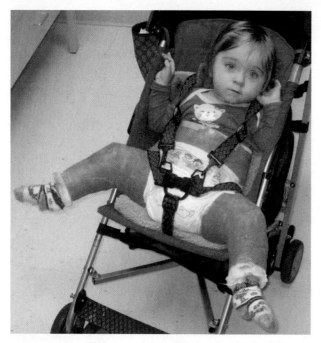

Figure 23-4 *A spica cast on a young toddler.*

Courtesy of International Hip Dysplasia Institute

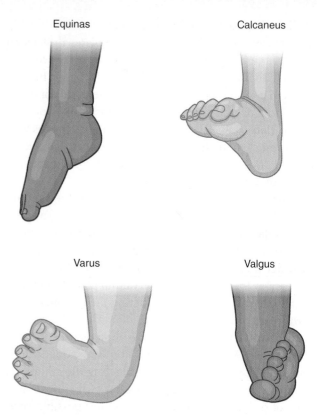

Figure 23-5 *Four forms of club foot: equinas, calcaneus, varus, and valgus.*

spinal column (posterior vertebral arches tail to fuse), which allows for either protrusion of the meninges and cerebral spinal fluid sac (meningocele) or protrusion of the meninges, cerebrospinal fluid, and a portion of the spinal cord nerve roots (myelomeningocele). Spina bifida is often accompanied by other debilitating neurologic conditions (e.g., hydrocephalus, cognitive impairment), but an especially important facet of this condition is that it leads to motor and sensory impairment, including bowel and bladder incontinence, below the level of the spinal lesion (Swaroop & Dias, 2015). Nursing care of the child with spina bifida focuses on improving mobility and function to the greatest degree possible and offering supportive care to the child and family in maximizing quality of life throughout the life span (Dicianno, Fairman, Juengst, Braun, & Zabel, 2010).

Club Foot

Club foot, in which the foot is twisted into an unusual position, is a relatively common congenital defect, being present in 1 in 1000 births (Dobbs & Gurnett, 2012). Although four distinct deformities are all diagnosed as club foot (**Figure 23-5**), the most common form of club foot is talipes equinovarus, which accounts for more than 95% of all childhood cases. In this case, the newborn presents with a foot that has inward and downward rotation, either unilaterally or bilaterally. This congenital condition is twice as common in boys as it is in girls. Although club foot is associated with several risk factors—such as

familial tendencies, improper intrauterine positioning, multiple fetuses, and neuromuscular pathologies—no exact, consistent etiology is known.

If treatment is initiated during the newborn period, a series of small casts that are changed weekly can be placed that slowly stretch the musculoskeletal structures into place. If not corrected in the newborn period, or if the condition is severe, the older infant or child may need to wear corrective splints or corrective shoes. Foot bone realignment surgery (with steel pins) will be required if splints, shoes, or casting is not successful.

Scoliosis

Scoliosis is a lateral curvature of the spine with no known etiology that is typically identified during the rapid growth period of adolescence, but in some instances manifests earlier and may be present from birth. It is typically classified into one of three categories: congenital, neuromuscular, and idiopathic. Many children have no symptoms, but their condition is identified during a routine health screening. Having a preteen or teenager bend forward will assist in the identification of the disorder, as it may be visualized as unequal shoulder height (rib hump), uneven hip alignment, and uneven scapula—all of which demonstrate an abnormal lateral curvature of the spine region (**Figure 23-6**).

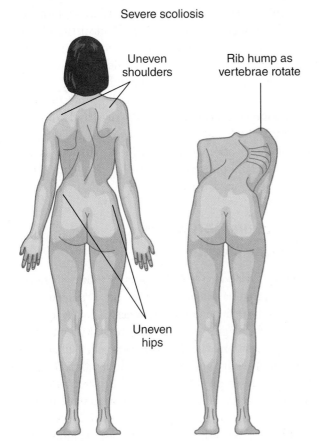

Severe scoliosis

Uneven shoulders

Rib hump as vertebrae rotate

Uneven hips

Figure 23-6 *Abnormal lateral curvature of the spine region may be visualized as unequal shoulder height (rib hump), uneven hip alignment, and uneven scapula.*

In case of mild to moderate scoliosis, the child will be custom-fitted with a plastic thoracic lumbar spinal orthotic (TLSO) or a Milwaukee brace, which needs to be worn up to 23 hours per day for 6 months to 2 years, with complete compliance required to achieve the best results (**Figure 23-7**). The brace should be removed only for bathing. Daily skin assessments are required to monitor for irritation, reddened areas, and breakdown from contact of the brace with the child's skin.

In severe scoliosis cases, such as with curvatures that cause pain or that impair ventilation or mobility, surgical correction with the placement of rods or wires via anterior and posterior thoracotomies will be required. The latest surgical techniques include the use of biological cement to secure the vertebral column in the desired straight alignment.

Acquired Issues with Mobility

Congenital issues represent one end of the spectrum of mobility disorders. At the other end, and by far more common, are acquired disorders. Musculoskeletal injuries, neurologic disease or damage, and nutritional deficits can all have long-term impacts on growth and development.

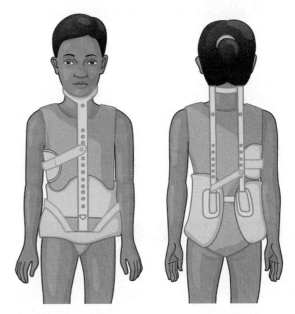

Figure 23-7 *A Milwaukee brace.*

Nutritional Deficiencies Affecting the Musculoskeletal System

Nutrition and bone, muscle, and joint health are closely related. For a child to have a healthy musculoskeletal system while growing and thriving during the developmental period, he or she must be provided with appropriate nutrition that supports the bones, muscles, and metabolic system. Metabolism, in general, influences the healthy growth of a child. The metabolic system, including healthy endocrine glands, also influences the maturation, regulation, and growth and development of the musculoskeletal system. In this way, it influences the achievement of locomotion mastery in infants and toddlers, and mobility status throughout childhood.

Nutritional deficits must be identified early, and professional counsel by a nutritionist must be secured for immediate interventions. Nutritional defects influencing musculoskeletal development and mobility include insufficient intake of the following nutrients:

- Vitamin D: Plays a critical role in accrual of bone mass, bone matrix, and bone geometry, and regulation of calcium. Adequate levels of vitamin D also influence the decreased proliferation of osteoclast precursors, which otherwise would cause bone destruction (Fuleihan & Vieth, 2007).
- Calcium: Provides the major building blocks of bone tissue.
- Magnesium: Plays a critical role in forming bone minerals.
- Vitamin K: Required for mineralization of bone tissue. Low levels have been associated with fractures.

- Zinc: Required for the renewal of bone tissue, especially after bone fractures or trauma. Low levels of zinc have been associated with impaired bone growth across childhood (International Osteoporosis Foundation, 2015).
- Protein: Essential in optimizing bone mass throughout childhood (International Osteoporosis Foundation, 2015). Protein can be found in lean meats, eggs, fish, and legumes (e.g., kidney beans and lentils), as well as grains, seeds, nuts, and tofu products.

RESEARCH EVIDENCE

Nutrition and Children's Physical Activity

According to Janssen (2007), children who have the nutritional disorder of obesity are at high risk for complications associated with their musculoskeletal system and mobility. Moderate to vigorous physical activity during childhood is required to positively influence an obese child's quantity of adiposity, development of metabolic syndromes, high-density lipoprotein (HDL) cholesterol and triglyceride levels, and childhood blood pressure readings. In a dose-response study conducted by Strong et al. (2005), the researchers found that aerobic exercise for 30 to 40 minutes, 3 to 5 days per week, is required to successfully reduce adipose levels in children.

Rickets

Another disorder stemming from nutritional inadequacy is rickets. Three major types of rickets are distinguished:

- Renal osteodystrophy, in which the kidneys fail to maintain blood levels of calcium and phosphorus
- Vitamin D–resistant or hypophosphatemic rickets, which is a genetic disorder characterized by low phosphate levels unrelated to intake or vitamin D status
- Nutritional rickets stemming from deficiency of intake of dietary vitamin D, calcium, and/or phosphate during childhood—the most common form (Chan & Roth, 2015)

Globally, rickets is most commonly found in children between 6 months and 24 months of age; it is uncommon in the United States. In this country, the vitamin D deficiency that predisposes most children to rickets is most frequently seen in overweight and obese children, particularly those who live in northern states, who are dark-skinned, and who spend little time outdoors (Turer, Lin, & Flores, 2013).

Rickets develops after prolonged and extreme nutritional deficiencies. Poor mineralization of bone tissue from deficient nutrient intake leads to several bony abnormalities from the weakening and softening of bone tissue. Findings associated with prolonged and extreme deficient intake typically include muscle weakness; delayed growth; pain in the legs, pelvis, and spine; and significant skeletal deformities. A child with rickets may display projection of the breastbone, thickened ankles and wrists, and bowed legs (**Figure 23-8**). Children with clinical signs and symptoms of rickets must have adequate nutrition, to include calcium, vitamin D, and phosphates, as well as sunlight exposure (Casey, Slawson, & Neal, 2010).

Injuries and Infections Affecting Mobility

Children may develop mobility issues for a variety of reasons, including trauma and other injuries, bone tissue infections (osteomyelitis), or bone, muscle, or nerve damage secondary to other pathologies (e.g., declining mobility with autoimmune destruction of peripheral nerves with Guillain-Barré syndrome). Four syndromes—cerebral palsy, Duchenne muscular dystrophy, dystonia, and Legg-Calvé-Perthes disease—that affect mobility via nontraumatic injury to muscles, bones, or nerves are described in this section as exemplars of secondary damage that affects mobility; the remainder of the section focuses on traumatic injuries.

Children with lifelong mobility issues (e.g., wheelchair-bound children and those who need multiple corrective surgeries) will require extensive interventions to assist the family with managing home care. Education around exercise and nutrition to prevent obesity, for example, is an important aspect of assisting families in caring for a

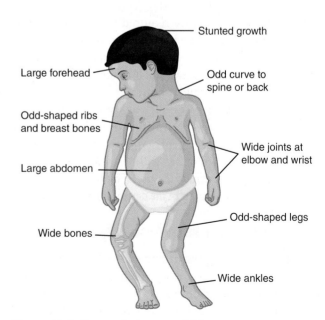

Figure 23-8 *Signs and symptoms of rickets.*

child with Duchenne muscular dystrophy (Christensen & Kockrow, 2013). Nursing interventions to ease caregiver burden are of significant importance.

Nontraumatic Musculoskeletal Disorders Affecting Mobility

Cerebral Palsy

Although generally categorized as a neuromuscular disorder, cerebral palsy is also associated with muscular disabilities. Cerebral palsy is defined as a nonprogressive central nervous disorder that impacts movement, muscular control, and often posture. Owing to a brain injury that occurs during or after birth, the child experiences a significant brain anoxia that leads to disrupted brain development. Growth failures, cognitive disabilities, feeding issues, speech delays or disorders, hearing and visual impairments, and possibly seizure disorders have all been associated with cerebral palsy. Risk factors for the development of cerebral palsy and subsequent musculoskeletal sequelae include birth asphyxia, postnatal hemorrhage, stroke, intrauterine infections, kernicterus, postnatal infection, and birth trauma.

In children with cerebral palsy, the musculoskeletal system can be affected by asymmetrical reflexes, exaggerated reflexes, hypertonicity, spasms, involuntary movements (dyskinesias), rigidity in the neck and back area (dystonia), scissoring of lower extremities, difficulty with gait, and poor control over arm and hand movements, especially when reaching for an object. Medical treatments for these musculoskeletal effects during childhood include surgical rhizotomy to reduce spasticity, surgery to muscle–tendon groups to increase limb movement, bracing and positioning devices, and injection of botulinum toxin (Botox) to decrease muscle spasticity.

Duchenne Muscular Dystrophy

Duchenne muscular dystrophy is the most common form of muscular dystrophy found in childhood. This recessive disorder is linked to a mutation on the X chromosome, and leads to progressive skeletal muscle abnormalities in children. The genetic mutation leads to an absence of the essential protein dystrophin, which then triggers a process of severe inflammation that induces muscle fiber necrosis.

The most typical age of clinical presentation of Duchenne muscular dystrophy is during the preschool period, from 3 to 4 years of age. Children who were previously mobile begin to display muscle weakness, especially in the muscles of the hip girdle. They may display the classic Gower's sign, in which the child, with great difficulty, uses arm muscles for assistance when rising from a supine position (**Figure 23-9**). Other musculoskeletal abnormalities include contractures, hypertrophy of lower limb (calf) muscles, tip-toe walking, waddling gait, and development of contractures. Muscle biopsies are performed to confirm the decreased production or absence of the protein dystrophin and subsequent infiltration of fatty material into the muscle areas.

Cardiomyopathy and respiratory failure are the leading causes of death in individuals with Duchenne muscular dystrophy, most of whom do not survive past age 20. Assisting families with coping, both in terms of acknowledging the clinical course and experiencing it, is an essential aspect of family-centered nursing care in such cases: Nearly 70% of family caregivers report significant mental health issues (Landfeldt et al., 2016).

Medical management of Duchenne muscular dystrophy includes surgical interventions for contractures, physical therapy, occupational therapy, braces and other mobility

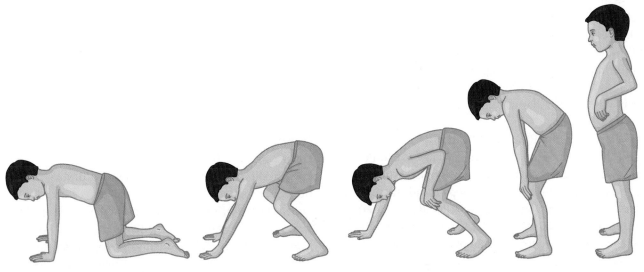

Figure 23-9 *Gower's sign.*

devices, and ventilation support as needed. Pharmacotherapy support includes corticosteroid administration to slow the muscle weakness progression, as well as angiotensin-converting enzyme (ACE) inhibitors and beta blockers to slow the progression of cardiomyopathy.

Dystonia

Children with a diagnosis of dystonia demonstrate sustained muscle contractions. They may display tense muscled, repetitive movements and, in older children, abnormal postures due to this muscle disorder. According to the Dystonia Society (2011), there is no single etiology for this condition; instead, researchers have associated it more generally with either a medical condition, such as severe trauma at birth, or a genetic predisposition. Determining the etiology in a specific case may require extensive workup, but it may be necessary because some causes of dystonia are treatable (Van Egmond et al., 2014).

The presence of dystonia is considered a physical disability, as a child's normal play, social, and academic experiences can be affected. Several types of dystonias are distinguished, with the most common being generalized dystonia (affecting most of the body), hemidystonia (affecting one side of the body), myoclonus dystonia (where the child displays jerking movements), paroxysmal dystonia (found anywhere on the body but lasts only brief moments), and dopa-responsive dystonia (a rare form that has been known to respond positively to the medication levodopa, which is also used in treating Parkinson's disease). Other categories of dystonia include "task-specific" types, such as musician's cramp and writer's cramp, and acquired dystonia, such as that associated with metabolic dysfunctions, drug-induced dystonia symptoms, brain injury dystonia, and cerebral palsy.

Legg-Calvé-Perthes Disease

Marked by avascular necrosis of the femoral head, **Legg-Calvé-Perthes disease** is considered a self-limiting disorder in childhood. Boys are affected by this disease four times more often than girls, and Caucasians are affected 10 times more often than African Americans. The cause of the avascular condition is unknown but may be related to trauma.

The more rapid the identification of the pathology and the beginning of treatment for Legg-Calvé-Perthes disease, the better the long-term prognosis. Typically, the child presents with a limp, aching pain and stiffness, and greater symptoms with activity and late-daytime periods. After diagnosis, the child is placed on bed rest, traction is applied to hold the structures in place, and eventually the application of non-weight-bearing devices such as casts and braces are applied while the tissues heal.

Common Childhood Injuries: Strains, Sprains, and Fractures

It is very common to see pediatric clients in healthcare settings for soft-tissue injuries that affect mobility or fractures. Sprains, strains, and overuse syndromes of joints and soft tissues are very common during the developmental period. Notably, child athletes and children who attempt a new sport or activity in which they stress their musculoskeletal system can experience a variety of injuries that affect mobility (**Table 23-1**). Nevertheless, the healthcare provider should never assume that fractures stem from common childhood accidents. Some fractures, such as spiral fractures in very young children, have a high index of suspicion for child maltreatment. Others may suggest an underlying "hidden" disorder such as osteomalacia or primary hyperparathyroidism (Ganie et al., 2016). If the etiology of a fracture seems questionable due to inconsistencies in the history or presentation, the nurse should keep in mind other possible etiologies and explore further.

Most injuries bring only short-term limitations in mobility. A child with a minor fracture from falling on a trampoline, for example, should return to full mobility in weeks or months, depending on how severe the injury is and how well the child and his or her caregivers follow the treatment plan. As described later in this chapter, teaching families how to correctly change dressings (in cases where a wrap dressing is used) and how to manage hard casts is an important part of ensuring rapid and thorough healing without complications.

Severe injuries or trauma involving multiple fractures can be considerably more challenging. Important considerations for nursing care include ensuring optimal pain management (children are often undertreated for pain), assessing skin integrity and avoiding bed sores for bedridden children, identifying the potential for long-term mobility issues (particularly in patients with spinal or head injuries), and assisting the family in providing for the child's continued well-being and education during what may be a protracted convalescence. Nursing care providers should be alert to signs of post-traumatic stress in children who have undergone severe physical trauma (Marsac et al., 2014).

Slipped Capital Femoral Epiphysis

Occurring most frequently during periods of very rapid growth, **slipped capital femoral epiphysis** develops when the upper section of the femoral epiphysis slips from its normal position, leading to an acute and painful slip of the femoral head at the site of the femoral head's epiphyseal growth plate. The child suddenly develops a painful limp, may complain of pain radiating down the affected leg, and cannot or refuses to bear weight. Treatment must be

TABLE 23-1	Types of Fractures		
› Simple closed		› Comminuted	
› Incomplete		› Greenstick	
› Complete		› Bend	
› Compound (open)		› Buckle	
› Compression		› Spiral	

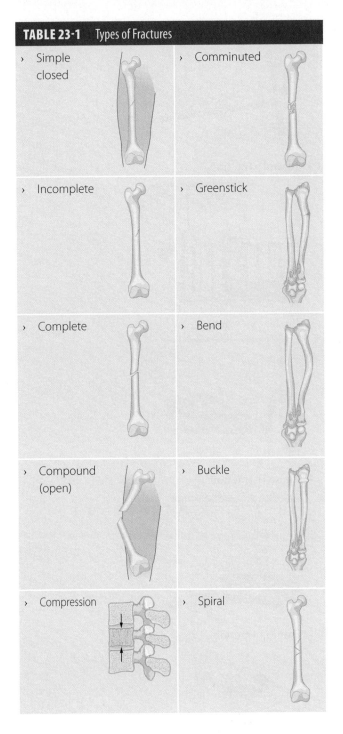

child abuse. Such an injury occurs when a rotating force is applied along the long axis of a child's bone; hence, spiral fractures are also referred to as torsion fractures.

Accidental spiral fractures often occur when the child is in motion, as one foot remains fixed on the floor or some stationary surface but the other extremities continue in motion. Such fractures can be seen in older infants and young children who experience falls (off countertops, changing tables, high chairs, and play structures) that fracture the tibia. Preschool children who fall from heights onto a leg that is extended can experience a spiral fracture.

When a pediatric healthcare team finds a spiral fracture in an infant or young toddler, intentional injury must always be ruled out. Notably, forceful twisting—such as picking up a young child by the ankle and causing a jerking, twisting motion, sometimes with impact—can cause spiral fractures (Lukefahr, 2008).

QUALITY AND SAFETY

Suspicious Fractures

Any fracture confirmed via radiography in children six months or younger should raise suspicion for an intentional child abuse injury. Due to these children's limited mobility, it is unlikely that they would fall from a distance sufficient to create enough impact to cause a significant fracture. Although such a scenario is possible, further history and physical examination should focus on identifying the possibility of child abuse.

Spiral fractures found in non-ambulatory young children are associated with intentional harm. The force required to produce this type of fracture in a non-ambulatory child would require holding the child by the knee, ankle, or elbow and causing a forceful twisting, with or without impact to a surface such as the floor or a wall.

Use of Traction in Children

Traction is often used as a treatment for young children and school-age children who present with a significant fracture. Traction can be used solely as a treatment, or it can be used preoperatively or postoperatively in preparation for surgical repair or after the application of surgical hardware to keep a limb immobile to promote healing. In general, there are three main purposes for applying traction: (1) to align the fractured limb or body part in preparation for casting, splinting, or surgical stabilization; (2) to reduce muscle spasms and tremors associated with bone fractures to promote healing and illicit fatigue of muscle groups that are having spasms; or (3) to place the fractured sites together to immobilize them and allow the ends to heal and strengthen.

initiated promptly, including immobility via bed rest until surgery is performed.

Child Abuse: Spiral Fractures

Although not always associated with child abuse, a classic spiral fracture finding via radiography on the upper limbs or, more commonly, on the lower limbs should prompt the pediatric healthcare team to conduct an expanded health history and physical exam assessing for further evidence of

The child's traction setup may provide three types of force. First, a forward pulling force may be used to reduce the dislocation of the fracture and realign the two surface sites. Second, a counter-force, also called backward pull, may use the child's weight as an anchor. Third, a frictional force may be established in which the child's body on the bed surface contributes to the stabilization of the traction setup.

Types of Traction

The type of traction ordered to treat a child's fracture depends on the child's size, age, and fracture experienced. In general, two types of traction are applied: skeletal or skin.

Skeletal traction is the surgical placement of anchoring devices such as pins, wires, plates, screws, and other metal hardware needed to hold fractured surfaces together to promote healing. Traction setups typically require a forward force, but using water bags, sand bags, or weights has also been determined to be sufficient to provide a pull to keep the fractured sites in place.

Skin traction uses stabilizing materials (dressings) to hold the fractured limb in preparation for the application of a traction setup. It is used with lesser degrees of fracture complexity and minimal displacement of fractured surfaces. In such a case, bandages are used to wrap the afflicted limb, thereby providing a pull on the skin, muscle, and overall limb.

Another way to remember traction types concerns where the fracture is located:

- Pelvic traction

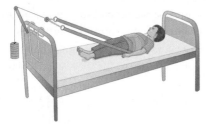

- Cervical traction

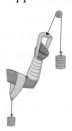

- Upper-extremity traction

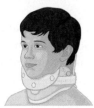

- Lower-extremity traction

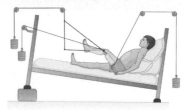

- Bryant's traction

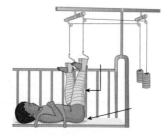

- Buck's extension

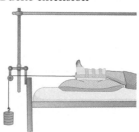

- Russell's traction

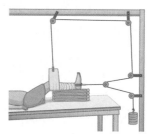

- Dunlop traction

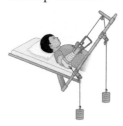

- Halo brace

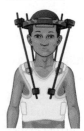

- 90-90 degree femoral traction

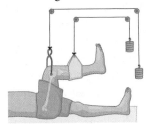

- External fixators such as the Ilizarov device

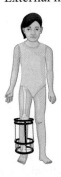

BEST PRACTICES

Assessment Findings Requiring Immediate Reporting

Children who, either verbally or nonverbally, demonstrate a change in neurologic or circulatory status while being treated for a fracture or other musculoskeletal disorder must have the change reported. Any change in clinical status should be reported to the responsible primary provider immediately. Evidence of the "five P's of neurologic or circulatory impairment" can denote serious complications of pressure, bleeding, or accumulation of secretions, all of which can lead to ischemia, necrosis, and tissue death:

- Pain
- Pallor
- Paralysis
- Pulselessness
- Paresthesias

Complications Associated with a Fracture During Childhood

Fractures are often seen as a common and almost expected childhood injury by many people. Nevertheless, they must be viewed as serious injuries with the potential for both mild and severe complications (**Box 23-1**). The pediatric nurse, while assisting in the application of casts, should monitor for appropriate alignment of the body part, adequate padding under the cast, and prevention of thermal injuries with cast saws.

Although considered the most frequently used orthopedic treatment for fractures, the application of casts on children is not without concerns. Casting a fracture during childhood requires meticulous assessments, care, and parent teaching. The five most common complications associated with casting are pain, skin abrasions, skin breakdown leading to ulcers, thermal injuries during application, and injuries to the afflicted sites neurologic system (Harp, 2005).

In rarer situations, the development of a deep vein thrombosis or compartment syndrome may occur. Measurement of compartment pressures is necessary if compartment syndrome is suspected. Children with acute-onset pain or changes in neurologic sensations at and distal to the site should be assessed for the development of bleeding or inflammatory fluids leaking into muscles bundles, thereby increasing pressure in those areas. Without intervention, compartment syndrome can lead to ischemia, necrosis, and loss of limb. Other extreme complications of extremity injuries associated with splinting, casting, and orthopedic treatments include toxic shock syndrome and necrotizing fasciitis (Delasobera, Place, Howell, & Davis, 2011).

Family Education for a Child in a Brace or Cast

With the variety of braces and casts that are used for pediatric patients who experience a fracture or musculoskeletal injury or disorder, family teaching will be required. Placement of the brace or cast is performed by the medical team, and the essential teaching on care of the child and his or her device is reinforced by the pediatric nurse. Seven key points should be covered before the family takes charge of the child's care, and it is imperative that appropriate language and level of health literacy be taken into account during this education so the child can experience a positive and timely healing process.

- Teach the family about *immediate care of the newly applied cast or brace*. If the cast has a plaster component, the family must be taught how to care for the device while it is drying. Healthcare professionals and family members should use only their palms, not their fingers, to move the child's drying cast. Typically, a fiberglass casts dries in less than 30 minutes, whereas a plaster cast does not completely set for 24 to 48 hours. If the child is placed in a brace, the healthcare team and family should assess for the child's immediate response to the placement of the device. Assessment for discomfort, distress, and compliance in the initial phase of application must be performed, and adjustments made when possible.
- The family should next be taught to *assess for deviations in neurovascular integrity*. If the child has new-onset pain or slowly increasing discomfort, or changes in sensation, movement, skin discoloration, distal-extremity temperature, or capillary refill time (all should be taught and demonstrated), the healthcare team must be immediately contacted. The family must know exactly how to contact the pediatric orthopedic team to report these deviations. Significant tissue damage from compartment syndrome must be avoided.
- Explain the importance of *assessing and reporting for symptoms of infection* when a child's musculoskeletal disorder requires a treatment that disrupts skin integrity (such as an open reduction and internal fixation [ORIF] device). The family should know how to assess for elevations in the affected extremity's temperature, elevations in the core body temperature, and local signs of infection such as redness, swelling, pain, purulent discharge, or any form of discharge and odor.
- Work with the family in *using a developmentally appropriate pain assessment method* for their child. Using family-preferred words for pain (e.g., "ouchie," "booboo"), the family should assess for sudden-onset pain, gradual pain, or intermittent pain. The family should know to contact the healthcare team if the child's discomfort does not respond to recommended pain management techniques, or

if concern arises that the cast or brace fits poorly, is too tight (possible swelling, edema, or accumulation of drainage), or needs an adjustment.
- Teach the family how to *assess the cast edges daily*. Look for drainage, presence of moisture, dirt, irritation, or blisters. Teach the family not to use lotions, powder, or any creams near the cast. Explain that the child must never put any object into the cast or brace, or use a stick or long object to scratch the skin under the device. The cast must be kept dry, and the cast edges may need to be covered with water-proof tape or plastic to keep moisture out.
- In the beginning of the cast or brace placement, teach the family to *adhere to any movement or activity restrictions*, such as weight bearing or use of a sling for support and immobilization.
- For certain musculoskeletal disorder treatments, such as serial casting for club foot or lengthy management via harnesses (e.g., spica casts or Pavlik harness for congenital hip dysplasia) or orthotics (e.g., thoracolumbosacral orthosis [TLSO] for scoliosis), the pediatric nurse must *teach the family exactly which follow-up appointments will be required*. Length of treatment must be understood and follow-up for any device issues or adjustments must be set.

RESEARCH EVIDENCE

Skin Complications with Spica Casting

According to research findings reported by DiFazio, Vessey, Zurakowski, Hresko, and Matheney in 2011, the incidence of skin complications associated with spica casting in young children with femur fractures (6 months to 6 years) is as high as 28% ($N = 297$, $n = 77$), with 31% of these patients requiring removal of the original spica cast and recasting. The most significant predictors for spica cast-related skin complications were being a victim of child maltreatment, having the cast on for more than 40 days, and being in a young developmental period. Pediatric nurses must work within an interdisciplinary team to ensure adequate assessment, teaching, parental follow-up for concerns, and immediate interventions for such skin complications.

Case Study

Dean, a 15-year-old boy, has been transferred to an acute care pediatric unit from a large urban medical center, where he had three surgeries and both critical care and acute care stays for a pedestrian-versus-motor vehicle accident that took place three weeks ago. The teen was riding without protective gear or a helmet on the back of a motorcycle being driven by an acquaintance; he was thrown off when the driver accelerated quickly. Dean was struck by a car following the motorcycle from which he was thrown. He sustained multiple fractures from the impact of the car. He had three open reduction and internal fixation (ORIF) procedures for his left femur, left humerus, and left ulna and radius. He also experienced five fractured ribs that did not require surgical intervention.

Dean has now been transferred to a hospital closer to the family's home and admitted to the pediatric unit for further nursing care and symptom management. Traction is no longer required. Upon initial assessment, his vital signs are stable, but he is tachycardic, with a heart rate of 118 beats/min. Upon admission, his current overall pain score is a 4 on a numerical pain scale. Laboratory findings upon arrival include the following:

Hemoglobin: 10.2 g/dL
Hematocrit: 31%
WBC: 7.1 per mcL
Platelets: 289,000 per mcL
Albumin: 2.9 g/dL
Calcium: 6.7 mg/dL
Magnesium: 1.2 mg/dL
C-reactive protein: 8.9 mg/L

Case Study Questions

1. What are three top-priority assessments that should be conducted during the admission process for this teen?
2. Which support services should be initiated for the family after admission?
3. Which developmental support can be offered to this teen, who will continue to have a lengthy hospitalization?
4. Which laboratory findings are of concern?

As the Case Evolves...

Dean has now been in long-term care for 6 weeks. Due to the extended time spent in traction and the severity of his injuries, this formerly athletic teen has experienced muscle wasting and has difficulty walking for more than a few minutes at a time without the aid of crutches. A physiotherapist has worked with him since he became strong enough to get out of bed, but in the past 2 days Dean has refused to cooperate and says he prefers to stay in his room and read. His mother approaches one of the nursing staff and states that she is worried because her son seems "withdrawn." She asks if there is some way to speed up his healing process and improve his motivation.

5. Which of the following interventions may be required for this teen?
   A. Referral to a nutritionist to develop a nutrition plan for optimal bone, muscle, and nerve regeneration
   B. Referral to a neurologist to assess for hidden nerve damage that could be impeding progress
   C. Referral to a psychotherapist to assess for depression or post-traumatic stress disorder
   D. No intervention is needed, as the patient's behavior is normal in this situation

Chapter Summary

- A child's musculoskeletal system's structures should be intact at birth. Through the process of maturation, cartilage is replaced with osteoblasts within bony structures, progressing outwardly from the diaphysis; this process continues until the child is in late adolescence, when skeletal maturation reaches completion.
- A young child's bones are more porous and less dense than adults' bones and, therefore, are more prone to fractures and trauma.

- After ossification, the bones grow via the epiphyseal plate (the growth plate). Muscles, as they mature through hypertrophy, provide greater stamina, coordination, and strength.
- The initial assessment of a newborn must include the assessment for birth trauma and congenital disorders such as club foot, congenital hip dysplasia, and limb-length discrepancies. A complete health history of the pregnancy and birth, followed by a thorough physical exam of the newborn, allows for early identification of such disorders.

- Assessments for evidence of child abuse, developmental motor delays, and abnormal bone structures and gait should be performed throughout childhood.
- Congenital disorders may develop in utero or occur during the birthing process. Disorders identified during childhood include congenital hip dysplasia, spina bifida, club foot, and scoliosis, among others.
- Nutritional defects influencing musculoskeletal development and mobility include insufficient intake of vitamin D, calcium, magnesium, vitamin K, zinc, and protein.
- When a child presents with a fracture, traction may be required to stabilize the site prior to or following surgical manipulation. Skeletal traction is used for fractures that require the placement of metal hardware for stability. Skin traction is used for more minor stabilization and uses only dressings to hold traction setups in place.

Bibliography

Casey, C. F., Slawson, D. C., & Neal, L. R. (2010). Vitamin D supplementation in infants, children, and adolescents. *American Family Physician, 81*(6), 745–748.

Chan, J. C. M., & Roth, K. S. (2015). Hypophosphatemic rickets. *Medscape.* Retrieved from http://emedicine.medscape.com/article/922305-overview

Christensen, B. L., & Kockrow, E .O. (2013). *Foundations of nursing.* Philadelphia, PA: Elsevier.

Delasobera, B. E., Place, R., Howell, J., & Davis, J. E. (2011). Serious infectious complications related to extremity cast/splint placement in children. *Journal of Emergency Medicine, 41*(1), 47–50.

Dicianno, B. E., Fairman, A. D., Juengst, S. B., Braun, P. G., & Zabel, T. A. (2010). Using the spina bifida life course model in clinical practice: An interdisciplinary approach. *Pediatric Clinics of North America, 57*, 945–957.

DiFazio, R., Vessey, J., Zurakowski, D., Hresko, M. T., & Matheney, T. (2011). Incidence of skin complications and associated charges in children treated with hip spica casts for femur fractures. *Journal of Pediatric Orthopedics, 31*(1), 17–22. doi:10.1097/BPO.0b013e3182032075.

Dobbs, M. B., & Gurnett, C. A. (2012). Genetics of clubfoot. *Journal of Pediatric Orthopedics B, 21*(1), 7–9.

Dystonia Society. (2011). Types of dystonia. Retrieved from http://www.dystonia.org.uk/index.php/about-dystonia/types-of-dystonia

Fuleihan, G. E-H., & Vieth, R. (2007). Vitamin D insufficiency and musculoskeletal health in children and adolescents. *International Congress Series, 1297*, 91–108. Retrieved from https://www.aub.edu.lb/fm/cmop/publications/16r.pdf

Ganie, M. A., Raizada, N., Chawla, H., Singh, A. K., Aggarwala, S., & Bal, C. S. (2016). Primary hyperparathyroidism may masquerade as rickets-osteomalacia in vitamin D replete children. *Journal of Pediatric Endocrinology and Metabolism, 29*(10), 1207–1213.

Harp, J. H. (2005). Complications from casting: Pitfall and pearls. Retrieved from http://www2.aaos.org/bulletin/dec05/rskman2.asp

International Osteoporosis Foundation (IOF). (2015). Nutrition and musculo-skeletal disorders. Retrieved from https://www.iofbonehealth.org/nutrition

Janssen, I. (2007). Physical activity guidelines for children and youth. *Applied Physiological Nutrition, 32*(suppl 2E), 2007; *Canadian Journal of Public Health, 98*(suppl 2), S109–S121.

Landfeldt, E., Lindgren, P., Bell, C. F., Guglieri, M., Straub, V., Lochmuller, H., & Bushby, K. (2016). Quantifying the burden of caregiving in Duchenne muscular dystrophy. *Journal of Neurology, 263*, 906.

Lukefahr, J. (2008). Abuse and neglect: Fractures. *Essentials of Pediatrics.* Retrieved from https://www.utmb.edu/pedi_ed/core/abuse/page_08.htm

Marsac, M. L., Kassam-Adams, N., Delahanty, D. L., Widaman, K., & Barakat, L.P. (2014) Posttraumatic stress following acute medical trauma in children: A proposed model of bio-psycho-social processes during the peri-trauma period. *Clinical Child and Family Psychology Review, 17*, 399–411.

Noordin, S., Umer, M., Hafeez, K., & Nawaz, H. (2010). Developmental dysplasia of the hip. *Orthopedic Reviews (Pavia), 2*(2), e19.

Strong, W. B., Malina, R. M., Blimkie, C. J., Daniels, S. R., Dishman, R. K., Gutin, B., . . . Trudeau, F. (2005). Evidence based physical activity for school-age youth. *Journal of Pediatrics, 146*, 732–737. Retrieved from http://www.nrcresearchpress.com/doi/pdfplus/10.1139/H07-109

Swaroop, V. T., & Dias, L. (2015). Orthopedic issues in myelomeningocele (spina bifida). *UpToDate.* Retrieved from http://www.uptodate.com/contents/orthopedic-issues-in-myelomeningocele-spina-bifida

Turer, C. B., Lin, H., & Flores, G. (2013). Prevalence of vitamin D deficiency among overweight and obese US children. *Pediatrics, 131*, e152–e161.

Van Egmond, M. E., Kulper, A., Eggink, H., Sinke, R. J., Brouwer, O. F., Verschuuren-Bemelmans, C. C., . . . de Koning, T. J. (2014). Dystonia in children and adolescents: A systematic review and a new diagnostic algorithm. *Journal of Neurology, Neurosurgery, and Psychiatry, 86*(7), 774–781, 8. doi:10.1136/jnnp-2014-309106

CHAPTER 24

Cognition and Mental Health

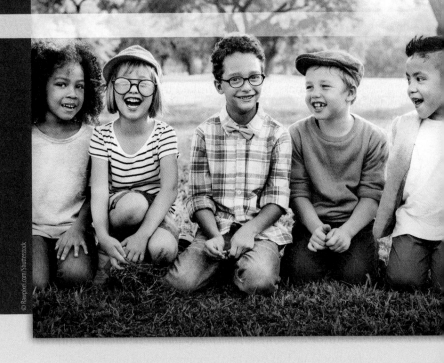

© Rawpixel.com/Shutterstock

LEARNING OBJECTIVES

1. Incorporate into nursing care the concepts of cognition and mental health.
2. Evaluate the levels of consciousness and variations in cognition for children in accordance with the various stages of the developmental period.
3. Analyze various aspects of cognitive impairment, including etiologies, assessments, management, family education, and nursing care.
4. Analyze the most common mental health issues affecting young children, school-age children, and adolescents in the United States today.
5. Assess children at risk of eating disorders, and critique the effectiveness of current treatments used to assist children and adolescents experiencing severe disordered eating.
6. Evaluate suicidal behaviors such as suicidal ideation, gestures, suicide attempts, and successful suicide.

KEY TERMS

Anxiety
Cognition
Cognitive development
Cognitive impairment
Depression
Pica
Suicidal ideation
Suicide attempt
Suicide gesture

Introduction

Cognition and mental health are grouped together as inter-related concepts. **Cognition**, or the child's mental capacity and awareness, is directly linked to the child's mental health state. Interwoven with mental health and cognitive processing is the child's thinking about the world and the meaning of his or her existence. Both of these concepts are discussed in this chapter.

Cognition

A child's cognition is loosely defined as his or her level of awareness. This term denotes a child's ability to take in and process sensory stimuli, and then react. A child's cognition can be considered to be based on several factors, including health state, developmental level (**Box 24-1**), presence of disease, intelligence quotient (IQ), personal challenges, and family dynamics. More generally, one can consider cognition as the child's ability to respond to external stimuli (sensory) such as pain and temperature and touch, as well as intellectual or developmental stimuli.

Many factors can lead to a decline in a child's cognitive status, including metabolic disease, altered brain chemistry, diabetes mellitus, uremia, alteration in serum sodium (hypernatremia or hyponatremia), drug toxicity, lead poisoning, changes in core body temperature, stroke, central nervous system infections, sepsis, after-seizure (postictal) state, and increased intracranial pressure. Social factors influencing child's delayed cognitive processing may include chronic stress, anxiety, a poorly stimulating environment, social isolation, and child maltreatment.

BEST PRACTICES

Any change of cognition, or consciousness, should be reported immediately and further diagnostics undertaken. Continued change in cognition can be a progressive and life-threatening event requiring medical evaluation and treatment. Any cognitive developmental delay must be referred for evaluation.

Assessments of a child's cognitive ability cover two general areas. First, assessment considers the ability to process sensory stimulation, where a child's level of consciousness can be determined (i.e., painful stimuli). Second, assessment addresses the child's intellectual ability or capacity. Tools for assessing the sensory-based level of cognition include reflexes, pain responses, ability to swallow and cough, and gag reflexes. Tools for assessing level of consciousness are varied but are based on the assessment of awareness and level of ability to respond to stimuli.

BOX 24-1 Piaget's Stages of Cognitive Development

According to Jean Piaget's theory of **cognitive development**, a child works through and masters a series of age-related phases in a sequential and orderly manner, with each phase comprising challenges of mastering increasingly difficult sets of tasks. Piaget's theory includes four stages:

- *Sensorimotor* (age 0–2): The child learns to move and interact with sensory stimuli over the first two years of life.
- *Preoperational* (age 2–7): The child's egocentric self moves to social awareness, animism (the attribution of a soul or consciousness or being to an inanimate object), and magical thinking.
- *Concrete operations* (age 7–11): The child learns about conservation of matter and the process of cause and effect.
- *Formal operations* (age 11–18): The child develops abstract thinking, achieves intellectual mental processing, and masters the ability to consider various outcomes to situations (which, in turn, greatly influences safety and adult decision making).

QUALITY AND SAFETY

Levels of Consciousness

As part of the concept of human awareness, determining a child's level of consciousness is a nurse's responsibility as a member of the healthcare team—and often the one who engages in the most prolonged child–team member interactions. The levels of a child's consciousness are presented here in order of increasing severity:

- Fully conscious and aware and alert
- Lethargy
- Obtunded
- Stupor
- Coma

As part of the cognitive assessment, the pediatric team may want to order a series of laboratory analyses, including a thyroid panel, electrolytes, serum glucose, urine drug screen, and lead levels. The team may also choose to have the child undergo computed tomography (CT) scan of the head, pulse oxygen monitoring, and arterial or capillary blood gas analysis. Both a cerebral bleed and meningitis should be ruled out by means of a lumbar puncture.

If a child's lower level of cognition is due to use of drugs that influence mental processing, such as narcotic use, or other drug toxicities, medications for reversal may need to be administered. For example, naloxone may be administered for narcotic reversal (**Figure 24-1**). Other

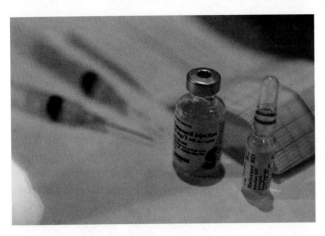

Figure 24-1 *Naloxone.*

B Christopher / Alamy Stock Photo

sources of support or reversal include the administration of oxygen, thiamine, and glucose, and chelation therapy for heavy metal poisoning.

Cognitive Impairment

The term **cognitive impairment** is used to describe a child's overall mental deficiency or mental difficulty. This broad term denotes many different lower-than-expected states of mental processing. Risk factors associated with cognitive impairment include brain trauma, microcephaly, metabolic disorders, chronic lead exposure, congenital rubella or syphilis, and fetal alcohol syndrome. Due to the social stigma attached to the previously used term "mental retardation," "cognitive impairment" is now the preferred terminology.

The diagnosis of cognitive impairment in a child is based on objective data collected to compare a child's current mental processing with the behaviors and mental processing expected for the child's age and developmental level. The clinical presentation of cognitive impairment can range from mild to quite severe. Parents, childcare providers, or health professionals may be the first to recognize a delay in expected motor and developmental milestones. Early clinical manifestations include decreased alertness, delay in gross motor development, delay or absence of language development, feeding issues, and abnormal responses to physical contact or eye contact. A child who displays any of these symptoms should be referred for professional assessment and the determination of the cause and severity of cognitive impairment.

Treatment for cognitive impairment is based on the etiology and probability for improvement. After the child's level of deficiency is determined, the family should immediately be referred to a regional early intervention program based on the child's level of development (not the child's age). Referrals for speech therapy, occupational therapy, and physical therapy should be made as appropriate. The

assistance of a social worker should be secured to help the family navigate resources, obtain financial assistance for the child's care as needed, and investigate supportive services such as transportation, housing (if needed), and support for siblings and family dynamics. A social worker can also assist with securing the best educational program for the child's level of impairment. The overall focus of treatment for the child is improving his or her social behaviors such as communication, social activities, and appropriate play. Families should help the child with self-care behaviors and the promotion of healthy relationships.

Mental Health Issues in Children

The incidence of mental health issues, concerns, and diagnoses is on the rise both in the United States and worldwide (Olfson, Blanco, Wang, Laje, & Correll, 2014). Today's children have more concerns with depression, anxiety, post-traumatic stress disorder, and other psychiatric disorders than their historical counterparts. The overall incidence of mental health issues in children is now 13% to 20% and is increasing (Centers for Disease Control and Prevention [CDC], 2013). Pediatric registered nurses, as part of an interdisciplinary team, can play an integral role in the early identification, referral, assessment, and treatment and management of children with mental health issues.

Levels of anxiety, depression, post-traumatic stress, and participation in risky behaviors are believed to be increasing due to the current social milieu, which includes the social pressures of bullying, pressure to participate in high-risk behaviors, violence in communities, economic concerns leading to unemployment, and stressors on families (Abma, Martinez, & Copen, 2010; CDC, 2010; Kirby & Lepore, 2007). Children are highly vulnerable to these pressures. They respond and react to their life experiences with keen awareness, such that stressors can greatly affect their mood and state of being. Children are also vulnerable to the influence of genetics, family tendencies, and family history of severe mental illnesses such as bipolar disorder, schizophrenia, and severe depressive disorders. During any pediatric healthcare interaction, members of the pediatric team must be aware of the child's cognitive, behavioral, and emotional states so that early detection of mental health issues will be ensured and treatment can be initiated.

The following organizations are three excellent sources of information on the wide variety of mental health issues during childhood:

- MentalHealth.gov: http://www.mentalhealth.gov
- National Institute of Mental Health (NIMH): http://www.nimh.nih.gov
- National Library of Medicine's *Medline Plus*: http://www.medlineplus.gov

Self-Esteem in Children

Self-esteem is defined as how one feels about oneself. Low or negative self-esteem can lead children to believe that they do not deserve love and support, and to perceive that they are generally not good at things when situations tend to work out poorly. Building self-esteem is a very crucial part of every child's development.

According to psychiatrist Heinz Kohut, the development of self-esteem is achieved, in part, through maternal "mirroring" of the young child. That is, the mother (or other parent/guardian) fulfills the child's innate need for approval and validation through the process of mirroring, helping to solidify the child's sense of self (Clark, 1999; "Heinz Kohut's Self Psychology: An Overview," 1987).

How children play, interact with other people, show confidence, admit mistakes, learn, and problem-solve are all influenced by their self-esteem. When children have low self-esteem, they tend to have no pride in their work, have a negative image of themselves on many levels, compare themselves (physically, emotionally, and intellectually) against others, and tend to struggle in making and keeping friends. Low self-esteem has been directly linked to depression, self-destructive and self-harm behaviors, anxiety, and other mental health issues (Orth & Robins, 2013; YoungMinds, 2016). Encouraging families to assess their child's emerging self-esteem, and being aware of how important self-esteem is to the child's current and long-term success in life, is important to the child's sense of well-being.

Depression

Depression—that is, sadness—is a normal part of life, often situational in nature and based on circumstances that warrant deep feelings of despair. A child who loses a parent, sibling, or best friend may fall into a depressive state. Even the loss of a treasured pet may cause a situational state of depression. These circumstances may elicit depressive signs and symptoms of a limited duration, followed eventually by a return to full functionality.

In contrast, the term **depression**, when used in reference to the clinically diagnosed mental health disorder, denotes a persistent mood disorder that is characterized by an ongoing state of sadness and loss of interest in life activities; for some children, it can profoundly impact their ability to function on a daily basis (**Figure 24-2**). Only a specialized medical professional can diagnose depression as a disorder in children. Children with a documented history of clinical depression require treatment. Counseling and sometimes the administration of antidepressant medications are required to assist a child battling depression.

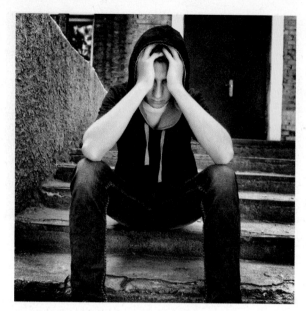

Figure 24-2 *For some children, depression can profoundly impact their ability to function on a daily basis.*
© Sabphoto/Shutterstock.

Many well-accepted, reliable, and valid tools are available to assess for depression in children, including the Children's Depression Rating Scale and the Children's Depression Inventory. The pediatric nurse should assess for the following symptoms and report their presence to the pediatric team, with immediate referral of the child for specialized mental health services:

- Depressed mood state
- Poor hygiene and/or a significant change in appearance, dress, and weight (gain or loss)
- Feelings of low self-worth
- Inability to feel joy or pleasure (anhedonia) and lack of desire for play and peer interaction
- Difficulty with academic performance or poor concentration
- Changes in relationships with family and friends
- Suicidal thoughts, **suicidal ideation** (preoccupation with suicide), **suicide gesture** (an attempt at self-harm that is suggestive of suicide, but in which the person does not intend to die), or **suicide attempt** (an unsuccessful attempt to commit suicide, in which the person survives)

Many associate the teenage period with concerns of suicidal thoughts and attempts, but the pediatric nurse must recognize that school-age children also experience suicidal thinking and acts. Most important, the pediatric nurse and all members of the healthcare team must be able to recognize the warning signs of suicide (**Table 24-1**). If the child is suspected of harboring thoughts of suicide, the pediatric nurse—no matter what the practice setting

TABLE 24-1	Classic Warning Signs of Suicide in Children

- › Depression
- › Major life stressors
- › Talking of taking one's life
- › Another suicide in the child's community
- › Academic failure
- › Severe mood swings
- › Change in personal appearance, hygiene, and eating behaviors
- › Significant losses (deaths) in the family or social community
- › Withdrawn behaviors, social isolation, change in behaviors and relationships
- › Giving away meaningful possessions

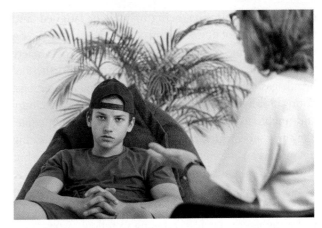

Figure 24-3 *Potential treatment modalities for a child's depression include various types of therapy.*

or healthcare institution—must immediately report the child's suicidal thoughts or behaviors to the interdisciplinary team and nursing administration, and then implement all safety precautions needed to protect the child from acting on suicidal impulses. An assessment of lethality should be conducted to determine if the child's suicidal plan has progressed to a time, place, and method. If the child is truly at risk for suicide, protective custody may be warranted.

Treatment for Depression

Due to the high-risk nature of this psychiatric condition, treatment of depression in children is addressed via a three-pronged approach. Children will need the services of a mental health counselor or therapist to help them determine the causes of their feelings of hopelessness, unhappiness, and possibly loneliness (feelings of dejection) in their lives and relationships, as well as to help them determine positive coping strategies to deal with each causative factor. Medication may be necessary if the depression is deep and prolonged. Finally, the family will need support to best understand their child's behaviors, feelings, and needs.

Because childhood depression can be short term, situational, or prolonged, a professional child mental health specialist should be involved in the assessment, management, and treatment of any child with depression. Ensuring the child's safety is imperative, and the progression of depression to suicidal behaviors must be evaluated. Potential treatment modalities for the child's depression include psychotherapy, family therapy, cognitive therapy, environmental therapy, psychiatric therapy with medication, and educational therapy concerning personal coping strategies and skill development (**Figure 24-3**).

PHARMACOLOGY

Warnings on Use of Antidepressant Medications in Children

Selective serotonin reuptake inhibitors (SSRIs) are the primary types of medications used for treatment and support of children with depression. Two SSRIs are specifically approved for pediatric use:

- Sertraline (Zoloft)
- Fluoxetine (Prozac)

Two other medications in this class, paroxetine (Paxil) and bupropion (Wellbutrin), are not approved for use in children because they carry a higher risk of suicidal thinking.

Family education on these medications includes the following points:

- Never stop the medication abruptly; talk to the prescribing pediatric specialist before taking the child off the medication.
- Understand the increased risk for suicidal ideation during the early phase of taking these medications; monitor for signs of suicide discussions, planning, or behaviors.
- Become familiar with the adverse side effects of the medications. Mild effects include headache, sleep problems, nausea, and restlessness. Severe side effects include suicidal thoughts and actions and the development of depression resistant to medications.
- Know when to expect therapeutic effectiveness to begin, as each medication has an average length of time before its full therapeutic value is seen.

Anxiety

Anxiety is the most common mental illness in children (Merikangas et al., 2010). Children with anxiety have the potential to display unique symptoms. Restlessness, difficulty concentrating, being irritable or fatigued, and feeling insecure or powerless are common descriptions of a child's experience of anxiety. Physical symptoms of anxiety may include headaches, tremors, shakiness, shortness of breath, gastrointestinal distress, sweating, and palpitations. Young children with anxiety disorder may be very clingy and unable to adapt to new situations and new people. They may show regressive behaviors such as thumb sucking not only as an attempt to soothe their emotional state but also to gain attention from caregivers (Field, McCabe, & Schneiderman, 2013). Other symptoms may develop that cause difficulty for those around the child with anxiety, including aggressiveness, refusing to follow instructions or behave, refusing to eat, and crying.

Anxiety is a mental health issue that requires assessment, treatment and management. The disorder can be so severe that children experience anxiety every time they leave their home, leading to academic failure; poor relationships with peers, teachers, and family; and physical sequelae. Tremendous feelings of doom can cause a child to experience significant palpitations and impairments of functioning. **Table 24-2** provides a list of anxiety disorders.

In adults, anxiety disorders are frequently treated with medications; however, most of the medications typically used for this purpose—such as lorazepam (Ativan), clonazepam (Klonopin), and chlordiazepoxide (Librium)—are not approved for this use (or at all) in children due to safety concerns. Psychotherapeutic methods such as cognitive-behavioral therapy are generally preferred over medications for this reason, but a combination of psychotherapy and medication is sometimes used (James, James, Cowdrey, Soler, & Choke, 2013).

RESEARCH EVIDENCE

Research at the University of Houston, funded by the National Institutes of Health, has linked a lack of quality sleep in children with a higher risk for an emotional disorder later in life. Inadequate sleep, or frequently disrupted sleep, during childhood has been shown to increase the incidence of anxiety disorders (Life Sciences and Medicine, 2016).

Autism

The diagnosis of autism in children is a complex process and does not definitively occur until after the child reaches one year of age. Considered a group of developmental disabilities with an unknown origin, autism spectrum disorder causes significant impairment in three domains: communication (social interactions), repetitive behaviors, and imaginative play. It becomes evident in almost all cases by a child's third birthday, but consensus on a well-accepted etiology of this mental disorder has not been achieved. Possible etiologies that are being investigated include biochemical influences,

TABLE 24-2	Anxiety Disorders and Their Associated Symptoms
Agoraphobia	Characterized by intense fear of places or situations that are perceived as leading to being "trapped" and unable to escape, such as being alone outside of the home; traveling in a car, bus, or airplane; or being in a crowded area.
Generalized anxiety disorder	Characterized by unwarranted or excessive worry or fear unrelated to events or circumstances. Symptoms include restlessness, sleep difficulties, muscle tension, and irritability.
Obsessive-compulsive disorder (OCD)	Characterized by recurring thoughts or repetitive behaviors (compulsions) that prevent the individual from functioning effectively.
Panic disorder	Characterized by recurrent, sudden-onset episodes of intense fear with no obvious cause. Symptoms may include tachycardia, sweating, trembling or shaking, dyspnea or a sensation of smothering or choking, and a perception of impending doom.
Post-traumatic stress disorder (PTSD)	An anxiety disorder that develops after a traumatic experience. To be diagnosed with PTSD, the patient's symptoms must last more than a month and include significant changes in mood and cognition, avoidance of situations similar to the original trauma, heightened arousal and reactivity, and episodes in which he or she re-experiences the initial episode (flashbacks, nightmares).
Social anxiety disorder	Characterized by significant fear of social situations and worry about being judged, humiliated, or rejected by others. Symptoms include avoiding social situations and experiencing shaking, sweating, or nausea when required to participate in social situations.

Data from National Institute of Mental Health. (n.d.). Mental health information: Mental disorders and mental health topics. Retrieved from https://www.nimh.nih.gov/health/topics/index.shtml

genetics, neurotransmitter dysfunction, central nervous system disorders, and brain metabolism malfunction. The prevalence of autism spectrum disorder is currently documented as 1 in every 68 children, with males presenting with the disorder at 4.5 times the rate in females (1 in 42 for males versus 1 in 189 for females) (CDC, 2016a). Females show the most severe symptoms. Children born to older parents are at a greater risk of developing autism (CDC, 2016a). The overall percentage of children with autism spectrum disorder appears to be increasing (CDC, 2016b).

Autism is considered a spectrum disorder, meaning a child's symptoms may range along a spectrum of severity (NIMH, 2015c) from mild (need for minimal supervision and interventions) to profound (self-abuse, safety issues, and destructive behaviors). Children with autism often display the following behaviors:

- Social withdrawal and lack of development of meaningful relationships; lack of separation anxiety as a toddler
- Inability to perform expected play behaviors and outcomes with peers
- Withdrawal from reality and from the activities of daily living and social interactions surrounding the child
- Aversion to affection, cuddling, and most forms of physical contact; may display mild to violent reactions to touch
- Appearance of cognitive impairment due to indifference, but may be highly intelligent, have strong memories, or demonstrate excellent intellectual potential
- Apathy, lack of eye contact, withdrawal, and lack of empathy for others' feelings, emotions, expressed concerns, or injuries
- Display of unpredictable and uncontrolled behaviors, including intense temper tantrums and verbal and physical aggression, especially when routines are changed
- Participation in repetitive behaviors, bizarre movements, echolalia (echoing words), and physical rituals (rocking, flapping arms, twirling, playing with an object for hours each day)
- Display of self-destructive behaviors such as slapping, head banging, or hand-biting

There is a range of early screening tools available to assess young children for autism. **Table 24-3** lists both autism-specific screening tools and social/communication screening tools that are often used to supplement diagnostic interviews. To make the diagnosis of autism, a child must have 8 of 16 identifying characteristics, and have characteristics in three categories: inability to relate, impaired communication skills, and limited activities or repetitive behaviors (**Figure 24-4**). Although there are no treatments to cure autism, early developmental interventions and psychotherapy, starting as early as 18 months, have been shown to improve a child's autistic behaviors (Bradshaw, Steiner, Gengoux, & Koegel, 2015). Medications that have been trialed for this disorder include lithium, neuroleptics, and stimulants.

The focus of care for children with autism is to assist them in their daily function. Current interventions include consistent routines, consistent environments, limit-setting for unacceptable behaviors, and encouragement of verbalization and eye contact. Goals of treatment are to maintain or improve social interaction and social growth, as well as to promote education, intellectual growth, and participation in activities of daily living (ADLs). It is imperative to support the family in creating a safe environment for the autistic child. Preventing self-destructive behaviors and preventing the child from wandering off or becoming lost is paramount. Pediatric healthcare team members must assist the family of a child with autism to identify local, regional, state, and national organizations that will provide assistance and referrals as needed.

TABLE 24-3 Autism Screening Tools

Autism-Specific Screening Tools	Social/Communication Screening Tools
Autism Diagnostic Interview—Revised Semi-structured clinician-led interview of parents/caregivers; 93-item interview; designed to screen children with mental age > 2.	*Behavior Rating Inventory of Executive Function* To be completed by parent/caregiver and teacher; rates executive functioning at both home and school; ages 5–18.
Autism Diagnostic Observation Schedule Semi-structured clinician assessment; observe child's social and communication skills through activities; designed for ages 2+.	*Brief Infant–Toddler Social and Emotional Assessment (BITSEA)* A 42-item parent report; screens for social-emotional-behavioral problems, as well as delays in social competence; designed for children ages 12–26 months.
Autism Spectrum Quotient Self-administered 50-item questionnaire; designed for adults, but an adolescent version is available; assesses personal preferences and habits.	*Children's Communication Checklist—2* To be completed by parent or caregiver; 70-item list that screens children on 10 subscales.
Childhood Autism Rating Scale Two 15-item clinician-led rating scales; screens for autism and rates symptom severity; additional parent/caregiver questionnaire; designed for ages 2+.	*Communication and Symbolic Behavior Scales Developmental Profile* Screens for language predictors; combination 24-item parent/caregiver questionnaire, with clinician observation (behavior sample); designed for children ages 6 months–6 years.
Modified Checklist for Autism in Toddlers—Revised/Follow-up Designed for low-risk toddlers, ages 16–30 months; 20 Y/N questions directed to parents or caregivers, with structured follow-up questions if toddler screens positively.	*Joseph Picture Self-Concept Scale* Interactive clinician-led interview designed for children ages 3–13; assesses nonverbal self-concept; childhood and adolescent versions available.
Screening Tool for Autism in Toddlers and Young Children A 12-item, interactive and observational screening tool; delivered by clinicians or community professionals; designed for children ages 24–36 months.	*Social Communication Disorder Checklist* 12-item scale with good reliability and validity
Social Communication Questionnaire Previously known as the Autism Screening Questionnaire; 40-item Y/N questionnaire for parents/caregivers; designed to screen children with mental age > 2.	
Social Responsiveness Scale To be completed by parent, caregiver or teacher; targets children ages 4–18; measures impairment on a scale of severity.	

Asperger's Syndrome

Considered a high-functioning variant of autism, Asperger's syndrome is marked by a level of higher function but ongoing social deficits, poor relationships with peers, struggles with transitioning between settings, and difficulty interpreting contextual cues (Stichter, O'Connor, Herzog, Lierheimer, & McGhee, 2012). Parents, who tend to see their children achieve high function in some areas and intellectual normalcy, can become quite frustrated when their child with Asperger's syndrome demonstrates social deficits. One predicament parents face is that their child may be high functioning in regard to typical autism interventions, but require more assistance and guidance than those children with classic learning disabilities. Children with Asperger's syndrome can demonstrate average or above-average intellectual functioning, yet experience continued social struggles with adults and peers.

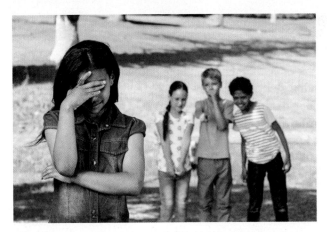

Figure 24-4 *Inability to relate is a category of characteristics of autism.*
© wavebreakmedia/Shutterstock

Attention-Deficit Disorder

Attention-deficit disorder (ADD) and attention-deficit/hyperactivity disorder (ADHD) are conditions in which a child displays three classic behaviors: impulsivity, inattentiveness, and hyperactivity. Typically diagnosed in the school-age period, the child with ADD/ADHD experiences struggles with learning, memorizing, behavioral challenges of attention, and social expectations for age. These disorders are considered developmentally inappropriate patterns of behavior in which symptoms appear before the seventh birthday and are present between the ages of 4 and 18 years. The child with ADD/ADHD also displays symptoms in more than one setting.

The prevalence of ADD/ADHD has been variously estimated to be 2.3 to 6 times higher in males than in females (DuPaul & Stoner, 2014; Ramtekkar, Reiersen, Todorov, & Todd, 2010). An estimated 11% of U.S. school-age children have received this diagnosis (CDC, 2016c). It is most commonly identified in the classroom by teachers (DuPaul & Stoner, 2014). The child's intelligence can be at or above average, yet the child struggles in completing tasks, studying, and staying quiet when expected. A cycle of behavior followed by negative reactions from peers and adults, followed by maladaptive behaviors, is common. Self-esteem and self-image can be affected, causing the child distress.

Physiologically, the child with ADD/ADHD may display abnormal levels of serotonin, norepinephrine, or dopamine. In some cases, there may be an alteration in the child's reticular activating system within the midbrain. With other children, ADD/ADHD is associated with an abusive home, a chaotic home, or a history of parental substance abuse, depression, or antisocial disorders.

Classic symptoms of ADD and ADHD include the following manifestations:

- Inattention to details in the classroom, when studying, and in other environments where instructions are given and performance expectations are present; avoids or dislikes activities where the child must demonstrate sustained mental effort
- Poor listening skills, inability to follow important instructions, ineffective work habits leading to lack of completion and losing academic assignments, paperwork, and other items needed for school; typically cannot wait for his or her turn in group situations
- Fidgety behaviors, difficulty in sitting, impulsivity, and increased motor function displayed in most situations
- Seems to be busy at all times and does not engage in quiet play
- Communicates poorly with excessive talking, inappropriate conversations, and interruptions; blurts out answers before being asked to provide one when questioned
- Physical complaints associated with decreased appetite and insomnia

Treatment for ADD/ADHD includes two approaches: Medications may be ordered to assist the child with improved attention, and behavioral modification may be provided through parental and teacher education and support. The medications used to treat attention disorders have side effects, so the decision to place a child on pharmacologic interventions should not be made lightly. **Table 24-4** identifies medications currently prescribed for ADD/ADHD, along with their trade names, mechanism of action, and side effects.

TABLE 24-4	Medications for Treatment of Attention-Deficit Disorders		
Medication	**Trade Name**	**Mechanism of Action**	**Common Side Effects**
Amphetamine mixture (dextroamphetamine and amphetamine)	Adderall	Has a similar chemical structure to brain neurotransmitters; boosts the effects of dopamine and norepinephrine in the brain, acting like a stimulant	Appetite suppression, weight loss, insomnia, nervousness, palpitations, tachycardia, headaches, bruxism
Dextroamphetamine	Dexedrine	Psychostimulant that increases dopamine and norepinephrine levels in the brain	Restlessness, dry mouth, diarrhea, constipation, appetite suppression, weight loss, insomnia, nervousness, dizziness, palpitations, tachycardia, headache
Methylphenidate	Ritalin	Psychostimulant that increases dopamine and norepinephrine levels; should be given 30 minutes before eating	Appetite suppression, weight loss, nervousness, palpitations, tachycardia, headache. Insomnia is also a concern. The last dose of the day should be given prior to late afternoon so sleep is not interrupted.
Atomoxetine	Strattera	Selective norepinephrine reuptake inhibitor	Dyspepsia, fatigue, decreased appetite, weight loss, dizziness, mood swings, constipation, dry mouth, insomnia. Monitor the child for suicidal ideation, as this is rare occurrence but a major concern.

Nursing care should support the family in understanding that successful management of a child with this disorder includes remaining calm and respectful, while being firm and providing clear expectations of desired behaviors. The adult should secure the child's full attention before giving the child feedback on behaviors. The child needs positive feedback, rewards for desired behaviors, and support; consistent negativity and frustration expressed by parents, siblings, peers, and teachers will not help the child's behaviors and coping. Whenever possible, safe play, chores, and academic activities should be planned so that the child can be up, be active, and use his or her energy.

Bipolar Disorder

Bipolar disorder manifests as a condition of intense and extreme mood behaviors. Classically, the child will demonstrate the mood swings of depression and manic behavior, with each phase often lasting at least seven days (NIMH, 2016b). Parents may receive feedback that their child is excessively "moody" and more excitable and responsive than other children of the same age and developmental level. Parents describe their children as showing highs and lows of emotional responses at a level that is more pronounced than their peers or siblings.

Bipolar disorder, which was previously known as manic-depressive illness, is a severe mental illness that requires treatment. It is marked by displays of behavior described as being very "up," with high energy, talkativeness, and active behaviors (manic episode), as well as by the opposite state, in which the child is "low" and displays behaviors of classic depression with low energy, social withdrawal, and sadness (depressive episode). The swings of emotion come with a wide variety of temporal factors. Each side of the mood swings can last for hours, days, weeks, or months. The extreme swings of "high" and "low" can be accompanied with short or long periods of "normal" or expected behaviors found in children without the disorder, or behaviors can be described as "mixed." The diagnosis of bipolar disorder is not representative of normal childhood mood swings; rather, it is a serious psychiatric disorder characterized by extremes in behaviors.

Other symptoms of bipolar disorder include changes in eating, sleeping, playing, and interacting with others. When in the manic phase, children can have a short temper, be very silly, or display unusual moods for their age. They have trouble focusing at home and at school, and may engage in a higher level and frequency of high-risk behaviors. When in the depressive phase of the mood extremes, children may be very quiet, withdrawn, and sad; have somatic complaints (headache, stomachache, cramps); sleep for prolonged periods; eat less; show low energy; and have suicidal ideations. Children and teens with bipolar disorder are at greater risk for self-harm, self-destructive behaviors, and suicidal behaviors (NIMH, Office of Science Policy, Planning and

Communications, 2015). Three comorbid conditions that often complicate the clinical picture are substance abuse, anxiety disorders, and ADD/ADHD (NIMH, Office of Science Policy, Planning and Communications, 2015).

Bipolar disorder can run in families, but no genetic link for this disorder has been confirmed. Scientists do not know what causes bipolar disorder (NIMH, Office of Science Policy, Planning and Communications, 2015). Treatment includes counseling, such as "talk" therapy with a psychotherapist who provides guidance, education, and support. Psychogenic medications such as lithium and other mood stabilizers or antidepressants may be required.

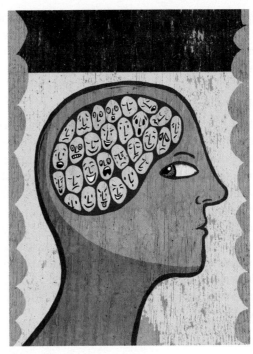

Figure 24-5 *A child with schizophrenia may have "positive symptoms"—that is, overt alterations in mentation, including delusional thinking, hallucinations, dysfunctional thought processing, and agitated movements of the body.*

© Alberto Ruggieri/Illustration Works/Getty Images

QUALITY AND SAFETY

Adults and peers who interact with a child with bipolar disorder must be prepared to call for immediate assistance in the event of extreme behaviors and mood swings. The child should not be left alone, and the child's doctor should be called immediately; the child should be transported to the nearest emergency services or 911 should be called for help. Families should have access to the National Suicide Prevention telephone line at 1-800-273-8255 (TALK).

Schizophrenia

Considered a severe chronic mental health disorder, schizophrenia affects all aspects of a child's mental processing, feelings, and behavior. This highly disabling disorder appears as though the person afflicted does not live in reality or has lost touch with reality. Cases in children are usually not confirmed until the child is 16 years or older. Only rarely do young children display the symptoms of this disorder.

Schizophrenia affects three main areas of cognitive and behavioral functioning. First, a child may display "cognitive symptoms," such as difficulty processing information, remembering, making decisions, and paying attention. Second, a child may have "positive symptoms"—that is, overt alterations in mentation, including delusional thinking, hallucinations, dysfunctional thought processing, and agitated movements of the body (**Figure 24-5**). Third, a child may have "negative symptoms," in which emotional and mental processes are greatly subdued, as indicated by a flat affect, reduced communication, and reduced pleasure in everyday life.

No exact etiology of schizophrenia in children has been identified, but research supports a relationship between genes, the child's environment, malnutrition, viral exposure, and several psychosocial factors. An imbalance of glutamate, dopamine, and other neurotransmitters may play a role in the development of this disorder, especially during puberty (NIMH, 2016c). Some evidence suggests a link between cannabis use and development of schizophrenia in individuals with a family history of the disorder (Radhakrishnan, Wilkinson, & D'Souza, 2014).

Treatment for schizophrenia initially focuses on finding the right medication to stabilize the child's symptoms. Psychotherapy follows pharmacologic therapy, and focuses on coping skills, life goals, academic achievement, and relationships. The most successful management of schizophrenia is achieved through a "coordinated specialty care" management program that integrates medications, education, therapy, family involvement, and academic or employment assistance through a multidisciplinary coordinated effort. Young people benefit highly from having a coordinated and sustained program to reduce what can be a very significant long-term mental disability (NIMH, 2016c).

Eating Disorders

Eating disorders cover both severe underweight and severe overweight, as well as abnormal eating behaviors. The incidence of eating disorders continues to rise in the United States (Wade, Keski-Rahkonen, & Hudson, 2011). Although females have a higher rate of eating disorders than males, the incidence in males is also increasing. Currently, the prevalence rate for obesity is 16.9% among children between 2 and 19 years of age (Ogden, Carroll, Kit, & Flegal, 2014). Restrictive eating disorders have an incidence of 3.8% of females and 1.5% of males (Merikangas et al., 2010; NIMH, 2016a). Eating disorders have the highest mortality rate of all psychiatric disorders (Arcelus, Mitchell, Wales, & Nielsen, 2011).

Anorexia and Bulimia

The etiology of restrictive eating disorders remains a controversial topic, but experts agree that they are serious and often life-threatening psychological disorders associated with an altered body image and extreme fear of obesity or overweight status. **Table 24-5** differentiates the features of two types of restrictive eating disorders—namely, bulimia and anorexia nervosa. Risk factors for the development of an eating disorder during the developmental period include depression, family predisposition (e.g., mother is anorexic), middle to upper socioeconomic class, dysfunctional family, excessive self-expectations, obsessive–compulsive behaviors, and sexual abuse.

Pica

Another eating disorder found across the developmental period is **pica**, or the consumption of material not associated with food substances. Pica behaviors include eating non-nutritive items such as house plants, paper, twigs, clay, carpet pieces, human hair, and other digestible and nondigestible household and environmental substances such as dirt, pebbles, and sand. Pica has been associated with anemia, autism, and developmental delay. It is found more commonly in young children than across the other stages of the life span (Katz & DeMaso, 2011).

One serious consequence of pica is the accumulation of a trapped mass of indigestible material in the digestive tract, called bezoar. The development of an intestinal blockage is considered a health emergency.

Treatment for Eating Disorders

The physiological consequences of eating disorders in children require attention by an interdisciplinary pediatric healthcare team. Nurses, physicians, child psychologists, pharmacists, family members, and teachers need to be involved in the early identification of the disorder and its treatment and management. A significant number of children—mostly teen girls—die each year in the United States due to the physiological consequences of extreme dietary restriction, purging, vomiting, and self-abuse. Estimating the true mortality rate is difficult, however, because a frequent cause of death (up to 25% in one study) in those with eating disorders is suicide (Franko et al., 2013). **Box 24-2** identifies moderately severe and life-threatening consequences of eating disorders.

TABLE 24-5 Bulimia Versus Anorexia Nervosa	
Bulimia	**Anorexia Nervosa**
› Altered body image, participation in activities aimed at the consumption of calories for weight loss, obsessive exercise	› Altered body image, participation in extreme eating restriction, and morbid fear of being "fat"
› Binge eating (sometimes thousands of kilocalories) followed by guilt, fear, and anxiety, leading to purging through self-induced vomiting, inappropriate use of laxatives and diuretics, and excessive and intense exercise	› Weight below or extremely below expectations for weight on national growth charts for age
› Weight may be near or at normal per national growth charts for expected weight for age	› The *Diagnostic and Statistical Manual of Mental Disorders*, fifth edition (*DSM-5*), changed one of the diagnostic criteria for anorexia from a patient needing to be 85% or less than expected body weight to a "restriction of energy intake" that leads to "significantly low body weight" (American Psychiatric Association, 2013)

BOX 24-2 Moderately Severe and Life-Threatening Consequences of Eating Disorders	
• Severe electrolyte imbalances • Body fluid imbalances • Nutritional deficiencies • Osteoporosis • Metabolic acidosis • Metabolic alkalosis (hypochloremia) • Dehydration • Hypotension and bradycardia • Thyroid dysfunction: low levels of T_4 and T_3 hormones • Side effects of laxative abuse (rectal hemorrhage, hemorrhoids)	• Loss of teeth, discoloration of teeth, gum disease, and severe dental caries from acid emesis • Amenorrhea • Delayed puberty • Altered sexuality pattern • Anemia • Stress ulcers • Cardiovascular complications such as mitral valve prolapse, dysrhythmia, and congestive heart failure

Treatment of eating disorders is complicated. The rate of relapse is reportedly as high as 41% for some types of disordered eating (Carter et al., 2012). Children and teens with eating disorders need treatment and management in three areas: psychological care, medical care (refeeding, prevention and treatment of complications), and family support/other support system. Initially, the child must be physiologically managed, with care including correction of acidosis, alkalosis, and electrolyte imbalances. Supervised refeeding is necessary to ensure adequate calories and nutrients are consumed. In moderate to severe cases, this process will occur in the hospital under supervision. Dehydration will need to be corrected and a nasogastric tube (NGT) placed. Total parenteral nutrition (TPN) may be warranted either by a central line or peripheral line (PPN). A team of specialists should be coordinated by the nurse, to include nutrition, medicine, child psychology, and family therapy specialists.

Case Study

A 15-year-old female has been received in the pediatric emergency room with recent consumption of forty-five 500-mg acetaminophen tablets. She has a long history of depression and sporadic treatment by a pediatric clinical psychologist, and attempted suicide at home after barricading herself in her younger sibling's room. The patient was found by her mother approximately 1 hour ago and was transported by paramedics. She was not currently taking, nor did she have a history of taking, antidepressant medications. Her mother stated she had a recent breakup with her boyfriend of two years and her best friend from elementary school recently moved to the East Coast. The patient has been demonstrating a slow decline in academic performance and was recently caught twice with marijuana.

The teen arrived in the emergency department appearing disheveled, with poor hygiene and very pale skin. She presented in a stupor. The pediatric emergency team noted that she had three linear scars on her right wrist. Her vital signs on arrival were blood pressure, 91/42 mm Hg; heart rate, 116 beats/min; respiratory rate, 36 breaths/min; oxygen saturation, 97% on room air; and axillary temperature, 98.2°F.

The patient's mother is currently on the phone with her employer, and the younger sibling is in the waiting room, playing. The mother is distressed, has been crying, and is interacting only minimally with the healthcare team. She provides a poor historical picture of her daughter's past health status and seems very reluctant to interact with the emergency staff.

Case Study Questions

1. What is the initial course of action to be taken in assessing and treating this child?
2. After the teen's condition is stabilized, which assessments and interventions are most appropriate?
3. How can the emergency department staff best support the mother and younger sibling?

As the Case Evolves...

This teenager has now been successfully treated for her attempted overdose and referred for psychiatric evaluation. During her initial intake, she is uncommunicative and sits hunched over, staring at the floor, when the psychiatric nurse attempts to talk to her during her intake. Her affect is flat and expressionless, but she fidgets and taps her foot during the session. She says nothing when asked questions. Although the nurse is unable to elicit any answers from her, the teen's facial expressions, restless fidgeting, and other body language assure the nurse that she is not catatonic and can hear the questions. At last, the girl turns to the nurse and says in a monotone, "If you want to talk to me, you really should turn down the music." There is no music playing in the room.

4. Which of the following behaviors displayed by the teen is clearly consistent with a diagnosis of schizophrenia?
   A. Flat affect and lack of expression
   B. Suicidality
   C. Auditory hallucinations
   D. Fidgeting

Chapter Summary

- Cognition, or the child's mental capacity and awareness, is directly linked to the child's mental health state. Mental health and cognitive processing are also intertwined with the child's thinking about the world and the meaning of his or her existence.

- Cognitive impairment denotes a variety of unusually low states of mental processing. Risk factors associated with the development of cognitive impairment include brain trauma, microcephaly, metabolic disorders, chronic lead exposure, congenital rubella or syphilis, and fetal alcohol syndrome.

- The incidence of mental health issues, concerns, and diagnoses is increasing both in the United States and worldwide. Children can present with depression, anxiety, post-traumatic stress disorder, and other psychiatric concerns. Pediatric nurses play an integral role in the early identification, referral, assessment, and treatment and management of children with mental health issues.

- Depression is a mental health disorder that, for some children, profoundly impacts their ability to function on a daily basis.

- Treatment of depression in children includes three aspects: (1) a mental health counselor or therapist to help children determine the causes of their feelings of hopelessness, unhappiness, and possible loneliness; (2) positive coping strategies to deal with these stressors; and (3) medications and family support.

- Attention-deficit disorder and attention-deficit/hyperactivity disorder are conditions diagnosed during the school-age period where a child displays three classic behaviors: impulsivity, inattentiveness, and hyperactivity. The child with ADD/ADHD experiences struggles with learning, memorization, behavioral challenges of attention, and social expectations for age.

- Other mental health conditions the pediatric nurse may encounter in children include autism, schizophrenia, bipolar disorder, and eating disorders.

Bibliography

Abma, J. C., Martinez, G. M., & Copen, C.E. (2010). Teenagers in the United States: Sexual activity, contraceptive use, and childbearing: National Survey of Family Growth 2006-2008. National Center for Health Statistics. *Vital and Health Statistics, 23*(30). Retrieved from http://www.cdc.gov/nchs/data/series/sr_23/sr23_030.pdf

American Foundation for Suicide Prevention. (2016). Suicide statistics. Retrieved from https://afsp.org/about-suicide/suicide-statistics/

American Psychiatric Association. (2013). *Diagnostic and statistical manual of mental disorders* (5th ed.). Arlington, VA: Author.

Arcelus, J., Mitchell A. J., Wales, J., & Nielsen, S. (2011). Mortality rates in patients with anorexia nervosa and other eating disorders. *Archives of General Psychiatry, 68*(7), 724–731.

Arnold, L. E., Lofthouse, N., & Hurt, E. (2012). Artificial food colors and attention-deficit/hyperactivity symptoms: Conclusions to dye for. *Neurotherapeutics, 9,* 599.

Aungst, J. (n.d.). *Evaluation of studies on artificial food colors and behavior disorders in children.* Silver Spring, MD: U.S. Food and Drug Administration.

Baron-Cohen, S., Hoekstra, R. A., Knickmeyer, R., & Wheelwright, S. (2006). The Autism-Spectrum Quotient (AQ)—Adolescent Version. *Journal of Autism and Developmental Disorders, 36*(3), 343–350.

Bishop, D. V. M. (1998). Development of the Children's Communication Checklist (CCC): A method for assessing qualitative aspects of communicative impairment in children. *Journal of Child Psychology and Psychiatry, 39*(6), 879–891. doi: 10.1111/1469-7610.00388

Bishop, D. (2013). Children's Communication Checklist (CCC-2). In F. R. Volkmar (Ed.), *Encyclopedia of autism spectrum disorders* (pp. 614–618). New York, NY: Springer.

Borelli, J. L., Rasmussen, H. F., St. John, H. K., West, J. L., & Piacentini, J. C. (2015). Parental reactivity and the link between parent and child anxiety symptoms. *Journal of Child and Family Studies, 24,* 3130–3144.

Bradshaw, J., Steiner, A. M., Gengoux, G., & Koegel, L. K. (2015). Feasibility and effectiveness of very early intervention for infants at-risk for autism spectrum disorder: A systematic review. *Journal of Autism and Developmental Disorders, 45*(3), 778–794.

Carter, J. C., Mercer-Lynn, K. B., Norwood, S. J., Bewell-Weiss, C. V., Crosby, R. D., Woodside, D. B., & Olmsted, M. P. (2012). A prospective study of predictors of relapse in anorexia nervosa: Implications for relapse prevention. *Psychiatry Research, 200,* 518–523.

Centers for Disease Control and Prevention (CDC). (2010). Youth Risk Behavior Surveillance Survey—United States, 2009. *MMWR Surveillance Summaries, 59*(SS-5). Retrieved from http://www.cdc.gov/mmwr/pdf/ss/ss5905.pdf

Centers for Disease Control and Prevention (CDC). (2013). Mental health surveillance among children 2005-2011. *Morbidity and Mortality Weekly, 62*(2), 1–35.

Centers for Disease Control and Prevention (CDC). (2016a). New data on autism: Five important factors to know. Retrieved from http://www.cdc.gov/features/new-autism-data/

Centers for Disease Control and Prevention (CDC). (2016b). Autism spectrum disorder (ASD): Data and statistics. Retrieved from http://www.cdc.gov/ncbddd/autism/data.html

Centers for Disease Control and Prevention (CDC). (2016c). Children with ADHD: Data and statistics. Retrieved from http://www.cdc.gov/ncbddd/adhd/data.html

Chandler, S., Charman, T., Baird, G., Simonoff, E., Loucas, T., Meldrum, D., . . . Pickles, A. (2007). Validation of the Social Communication Questionnaire in a population cohort of children with autism spectrum disorders. *Journal of the American Academy of Child & Adolescent Psychiatry, 46*(10), 1324–1332.

Child Trends. (2010). Child Trends databank: Dating. Retrieved from https://www.childtrends.org/indicators/dating/

Clark, R. (1999). The parent–child early relational assessment: A factorial validity study. *Educational and Psychological Measurement, 59*(5), 821–846.

DuPaul, G. J., & Stoner, G. (2014). *ADHD in the schools: Assessment and intervention strategies.* New York, NY: Guilford Press.

Estes, A., Munson, J., Rogers, S. J., Greenson, J., Winter, J., & Dawson, G. (2015). Long-term outcomes of early intervention in 6-year-old children with autism spectrum disorder. *Journal of the American Academy of Child & Adolescent Psychiatry, 54*(7), 580–587.

Field, T. M., McCabe, P., & Schneiderman N. (2013). *Stress and coping across development.* London, UK: Psychology Press.

Franko, D. L., Keshaviah, A., Eddy, K. T., Krishna, M., Davis, M. C., Keel, P. K., & Herzog, D. B. (2013). A longitudinal investigation of mortality in anorexia nervosa and bulimia nervosa. *American Journal of Psychiatry, 170*, 917–925.

Heinz Kohut's self psychology: An overview. (1987). *American Journal of Psychiatry, 144*(1), 1–9.

James, A. C., James, G., Cowdrey, F. A., Soler, A., & Choke, A. (2013). Cognitive behavioural therapy for anxiety disorders in children and adolescents. *Cochrane Database of Systematic Reviews, 6*, 1–107.

Katz, E. R., & DeMaso, D. R. (2011). Pica. In R. M. Kliegman, R. E. Behrman, H. B. Jenson, & B. F. Stanton (Eds.), *Nelson textbook of pediatrics* (19th ed., chapter 21.2). Philadelphia, PA: Elsevier Saunders.

Kim, S. H., Hus, V., & Lord, C. (2013). Autism Diagnostic Interview—Revised. In F. R. Volkmar (Ed.), *Encyclopedia of autism spectrum disorders* (pp. 345–349). New York, NY: Springer.

Kirby, D., & Lepore, G. (2007). *Sexual risk and protective factors: Factors affecting teen sexual behavior, pregnancy, childbearing and sexually transmitted disease.* Washington, DC: ETR Associates and the National Campaign to Prevent Teen and Unplanned Pregnancy. Retrieved from https://thenationalcampaign.org/resource/sexual-risk-and-protective-factors%E2%80%94full-report

Kruizinga, I., Visser, J. C., van Batenburg-Eddes, T., Carter, A. S., Jansen, W., & Raat, H. (2014). Screening for autism spectrum disorders with the Brief Infant–Toddler Social and Emotional Assessment. *PLoS ONE, 9*(5), e97630. Retrieved from https://doi.org/10.1371/journal.pone.0097630

Landa, R. (2013). Pragmatic Rating Scale. In In F. R. Volkmar (Ed.), *Encyclopedia of autism spectrum disorders* (pp. 2327–2331). New York, NY: Springer.

Life Sciences and Medicine. (2016, July 22). Children who experience inadequate sleep are more likely to develop depression and anxiety later in life. *Medical News.* Retrieved from http://www.news-medical.net/news/20160722/Children-who-experience-inadequate-sleep-more-likely-to-develop-depression-anxiety-later-in-life.aspx

Lord, C., Rutter, M., & Couteur, A. L. (1994). Autism Diagnostic Interview—Revised: A revised version of a diagnostic interview for caregivers of individuals with possible pervasive developmental disorders. *Journal of Autism and Developmental Disorders, 24*(5), 659–685.

Merikangas, K. H., He, J., Burstein, M., Swanson, S. A., Avenevoli, S., Cui, L., . . . Swendsen, J. (2010). Lifetime prevalence of mental disorders in US adolescents: Results from the National Co-Morbidity Study—Adolescent Supplement (NCS-A). *Journal of the American Academy of Child and Adolescent Psychiatry, 49*(10), 980–989.

Morris, A. S., Silk, J. S., Steinberg, L., Myers, S. S., & Robinson, L. R. (2007). The role of the family context in the development of emotion regulation. *Social Development, 16*(2), 361–388.

National Eating Disorders Organization. (2016). Recovery. Retrieved from https://www.nationaleatingdisorders.org/learn/general-information/recovery

National Institute of Mental Health (NIMH). (2015a). Antidepressant medications for children and adolescents: Information for parents and caregivers. Retrieved from http://www.nimh.nih.gov/health/topics/child-and-adolescent-mental-health/antidepressant-medications-for-children-and-adolescents-information-for-parents-and-caregivers.shtml

National Institute of Mental Health (NIMH). (2015b). Attention deficit hyperactivity disorder. Retrieved from https://www.nimh.nih.gov/health/topics/attention-deficit-hyperactivity-disorder-adhd/index.shtml

National Institute of Mental Health (NIMH). (2015c). Autism spectrum disorder. Retrieved from https://www.nimh.nih.gov/health/publications/autism-spectrum-disorder/index.shtml

National Institute of Mental Health (NIMH). (2016a) Anxiety disorders. Retrieved from https://www.nimh.nih.gov/health/topics/anxiety-disorders/index.shtml

National Institute of Mental Health (NIMH). (2016b). Bipolar disorder. Retrieved from http://www.nimh.nih.gov/health/topics/bipolar-disorder/index.shtml

National Institute of Mental Health (NIMH). (2016c). Schizophrenia. Retrieved from http://www.nimh.nih.gov/health/topics/schizophrenia/index.shtml

National Institute of Mental Health (NIMH). (n.d.) Agoraphobia among children. Retrieved from https://www.nimh.nih.gov/health/statistics/prevalence/agoraphobia-among-children.shtml

National Institute of Mental Health (NIMH), Office of Science Policy, Planning and Communications. (2015). Bipolar disorder in children and teens. Retrieved from https://www.nimh.nih.gov/health/publications/bipolar-disorder-in-children-and-teens/index.shtml

Ogden, C. L., Carroll, M. D., Kit, B. K., & Flegal, K. M. (2014). Prevalence of childhood and adult obesity in the United States, 2011–2012. *Journal of the American Medical Association, 311*(8), 806–814.

Olfson, M., Blanco, C., Wang, S., Laje, G., & Correll, C. U. (2014). National trends in the mental health care of children, adolescents, and adults by office-based physicians. *JAMA Psychiatry, 71*(1), 81–90.

Orth, U., & Robins, R. W. (2013). Understanding the link between low self-esteem and depression. *Current Directions in Psychological Science, 22*(6), 455–460.

Radhakrishnan, R., Wilkinson, S. T., & D'Souza, D. C. (2014). Gone to pot: A review of the association between cannabis and psychosis. *Frontiers in Psychiatry, 5*, 54.

Ramtekkar, U. P., Reiersen, A. M., Todorov, A. A., & Todd, R. D. (2010). Sex and age differences in attention-deficit/hyperactivity disorder symptoms and diagnoses: Implications for *DSM-V* and

ICD-11. *Journal of the American Academy of Child and Adolescent Psychiatry, 49*(3), 217–28.e1–3.

Robins, D. L., Casagrande, K, Barton, M., Chen, C.-M. A., Dumont-Mathieu, T., & Fein, D. (2014). Validation of the Modified Checklist for Autism in Toddlers, Revised with Follow-up (M-CHAT-R/F). *Pediatrics, 133*(1), 37–45.

Ruzich, E., Allison, C., Smith, P., Watson, P. Auyeung, B., Ring, H., Baron-Cohen, S. (2015). Measuring autistic traits in the general population: a systematic review of the Autism-Spectrum Quotient (AQ) in a nonclinical population sample of 6,900 typical adult males and females. Molecular Autism. 6(2). doi: 10.1186/2040-2392-6-2.

Schopler, E. Reichler, R. J., DeVellis, R. F., & Daly, K. (1980). Toward objective classification of childhood autism: Childhood Autism Rating Scale (CARS). *Journal of Autism and Developmental Disorders, 10*(1), 91–103.

Skuse, D. H., Mandy, W. P. L., Scourfield, J. (2005). Measuring autistic traits: heritability, reliability and validity of the Social and Communication Disorders Checklist. *The British Journal of Psychiatry, 187*(6), 568–572. doi: 10.1192/bjp.187.6.568

Stichter, J. P., O'Connor, K. V., Herzog, M. J., Lierheimer, K., & McGhee, S. D. (2012). Social competence intervention for elementary students with Aspergers syndrome and high functioning autism. *Journal of Autism and Developmental Disorders, 42,* 354–366.

Stone, W. L., McMahon, C. R., & Henderson, L. M. (2008). Use of the Screening Tool for Autism in Two-Year-Olds (STAT) for children under 24 months. *Autism, 12*(5), 557–573.

Suicide.org. (2016). International suicide statistics: Teen suicide and youth suicide. Retrieved from http://www.suicide.org/international-suicide-statistics.html

Teen Suicide Statistics. (2016). Teen suicide facts. Retrieved from http://www.teensuicidestatistics.com/statistics-facts.html

Wade, T. D., Keski-Rahkonen, A., & Hudson, J. (2011). Epidemiology of eating disorders. In M. Tsuang & M. Tohen (Eds.), *Textbook in psychiatric epidemiology* (3rd ed., pp. 343–360). New York, NY: Wiley.

YoungMinds. (2016). About self esteem. Retrieved from http://www.youngminds.org.uk/for_parents/whats_worrying_you_about_your_child/self-esteem/about_self-esteem

Zwaigenbaum, L. Bauman, M. L., Choueiri, R., Kasari, C., Carter, A., Granpeesheh, D., . . . Natowicz, M. R. (2015). Early intervention for children with autism spectrum disorder under 3 years of age: Recommendations for practice and research. *Pediatrics, 136*(Suppl. 1), S60–S81.

CHAPTER 25

Immune System Disorders

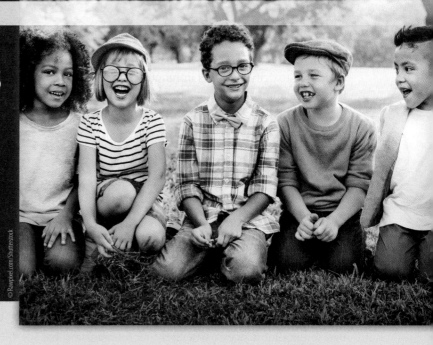

© Rawpixel.com/Shutterstock

LEARNING OBJECTIVES

1. Apply nursing concepts in the care of children with immune deficiencies, immune hyper-responsiveness, and autoimmune disorders.
2. Identify how the processes of natural and acquired immunity malfunction in immune system disorders.
3. Incorporate understanding of immune system defects into care plans for children with immune deficiencies, hyper-responsiveness, and autoimmune diseases.
4. Link clinical exemplars—systemic allergic reaction, idiopathic thrombocytopenia purpura, and juvenile idiopathic arthritis—to the concept of immunity.
5. Analyze how the care of children with immune-related conditions differs from the care of immunocompetent children.

KEY TERMS

Acquired immunity
Active immunity
Adaptive immunity
Autoimmune response
Hyper-responsiveness
Impaired immunocompetence
Innate immunity
Intravenous immunoglobulins
Natural immunity
Passive immunity

Introduction

The concept of immunity refers to the ability of the human body to defend against organisms and antigens that cause disease or toxicity. A child's immunity status determines the child's ability to fight against childhood infectious disease as well as the child's susceptibility to routinely encountered allergens such as pollen, dust, and other substances. Because children are progressively exposed to infectious organisms in their environment, they are at risk for developing diseases from these pathogenic sources. The administration of childhood immunizations is encouraged to prevent a child from developing certain infectious diseases that range from relatively mild (i.e., chickenpox) to severe enough to be potentially life threatening.

Immune System Function

The human body has the capability to identify and eliminate foreign substances, particularly microorganisms that enter the body and cause infection there. The immune system includes both specific and nonspecific components, including barriers, eliminators, and antigenic specificity. The most obvious immune barrier is the skin, but mucosal surfaces of the gastrointestinal tract, eyes, inner ears, and urogenital tract also offer protection against invaders (Dwivedy & Aich, 2011). **Innate immunity** consists of cells and proteins—such as macrophages, neutrophils, and natural killer cells—that are programmed to quickly identify and react to the invasion of microorganisms. **Adaptive immunity** refers to components of the lymph system (lymphocytes) that are responsible for identifying self versus non-self, and therefore that do not react until activated by a foreign invader. This system is called *adaptive* because, unlike the components of the innate immune system, the cells of the adaptive immune system (such as T and B lymphocytes) change in response to exposures so that they can respond more rapidly and aggressively to a repeat exposure. Thus, once exposed to various disease-causing pathogens through either infection or vaccination, the child is subsequently less susceptible to infection by that pathogen. The adaptive immune system is the "memory" of immunity (**Figure 25-1**).

Acquired Versus Natural Adaptive Immunity

Adaptive immunity comes in four intersecting types: **natural** (immunity developed through contact with an agent in the environment) and **acquired** (immunity that is not inherited), and **active** (immunity developed through contact with a disease-causing agent) and **passive** (immunity developed through exposure to antibodies, such as through breast milk).

- *Natural active immunity* occurs when a child comes into contact with an agent that has the potential to cause disease but was not deliberately introduced. The encounter with the antigen may or may not result in a symptomatic response—for example, release of histamine, inflammation, or fever—but in either instance it results in the creation of memory

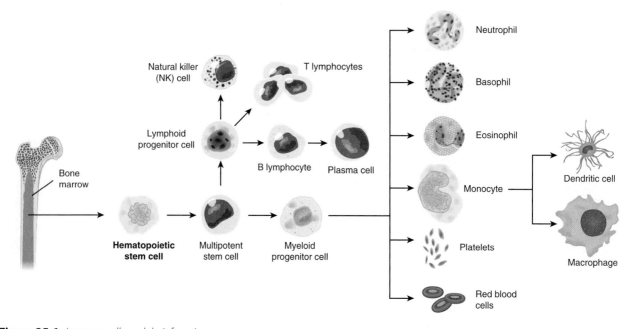

Figure 25-1 *Immune cells and their functions.*

T cells, which allow the immune system to recognize that antigen at a later date.

- *Acquired active immunity*, also called nonspecific immunity, develops when a child is deliberately exposed to an antigen via a *vaccine* or *immunization* intended to produce memory T cells without causing disease.
- *Natural passive immunity* develops from the passage of maternal antibodies across the placenta from mother to the fetus, or during breastfeeding.
- *Artificial or intentional passive immunity* is derived from actively administering antibodies to a non-immune child, such as via plasma with pooled antibodies called **intravenous immunoglobulins** (IVIG) or intramuscular injections (IM) or by monoclonal antibodies (mAb).

Immune System Malfunctions

There are a number of circumstances in which the immune system may function incorrectly or inadequately. Immune deficiency disorders represent situations in which the appropriate types or amounts of immune cells are not present, are present in insufficient amounts to perform their function, or are altered in some way such that they cannot function properly. These disorders include primary immunodeficiency diseases such as chronic granulomatous disease, which results in defective monocytes, macrophages, and neutrophils (making the child susceptible to *Staphylococcus* and fungal infections), and severe combined immunodeficiency (SCID), in which both T and B cells are absent, leaving the child vulnerable to any form of microbial infection (Delves, Martin, Burton, & Roitt, 2011). Immune deficiency may also be acquired via infectious diseases, of which human immunodeficiency virus (HIV) is among the best known, or it may develop due to blood cancers (leukemia) that cause immature, nonfunctional lymphocytes to proliferate at the expense of normal cells. In these situations, the child develops **impaired immunocompetence**—that is, he or she is left with reduced ability to fight off infections so that even minor microbial encounters can become extremely serious.

In contrast to deficiency disorders, in which immune system function is inadequate, other immune disorders may develop in which the immune system either overreacts against a genuine foreign body (**hyper-responsiveness** or hyper-reactivity response, also known as allergy), or else reacts against a "self" antigen on normal body tissues that it is supposed to ignore (**autoimmune response**) (Delves et al., 2011). Allergy can range in severity from annoying—sneezing and runny nose in response to spring pollen, for example—to life-threatening anaphylactic reactions to foods, chemicals, or insect venom. A hyper-reactive immune system may overreact only to very specific triggers, such as animal dander or a particular species of pollen, or a child may have multiple allergies. Autoimmune response may target particular tissues, as in type 1 (autoimmune) diabetes or Graves's thyroiditis, or it may cause system-wide immune attacks on normal tissues, as in systemic lupus erythematosus. In autoimmune disease, the immune system usually responds appropriately in the presence of infectious agents, but its effects on body tissues can range from progressively debilitating (as in rheumatoid arthritis) to acutely life-threatening (as in type 1 diabetes).

Assessments of the Immune System

There are limited means to assess the immune system. Laboratory values provide the most consistent and accurate information about a child's ability to fight infection. Specific symptoms associated with immune system dysfunction or immune pathologies can assist in making a definitive diagnosis in case of immune-related disorders. The following laboratory assessments are used to determine immune function, status, and disease (UCLA Pathology and Laboratory Medicine, 2015):

- Complete blood cell counts with white blood cell differentiation (neutrophils, basophils, eosinophils, megakaryocytes) (**Figure 25-2**)
- Quantification of global cell-mediated immunity
- Lymphocytes (CD4 T-helper cells)

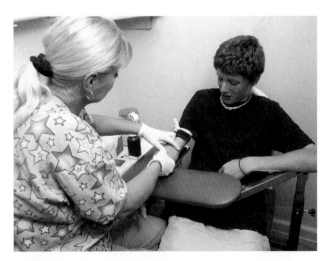

Figure 25-2 *A complete blood cell count is one of the laboratory assessments that can help determine immune function, status, and disease.*

© JSABBOTT/E+/Getty Images

- Immunoglobulin identification and levels (IgM, IgG, IgA, IgE, and IgD)
- Biomarkers of immune reactivity
- Flow cytometry immunophenotyping
- DNA or RNA assays to particular pathogens such as HIV
- Sequential analysis using assays that measure distinct immune functions

Immunity Concept Exemplars

This section outlines three exemplars for the concept of immunity. Understanding the concept as it relates to the general principles of immunity, immune response, autoimmunity, and nursing provides a foundation for care.

Systemic Allergic Reactions

When a child is exposed to an allergen, IgE antibodies are quickly synthesized and attach themselves to the cell walls of mast cells and basophils. These cells release large quantities of histamines and inflammatory mediators, causing rapid vasodilation, increased capillary permeability and fluid leakage, and bronchoconstriction. In severe cases, a rapid onset of life-threatening symptoms (anaphylaxis) occurs (**Table 25-1**). Food allergies, insect venom, drugs, latex, and environmental allergens can all potentially trigger a systemic allergic reaction in highly susceptible children. In most cases, avoidance of the allergen, once it is identified, is the best way to prevent reactions.

Diagnosis

The diagnosis of systemic allergic reactions can be made by visual inspection. The child may present with itching, flushing, hives, stridor, wheezing, dyspnea, nausea, abdominal pain, dizziness, hypotension, and finally shock (**Box 25-1**; **Figure 25-3**).

Risk Factors

Knowing and communicating a child's risk factors to all adults involved with a child's care is imperative. Risk factors include medical history, family history, concurrent asthma or atopy, and elevated allergen-specific IgE levels.

Medical Treatment

Rapid medical treatment for systemic allergic reactions is based on the progression of the condition and prevention of shock. The child should be managed by an experienced code blue or rapid response team, and should be transferred to a pediatric intensive care environment for observation.

TABLE 25-1 Anaphylaxis
Anaphylaxis is a severe allergic reaction that is a rare but important side effect of childhood immunization administration.
Symptoms
Bronchial edema
Laryngeal spasms
Hypotension
Poor perfusion
Rapid change in level of consciousness
Treatments
Rapid identification of the onset
Administration of epinephrine subcutaneously (SQ) or intramuscularly (IM)
Administration of an antihistamine
Airway support and cardiopulmonary resuscitation as needed
Administration of oxygen
Transfer to a high level of care such as an emergency department or an intensive care unit

BOX 25-1 Early Symptoms of a Severe Allergic Reaction
• Swelling of the airway • Increased work of breathing • Feeling of restlessness or feelings of doom • Tachycardia • Swelling and redness of the face • Change in level of consciousness

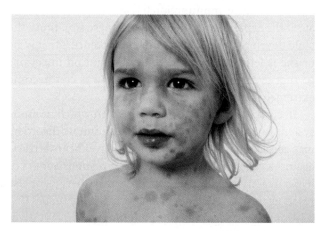

Figure 25-3 *A child experiencing an allergic reaction might present with hives.*

© DIGIcal/iStock/Getty Images Plus/Getty

Administration of the following medications complements a team effort for resuscitation and vascular support:

- Epinephrine
- Rapid-acting bronchodilator such as albuterol
- Diphenhydramine (Benadryl)
- Systemic corticosteroid anti-inflammatory agent (Solu-Medrol)

QUALITY AND SAFETY

Preparing for Anaphylaxis

Pediatric nurses who knowingly administer a medication that has the potential to cause a severe allergic reaction should be prepared to respond quickly if the patient develops anaphylaxis. Having access to a code cart and the following medications and supplies is imperative:

- Epinephrine
- Antihistamine
- Steroid anti-inflammatory agent
- Intravenous fluid boluses
- Oxygen

Nursing Care

Children who are at risk for or who have a confirmed experience with systemic allergic reactions should wear medical alert jewelry, should have an EpiPen (**Figure 25-4**) available at all times, should know what their triggers are, and should have an emergency action plan that the child, family, school, caregivers, and coaches understand and feel confident in implementing. The nursing team should confirm that the child's medical records highlight the allergies and the severe reactions associated. Education and reinforcement of an emergency plan with available, unexpired medications is the most important component of the nursing care.

Idiopathic Thrombocytopenic Purpura

Also known as immune thrombocytopenic purpura, idiopathic thrombocytopenic purpura (ITP) is an acquired immune deficiency disorder in which a child presents with easy or excessive bleeding and bruising due to low circulating platelets. A normal platelet count for children is between 150,000 to 300,000; however, children with ITP have platelet counts less than 100,000. This condition is caused by an autoimmune response in which antibodies are produced against the child's own platelets. Consequently, the child cannot produce clots sufficient to stop bleeding episodes. In children, ITP is associated with recovery from a viral illness; in such a case, the child will usually fully recover from ITP. If a child's platelet count falls dangerously low, the child is at risk for intracranial hemorrhage and other serious consequences.

Diagnosis

A diagnosis of ITP is made by identifying the symptoms of bleeding into the skin (petechial rash), easy bruising, nosebleeds, or bleeding from the mouth (**Figure 25-5**). Laboratory evaluation of the child's platelets will demonstrate a low count, but a bone marrow aspiration or biopsy may be required in clinical situations where the child's condition is not improving on its own.

Risk Factors

The only known risk factor is a viral infection prior to the presentation of low platelets. This condition is not common and cannot be prevented or identified via genetic testing.

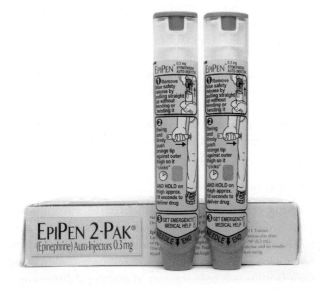

Figure 25-4 *An EpiPen.*

© Amy Kerkemeyer/Shutterstock

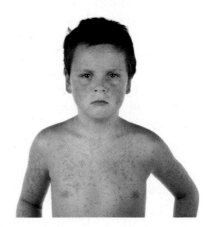

Figure 25-5 *Petechial rash is a symptom of idiopathic thrombocytopenic purpura.*

© Stacy Barnett/Shutterstock

Medical Treatment

A child's condition may warrant medical treatment. Steroidal anti-inflammatory drugs are the first-line treatment. If the platelet count does not improve with this therapy, the child may need to be given intravenous infusions of high-dose gamma-globulins, danazol (oral), or other drugs that suppress the immune system's production of antiplatelet antibodies.

Nursing Care

Safety is paramount to the care of a child with ITP. The child should be placed on bleeding precautions, and the family must be taught how to minimize the chances of bleeding. Discuss how to keep the child quiet and engaged in nonharmful activities. Teach the family the importance of the medication regimen and when to report worsening conditions.

Juvenile Rheumatoid Arthritis and Juvenile Idiopathic Arthritis

As their names imply, both forms of juvenile arthritis affect children younger than the age of 16. Juvenile rheumatoid arthritis (JRA) is an autoimmune condition in which the child's immune system attacks the cells surrounding the synovial membranes of the joints, causing persistent and painful joint injury, swelling, stiffness, and decreased range of motion. Juvenile idiopathic arthritis (JIA) is slightly different: It is an "autoinflammatory" condition in which the cells responsible for the normal inflammatory response are triggered by encounters with the body's "self" antigens. In this case, inflammation arises but the tissues of the body are not actually destroyed (National Institute of Arthritis and Musculoskeletal and Skin Diseases [NIAMSD], 2015). Nevertheless, the symptoms of pain, swelling, and stiffness are very similar, and the only distinguishing factor is whether autoantibodies are present (they are present in JRA, and absent in JIA).

Some children diagnosed with JRA or JIA have continual symptoms lasting only a few months, while others have exacerbations that last an entire lifetime. The location of the joints and the number of joints affected vary per child. For some children with JRA/JIA, systemic symptoms occur, including significant skin rashes, high fever spikes, uveitis or iritis, and lymphadenopathy. Both environmental factors and viral exposures may trigger an exacerbation (NIAMSD, 2015).

Diagnosis

The American College of Rheumatology (2010) encourages the use of the following criteria to diagnose JRA:

1. Morning stiffness, joint pain
2. Swelling or fluid around three or more joints simultaneously, with at least one being in the fingers, wrist, or hand area
3. Symmetry (arthritis is present on both sides of the body)
4. Presence of rheumatoid nodules
5. Specific factors isolated in the child's blood: anti-cyclic citrullinated peptide (anti-CCP) antibodies, rheumatoid factor (RF), and antinuclear antibodies (ANAs)
6. Measurement of the red blood cell (erythrocyte) sedimentation rate (ESR)
7. Radiography-demonstrated rheumatoid arthritis including bone destruction around the joint area (late-stage disease)

Risk Factors

Risk factors for JRA/JIA include familial tendencies toward autoimmune disorders. JRA occurs more often in female children than in male children.

Medical Treatment

Treatment for JRA focuses on managing symptoms such as pain, swelling, and stiffness, and on preventing exacerbations. There is no cure for JRA/JIA. The care for a child with JRA/JIA should be a coordinated effort and include rheumatologists, physical and occupational therapists, and pediatric nursing care. Medications used as treatments include the following:

- Nonsteroidal anti-inflammatory drugs (NSAIDs) as first-line treatment.
- Steroids for children with moderate or severe arthritis or nonarthritic inflammatory consequences of JRA. The lowest possible dosing is prioritized due to the severe side effects of steroids.
- Antirheumatic medications such as cyclosporine (Sandimmune), sulfasalazine (Azulfidine), methotrexate (gold standard), and azathioprine (Imuran). The greatest risk identified with antirheumatics is immune suppression, which is accompanied by increased risk for infections. Tumor necrosis factor alpha (TNF-α) inhibitors are also used to treat JRA/JIA.
- Autologous stem cell transplantation is reserved for children with JRA for whom all other treatment options have failed.

Nursing Care

Nursing care for children with JRA/JIA encompasses both prevention and support. It includes education on adherence to medicines, follow-up appointments, therapy, home care, and, as the child grows, self-care. Children and their families will need support, as emotional distress over JRA's tendency to cause significant pain and disabilities can occur. Clinically significant pain, even with medical treatment, can influence the child's functioning, social life, emotional health, and role functions (Stinson & Luca, 2012). Teaching families to supplement medical treatment with nonpharmacologic interventions has been shown to decrease symptoms. Research has shown warm baths and compresses before school, gentle daily range-of-motion exercises, swimming, low- and high-intensity exercises, splinting and orthoses, sleep hygiene, and Internet support interventions to be effective palliative treatments (Stinson & Luca, 2012). Nursing care must focus on preventing complications of JRA/JIA, including significant joint damage with deformity, osteoporosis, emotional distress, and growth abnormalities. Opioid therapy may be required for children with refractory joint pain (Connelly & Schanberg, 2008).

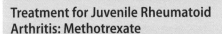

PHARMACOLOGY

Treatment for Juvenile Rheumatoid Arthritis: Methotrexate

Many children with JRA affecting several joints will be placed on oral methotrexate, a type of antineoplastic used in many childhood cancer treatment protocols. Methotrexate works by depleting the folinic acid from dividing cells. In small doses, the drug will suppress the child's immune system to decrease or prevent autoimmune joint erosion. The child will be on six days of oral methotrexate, followed by a day of oral folinic (vitamin B) supplements. Adherence to this "rescue" dose is imperative. The pediatric nurse must reinforce family teaching on these medications.

FAMILY EDUCATION

In a study by Cespedes-Cruz et al. (2008), 521 children with JRA were treated with methotrexate. The researchers' findings showed that over the course of 6 months, the children reported dramatic reductions in pain, and increased physical activity and function.

Human Immunodeficiency Virus and Acquired Immunodeficiency Syndrome

The human immunodeficiency virus (HIV) is the viral organism that causes acquired immunodeficiency syndrome (AIDS). HIV is transmitted by direct contact with an infected person's body fluids, secretions, or blood. The virus enters the body and binds to the CD4 receptor located on the cell membrane of the T-lymphocyte cell. The viral DNA attaches to the T cell's DNA and reproduces new viral material as the T cell replicates. This process, called reverse transcription, results in the gradual suppression of cell-mediated immunity, causing the lymph organs to become infected. The child's immune system function is altered, leaving the child susceptible to infections.

HIV and AIDS may be transmitted to children via the following routes:

- Infants: Transmission from an infected mother, either in utero or via breastfeeding
- Adolescents: Unprotected sex with an infected sexual partner or injection drug use
- Any age: Transfusion of HIV-infected blood products when product screening is inadequate

Diagnosis

The diagnosis of AIDS requires an extremely low total CD4 cell count (**Table 25-2**) and the development of an AIDS-defining illness such as the following conditions:

- Lymphoid interstitial pneumonitis
- Recurrent bacterial infections
- *Pneumocystis jirovecii* pneumonia
- Cryptosporidiosis
- Herpes simplex virus
- Severe yeast infections, especially in the esophageal or pulmonary tissues
- *Mycobacterium avium-intracellulare* complex infection
- Cytomegalovirus infections
- Kaposi's sarcoma

Medical Treatment

Highly active antiretroviral therapy (HAART) remains the gold-standard treatment for HIV-positive children.

TABLE 25-2 HIV Stages of Infection
Acute retroviral syndrome: Develops within a few days of infection or a few weeks. Symptoms range from mild to severe; mimics symptoms of mononucleosis infection.
Stage 1: No AIDS-related conditions or infections, CD4+ count is at or above 500 cells/mcL, and CD4+ cells represent at least 29% of entire lymphocyte count.
Stage 2: No AIDS-related conditions or infections, CD4+ count is between 200 and 499 cells/mcL, and CD4+ cells represent between 14% and 28% of all lymphocytes.
Stage 3: AIDS is present; CD4+ count is less than 200 cells/mcL and CD4+ cells represent less than 14% of all lymphocytes.

Modified from Centers for Disease Control and Prevention. (2013). Diagnosis of HIV Infection in the United States and Dependent Areas, 2013. Retrieved from https://www.cdc.gov/hiv/pdf/library/reports/surveillance/cdc-hiv-surveillance-report-2013-vol-25.pdf

Unique Aspects of HIV and AIDS in Young Children

Almost all children under the age of 13 years old become infected during the mother's pregnancy, birthing process, or breastfeeding.

Highly reliable testing for HIV antibodies is difficult during the newborn period and early infancy. Maternal antibodies can stay in the infant's blood system for as long as 18 months. Specific laboratory tests that identify the presence of HIV must use an amplification process in order to detect small amounts of the virus.

As many as 20% of children in their first year of life will develop a significant opportunistic infection.

Normal and expected motor developmental milestones are often delayed in young children with HIV and AIDS.

Many young children with HIV develop more frequent and more severe childhood infections.

Data from AIDS.gov (2009). Children. Children and HIV. Retrieved from www.aids.gov/hiv.aids-basic/just-diagnosed-with-hiv-aids/overview/children/

The standard treatment consists of at least three antiretroviral drugs within at least two of the following drug classes:

- Nucleoside reverse transcriptase inhibitors, to prematurely end viral DNA replication
- Protease inhibitors, to inhibit replication of viral material later in the replication process
- Non-nucleoside reverse transcriptase inhibitors, to inhibit reverse transcriptase production

Nursing Care

Several important nursing care concerns should be addressed when caring for a child infected with HIV or who presents with AIDS. Nutritional support, rest, medication adherence, prevention of transmission of the virus, identification of disease progression and when to seek treatment, prevention of opportunistic infections, emotional support, and education are all necessary components of holistic care of the child and family. Keeping the family integrated in the healthcare system through regular assessments of lab data, medication supervision, and emotional support can be lifesaving.

Prophylactic medications are administered to children with AIDS to prevent life-threatening infections:

- Isoniazid or rifampin prophylaxis for *Mycobacterium tuberculosis* infections with a positive skin test or confirmed tuberculosis contact
- Trimethoprim/sulfamethoxazole (TMP/SMX; Bactrim, Septra) prophylaxis for *Pneumocystis jirovecii* infections
- Clarithromycin or azithromycin prophylaxis for *Mycobacterium avium-intracellulare* complex infections

Case Study

A 17-month-old boy is brought to his pediatrician with symptoms of fussiness, excessive thirst, and frequent urination. The results of urinalysis show that the child has both glucosuria and ketonuria, and he is given a preliminary diagnosis of type 1 (autoimmune) diabetes. The family is sent to the emergency department of a nearby medical center, where they are met at the door by a pediatric endocrinologist and pediatric nursing team. The child's blood glucose level is measured at 590, and his blood pH is 7.2 with a serum bicarbonate of 12 mEq/L.

His family history is notable for Hashimoto's thyroiditis in his mother, rheumatoid arthritis in his maternal grandfather, and diabetes of unknown type in his paternal grandfather. The child also has a recent 6-month history of repeated viral infections characterized by high fevers. These fevers were frequent and severe enough that his pediatrician's notes include a comment that the child's first measles/mumps/rubella (MMR) immunization, which he should have received by 15 months of age, had been postponed to 18 months of

(continues)

Case Study *(continued)*

age to ensure he was completely well before his immune system was challenged by the vaccine.

Case Study Questions

1. In general terms, how do autoimmune diseases like type 1 diabetes originate?
2. What is the significance of (a) the family history and (b) the recurrent viral infections in the etiology of this child's autoimmune disease?
3. Evaluate the physician's decision to delay vaccination in this child in the months preceding his diabetes diagnosis. What are the pros and cons of the delay? At which point, if at all, should a child with an autoimmune disorder be given routine childhood immunizations?

As the Case Evolves...

The toddler has now been stabilized and transferred from the pediatric intensive care unit into the regular pediatric ward.

His parents are given instructions on his care by the staff so that their son can be discharged from the hospital. During the final meeting before discharge, the child's father asks the pediatric nurse whether his son is at risk of any other immune system diseases as a result of his type 1 diabetes diagnosis.

4. Which of the following is the most appropriate response?
   A. "Your son's immune system is targeting only his pancreas, so there's no risk to his other organs or systems."
   B. "There is a specific risk of autoimmune thyroid disease and celiac disease, and in general he is at higher risk of other autoimmune disorders, too."
   C. "There is a specific risk of rheumatoid arthritis and systemic lupus erythematosus, and in general he is at risk of other autoimmune disorders, too."
   D. "His immune system is extremely hyper-responsive, so we need to suppress his immunity to prevent him developing other autoimmune disorders."

Chapter Summary

- Immunity refers to the ability of the human body to fight against organisms that cause disease or allergens; it may be either natural or acquired.
- A child's immunity status determines the ability to fight off infectious diseases encountered during childhood. Although children have innate immunity, their adaptive immune systems are still immature; thus, they are at increased risk for developing diseases.
- Malfunctions in the immune system can include immune deficiency, immune hyper-reactivity, and autoimmunity.
- Immune deficiency disorders may be congenital or acquired. Congenital immune deficiency may include an inability to produce one or more types of immune cells, leaving the child vulnerable to infection. Acquired immune deficiency may be caused by viral pathogens such as HIV.
- Immune hyper-reactivity or allergy is an overreaction by the immune system to certain antigens. The response can range from mild symptoms such as rhinitis to life-threatening anaphylaxis. Nurses should be aware of children's history of allergic responses and triggers and have the tools and supplies necessary for averting anaphylaxis readily available.
- Autoimmunity occurs when the immune system fails to distinguish "self" antigens from foreign antigens and attacks the body's own tissues. Autoimmune disorders

may target specific organs or tissues, or they may be systemic, attacking a range of tissues.

- Clinical exemplars of the concept of immunity include systemic hypersensitivity response (anaphylaxis), idiopathic thrombocytopenia purpura, juvenile rheumatoid arthritis, and HIV/AIDS.
- Care of children with immune-related conditions is often considered chronic care and focuses on both the prevention of exacerbations and complications and the restoration of health to prevent progression.

Bibliography

American College of Rheumatology. (2010). Classification criteria for rheumatic diseases. Retrieved from https://www.rheumatology.org/Practice/Clinical/Classification/Classification_Criteria_for_Rheumatic_Diseases/

Biology On-Line. (2015). Viral research tools: Passive and active types of immunity. Retrieved from http://www.biology-online.org/1/11_cell_defense_2.htm

Centers for Disease Control and Prevention. (2015). HIV risk reduction tool. HIV beta version. Retrieved from https://wwwn.cdc.gov/hivrisk/what_is/stages_hiv_infection.html

Centers for Disease Control and Prevention. (2017). About HIV/AIDS. Retrieved from https://www.cdc.gov/hiv/basics/whatishiv.html

Cespedes-Cruz, A., Gutierrez-Suarez, R., Pistorio, A., Loy, A., Murray, K. J., Gertoni, M. V., . . . Ruperto, N. (2008). Methotrexate improves the health-related quality of life of children with juvenile idiopathic arthritis. *Annals of the Rheumatic Diseases, 67*, 309–314.

Connelly, M., & Schanberg, L. (2008). Opioid therapy for the treatment of refractory pain in children with juvenile rheumatoid arthritis. *Nature: Clinical Practice Rheumatology, 2*(12), 636–637.

Delves, P. J., Martin, S. J., Burton, D. R., & Roitt, I. M. (2011). *Roitt's essential immunology* (12th ed.). Chichester, UK: Wiley-Blackwell.

Dwivedy, A., & Aich, P. (2011). Importance of innate mucosal immunity and the promises it holds. *International Journal of General Medicine, 4*, 299–311.

Ercolini, A. M., & Miller, S. D. (2009). The role of infections in autoimmune disease. *Clinical & Experimental Immunology, 155*(1), 1–15.

National Institute of Arthritis and Musculoskeletal and Skin Diseases (NIAMSD). (2015). Questions and answers about juvenile arthritis. Retrieved from http://www.niams.nih.gov/health_info/juv_arthritis/

Stinson, J., & Luca, N. (2012). Assessment and management of pain in juvenile idiopathic arthritis. *Pulsus: Pain Research & Management, 17*(6), 391–396.

UCLA Pathology and Laboratory Medicine. (2015). UCLA Health: Immune assessment. Retrieved from http://www.pathology.ucla.edu/body.cfm?id=179

University of Rochester Medical Center. (2015). Disorders of the immune system. *Health Encyclopedia.* Retrieved from https://www.urmc.rochester.edu/encyclopedia/content.aspx?ContentTypeID=134&ContentID=123

CHAPTER 26

Infection and Communicable Diseases in Childhood

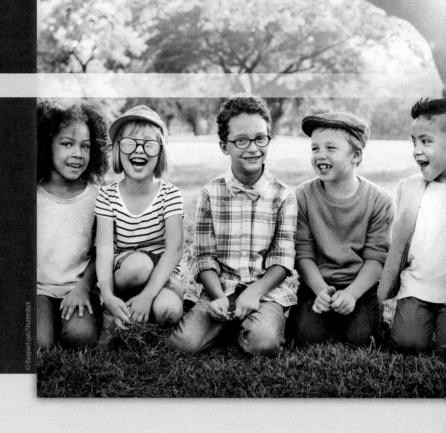

© Rawpixel.com/Shutterstock

LEARNING OBJECTIVES

1. Apply nursing concepts to the management of infection and communicable diseases during childhood.
2. Evaluate symptoms and laboratory tests to identify various types of microbes as the source of infection.
3. Apply nursing considerations with each of the common categories of antimicrobial agents and common infections treated with these antimicrobial agent categories.
4. Assess and treat common infections during childhood.
5. Analyze the complexities of immunizations, including parental refusal due to cultural beliefs, religious beliefs, and fears as cited by parents.
6. Critically evaluate elements of the developmental period that leave a child more susceptible to infections.
7. Evaluate the various hospital-acquired infections and the risk factors associated with each.

KEY TERMS

Bacteria
Carriage
Carrier
Contagious
Endemic
Epidemic
Fungi
Infection
Macroparasites
Normal inhabitants
Pandemic
Pathogen
Prions
Vaccination
Viruses

Introduction

When one thinks about young children, it is common to associate infectious diseases or communicable diseases with them during the developmental years. The most frequently seen illness in childhood is the common cold, which can be caused by any one of a variety of viruses (Centers for Disease Control and Prevention [CDC], 2016a). A common reason for hospitalization of infants is the severity of clinical presentation and complications associated with respiratory syncytial virus (RSV) infection, which may lead to significant bronchiolitis requiring clinical support. Young children and infants are prone to contracting infections due to their immature immune systems (**Table 26-1**). Children entering childcare facilities and school environments become rapidly exposed to infectious materials due to their increased socialization in this setting and their encounters with other children who may be under-immunized or infected due to older siblings' exposure. Pediatric nurses will undoubtedly find themselves caring for and treating children with an abundance of infectious diseases. For the purpose of this chapter, the terms "communicable diseases" and "infectious diseases of childhood" will be used interchangeably to describe these illnesses.

Although childhood infectious diseases are associated with microbial pathogens, not all microbes cause childhood illness. Sometimes the germ causes illness, but at other times it is the process of intoxication, or exposure to the pathogen's toxins, that causes disease.

The bacteria that make up the normal flora on a child's skin do not cause the child to experience an **infection** (i.e., invasion by microorganisms, which then reproduce in the body) unless there is a breach in skin integrity and the conditions are right for the microbe to flourish. The term *normal flora* is used to denote the billions of bacteria found on the skin of a child, also known as the **normal inhabitants**. The normal flora on a child's skin provide protection from disease-causing fungi and bacteria. The normal flora found throughout a child's intestines provides a first line of protection from disease-producing bacteria, help to manufacture vitamin K (essential for clotting factors), and assist in the breakdown and digestion of food. Breaches in the protective layer of normal flora are associated with breaks in skin integrity, infectious invasion of harmful microbes, or the use of antibiotics that destroy the "good" bacteria. If microbes exist without causing illness, their presence is called **carriage** of the microbe and the child is considered a **carrier**—asymptomatic and well, but capable of spreading the pathogen to others.

Scientists continue to try to determine why some children develop illness, others develop serious infections, and still other children become carriers without developing infection. Influencing factors associated with the development of childhood infections include genetics, family hygiene practices, the child's age, immunity status, nutritional status, chronic disorders such as diabetes, and overall general health. Developmental stage highly influences a child's transmission and reception of infectious materials. For example, the youngest children have an oral fixation such as mouthing objects and inability to control secretions. By the age of 3 years, children should be able to effectively wash their hands with minimal supervision (**Figure 26-1**). Positive reinforcement of such behaviors is key, as young children will not be able to comprehend germ theory and the interrelation of hand hygiene, secretion control, and microbial transmission factors.

Infectious Microbes Found During Childhood

Pediatric nurses should associate the care of children with the treatment of common infections. Most children do not require intensive treatment or management, but rather supportive care including rest, hydration, symptom management, and sometimes oral antibiotics if the microbe is bacterial

---

TABLE 26-1 Germs (Microbes) That Cause Childhood Infectious Diseases

› **Prions**: The smallest known disease-causing agents. They are made of infectious protein, but lack DNA and RNA (which distinguishes them from viruses). An example of a prion-caused disease is Creutzfeldt–Jakob disease.

› **Viruses**: Noncellular organisms composed of a protein capsule surrounding genetic material that can cause illness by taking over a human cell and reproducing themselves. An example of a viral disease is the common cold.

› **Bacteria**: Single-cell organisms capable of causing infection. An example of a bacterial disease is a *Streptococcus* throat infection ("strep throat").

› **Fungi**: Yeasts and molds capable of causing infection. An example of a fungal infection is thrush (*Candida albicans*).

› Protozoa: A phylum of single-celled organisms including sporazoans, flagellates, amoebas, and ciliates. An example of a protozoal disease is giardiasis (*Giardia lamblia*).

› **Macroparasites**: Organisms visible to the naked eye, such as nematodes (worms) or arthropods (insects), that live in and feed on other organisms' tissues. Examples include pinworms, mites, and lice.

in nature or oral antiviral medication if required. Infections in childhood can be classified in four distinct ways:

- Single case: Isolated case where exposure source is unknown or not identifiable.

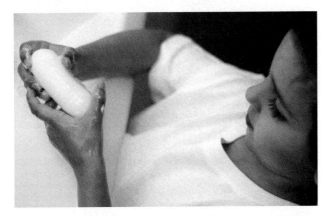

Figure 26-1 *By the age of 3 years, children should be able to effectively wash their hands with minimal supervision.*

- **Epidemic**: A widespread occurrence of an infectious disease within a community found at a particular time.
- **Endemic**: A more widely spread occurrence of an infectious disease within a larger geographical area or beyond a particular community.
- **Pandemic**: The presence of an infectious disease breakout within a large or wide geographical area such as across a country, a continent, or the world.

A major role of the pediatric nurse working in any clinical setting is to understand the clinical presentations of common childhood infectious diseases (**Table 26-2**), report findings for confirmation and treatment, and teach families about prevention and control. Adults working with children in daycare or school settings should also understand which signs and symptoms to assess children for. Providing clean water, frequently cleansed food preparation and eating surfaces, frequent hand washing, control of fecal contamination for daycare programs with diapered children, and control over bodily secretions (mucus and

TABLE 26-2 Common Infections Caused by Microbes Found Across Childhood

› Herpesviruses: Stay in the body for life. These viruses include herpes simplex, cytomegalovirus, varicella, Epstein-Barr virus, and herpesvirus 6 and 7, all of which cause infection.

› Measles: An acute viral infection characterized by inflamed eyes, cough, rash, sore throat, and fevers. It is one of the leading causes of death in young children worldwide despite being preventable with vaccines (World Health Organization, 2017).

› Mumps: Also known as parotitis due to the acute swelling of the parotid glands (salivary). This viral infection can infect the testes and the pancreas as well.

› Norovirus: Causes rapid-onset acute diarrhea. The viral infection is highly contagious and can be acquired through touching contaminated surfaces, water, or food.

› Pertussis: Also called whooping cough. The bacterium *Bordetella pertussis* causes a highly contagious, acute lung infection that leads to severe episodes of coughing and requires antibiotic therapy (CDC, 2015c).

› Pneumonia: An acute lung inflammation, congestion, and consolidation. Infections can be caused by a variety of viruses, bacteria, and fungi, and are associated with fever, cough, and dyspnea.

› Respiratory syncytial virus: Cause of acute lung infections leading to bronchiolitis. This infection can be very severe in infants, requiring hospitalization for clinical support.

› Rotavirus: Associated with acute diarrhea. This virus is a very common cause of diarrhea in young children around the world.

› Rubella: A contagious viral infection caused by the rubella virus and spread through droplets that is associated with a rash, fever, fatigue, and sore throat; sometimes called "German measles."

› Staph infections: Bacterial infections (usually *Staphylococcus aureus*) that are commonly found on the skin and can cause boils or secondary infections through breaches in skin integrity.

› Strep infections: Infections (usually Group A *Streptococcus* bacteria) that are commonly found on the skin. They can be serious, with complications including glomerulonephritis and severe throat infections.

› Tetanus: A bacterial infection associated with exposure to contaminated puncture wounds, which leads to painful and involuntary contractions of the muscles of the jaw ("lockjaw").

› Varicella zoster: Also known as chickenpox; a highly contagious viral infection that is spread by contact and airborne means. It causes a classic raised rash with honey-color exudates that weep and crust.

respiratory secretions) are the most important areas in which to provide preventive education.

Ancillary healthcare providers and childcare providers must understand the basic clinical presentation of common childhood infections. Early identification of urinary tract infections, respiratory tract infections, communicable skins lesions, otitis media, gastrointestinal infections, and other common childhood infections will assist in rapid clinical management and prevention of disease transmission. For instance, bacterial urinary tract infections are very common in diapered infants and young children, as well as in toddlers who are being potty trained (**Box 26-1**). Identification of early signs and symptoms of this infection across these developmental periods should elicit rapid assessments, early treatment, and prevention of possible longer-term complications.

BOX 26-1 Common Bacterial Strains Causing Urinary Tract Infections
• *Escherichia coli* from the intestines; children wiping from back to front • *Staphylococcus saprophyticus* • *Klebsiella* • *Enterococcus* • *Proteus mirabilis*

Childhood Immunizations

As a child grows and develops, he or she is exposed to more and more environments that inherently have germs and potential pathogens. When a germ enters a child's body, the immune system will recognize it as a foreign substance known as an antigen. The child's immune system launches a fight against antigens by producing massive quantities of antibodies. When a child is given a vaccine, the dead or weakened antigen triggers the production of antibodies that provide protection to the child if he or she is ever again exposed to that particular communicable disease or pathogen. A vaccine does not and cannot produce the disease itself; instead, it stimulates the child's immune system to create disease-fighting antibodies. The small risk of side effects associated with a vaccine outweighs the risk of the child developing a disease that might potentially cause serious illness or death (**Figure 26-2**). Mild side effects can occur with administration of vaccines, such as tenderness at the injection site, soreness, fever, and fussiness; serious side effects are very rare. Children with chronic illnesses, with certain forms of childhood cancer, or who are taking immunosuppressive drugs may not be able to tolerate vaccines for a period of time, and sometimes forever.

Compliance with timely and complete childhood immunization schedules has been credited with the near-elimination

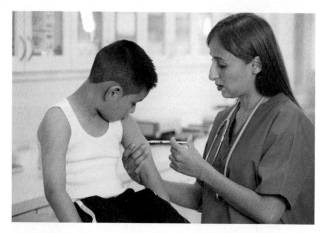

Figure 26-2 *The small risk of side effects associated with a vaccine outweighs the risk of the child developing a disease that might potentially cause serious illness or death.*

© Ariel Skelley/Blend Images/Getty Images

of many complex childhood infectious diseases, such as polio and diphtheria, that have caused significant morbidity and mortality in the past. Immunization schedules are updated regularly and are based on the needs of a population. In the United States, immunization schedules are recommended by the Centers for Disease Control and Prevention, which provides specific guidelines for healthcare providers across settings who provide **vaccinations** (i.e., administration of weakened or dead pathogens; the vaccine is intended to provoke the production of antibodies that confer immunity against the full-blown disease) to patients across the developmental period (CDC, 2015a) (**Table 26-3**). If a child experiences a medical condition or a life circumstance (e.g., travel or immigration) that leads to a delay or incomplete participation in the usual immunization schedule, "catch-up" and alternative schedules are available that can be used to determine best practices for the individual child. Children who are partially immunized or do not start immunizations until later in childhood for other reasons should also follow alternative schedules; these schedules may be found on the CDC and National Institutes of Health (NIH) websites.

Families must be taught to maintain accurate records so that children entering school have the immunization documentation required for enrollment. Some states have also passed laws preventing children from attending private and public schools if immunization schedules are not complete according to the child's age.

Family education is needed concerning the circumstances in which a child cannot be administered a vaccine. Minor illnesses are typically not a reason to withhold administration. If a required and scheduled vaccine is not administered, the next appointment should be made and the family should receive clear guidelines on the importance of keeping the child's immunization on track.

TABLE 26-3   Recommended Childhood Immunizations

DTaP Vaccine (All bacteria; diphtheria, tetanus, and pertussis)

› Administered intramuscularly (IM)

› Maximal effects occur if the immunization is administered with a time lapse of 8 weeks between doses

› Acetaminophen can be administered at 4 and 8 hours after the injection to decrease local responses and febrile incidents

› Tdap is recommended to be administered to children older than 7 years of age; DTaP is recommended for children younger than 7 years

Measles Vaccine

› Administered subcutaneously (SQ)

› First dose is given between 12 and 16 months of age; second dose is given between 4 and 6 years of age

› Post-immunization mild reactions include transient rashes and fever up to two weeks after the injection

Mumps Vaccine

› Administered SQ

› Given in combination with measles and rubella at 12–16 months of age

› A second dose is definitely required based on the number of mumps cases that have occurred in recent years

Rubella Vaccine

› Administered SQ

› Important to immunize postpubertal children

› Pregnancy should be avoided within 3 months of the vaccine's administration due to a theoretical risk to the fetus

Polio Vaccine

› Administered IM or SQ

› CDC recommends exclusive use of inactivated polio vaccine (IPV) and not oral polio vaccine (OPV); live organisms from OPV are shed in stool for up to 1 month

Hepatitis B Vaccine

› Administered IM

› Infants born to mothers who test negative for hepatitis B surface antigen should follow the routine immunization schedule

› Infants born to mothers who test positive for hepatitis B surface antigen should follow the alternative immunization schedule, which includes vaccine within 12 hours of birth and hepatitis B immunoglobulin infusion; contact the CDC for more information

› First dose is given during the neonatal period up to 2 months of age; the second dose is given 1–2 months later; the third dose is given at 6 months of age

Pneumococcal Vaccine

› There are two types: PCV7/Prevnar (administered IM) and PPV/Pneumovax (administered IM or SQ)

› PPV is recommended for children 2–5 years old with high risks, such as sickle cell disease, HIV, asplenia, nephrotic syndrome, and other immunosuppressive disorders

Varicella Vaccine

› Administered SQ

› Considered live, attenuated viral vaccine

› Approved for children older than 12 months of age

› First dose is given at 12–16 months of age; second dose is given at 4–6 years of age or at least 3 months after the first dose

Data from Pediatric Primary Care retrieved from http://ovidsp.tx.ovid.com/sp-3.10.0b/ovidweb.cgi?targetFrame=1&S=MLPIFPCKDPDD (2013) on December 1st, 2014

Pediatric healthcare teams must be prepared to offer families written information about childhood immunizations. This material should include information about which disease the immunization covers, what the common side effects are, what to report to whom, and how to care for symptoms. Downloadable childhood immunization information sheets can be found at the CDC website (https://www.cdc.gov). The healthcare team is responsible for providing written information in languages commonly used in the community so that all parents can be educated.

Pediatric nurses are in the perfect position to deliver effective anticipatory guidance for the families whom they serve. Preventing infections and communicable diseases is part of an important teaching plan for families, both to help them recognize warning signs and so that they will know what to expect over the course of the child's development. Most important, the nurse needs to teach families how to participate in prevention of illnesses for their children. The most important topics to discuss with families of infants and children as means to prevent illnesses are good nutrition, adequate rest, personal hand hygiene to prevent the spread or acquisition of communicable diseases, and completion of the childhood immunization schedule.

FAMILY EDUCATION

The Concept of "Herd Immunity" with Childhood Immunizations

Immunization rates vary widely across diverse geographic locations. In some areas with low childhood immunization rates, some parents have a false sense of security about their children's health, based on the erroneous belief that their unimmunized or under-immunized child will be protected through the concept known as "herd immunity," "herd protection," or "social/population immunity." This concept relates to a form of indirect protection from infectious diseases that arises because a large percentage of a given population has been vaccinated against a particular infection. Thus, there is little likelihood of a disease outbreak, which in turn protects those who were not vaccinated. This idea creates a false sense of security and puts children at risk if an exposure occurs.

Annual Recommended Schedules

Pediatric nurses should stay up-to-date with any changes to the proposed immunization schedule and keep the information handy. In general, childhood immunizations address the following diseases:

- *Haemophilus influenzae* type b (Hib): meningitis, severe throat infections and pneumonia (3- or 4-shot series)
- Varicella: chickenpox (2 shots)
- *Clostridium tetanus* and diphtheria (Td) or diphtheria, tetanus, and pertussis (DTaP): severe systemic and airway infections; requires booster every 10 years (3 shots)
- Polio (inactivated poliovirus vaccine [IPV]): muscle pain, paralysis, and death (4 shots)
- Hepatitis B (HepB): liver inflammation and fatal complications (cirrhosis, hepatic carcinoma) (3 or 4 shots)
- Pneumococcal infections (pneumococcal conjugate PCV13): bacteremia and meningitis (4 doses)
- Measles, mumps, and rubella (MMR): rash, pneumonia, meningitis, painful swollen saliva glands, and ear infections (2 shots)
- *Neisseria meningitidis* (meningococcal conjugate MCV4): serious bacterial infection of the bloodstream (2 shots)
- Influenza (flu vaccine—optional): various types of influenza infections, primarily in the winter months (annual shot for children older than 2 years)

Vaccine Administration Considerations

- Ensure strict adherence to the vaccine manufacturer's handling, storage, and administration recommendations. Do not allow the vaccine's potency to diminish.
- Make sure all healthcare professionals who are administering childhood vaccines are immunized to measles, mumps, hepatitis B, influenza, rubella, pertussis, tetanus, polio, and diphtheria.
- Use sterile, disposable needles with safety devices on the syringes to prevent needle sticks; never recap needles; and keep a red biohazard container for syringe disposal within reach.
- Wear gloves when giving immunizations to children, as they may be challenging to hold, which increases the risk for body fluid exposure.
- Provide written vaccine information to the family prior to administering the medication.
- Routine childhood vaccines can be safely administered simultaneously.

Contraindications to Immunization

It is important for the healthcare team to fully understand and verify the rationale when making the decision to withhold the administration of required immunizations to a child. The following conditions are most commonly regarded as appropriate reasons for not immunizing a child or waiting to immunize a child:

- Acute childhood illnesses that cause high-grade fever
- Serious cases of diarrhea
- Reactions to previous DTaP or other immunizations that involved neurologic sequelae
- Extreme prematurity
- Children on high doses of steroids for more than 14 days
- Allergies to eggs (pediatric healthcare professionals should contact the CDC for guidelines and alternatives)
- Serious exacerbations of immune-based chronic inflammatory diseases
- Recent administration of immunoglobulin preparations that can interfere with the desired serologic response

FAMILY EDUCATION

Tips for Talking to Parents About Immunizations to Prevent Childhood Communicable Diseases

- Present verbal and written information about each vaccine the child will receive and document that the information was provided in the appropriate language for each family's comprehension and linguistic need.
- Take a health history, inquiring whether the child has experienced a reaction to or side effect from vaccines in the past.
- Assess for the presence of any contraindication to immunization, including use of immunosuppressants, use of chemotherapeutics, allergies to components of various vaccines (including eggs), moderate to severe febrile illnesses or conditions, previous severe reactions such as anaphylactic reactions to the vaccine or vaccine constituents, recent intravenous immune globulin administration, or seizures within three days or fevers greater than 40.4°C (104.7°F) within 48 hours of previous vaccine administrations.
- Reinforce the need to adhere to the national guidelines on childhood immunizations schedules. On an annual basis, check for updated guidelines and schedules on either the CDC or NIH website.

Misconceptions About Vaccines

Many misconceptions exist regarding childhood immunizations. Overall immunization rates vary by geography, but range from 83% to 93%, on average (CDC, 2015b). Parental concerns, misconceptions, and inadequate education all influence national immunization rates. The following list gives examples of common misconceptions:

- *MMR vaccines and vaccines containing the preservative thimerosal cause autism.* Extensive scientific research shows that neither the MMR vaccine nor vaccines in general, with or without thimerosal, cause autism (Hurley, Tadrous, & Miller, 2010; Jain et al., 2015; Taylor, Swerdfeger, & Eslick, 2014).
- *The rotavirus vaccine is dangerous.* There is a slight association between the rotavirus vaccine and intussusception, but this outcome is rare and not considered dangerous enough to justify withholding immunization.
- *Vaccine ingredients are toxic and contain mercury, formaldehyde, and aluminum.* Some substances within vaccines can be toxic, but only when taken in much larger amounts than are present in a vaccine dose. Thimerosal—the preservative that is frequently cited as a "danger" because it contains mercury—was eliminated from most vaccines as of 1999; it is present in trace amounts in a small number of vaccines (Food and Drug Administration, 2015; Hurley et al., 2010). Vaccines are generally safe, and their benefits outweigh the risks.
- *Vaccines can fail and not cause immunity.* Only in 1% to 5% of cases will children fail to develop the relevant antibodies. When appropriate, serum antibody titers can be assessed and subsequent vaccine boosters can be administered.
- *Vaccines cause the disease.* With inactive (killed) childhood vaccines, it is not possible to get the infection or disease from the vaccine. Live, attenuated vaccines can cause a very mild case of the disease, but will still protect from a severe case. Live oral polio vaccine, known in the past to cause a risk of infection, is no longer used in the United States.
- *Parents can decline immunizations for their child if they want.* In each state, both medical and religious exemptions for immunizations are available; conversely, few states allow philosophic exemptions. Unvaccinated students may not be allowed to attend public or private schools, especially if there is an epidemic or pandemic occurring.

RESEARCH EVIDENCE

Does the Influenza Vaccine Cause Febrile Seizures?

The influenza vaccine has been recommended for all infants since 1973. Although the risk is only slightly higher, infants who receive the trivalent inactivated influenza vaccine concomitantly when they receive the pneumococcal (PCV13 or PCV7) or DTaP vaccine are at an increased risk for febrile seizures. Research suggests that the risk of a febrile seizure during the first few days after the vaccines are administered is less of a concern than the risk of febrile seizures for children who are not vaccinated for the host of childhood infectious and communicable diseases, some of which have a potential to be life threatening (Duffy et al., 2016).

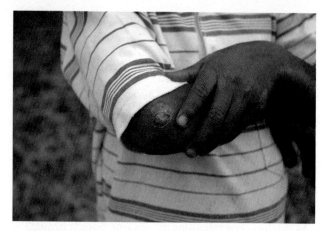

Figure 26-3 *If the wound is deep or concerning, the child should be evaluated.*

© Sean_Warren/iStock /Getty Images Plus/Getty

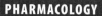
Wound Infections

In addition to infections via communicable diseases, children are prone to experiencing significant skin scrapes, excoriations, and open wounds. If the wound is deep or concerning, the child should be evaluated for wound cleansing, stitches to promote healing, and possible oral antibiotics if infection is present or suspected (**Figure 26-3**).

Typical small wounds, such as scrapes, abrasions, and shallow cuts, should be managed at home; parents can be taught to follow basic wound care guidelines. For wounds seen in the clinic, the following process should be used:

1. Always clean hands thoroughly before touching a child's open wound. In a healthcare setting, wear gloves and assume contamination requiring contact isolation.
2. If dressing a wound that has previously been treated, remove any old dressing or tape, and wash hands again.
3. Use normal saline to irrigate the wound, or wash it with mild soap and lukewarm water. If available, use a syringe to wash the wound and remove any pus or drainage.
4. Gently dab the skin with clean gauze or very clean soft cloth.
5. Do not use alcohol, detergents, hydrogen peroxide, or iodine on the wound, as these products may delay wound healing through epithelialization.
6. In fresh wounds, assess the wound carefully for pebbles, dirt, debris, clots, or any material that may delay wound healing. In previously treated wounds, assess for sloughing tissue and eschar; the presence of both can delay wound healing.
7. Assess the need for stitches. Absorbable or natural material such as catgut should be used to close the inner layers of a deep wound and will absorb completely within two months. Non-absorbable sutures, which are used for top-layer closure, are made of a thread material such as silk or synthetic fibers and must be removed when the wound has healed.
8. Pat the wound dry with clean gauze or a new section of the very clean cloth.
9. Dress the wound as needed to provide a barrier cover to prevent microbial contamination.

Once the initial phases of fresh wound healing begin, a child's wound should heal rapidly and without complications. These phases include hemostasis (vascular spasms to constrict vessels, platelet plug formation followed by blood coagulation), then inflammation (mobilization of nutrients, antibodies, migration of white blood cells [WBCs]), and finally proliferation (rebuilding of the wound with new healthy granulation tissue from leap-frogging epithelial cell migration).

Nursing Care for Children with Infections or Communicable Diseases

Care of a child with an infection or communicable disease is based on a series of critical thinking factors. The pediatric nurse should recall the unique aspects of caring for children; the care of a child with an infection also requires thoughtful consideration and prospective care planning. In particular, the nurse should keep in mind the following factors:

- The location, extent, severity, and clinical presentation of the wound or infectious process
- Sensitivity of the microorganism to antimicrobial therapy, including the minimal bactericidal concentration (MBC), which determines the amount of therapy needed to achieve 99.9% bacterial kill
- Age of the child and ability to participate in and comply with therapy, including leaving the wound alone to heal without picking, scraping, or chewing off dressings
- The child's immune system, nutritional status, and overall general health—presence of comorbidities may reduce the ability of the child's immune system to launch an effective healing process
- Presence of allergies, history of allergic reactions, and development of tolerance to the therapy (development of nausea, antimicrobial-associated diarrhea, and rashes or skin reactions)

Pediatric nurses are often requested to provide anticipatory guidance and teaching on childhood infections, including their transmission, incubation periods, classical signs and associated symptoms, treatments, and academic attendance guidelines.

Most children with infections are managed outside the hospital setting. Common childhood infections such as otitis media, impetigo, cellulitis, and small wound infections may need to be initially assessed in a pediatric healthcare setting, then subsequently treated and managed at home. In contrast, children who present with immune immaturity or immune compromise, or who have a complicated infectious process, will most likely be hospitalized for intravenous antimicrobial therapy.

Concept Exemplars

The following infectious diseases are used as concept exemplars: conjunctivitis, fifth disease, thrush, and impetigo.

Conjunctivitis

Conjunctivitis, or "pink eye," is an infection of the membrane covering the white of the eye. It is a common condition in children of all ages, including newborns, although the causes in newborns may be slightly different. Causes of conjunctivitis vary, with infection by bacterial and viral pathogens at one end of the spectrum and airborne chemicals or allergens (e.g., pollen) at the other.

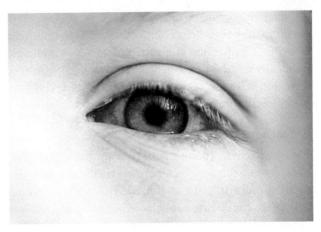

Figure 26-4 *Conjuctivitis is easy to identify by its symptoms of redness, swelling, and discharge.*
© Sharon Mccutcheon /EyeEm/Getty Images

Diagnosis

Conjunctivitis is easy to spot, as it involves noticeable redness, swelling, discharge, and often pain in the eyes (**Figure 26-4**). The cause of conjunctivitis may be more difficult to determine, as bacterial and viral infections have almost identical symptoms, and even allergic response can closely resemble an infection; foreign bodies such as eyelashes, dust, or pollutants in the air can also cause conjunctivitis. Common cues as to the cause are co-occurring infections and the appearance of discharge (CDC, 2016b): Viral conjunctivitis usually has watery discharge and coincides with respiratory infections; bacterial conjunctivitis discharge is generally thick rather than watery and coincides with otitis media; foreign bodies present with heavy tear production and a sensation of "grit" in the eye; and allergic conjunctivitis is usually seasonal, accompanied by intense itching of the eyes, and often occurs in children who have other allergic or atopic conditions (e.g., eczema). In severe cases or cases with complicating factors such as immune deficiency, contact lens use, or treatment failure, laboratory evaluation of exudate may be necessary to determine appropriate treatment (Cronau, Kankanala, & Mauger, 2010). In neonates, maternally transmitted infections such as chlamydia, herpesvirus, or other bacterial contaminants acquired during birth can be the cause; alternatively, blocked tear ducts or (ironically) topical medications used for prevention of bacterial conjunctivitis can cause the condition.

Risk Factors

Both viral and bacterial conjunctivitis are extremely **contagious** (readily spread through direct and indirect contact), and contact with another child who has conjunctivitis should raise suspicion for transmission via droplets or hand–eye contact. Presence of certain infections in the mother (gonorrhea, chlamydia) raises the risk of neonatal conjunctivitis. Children older than 5 years have lower risk of contracting infectious conjunctivitis due to improved hygiene. Allergies and atopy are risk factors for allergic conjunctivitis. Children with blepharitis—an inflammatory condition that supports bacterial growth in the eyelid—are at risk of chronic or recurrent infection (CDC, 2016b).

Medical Treatment

Treatment of viral conjunctivitis is supportive and emphasizes hand washing, cold compresses on the eye to reduce swelling, and artificial tears if needed to soothe irritation. Otherwise, the disease is usually self-limiting and resolves in 7 to 10 days without intervention (Cronau et al., 2010). Cases that last longer may need ocular steroid therapy and should be referred to an ophthalmologist.

Acute bacterial conjunctivitis follows the same treatment protocol as viral conjunctivitis, but is additionally treated with ocular antibiotic ointment. Treatment of bacterial infections may be handled by primary care practitioners, but chronic (recurring for at least 4 weeks) and hyperacute (sudden-onset with excessive, purulent discharge) infections should be referred to an ophthalmologist.

Allergic conjunctivitis is managed using antihistamines (either oral or topical), allergen avoidance, and artificial tears. Foreign body-related conjunctivitis should prompt evaluation for corneal abrasion, including assessing for the presence of a retained foreign body adhering to the eyelid (Cronau et al., 2010). In neonates, blocked tear ducts are managed with gentle rubbing of the eye to dislodge the blockage, but if the problem continues beyond 1 year of age, surgical intervention may be needed (CDC, 2016b).

Nursing Care

Nursing care should focus on primary prevention practices. Good hand hygiene and avoidance of hand-eye contact is essential for conjunctivitis prevention. Young children must be taught and then reminded to participate in adequate hand hygiene, and family members need to role model best practices.

If the cause of the conjunctivitis is bacterial, the family should be reminded to use the full dose of antibiotic ointment as prescribed to limit microbial resistance. If the cause is allergic, teaching should include allergen avoidance.

Fifth Disease (Erythema Infectiosum)

Fifth disease, also called erythema infectiosum, is a common viral infection caused by parvovirus B19 (CDC, 2015e). It got its name by virtue of being traditionally listed fifth in classifications of illnesses that frequently cause skin rash in children.

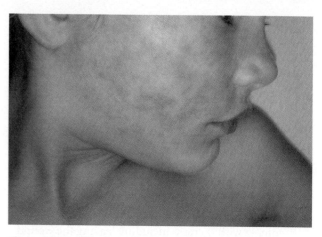

Figure 26-5 *Fifth disease is characterized by the "slapped cheek" facial rash.*

© Diomedia/ISM

Diagnosis

Fifth disease typically starts as a nonspecific set of symptoms: fever, runny nose, and headache. After several days, the "slapped cheek" facial rash that is characteristic of this infection develops, followed by a more generalized, sometimes itchy, rash on the rest of the body (**Figure 26-5**). Total duration of the infection from onset to disappearance of the rash is generally 10 to 14 days. Joint pain, which sometimes accompanies parvovirus B19 infections in adults, is rare in children.

Because most children with healthy immune response develop full immunity, the infection is usually a one-time occurrence. Children with immune deficiency, however, may not develop full immunity and are vulnerable to re-infection (CDC, 2015e).

Risk Factors

Children who attend school or daycare programs are most likely to be exposed to parvovirus B19. Children who have had fifth disease already are at low risk unless they have an immune defect. Once the rash develops, the child is no longer contagious (CDC, 2015e).

Medical Treatment and Nursing Care

Treatment is supportive and focused on symptom relief, as the disease is self-limiting, except in those children at risk of complications due to immune deficiency. Nursing care should focus on primary prevention practices and teaching about management of symptoms. Appropriate administration of analgesics and fever reducers to prevent overdose should be emphasized, particularly in very young children. Good hand hygiene, avoidance of hand-eye contact, and covering the nose and mouth when sneezing or coughing are important practices to prevent transmission. Young children must be taught and then reminded to participate in adequate hand hygiene, and family members need to role model best practices.

Thrush (Candidiasis)

Thrush (candidiasis) in children may be either an oropharyngeal or urogenital infection with the yeast *Candida albicans*. Oropharyngeal infections occur primarily in infants. Urogenital infections occur in infants and toddlers (diaper dermatitis) or in adolescent girls ("yeast infections"). Intertrigo—candidiasis of the skin folds of the groin, armpits, and torso—may also occur in overweight children, particularly if poor hygiene practices are present.

Diagnosis

Oral candidiasis presents as white plaques in the mouth that resemble cottage cheese (Jain, Jain, & Rawat, 2010). If the plaques are scraped away, the mucosa beneath is reddened and sore, and may bleed (**Figure 26-6**). Cracking in the corners of the mouth (angular cheilitis) is a concomitant symptom. Oral candidiasis is most common in infants, but may occur in children who have been recently treated with antibiotics and steroids due to the effects of the medications on the normal oral flora.

Urogenital candidiasis in infants presents as a red rash with a clearly defined border that is deepest in the folds of the groin and buttocks; suspicion of candidiasis should be raised by any significant diaper rash lasting more than 2 or 3 days with treatment (Jain et al., 2010). Vaginal candidiasis in adolescents is characterized by intense itching of the genitals; thick, white discharge; and redness in the groin area.

Risk Factors

Oral and urogenital thrush are not unusual in infants, particularly newborns. Urogenital thrush in adolescents is more common with sexual activity. Urogenital thrush and intertrigo may also be a product of poor hygiene and use of towels or clothing belonging to others.

Medical Treatment and Nursing Care

In infants, oral thrush is self-limiting. Urogenital thrush can be managed with appropriate hygiene and management to limit moisture in the diaper area (e.g., more frequent diaper changes). Diaper rash creams can be used to alleviate irritation. Vaginal candidiasis and intertrigo may be treated with topical or systemic antifungal medications.

Nursing care includes teaching new parents how to manage diaper rash and educating adolescents about hygiene and prevention. In sexually active teens, discussion of the importance of preventing other sexually transmitted diseases (STDs) may be an important facet of nursing care for urogenital candidiasis.

Impetigo

Impetigo is the most common bacterial skin infection in children (Cole & Gazewood, 2007). It is most frequently caused by bacteria such as *Staphylococcus aureus* and, less frequently, *Streptococcus pyogenes*, which are commonly present on the skin's surface. Impetigo is generally not serious except when it develops in concert with scabies (a parasitic mite, *Sarcoptes scabiei*, that burrows in the skin), in which case it can lead to serious complications (Romani, Steer, Whitfield, & Kaldor, 2015).

Two forms of impetigo are distinguished: bullous and nonbullous. The former presents as perioral or perinasal vesicles that rupture to form a dark yellow crust, while the latter presents as fragile, transparent bullae that may appear anywhere on the body (Lewis, 2016) (**Figure 26-7**). Nonbullous impetigo is highly contagious and usually resolves on its own in about 2 weeks. Bullous impetigo

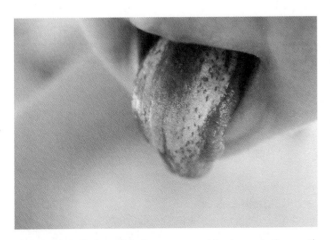

Figure 26-6 *Oral candidiasis presents as white plaques in the mouth that resemble cottage cheese.*

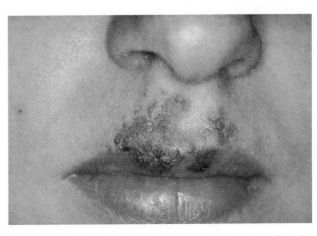

Figure 26-7 *Bullous impetigo presents as perioral or perinasal vesicles that rupture to form a dark yellow crust.*

is less contagious but may provoke systemic symptoms if lesions are widespread (Lewis, 2016). Approximately 70% of cases are nonbullous impetigo; the majority of bullous impetigo cases occur in infants.

Diagnosis

Diagnosis is based on clinical appearance and history. In situations where outbreaks are common or if the child has recently been hospitalized, culture of exudate beneath scabbed-over lesions may be needed to rule out possible methicillin-resistant *S. aureus* (MRSA) infection (Lewis, 2016).

Risk Factors

Impetigo may develop in children who have a history of minor trauma, insect bites, scabies, eczema, or any other condition that promotes an itchy rash; abrasions due to scratching are often a cause of infection. Risk is increased in children with a family member or close associate who has a streptococcal or staphylococcal infection. Poor hygiene; hot, humid living conditions; and crowded living quarters can put children at risk.

Medical Treatment and Nursing Care

Treatment of impetigo involves direct wound care of the lesions plus appropriate antibiotic therapy with an agent that is active against both *S. aureus* and *S. pyogenes*. Topical mupirocin or retapamulin are preferred agents for nonbullous impetigo that presents with single lesions, but systemic antibiotics are used when there is extensive skin involvement or when an outbreak occurs in a family, on an athletic team, or in a daycare setting. In infants with widespread bullous impetigo that has multiple ruptured lesions, dehydration and sepsis are concerns and inpatient treatment is warranted (Lewis, 2016).

As with other infectious processes, nursing care should initially focus on primary prevention practices. Good hygiene—particularly hand washing—is the key to infection prevention. Young children must be taught and then reminded to participate in adequate hand hygiene, and family members need to role model best practices.

When a child presents with an infection, nursing care includes determining the severity of the infection and communicating assessments to the medical team for treatment. Discharge teaching from a pediatric clinic or hospital should include the following points:

- Fill the child's antimicrobial prescriptions immediately.
- Plan on the same schedule of administration as started in the healthcare setting to ensure consistent serum plasma of the antimicrobial for maximal efficacy.
- Administer the medication completely. Stopping when the child feels better, no longer has fevers (if present), or appears to be well or free of infection symptoms contributes to the development of resistant strains and may cause a reinfection if the microbe is still present and not completely treated.
- Report a wound, rash, or infection that does not respond to medications or heals more slowly than expected.
- Prevent secondary infections in infants and young children by preventing children from scratching their wounds and contaminating them with dirt, feces, or other contaminates.

Hospital-Acquired Infections

When hospitalized, children have an increased vulnerability to experiencing infection with a variety of microbes. Children who undergo surgical manipulation may show signs of infection within 16 hours of a surgical procedure. The presence of urinary catheters, peripheral or central venous catheters, endotracheal (ET) tubes, or other lines where normal protective mechanisms are breached creates a vulnerability to nosocomial infection, also known as hospital-acquired infection (HAI).

The likelihood of contracting a HAI depends on the presence of invasive tubes, length of stay in the hospital environment, type of surgical procedure, use or overuse of antibiotics (**Table 26-4**), presence of a wound, hand hygiene of caregivers, and the location in the hospital where the child stays. Hospital days spent in a pediatric intensive care unit (PICU) increase a child's vulnerability to HAI. The infections most typically acquired in hospitals are hospital-acquired pneumonia (HAP), catheter-associated urinary tract infections (CAUTI), wound infections, and hospital-acquired bloodstream infections (HABSI) (CDC. gov, 2016c).

PHARMACOLOGY

Medications That Increase Risk for Infection in Children

- Corticosteroid use (lengthy course):
  - Cortisone
  - Dexamethasone
  - Hydrocortisone
  - Methylprednisolone
  - Prednisone
  - Triamcinolone
- Chemotherapeutic medications to treat cancer
- Tumor necrosis factor (TNF) inhibitors
- Immunosuppressants for organ transplantation or bone marrow transplantation

TABLE 26-4 Antimicrobial Therapy for Common Childhood Infectious Diseases

Antimicrobial therapy works via one of three mechanisms of action:

1. Inhibition of enzyme conversion required for the microbes' survival
2. Destruction of the microbial cell wall
3. Impairment of microbial protein synthesis

After laboratory testing such as sputum, urine, blood or wound base/drainage, a Gram stain may be performed to visually identify the infectious organism, or a culture may be grown to positively identify the culprit. Never administer antibiotic therapy until specimens have been collected, so that accurate identification of the microbial agent can be made in the cultures without the influence of antimicrobial effect of medications.

Common Antibiotics Used in the Treatment of Infectious Conditions and Communicable Diseases (Bacterial)

Penicillins

› Weaken or destroy the cell wall
› Nursing considerations:
  • Assess for previous allergic reactions
  • May affect kidney function at higher doses so monitor the child's input and output (I&O)
  • Amoxicillin, amoxicillin–clavulanate, and penicillin V may be taken with food; all others should be given with water on an empty stomach
  • Often given for streptococcal pneumonia, meningitis, and pharyngitis

Cephalosporins (First Through Fourth Generations)

› Weaken or destroy the cell wall
› Nursing considerations:
  • Can reach cerebrospinal fluid
  • Used for treatment of gram-negative organisms and anaerobes
  • Considered broad-spectrum antibiotics
  • Used to treat urinary tract infections, postoperative infections, and pelvic infections

Carbapenems

› Weaken or destroy the cell wall
› Nursing considerations:
  • Considered a beta-lactam antibiotic (e.g., imipenem–cilastatin or meropenem)
  • Should be taken with food
  • Used to treat pneumonia, urinary tract infections, and both gram-positive and gram-negative cocci

Tetracyclines

› Inhibit protein synthesis
› Nursing considerations:
  • Considered broad-spectrum antibiotics
  • Given for mycoplasma pneumonia, Lyme disease, and gastrointestinal infections
  • May cause tooth discoloration and photosensitivity

(continues)

Macrolides

› Inhibit protein synthesis

› Nursing considerations:

  • Prototypes include erythromycin and azithromycin

  • Often given if the child is allergic to penicillins

  • Macrolides should be taken on an empty stomach for greatest efficacy; the exception is azithromycin, which may be taken with food

  • Can be ototoxic at high doses

  • Monitor liver function tests if taken longer than 2 weeks

Aminoglycosides

› Inhibit protein synthesis

› Nursing considerations:

  • May require serum troughs (peaks are no longer typically monitored) to maintain therapeutic index and prevent toxicity; samples should be drawn 30 minutes after the administration (check and follow institutional policy)

  • Often used for *E. coli* infections

  • Monitor for ototoxicity, nephrotoxicity, and rash

Antibiotic-Resistant Microbes

Several microbes that were treated in the past with first-generation antibiotics are now becoming resistant to traditional therapies (**Box 26-2**). *Resistance* refers to the ability of a microbe to adapt to the presence of the antimicrobial without stopping its growth, reproduction, or life span. Although most microbes on a child's body remain harmless, those that are categorized as **pathogens** have the potential to cause infections. According to the CDC (2015d), the single greatest contributor to the development of resistant microbial strains is the overuse of antibiotics. This problem occurs when antibiotics are given in situations where they are not needed (such as trying to treat viral otitis media with oral antibiotics), when patients do not complete the full course of treatment (such as stopping the medication when symptoms abate after 4 days of therapy instead of the 10 days required by the prescription), not prescribing the correct antibiotic for the microbe involved, or not

BOX 26-2   Examples of Resistant Strains Currently Affecting U.S. Hospital Systems

Due to several factors, including incomplete antimicrobial prescription adherence, some bacteria have evolved the ability to evade common antibiotics (CDC, 2015d):

  • Methicillin-resistant *Staphylococcus aureus* (MRSA)
  • Carbapenem-resistant Enterobacteriaceae (CRE)
  • Vancomycin-resistant *Enterococcus* (VRE)
  • Other: *Klebsiella, Acinetobacter, Pseudomonas*, tuberculosis, and gonorrhea

prescribing the correct length of treatment. Furthermore, the indiscriminate use of antibiotics to prevent infections in farm animals has been documented to contribute to the development of resistant strains. Some microbes have developed the capacity to share drug resistance genetically (CDC, 2015d).

Case Study

The family of a 6-week-old infant girl brought her into the pediatric emergency department (ED) for symptoms of fever, fussiness, nasal congestion and discharge, persistent dry cough, lethargy, and poor feeding. The infant has a 3-year-old sibling who was not immunized for any childhood infectious diseases. The ED team determined the infant's symptoms resembled

(continues)

Case Study *(continued)*

pertussis and took a rapid pertussis swab. Once the child was stabilized with oxygen and IV fluid boluses, she was transferred to the PICU with a diagnosis of pertussis requiring antibiotics (erythromycin, azithromycin, or clarithromycin), respiratory therapy, and frequent nursing observation. The infant continued to have deep, persistent coughing spells that resulted in low oxygen saturation, poor feeding, and decreased level of consciousness.

Case Study Questions

1. How might the infant have become infected with pertussis?
2. What are the stages of a pertussis infection?
3. Why did this infant display severe symptoms of respiratory distress?
4. What is the best laboratory assessment of an infection of pertussis?
5. If a child receives an immunization for pertussis, which type of immunity is the immunization considered?

As the Case Evolves...

The parents of this 6-week-old infant are giving the child's history to the nurse in the pediatric ward. During the discussion,

the nurse asks why their daughter's 3-year-old brother has not been vaccinated against pertussis and other childhood infectious diseases.

6. Parents' reasons for failing to immunize their children are often concerns based on the following: (Select all that apply)
   A. Presence of thimerosal in vaccines
   B. Association of vaccines with autism
   C. Fear of deafness from vaccines
   D. Concerns with immune system health
   E. Cost of the vaccines
7. Suppose that the parents of this child express all the concerns listed in Question 6 when talking to the nurse. Which of these concerns may be regarded as valid and, therefore, require no further teaching to correct misunderstandings?
   A. Presence of thimerosal in vaccines
   B. Association of vaccines with autism
   C. Fear of deafness from vaccines
   D. Concerns with immune system health
   E. Cost of the vaccines

Chapter Summary

- Infectious diseases and communicable diseases are commonly associated with the developmental years. Young children and infants are prone to contracting infections due to their immature immune systems. Children entering childcare facilities and school environments become rapidly exposed to infectious materials due to their increased socialization in these settings and encounters with other children who may be under-immunized or infected due to older siblings' exposure.

- The normal flora on a child's skin and intestines provide a first line of protection from disease-causing fungi and bacteria, help to manufacture vitamin K (essential for clotting factors), and assist in the breakdown and digestion of food. Breaches in the protective layer of normal flora are caused by breaks in skin integrity, allowing for infectious invasion of harmful microbes.

- Factors associated with the development of childhood infections include genetics, family hygiene practices, the child's age, immunity status, nutritional status, chronic disorders such as diabetes, and overall general health. The youngest children's developmental stage highly influences transmission and reception of infectious materials due to their oral fixation and inability to control secretions.

- Immunizations administered during childhood include the DTaP, MMR, polio, hepatitis B, pneumococcal, and varicella vaccines. Other childhood vaccines include the annual influenza and rotavirus vaccines, as indicated.

- The pediatric nurse's role in childhood immunizations includes accurate administration of the correct vaccine, in the correct dose, at the correct site, and with the correct timing; parent/guardian education on aspects of the immunization being administered; assessment for contraindications to administration; and assessment of side effects or reactions.

- Several complexities surround childhood immunizations, including parental refusal of vaccines due to cultural beliefs, religious beliefs, and fears about the vaccines. Although state laws vary, childhood vaccine exemptions are generally categorized as medical, religious, or philosophical.

- Infections during childhood can be caused by a variety of macroparasites and microbial agents, including bacteria, viruses, fungi, protozoa, and prions.

- A major role of the pediatric nurse working in any clinical setting is to understand the clinical presentations of common childhood infectious diseases, report findings for confirmation and treatment, and teach families about prevention and control.
- Teaching families, and providing follow-up, on the importance of adhering to not only a complete course of antibiotic therapy for bacterial infections, but also the specified timing of administration, makes an important contribution in reducing the development of resistant pathogen strains.

Bibliography

American Academy of Pediatrics. (2015). Overview of infectious diseases. Retrieved from https://www.healthychildren.org /English/health-issues/conditions/infections/Pages/Overview -of-Infectious-Diseases.aspx

Centers for Disease Control and Prevention (CDC). (2015a). Immunization schedules: For health care professionals. Retrieved from http://www.cdc.gov/vaccines/schedules/hcp/index .html?s_cid=cs_000

Centers for Disease Control and Prevention (CDC). (2015b). Immunization FastStats: 2012 data for the U.S. Retrieved from http://www.cdc.gov/nchs/fastats/immunize.htm

Centers for Disease Control and Prevention (CDC). (2015c). Whooping cough or pertussis. Retrieved from http://www.cdc.gov/nchs /fastats/whooping-cough.htm

Centers for Disease Control and Prevention (CDC). (2015d). Antibiotic/antimicrobial resistance. Retrieved from https:// www.cdc.gov/drugresistance

Centers for Disease Control and Prevention (CDC). (2015e). Fifth disease. Retrieved from http://www.cdc.gov/parvovirusb19 /fifth-disease.html

Centers for Disease Control and Prevention (CDC). (2016a). Common colds: Protect yourself and others. Retrieved from https:// www.cdc.gov/dotw/common-cold/index.html

Centers for Disease Control and Prevention (CDC). (2016b). Conjunctivitis (pink eye). Retrieved from https://www.cdc.gov /conjunctivitis/index.html

Centers for Disease Control and Prevention (CDC). (2016c). HAI Data and Statistics. Retrieved from https://www.cdc.gov/hai /surveillance

Cole, C., & Gazewood, J. (2007). Diagnosis and treatment of impetigo. *American Family Physician, 75*(6), 859–864.

Cronau, H., Kankanala, R. R., & Mauger, T. (2010). Diagnosis and management of red eye in primary care. *American Family Physician, 81*(2), 137–144.

Duffy, J., Weintraub, E., Hambidge, S. J., Jackson, L. A., Kharbanda, E. O., Klein, N. P., . . . DeStefano, F. (2016). Febrile seizure risk after vaccination in children 6–23 months. *Pediatrics, 138*(1), 1–12. doi: 10.1542/peds.2016-0320

Food and Drug Administration. (2015). Thimerosal in vaccines. Retrieved from http://www.fda.gov/BiologicsBloodVaccines /SafetyAvailability/VaccineSafety/UCM096228#toc

Hurley, A. M., Tadrous, M., & Miller, E. S. (2010). Thimerosal-containing vaccines and autism: A review of recent epidemiologic studies. *Journal of Pediatric Pharmacology and Therapeutics, 15*(3), 173–181.

Jain A., Jain S., & Rawat S. (2010). Emerging fungal infections among children: A review on its clinical manifestations, diagnosis, and prevention. *Bioallied Sciences, 2*(4), 314–320.

Jain, A., Marshall, J., Buikema, A., Bancroft, T., Kelly, J. P., & Newschaffer, C. J. (2015). Autism occurrence by MMR vaccine status among US children with older siblings with and without autism. *Journal of the American Medical Association, 313*(15), 1534-1540.

Lewis, L. S. (2016). Impetigo treatment and management. *Medscape.* Retrieved from http://emedicine.medscape.com /article/965254-overview

Romani, L., Steer, A. C., Whitfield, M. J., & Kaldor, J. M. (2015). Prevalence of scabies and impetigo worldwide: A systematic review. *Lancet Infectious Diseases, 15*(8), 960–967.

Taylor, L. E., Swerdfeger, A. L., & Eslick, G. D. (2014). Vaccines are not associated with autism: An evidence-based meta-analysis of case-control and cohort studies. *Vaccine, 32*(29), 3623–3629.

World Health Organization. (2017). Measles. Retrieved from http:// www.who.int/topics/measles/en

Implementing Principles of Safe Care

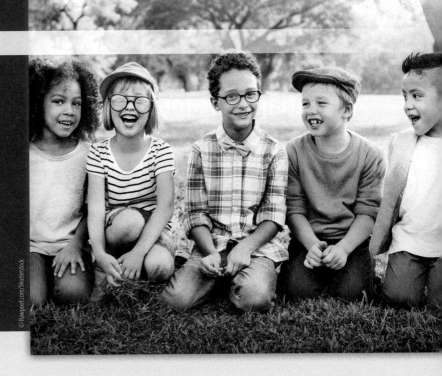

CHAPTER 27

Essential Skills for Pediatric Nursing

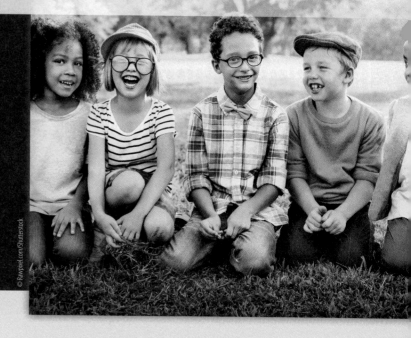

© Rawpixel.com/Shutterstock

LEARNING OBJECTIVES

1. Apply the essentials skills required of a pediatric nurse to provide safe care to children across the developmental stage.
2. Analyze the differences in skill equipment sizes and skill procedures for children of various ages, heights, and weights.
3. Compare the emotional, educational, and cognitive preparation of skills procedures for each of the developmental stages.
4. Analyze the differences between and merits of various forms of distraction and pain control during essential pediatric nursing skills that cause fear and discomfort.
5. Evaluate the team approach needed to perform essential skills in uncooperative young children.
6. Apply safe techniques to the various math calculations required for clinical care of children, and apply safe medication administration techniques to children from infancy through older childhood.

KEY TERMS

Fluid maintenance
Mummy wrap
Oral rehydration therapy
Osmolality
Scalp veins
Syringe pump
Venous access

Introduction

The pediatric registered nurse will perform skills on children ranging in age from the premature infant to the young adult. It is imperative that the nurse be aware of essential skills requiring adaptation for children. This chapter outlines important tips and information needed to safely and effectively apply skills to children of varying ages. The skills discussed here have been selected based on their frequency of use in pediatric acute care, home care, and clinic settings. If you are new to pediatrics, seek the assistance of an experienced nurse who is accustomed to adapting equipment to children, or who is familiar with applying principles of child development consideration to the application of skills. Important aspects of safely and accurately implementing nursing skills to children who may not be cooperative during skills procedures include preparedness and confidence.

Whenever possible, elicit the help of a Child Life team member. These specialists are highly trained in developmentally educating and preparing a child for a skill or procedure. They are well equipped to provide distraction during the procedure, and can help with the patient's physical and emotional recovery after a procedure that causes fear, anxiety, or discomfort.

Pain assessment and control are essential during procedures. Investigate policies and practices surrounding institutional pain control measures for invasive procedures. Offer and encourage the pain-reducing intervention of EMLA (eutectic mixture of local anesthetics) or 4% lidocaine cream topically for invasive needle-based procedures such as intravenous (IV) line placements, intramuscular (IM) and subcutaneous (SQ) injections, and skin biopsies. Offer a vibrating device such as the Buzzy (**Figure 27-1**) to provide nerve distraction during painful procedures. In general, if possible, plan ahead, create a plan of action, provide education, take child developmental considerations into account, and assemble equipment that will promote comfort during a skill procedure that might be frightening or cause discomfort.

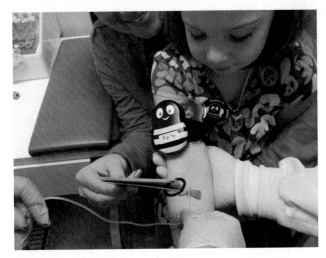

Figure 27-1 *Vibrating devices, such as the Buzzy, provide nerve distraction during painful procedures.*

Potts, D., Davis, K. F., & Fein, J. (2017). A vibrating cold device to reduce pain in the pediatric emergency department: A randomized clinical trial. *Pediatric Emergency Care*, 2017 Jan 24. [Epub ahead of print]. https://www.ncbi.nlm.nih.gov/pubmed/28121978. Photo courtesy of MMJ Labs.

QUALITY AND SAFETY

Know your scope of practice! Do not perform skills or procedures on children without a direct physician's or primary healthcare provider's written (or electronic) order set. Pediatric registered nurses must be competent in skills performance but should always practice with safety, knowledge of scope of practice within the state they are practicing, and a skills competency checklist.

QUALITY AND SAFETY

Do not perform any skill on a child unless specific institutional protocols and procedures are followed. Healthcare institutions vary in their skills procedures, physician orders, monitoring requirements, and equipment. The information in this chapter is based on the usual norms and evidence-based practice, but should not be used in place of your institution's protocols and procedures. Do not deviate in terms of your skills performance or choice of equipment from the set and approved institutional policies.

Whenever possible, a parent should stay with a child during a skills procedure. The performance of a skill that produces discomfort should be done in a pediatric treatment room. The parent should be encouraged to stay in this room and provide comfort to the child. The parent should be outside the area where the team is performing the skill, but close enough to provide visual contact and soothing support to the child. If the child is reasonably relaxed, having him or her sit on the parent's lap or lie on the parent's chest (**Figure 27-2**) may be less traumatic, but only in limited situations (e.g., injections). It should not be attempted for more invasive procedures such as blood draws, placement of IV lines, and so forth, because having the parent hold the child during a venipuncture or procedure to start an IV increases the risk that the nurse will get accidentally stuck with the needle as well as the risk that the child will need to be stuck multiple times because the parent inadvertently impedes the nurse's line of sight or fails to hold the child tightly enough. In such situations, another nurse or a physician's assistant who knows the correct techniques for restraining a child should be summoned to assist.

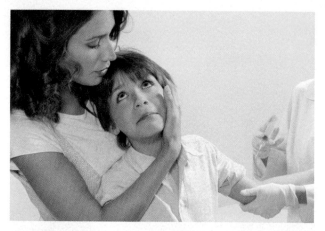

Figure 27-2 *A child can sit on the parent's lap or lie on the parent's chest during a skills procedure if he or she is reasonably relaxed.*

© Glow Wellness/Glow/Getty Images

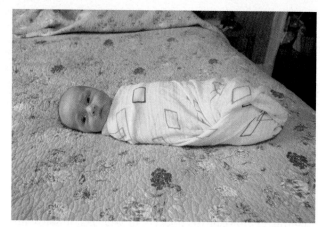

Figure 27-3 *A mummy wrap offers gentle restraint to help an infant or small child feel more secure.*

If the child is frightened and is likely to fight against the parent, nurse, and team during the procedure, it may be appropriate and safe to wrap the child in a **mummy wrap**. With this precaution, the child feels the security of the wrap and the team is able to place a gentle restraint on all of the child's extremities but the one required for the skill procedure (**Figure 27-3**).

Taking Vital Signs in Children

Respiratory Rate

A respiratory rate should be counted for one full minute whenever possible. Newborns and young infants have variable respiratory rates and patterns. Accuracy is achieved with a full minute count of breaths.

Heart Rate

Heart rates should be taken apically using the diaphragm of a pediatric stethoscope and counted for a full minute.

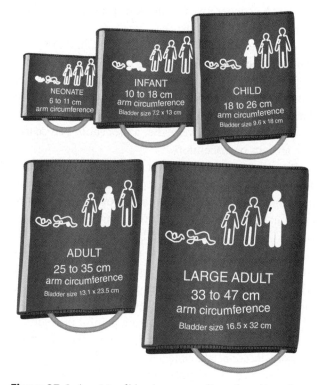

Figure 27-4 *A variety of blood pressure cuffs are found in pediatric nursing care.*

Nurses should avoid taking this vital sign from a heart rate monitor, as accuracy can be greatly compromised with this approach.

Blood Pressure

A variety of blood pressure cuffs are found in pediatric nursing care (**Figure 27-4**). It is important to measure the distance between the shoulder (acromion process) and the antecubital space in the inner elbow the first time a blood pressure is taken. The cuff should cover two-thirds of the distance between these two points. If the cuff is too small, the blood pressure reading will be falsely elevated. If the cuff is too big, the blood pressure reading may be too low.

Oxygen Saturation

Oxygen saturation readings provide information on the indirect measurement of the percentage of circulating red blood cells that are saturated with oxygen molecules. Direct measurements are taken in the form of arterial blood gas readings. Infants and toddlers do well with having the oxygen probe placed on a toe and then covered with a sock. For active young children, reinforcement with tape may be required to keep the pulse oximeter probe in place. Older children can easily keep a finger oxygen saturation probe in place.

Monitor saturation readings carefully after each change in oxygen therapy. Saturation readings may take a few minutes to display accurate saturations after any change in oxygen delivery quantity. The exact time to accurate reading depends on the probe location, probe adherence, and hemodynamic stability of the child.

Temperature

The most common means to measure temperatures are axillary readings in young children and oral readings in older children. Rectal temperatures are rarely taken due to the risk of injury from perforation. An older child, with guidance, can have an oral temperature taken; instructions should be to place the tip of the probe under the tongue or along the inner cheek, without biting, and to close the lips entirely. Do not use glass/mercury thermometers orally in children, especially if they are developmentally delayed or cognitively impaired. A child who bites down on a glass thermometer risks severe injury and mercury exposure.

RESEARCH EVIDENCE

The goal of measuring a child's temperature is to ascertain an accurate core body temperature, indicating the temperature of blood that bathes the tissues of the brain's hypothalamus. Research has shown that many variables influence the accuracy of temperature measurements in children (Robinson, 2004). The following body sites are currently used to take temperatures in the United States:

- *Axillary:* The probe must be placed over the axillary artery. All variations of thermometers read axillary temperatures below core body temperatures, leading to possibly inaccurate readings.
- *Rectal:* Readings taken at this site measure temperatures at a great distance from the hypothalamus; thus, changes in body temperature are often not rapidly detected in this anatomic area. Children are resistant

to this form of temperature reading, and it is not safe in patients with neutropenia or thrombocytopenia. Rectal temperature measurements are also inaccurate in the presence of large amounts of stool.
- *Tympanic:* This type of reading is not affected by either otitis media infections or the presence of cerumen. If the light on the probe is accurately shone on the tympanic membrane, the resulting measurement is considered more accurate than rectal measurement of temperature (Paes, Vermeulen, Brohet, van der Ploeg, & de Winter, 2010).
- *Oral:* Children who recently consumed fluids or foods prior to oral readings can influence the measurement. The presence of oxygen delivery has also been shown to influence the accuracy of oral temperature measurement.
- *Skin:* Research has shown a variability of 28% to 90% in the accuracy of temperature measurement using a skin-applied color-coded flat thermometer. This technique should not be used in critically ill children, children with neutropenia, or children with skin lesions or conditions.

Essential Calculations

Pediatric nurses require knowledge of child-specific calculations. The following sections present common calculations required for safe care.

Fluid Maintenance

Sick children are at risk for inadequate consumption of oral fluids. Because the amount of fluid needed differs depending on the child's weight, a pediatric nurse will calculate a safe quantity of fluid unique for the child to provide **fluid maintenance**; correction of fluid deficits with conditions such as dehydration requires a separate calculation. Fluid needs are determined in milliliters per kilogram of body weight, which must then be converted to identify the appropriate dose rate to provide the needed amount per unit of time, usually 1 hour. With oral fluids, the dose for 1 or more hours may be given in a marked cup or bottle so that the nurse can track how much the child is actually drinking during that time frame (and encourage the child to drink more if he or she is consuming too little). Fluid maintenance doses are also often calculated to determine the rate of infusion of the initial IV therapy in units of milliliters per hour. A nurse may be given a specific IV fluid and then an order to run the fluid at "one times maintenance" rate or "half maintenance" rate if there is concern with overhydration. In a specific circumstance in which the child needs to have extra fluids, such as in preparation for chemotherapy, the physician may order "two times maintenance," allowing for a larger volume to lower the child's urine specific gravity, hydrate the child well, and prepare for the administration of a nephrotoxic drug.

Fluid Maintenance Calculation

Weight in kilograms	Multiply by mL/day
First 10 kg (0–10 kg)	100 mL
Second 10 kg (11–20)	1000 mL plus 50 mL more for each kg between 11 and 20 kg
21–70 kg	1500 mL plus 20 mL for each kg between 21 and 70 kg

Examples:

Patient weight	Calculation
6 kg	100 mL × 6 = 600 mL/day *or* 600 mL ÷ 24 hr = 25 mL/hr
13.5 kg	1000 mL + (3.5 × 50 mL) = 1175 mL/day *or* 1175 mL ÷ 24 hr = 48.9 mL/hr
27 kg	1500 mL + (7 × 20 mL) = 1640 mL/day *or* 1640 mL ÷ 24 hr = 68.3 mL/hr

Oral Rehydration Therapy

Children who are able to take oral (PO) fluids (i.e., children who are not vomiting) should have their dehydration or fluid losses replaced through **oral rehydration therapy** (ORT). ORT is typically used in young children with acute gastroenteritis—a common viral infection leading to significant watery stool loss. Most orders will include the administration of an electrolyte solution such as Pedialyte. Do not use sugary drinks, juices, or soda to replace fluids orally; they contain sugar, which will draw fluids to the bowel and cause the child to have more stool loss.

ORT is calculated as follows:

- Children older than 1 year of age: 30–60 mL of electrolyte solution PO every hour as tolerated.
- Younger infants: Introduce 15 mL of electrolyte solution in a bottle every 2 hours.
- Older infants: Introduce 15–30 mL electrolyte solution in a bottle every 2 hours.

Body Surface Area Calculation

Body surface area (BSA), or meters squared (m^2), is used to determine the dose of specific medications. Intravenous immunoglobulins and chemotherapy medications are typically given in a dose related to the child's BSA. The following calculation is used to determine BSA:

1. Weight (in kilograms) multiplied by height (in centimeters)
2. Divided by 3600
3. Find the square root of the number

$$BSA = \sqrt{\frac{W \times H}{3600}}$$

Body Mass Index Calculation

The child's body mass index (BMI) is calculated as follows:

Child's weight (in kilograms) ÷ child's height (in meters squared) [or BSA]

or

[Child's weight (in pounds) × 703] ÷ child's height (in inches squared)

Kilocalorie Calculation

Pediatric nursing spans the care of children across the developmental period, from prematurity through late adolescence and sometimes into young adulthood. The determination of how many calories are needed for adequate growth and development in children across the developmental period depends on the child's age and weight. In older children (older than 9 years), sex is also taken into account, as caloric needs for girls are slightly lower from about age 9 onward (U.S. Department of Agriculture & U.S. Department of Health and Human Services, 2010).

Families often want to know how many calories, on average, their child should consume daily. A standard calculation can assist in that common question. One must take into consideration the child's overall activity level, age, and sex, and make allowances for overweight or underweight status. Children who are athletes and play on one or more sports teams will need to adjust the kilocalorie requirement upward to provide adequate energy. Although several kilocalorie calculations can be used, all of which produce similar findings, the following calculation is commonly used across pediatric nursing:

- 0–30 days: 100–110 kcal/kg/day.
- 1–4 months: 90–100 kcal/kg/day.
- 5 months to 5 years: 70–90 kcal/kg/day.
- Older than 5 years: 1500 kcal for the first 20 kg of weight, then an additional 25 kcal for each additional 1 kg of weight greater than 20 kg. Thus, to calculate an older child's daily caloric intake, the following formula is used: 1500 kcal + ([weight in kg – 20 kg] × 25 kcal) = total caloric need per day.

In an overweight or obese child, the total amount of kilocalories needed may exceed what would normally be considered adequate for a child of that age. For example, a 4 foot 10 inch, 11-year-old boy who weighs 130 pounds (approximately 59 kg) is considered overweight, with a BMI of 26.3; according to the formula, he would require 2475 kcal per day—within the acceptable range of 2000–2600 kcal suggested by the National Heart, Blood, and Lung Institute (2013) if the child is very active, but excessive (and therefore exacerbating his weight concerns) if he is sedentary. The opposite is true of an underweight child, who may need additional caloric support beyond the amount suggested by the calculation to encourage weight gain.

Caloric Intake in Infants

Standard over-the-counter infant formulas provide 20 kcal/ounce once prepared. It is easy to determine how many ounces of formula the infant should consume: Simply divide the total kilocalorie daily requirement by 20, which would then give the number of ounces needed.

As an example of calculating the kilocalorie needs and formula needs for an infant, consider a 2-month old infant weighing 9.57 pounds (4.35 kg):

- 4.35 × 90–100 kcal range = 391.5–435 kcal required per day.
- 391 ÷ 20 = 19.6 ounces of formula needed per day. Thus, if the child eats every 4 hours, she would require 3–4 ounces of formula per feeding.
- 435 ÷ 20 = 21.75 ounces of formula needed per day. Thus, if the child eats every 4 hours, she would require 3.6 ounces of formula per feeding.

Note that these calculations are averages. Each child has its own unique feeding habits.

Fluid Bolus Calculation

To rapidly replace intravascular fluid deficits, the pediatric nurse calculates the quantity of sterile crystalloid IV solution to administer. The calculation assumes 20 mL of IV fluid is needed for each kilogram of weight. For instance, if a toddler is seen in the pediatric oncology clinic with mucositis from chemotherapy and presents with tachycardia, no tears, and dry mucous membranes, the pediatric nurse should expect to receive orders for IV fluid boluses of 0.9% normal saline (NS). For a toddler weighing 28 pounds, the following example demonstrates the bolus calculation:

$$28 \text{ lb} = 12.73 \text{ kg}$$
$$12.73 \times 20 \text{ mL} = 255 \text{ mL of IV fluid per bolus}$$

If the child's vital signs are not what might be expected given the child's age, the nurse can expect to give more than one bolus. Take vital signs and conduct an assessment between each bolus. Report when urine output has been restored.

Minimum Urine Output Calculation

The minimum urine output (UOP) calculation must not be used as a measure of adequate hydration in children. Rather, it designates that the child's kidney function is intact—not that the child has adequate daily hydration. The goal of urine output is much higher. The calculation for minimum UOP is as follows:

- Infants: 2 mL/kg/hr
- Children (1–12 years): 1 mL/kg/hr
- Adolescents (13–19 years): 0.5–1 mL/kg/hr

Burn Fluid Resuscitation Calculation

Children who suffer significant burns usually require a fluid resuscitation calculation. The post-burn resuscitation calculations require the previously determined percentage of body surface area burned. Using a standard chart, the nurse will assist the emergency care team to determine this percentage, typically by using the Lund-Brower chart. Two examples of these calculations are found in **Table 27-1**.

BEST PRACTICES

Children who are tethered to lines, tubes, and electrical equipment require frequent assessments. Older infants and toddlers have died from unintentional strangulation by medical equipment used in hospital cribs. Always try to guide tubes away from a child's line of vision (e.g., by securely taping central line tubing or nasogastric tubing away from the child's visual field and extending down the child's back).

Whenever performing skills on a child that require the placement of tubes or lines, communicate their presence to members of the healthcare team by labeling the line. Write your initials, the date, and the time of insertion, and securely wrap the label around the line away from the child's reach. This form of safe communication allows team members to know when a line or tube was placed so that they can change lines (nasogastric tubes, central lines, central line dressing changes, IV tubing, and chest tube draining systems) according to the schedule set by institutional policy. This communication reduces the expensive waste of equipment that occurs when lines are changed earlier than necessary, and reduces the risk of injury, infection, or skin trauma that increases when lines, tubes, or dressings are left in place longer than intended due to confusion about when they were originally placed.

Blood Transfusion Dose Quantity Calculation

Blood transfusions are administered to children as a dose of blood rather than as units of blood. Adults receive units that contain variations in total volume, often ranging from 250 mL to 500 mL. Since children's bodies are smaller and

TABLE 27-1	Formulas for Calculating Post-Burn Fluid Resuscitation	
Parkland Formula	**Brooke Formula**
First 24-hour period post burn:	**First 24-hour period post burn:**
Administer 4 mL/kg/% of BSA burned.	1.5 mL/kg/% of BSA burned: crystalloid IV administration
Administer in the form of an intravenous crystalloid. IV fluids should not include a source of dextrose and should not be a colloid. The child may need dextrose-rich total parenteral nutrition and blood products (colloids).	0.5 mL/kg/% of BSA burned: colloid 2000 mL dextrose water IV infusion
Second 24-hour period post burn:	**Second 24-hour period post burn:**
Administer 50% to 75% of the first 24-hour fluid resuscitation calculation (above).	0.75–1.124 mL/kg/% of BSA burned: crystalloid IV administration
Administer albumin infusions to maintain serum albumin at more than 2 g/dL.	0.25–0.375 mL/kg/% of BSA burned: colloid 2000 mL dextrose water IV infusion

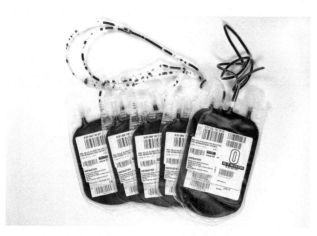

Figure 27-5 *A single adult unit of blood can be divided into four small units called aliquots.*

more vulnerable, they are given doses of blood transfusions. Packed red blood cells (PRBC) is the most commonly administered blood product. The following calculation is used to determine a safe PRBC transfusion dose:

- Determine the child's pre-transfusion hemoglobin and hematocrit. On average, a transfused dose of blood will raise a child's hemoglobin by 1 mg/dL and the child's hematocrit by 3%.
- Multiply the child's weight in kilograms by 10–15 mL per dose of blood.
- Request only the safe quantity from the blood bank.
- You may request that a single adult unit of blood be divided into four small units called aliquots (**Figure 27-5**). This practice allows for four

different doses of blood to be administered, if deemed needed, without exposure to multiple donors.

For example, a child requiring a blood transfusion for a hemoglobin of 7.7 may need more than one dose. If the child weighs 26.5 kg, the transfused dose should be between 265 mL and 397 mL of blood. An IV pump can be set to administer only the required dose to maintain safety over the 2 to 4 hours of the transfusion.

Absolute Neutrophil Count Calculation

Children who have medical conditions that affect immune status may have their absolute neutrophil count (ANC) calculated. An accurate ANC is used to make decisions concerning nursing care. An ANC of less than 500 cells/mcL requires implementation of neutropenic precautions. A complete blood cell count (CBC) with differentiation of the various white blood cells (WBC) is required to calculate the ANC. The calculation to determine ANC is as follows:

1. Add the segmented neutrophils (mature) to the band neutrophils (immature) as a total percentage.
2. Multiply the percentage of neutrophils by the total WBC count.

Example:

WBC = 1400
Segmented neutrophils = 13%
Band neutrophils = 3%
Add 0.13 + 0.03 = 0.16
0.16 × 1400 = ANC = 224 cells/mcL (very low finding—requires neutropenic precautions)

TABLE 27-2	FAO Recommendations for Pediatric Protein Intake
Age	Average Protein Intake per Day
0–4 months	2.40 g/kg at birth to 1.64 g/kg at 4 months
4–12 months	1.47 g/kg for 4-month-old to 1.15 g/kg for 12-month-old
1–2 years	1.26 g/kg
5–6 years	1.00 g/kg
9–10 years	0.83 g/kg

Data from Joint FAO/WHO/UNU Expert Consultation. (1985). Energy and protein requirements. Infants, children, and adolescents. Retrieved from http://www.fao.org/docrep/003/aa040e/AA040E07.htm

Protein Needs Across Childhood Calculation

Protein is a building block of growth and maturation in children. Requirements for protein intake depend on the child's age and weight. Breast milk has approximately 1.15 g of protein per 100 mL of fluid. **Table 27-2** shows the recommendations of the Food and Agriculture Organization of the United Nations (n.d.) for daily pediatric protein intake.

Maintaining Airway Patency

When assessing a child with a respiratory condition or a neurologic condition that adversely affects the child's ability to maintain a patent airway (e.g., head trauma with edema and pressure to the brain stem and thalamus), the nurse should take the following steps:

1. Place the child in an upright position.
2. Place the nose up in a sniffing position.
3. Assess for the need to suction the child by looking at the patency of each nare.
4. Suction using the correct suction device needed: bulb syringe, olive tip attached to suction device, tonsil tip for oral pharynx, or sterile deep suction for severe cases.
5. Determine if further interventions are required, such as oxygen administration, oral airway placement, or intubation for respiratory emergencies.

Use of a Length-Based Resuscitation Tape

Length-based resuscitation tape is used during emergencies when the child's actual age and weight are not known and the response team must act quickly. In circumstances where a child is brought into the emergency room or there is an emergency medical technician (EMT) or paramedic response to a severely injured child, the length-based tape can be used to determine safe equipment size, medication dosing, and other emergency responses. This kind of tape is color-coded to denote ranges in a child's height that correspond with average weight. For instance, measurement of an infant's length that falls under the pink color-coded section suggests that the average-size child's weight will be somewhere between 6 and 9 kg. The response team can then use all the information on the tape that is color-coded pink and be within safe limits for equipment size and medication administration based on the 6–9 kg weight range (**Table 27-3**).

Collecting Respiratory System Specimens

Sputum and Nasal Washing

Collecting specimens from the respiratory system is common in young children, as they frequently present to clinic, urgent care, or emergency room environments with increased work of breathing or respiratory distress requiring diagnosis of the microbial culprit causing the symptoms. Determining whether the child has a viral, bacterial, or fungal infection is crucial.

The pediatric nurse assists the team in collecting specimens for laboratory analysis and possible cultures. **Figure 27-6** illustrates a sputum collection device. The pediatric nurse must always understand the isolation precautions required for each respiratory illness, such as airborne and droplet precautions, and adhere to these precautions when collecting respiratory secretions.

Suctioning Devices and Tips

Many common pediatric upper respiratory infections produce copious nasal secretions that inhibit breastfeeding, bottle feeding, drinking from a cup, and sleeping. Rapid removal of secretions is an important skill for both the pediatric nurse and the parents. Several devices are commonly used for this purpose:

- *Bulb syringe:* The nurse teaches the family to compress the bulb prior to placing into the child's nose for secretion removal.
- *Olive tip suctioning:* This approach involves instilling a few drops of 0.9% normal saline into the nare, allowing the solution to dwell for a few seconds, and then removing the secretions. An olive tip suction device has a hole (suction outlet) for the

TABLE 27-3 Cardiopulmonary Resuscitation

	Infants	Children	Teens/Adults
Compressions	Check for brachial HR for 10 seconds. If HR < 90 beats/min, begin compressions with two-finger chest compression over the lower half of the sternum (just below the nipple line) with one rescuer, or two-thumb encircling hands technique with two rescuers. Activate the emergency response system if not already done after 2 minutes of CPR. Continue for 30 compressions before checking the airway.	Check for carotid or femoral HR for 10 seconds. If HR < 60 beats/min, begin compressions with one hand to one-third to one-half depth of the chest. Rate of compressions should be at least 100 compressions per minute. Activate the emergency response system if not already done after 2 minutes of CPR. Continue for 30 compressions before checking the airway.	Check for carotid or femoral HR for 10 seconds. If HR < 60 beats/min, begin compressions using the heel of one hand over the center of the chest, right between the nipples. Place one hand over the top of the other, with elbows straight and shoulders directly over hands. Use the upper body weight to compress the patient's chest at least 2 inches (5 cm) at a rate of 100 compressions per minute. Continue for 30 compressions before checking the airway.
Airway	After the first set of compressions, open the airway using the head tilt–chin lift maneuver unless the infant has a suspected head or neck injury. Check for normal breathing. Look for chest motion, listen with your ear for breath sounds, and feel for the infant's breath on your cheek. Take no more than 10 seconds.	After the first set of compressions, open the airway using the head tilt–chin lift maneuver unless the child has a suspected head or neck injury. Check for normal breathing. Look for chest motion, listen with your ear for breath sounds, and feel for the child's breath on your cheek. Take no more than 10 seconds.	After the first set of compressions, open the airway using the head tilt–chin lift maneuver unless the person has a suspected head or neck injury. Check for normal breathing. Look for chest motion, listen with your ear for breath sounds, and feel for the teen's breath on your cheek. Take no more than 10 seconds.
Breathing	Using a mask, give 1 breath and assess whether the chest rises. Then give 1 breath every 3–5 seconds or 12–20 breaths per minute. One rescuer: 2 breaths per 30 compressions. Two rescuers: 1 breath per 15 compressions.	Using a mask, give 1 breath and assess whether the chest rises. Then give 1 breath every 3–5 seconds or 12–20 breaths per minute. One rescuer: 2 breaths per 30 compressions. Two rescuers: 1 breath per 15 compressions.	Using a mask, give 1 breath and assess whether the chest rises. Then give 1 breath every 3–5 seconds or 12–20 breaths per minute. One rescuer: 2 breaths per 30 compressions. Two rescuers: 1 breath per 15 compressions.

Abbreviations: CPR, cardiopulmonary resuscitation; HR, heart rate.
Data from Atkins, D. L., Berger, S., Duff, J. P., Gonzales, J. C., Hunt, E. A., Joyner, B. L., . . . Schexnayder, S. M. (2015). Pediatric basic life support and cardiopulmonary resuscitation quality. 2015 American Heart Association guidelines update for cardiopulmonary resuscitation and emergency cardiovascular care, Part 11. *Circulation, 132,* S519–S525.

application of suction with one finger; typically the thumb. Enter the nose with the hole uncovered, and then apply suction to remove the secretions while moving the thumb up and down to add and delete suction during collection. A wall-mounted suction canister and device are required for olive tip suctioning.

- *Deep sterile suctioning:* This approach is rarely needed in pediatric patients unless the child has copious secretions in the mid and lower airways and is unable to cough and expectorate. Children with new tracheostomies and children with neurologic impairment whose cough is diminished may require deep sterile suctioning.

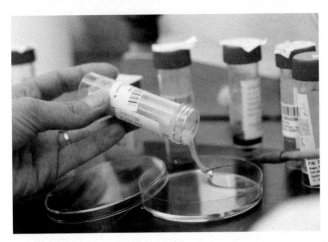

Figure 27-6 *A sputum collection device.*

© Arno Massee / Science Source

Chest Tube Drainage Systems

Chest tube drains, also referred to as underwater-sealed drains, are inserted to promote removal of inflammatory fluids, lymph fluid (chylothorax), blood (hemothorax), air (pneumothorax), or collapse (tension pneumothorax) in the pleural space using a one-way valve draining system (**Figure 27-7**). This removal allows for expansion of the child's lungs and restores the required negative pressure needed in the child's thoracic cavity for breathing and ventilation. Chest tubes are placed in the pediatric intensive care unit (PICU), neonatal intensive care unit (NICU), and emergency department (ED). When needed, they can be placed on the pediatric hospital unit, preferably in the pediatric treatment room, rather than in the child's bed.

Chest tube drainage systems in pediatrics have the same components as the systems used in adults: three chambers of water seal, suction control, and collection and measurement of drainage. A flutter valve, also known as a Heimlich valve or a pneumostat, prevents the backflow of air or drainage into the pleural cavity.

Whatever their type, such systems have the same purpose (dry or wet drainage), setup, and nursing care. Typical nursing care concerns include the following issues:

- Adhering to strict hand hygiene and infection prevention measures.
- Maintaining the equipment in an upright position to accurately determine fluid output. Children produce small volumes of fluid, pus, or blood; therefore, the equipment should be taped to the floor to prevent accidental falls.
- Maintaining the equipment lower than the child's chest level to ensure continuous drainage.
- Maintaining a sealed dressing over the chest tube insertion site to prevent air from entering and potentially causing a pneumothorax. A tight seal

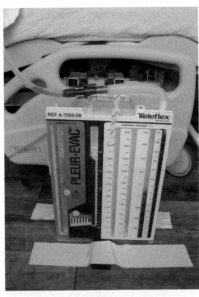

Figure 27-7 *A chest tube drainage system.*

© Diomedia/Barry Slaven, MD, PhD

around the skin's exit site prevents the loss of the suction provided by the setup.

- Monitoring the tubing for debris, clots, or kinks that would prevent proper drainage.
- Securing the tubing to the bed with the provided clamp so that as the child moves around, the tubing stays in a safe place.
- Providing adequate pain control measure during the insertion and maintenance of the chest tube drainage system.
- Ensuring that no part of the system is ever clamped. This concern is especially important when there is an air leak, which puts the child at risk for a tension pneumothorax.
- Assessing the child's lung sounds frequently to ensure bilateral breath sounds are consistently present.
- Teaching the family about the purpose of the chest tube, communicating how to keep the equipment safe and upright, and providing support during the length of treatment.
- Troubleshooting complications:
  - Sudden decrease in the child's oxygen saturation, increased work of breathing, chest pain, tachycardia, bradycardia, or hypotension—all of these symptoms denote the development of a pneumothorax. If this occurs, notify the medical staff immediately; plan for an immediate portable chest radiograph; place a new occlusive dressing over the existing one; assess for leaks, kinks, or blockages of the tubing; and prepare new sterile equipment for a replacement of the system.
  - Presence of bleeding, which requires occlusive dressings, pressure, notification of medical team,

and preparation for the assessment of the child's coagulation laboratory analysis.

- Temperature increases, which indicate the development or presence of infection, requiring site cultures by swab and blood cultures.
- Accidental dislodgement of the chest tube or its removal, requiring rapid application of an occlusive dressing to seal the chest.

Medication Administration

Preventing medication errors is essential in pediatric nursing care. Children are vulnerable to such errors, and families need astute professional guidance on proper medication administration, safe storage, and accurate dosing.

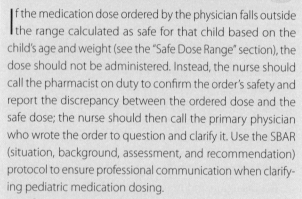

PHARMACOLOGY

If the medication dose ordered by the physician falls outside the range calculated as safe for that child based on the child's age and weight (see the "Safe Dose Range" section), the dose should not be administered. Instead, the nurse should call the pharmacist on duty to confirm the order's safety and report the discrepancy between the ordered dose and the safe dose; the nurse should then call the primary physician who wrote the order to question and clarify it. Use the SBAR (situation, background, assessment, and recommendation) protocol to ensure professional communication when clarifying pediatric medication dosing.

Infants and young children are particularly susceptible to adverse consequences of medication errors in which a larger-than-recommended dose is administered due to the following differences in their pharmacodynamics (absorption), pharmacokinetics (distribution), and drug excretion:

- Their immature liver leads to slower drug metabolism and longer drug exposure.
- Medications rapidly cross their blood–brain barrier.
- Their immature kidney function leads to delayed drug excretion.

Calculating Medication Doses Based on Weight

Safe doses of medications for children, regardless of the administration route, are calculated in terms of milligrams of medication per kilogram of weight. It is important to have a recent and accurate weight of a child to ascertain that the medication to be administered is safe for the specific child. Most medications are dispensed in either unit doses, multiple doses, or prefilled cups, syringes, or IV bags. Double-check that the medication dose in the prefilled syringe, cup, or IV bag is within the safe dose range for the child. The nurse is the last person in the line for safety checks, and is in a good position to prevent medication errors in children.

Safe Dose Range

Most medications administered to children are calculated by determining the safe dose range and confirming that the medication dose ordered falls within that range. For instance, amoxicillin, an oral medication often given for infectious processes such as bacterial otitis media, has the following safe dose range for mild to moderate ear, nose, and throat infections (GlaxoSmithKline, 2006; *Medscape*, 2016):

- Birth to 3 months: $\leq$ 30 mg/kg/day PO divided every 12 hours for 48–72 hours; to be given for $\geq$ 10 days
- 3 months and weight up to 40 kg: 20–40 mg/kg/day, divided into 3 doses every 8 hours; 25–45 mg/kg/day PO divided every 12 hours
- Weight greater than 40 kg: 500 mg PO every 12 hours or 250 mg PO every 8 hours for 10–14 days, up to 875 mg every 12 hours

Determining the Volume to Draw from the Available Packaging

After confirming the accuracy of the received medication order, double-checking the mg/kg dose, and determining the safe dose range, the pediatric nurse next determines the process and quantity of drawing up the medication. For instance, suppose the nurse receives an order for 22 mg of methylprednisolone. This dose is confirmed to be safe for the child's weight and the dose falls within the safe dose range. The nurse, upon opening an electronic medication dispensing machine, notes that the medication comes as a powder in a vial. The instructions state to push the sterile fluid attached to the vial into the medication to produce 40 mg of methylprednisolone for 1 mL of sterile fluid. The nurse then calculates the safe quantity to draw up out of the vial. In this example, the total amount that should be drawn up is 0.55 mL.

Intramuscular, Subcutaneous, and Intradermal Injections

When oral or other options are available for administering medications, injections may be avoided in children. When an injection or IV is required, however, pain control is essential to minimize children's distress. For routine intramuscular or subcutaneous injections, such as immunizations, distraction or use of a vibrating pain-reducing device such as the Buzzy is appropriate, or a rapid-acting (but short-lived) topical spray anesthetic such as Pain Ease can be used. For blood draws, infusions, IV placement, or any other procedure that requires insertion of a needle or cannula through the skin, it is appropriate to use 4% lidocaine cream or EMLA, which take longer to reach full effect but provide a longer-lasting and deeper anesthetic response. **Table 27-4** offers tips on medication administration across the developmental period.

TABLE 27-4 Tips for Medication Administration Across the Developmental Period

	Newborn	Young Infant	Older Infant	Toddler	Preschooler	School Age and Adolescent
Oral (PO)	Use the smallest quantity (mL) of medication possible to prevent choking. Place the medication in a nipple and have the newborn suck the liquid medication through the nipple. If adding to breast milk or formula, mix in a few milliliters of fluid and give the medication to the newborn when hungry, before giving the rest of the bottle. If exclusively breastfeeding, carefully administer the medication in an oral syringe in small quantities into the cheek, allowing the child to swallow after each small pulse of medication.	Use the smallest quantity (mL) of medication possible. May mix with 1–2 mL of flavored syrup. Do not administer medications to a crying infant, as there is a risk of aspiration.	Use the smallest quantity of medication possible. Use playfulness during medication administration. Show appreciation and smiles after the medication is taken. If the older infant protrudes the tongue and spits the medication out, do not administer more unless directed to do so by the prescribing practitioner.	Whenever possible, give the toddler two choices, such as two different-flavored syrups in which to mix the medication. Give praise and, if appropriate, a small prize such as a colorful sticker.	Provide the opportunity for the child to self-administer the medication. Try both an oral syringe and a small 1-ounce medication cup to assess which one is easier for the child.	Allow the older child to self-administer the medication. Provide positive feedback for being on time and cooperative. Prevent the older child from participating in stalling behaviors.
Rectal (PR)	Lubricate the suppository and insert it gently with the little finger.	Lubricate the suppository and insert it gently with the little finger.	Lubricate the suppository and insert it gently with the little finger.	Lubricate the suppository and insert it gently with the little finger. The toddler will need to be in a comfort hold, as there is typically great resistance.	Lubricate the suppository and insert it gently. With fears of genital mutilation now being common, the preschooler will typically be very resistant. The process may require two nurses to provide a comfort hold.	Explain the need for the medication and allow the older child to ask questions and have time to prepare. Lubricate the suppository and insert it gently. Provide privacy and uncover the anal area only briefly.

(continues)

TABLE 27-4 Tips for Medication Administration Across the Developmental Period *(continued)*

	Newborn	Young Infant	Older Infant	Toddler	Preschooler	School Age and Adolescent
Ophthalmic **(Figure 27-8)**	Use aseptic technique. Place drops into the center of the eye, and ointment in the inner lower canthus.	Use aseptic technique. Place drops into the center of the eye, and ointment in the inner lower canthus.	May require two nurses to provide comfort hold of the child's head. Use aseptic technique. Place drops into the center of the eye, and ointment in the inner lower canthus.	Toddlers will require a firm comfort hold of the body and the head. Use aseptic technique. Place drops into the center of the eye, and ointment in the inner lower canthus.	Preschool children may be quite resistant at first, but can learn to accept this route of administration. Use aseptic technique. Place drops into the center of the eye, and ointment in the inner lower canthus.	Teach older children or teens how to wash their hands and self-administer the medication if appropriate.
Otic **(Figure 27-9)**	Place newborns on their side. Instill room-temperature otic drops as ordered.	Place young infants on their side. Instill room-temperature otic drops as ordered. Provide distraction while the medication dwells.	Place older infants on their side. Instill room-temperature otic drops as ordered. Provide distraction while the medication dwells.	Place toddlers on their side. Instill room-temperature otic drops as ordered. Provide distraction while the medication dwells. May require a comfort hold.	Place preschoolers in high Fowler's position. Instill room-temperature otic drops as ordered. Provide distraction while the medication dwells.	Place older children in high Fowler's position, with head tilted. Instill room-temperature otic drops as ordered.
Inhaler	Inhalers are not used on newborns.	Use a small mask attached to the chamber.	Use a small mask attached to the chamber.	Use a well-fitting mask attached to the chamber. Toddlers may cry and be resistant during administration. Provide positive reinforcement for cooperation.	Use a well-fitting mask attached to the chamber. Older preschoolers may be able to self-administer the inhaler with supervision and encouragement.	Allow older children to perform their own inhaled medication administration. Use of a spacer device is recommended, but a mask is not necessary.

EMLA stands for "**e**utectic **m**ix of **l**ocal **a**nesthetics." It is a mix of two drugs, lidocaine (2.5%) and prilocaine (2.5%), and comes in the form of a cream, gel, or patch. The cream and patch are approved for use in children having dermal procedures, whether minor (injection or blood draw) or major (skin grafting). The patch tends to be more useful in minor procedures because of the limited area of coverage it provides. The cream can also be used for smaller areas (e.g., an injection site) if taped to the location with an occlusive dressing such as Tegaderm, which improves absorption in the site. Numbing of the skin occurs in approximately 45 to 60 minutes, and lasts an hour or two after the medication is wiped from the skin, although a shorter duration of effect may occur in more vascular areas. Blanching or reddening of the skin may occur but is harmless. Manufacturer-recommended dosing is as follows:

- 0–3 months or weight < 5 kg: 1 g over 10 cm^2 skin surface per ≤ 1 hour
- 3–12 months and weight > 5 kg: 2 g over 20 cm^2 skin surface per ≤ 4 hours
- 1–6 years and weight > 10 kg: 10 g over 100 cm^2 skin surface per ≤ 4 hours
- 7–12 years and weight > 20 kg: 20 g cm^2 skin surface per ≤ 4 hours

Use of EMLA should be avoided in infants of gestational age less than 37 weeks or infants younger than 12 months who are being treated with phenytoin or acetaminophen. This medication should be used with caution in children at risk of methemoglobinemia.

Data from Pesaturo, K. A., & Matthews, M. (2009). Topical anesthesia use in children. *US Pharmacist, 34*(3), HS-4–HS-7. Retrieved from http://www.medscape.com/viewarticle/704761_2

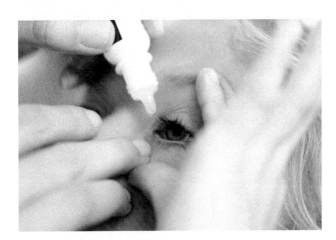

Figure 27-8 *Administration of ophthalmic medication.*
© Sharon Pruitt/ EyeEm/Getty Images

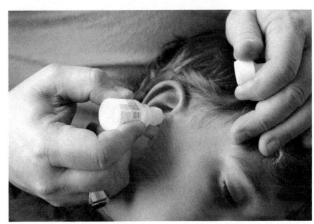

Figure 27-9 *Administration of otic medication.*
© ftwitty/E+/Getty Images

Intravenous Therapy

Many children who present with acute or severe injuries or illnesses will require IV therapy, including fluid replacement (**Table 27-5**). For safety, infants and children should not have their IV fluids or IV medications administered without an IV pump. In extreme emergencies such as trauma triage, disasters, or electrical failures with an exhausted battery supply, the pediatric nurse will use drip factors to calculate the IV fluid rates.

Principles of Pump Function

The latest technological advancements in IV pump therapy have both increased the safety and reduced errors with this mode of medication administration. Pumps now have multiple safety-oriented features, such as automatic tube clamping when the door of the pump opens and tubing is removed. Internal data collection and analysis allows for pumps to be set with safety features such as maximum fluid rates for newborns and young infants, maximum fluid bolus rates, and automatic dosing and rate suggestions for medications preprogrammed into the pump device. Many new pumps enable the pediatric nurse to administer medication doses measured in tenths and hundredths of a milliliter, allowing for precision in dosing of fluids and medications.

Administration of IV Fluids

The pediatric nurse must be vigilant in applying the principles of safe IV therapy administration when providing IV fluids (IVF). Double check-orders and determine safety of the fluids ordered, keeping in mind the precautions,

TABLE 27-5	Fluid Replacement Solutions and Agents

Crystalloids: Used for volume replacement; readily leaves blood and enters cells

› 0.9% normal saline (NS)

› Lactated Ringer's solution

› 0.5% dextrose in water (D_5W)

› Plasma-Lyte

› Hypertonic saline 3%

Colloids: Increase plasma oncotic pressure and draw fluid out of the cells and tissues and into the vasculature

› Serum albumin, human

› Plasma protein fraction

› Dextran 40 or dextran 70*

› Hetastarch*

› Fresh frozen plasma

› Serum globulins

Blood products: Used for replacement of blood loss

› Packed red blood cells (PRBC)

› Whole blood (red blood cells [RBCs] and plasma; rarely given due to the potential for reactions)

› Fresh frozen plasma

› Plasma protein fraction

› Granulocytes (rarely given due to the potential for severe reactions)

* Agents used for vascular volume support after massive hemorrhage.

reactions, mechanism of action, and appropriateness of ordered IVF for the child's condition.

The two most important aspects of IVF are the **osmolality** (the number of dissolved particles in 1 liter of fluid) and tonicity (the ability of a solution to move water across a membrane). The movement of fluids across membranes is due to osmotic forces of the fluids. Osmosis means that fluids will move from areas with less solutes (low solute concentrations) to areas of with more solutes (higher solute concentrations). Both osmolality and tonicity influence how water and body fluids shift through the child's body. Sodium—the most abundant electrolyte in the body—has a significant role in maintaining appropriate osmolality in the child's body.

The following definitions are important for the pediatric nurse who is administering IVF therapy:

- *Hypertonic solutions:* Contain more solutes than plasma; they cause water to leave the cells and tissues to dilute the hypertonicity of the plasma.
  - Hypertonic saline (3% NaCl)
  - 5% dextrose in normal saline (D_5NS)
  - 5% dextrose in lactated Ringer's solution (D_5LR)
  - 5% dextrose in Plasma-Lyte 56
- *Hypotonic solutions:* Contain fewer solutes than plasma; they cause water to enter the cells and tissues, moving fluids toward the higher osmolality (solutes) found in the cells and tissues.
  - Hypotonic saline (0.45% NS)
  - Plasma-Lyte 56
- *Isotonic solutions:* Freely cross cell membranes.
  - Normal plasma
  - 0.9% NS
  - Lactated Ringer's solution
  - Plasma-Lyte 148
  - 5% dextrose in water (D_5W)
  - 5% dextrose in 0.2% saline

Central Lines: Types, Functions, and Nursing Care

When children have long-term intravenous fluid and medication administration needs, it is common for a pediatric surgeon to place a central venous catheter (**Figure 27-10**). This line, which provides easy access without requiring multiple **venous access** sticks (i.e., insertion of a needle into a vein), assures that the child is more comfortable. Having readily available access also increases safety during emergencies such as treatment of

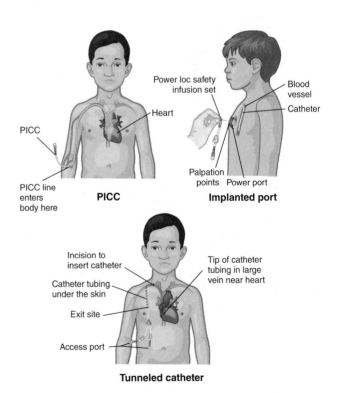

Figure 27-10 *Three types of central lines: PICC line, implanted port, tunneled catheter.*

a high fever with rapidly administered antibiotics and with fluids administration in a child with cancer who is immunocompromised. When a child with a central venous catheter device experiences a fever, blood cultures are drawn from the device.

Central lines are distinguished based on how long they are intended to stay in place:

- Shorter term; up to 90 days in certain conditions
  - Peripherally inserted central catheters (PICCs)
- Longer term: may be maintained for years
  - Implanted ports (mediports): accessed with a specialized non-coring needle set
  - Tunneled catheters (e.g., Broviac, Hickman, Groshong)

Preferred Sites for Venous Access in Infants

Due to young children's unique feature of small veins, great skill is needed to access sites for IV insertion or blood draws. **Scalp veins** can be used for this purpose, but must be protected with devices to prevent dislodgment. Foot veins in standing and walking children should be avoided. Use of IV protection, such as pediatric "no-no" arm restraints, is recommended to avoid accidental dislodgment of the site.

Syringe Pumps

Syringe pumps—a type of small infusion pump—are often used in the care of children (**Figure 27-11**). For premature infants, neonates, infants, and young children, syringe pump infusions allow for the safest minimal volumes to be infused via an IV pump system that holds syringes rather than IV fluid bags. The smallest syringe accepted by most syringe pumps is 3 mL, and the largest is 60 mL.

Syringe pumps provide for control of volume and rate of infusion, along with safety alarms indicating increasing pressure caused by occlusion. These devices can be used alone, with specific syringe pump tubing being directly attached to the child's peripheral or central venous catheter, or they can be inserted (Y-ed) into a child's existing IV line. In new syringe pump technology, medication dosing is determined by preset safety calculation programs based on the child's weight. If a pediatric nurse mistakenly programs the syringe pump to administer a specific medication at an unsafe rate (too rapidly), the syringe pump technology will alarm and display a caution message.

Patient-Controlled Analgesia in Pediatrics

Children in acute or chronic pain may benefit from the use of patient-controlled analgesia (PCA). With this type of therapy, the IV PCA pump is programmed to deliver opioid medication either at a continuous (basal) rate or a dose determined by the patient's control of the administration button; alternatively, it may accommodate both types of doses. Although PCA is most commonly used in school-age or older patients, some children as young as 4 years have learned to use PCA appropriately. Children's ability to use a PCA machine is influenced by their developmental level, age, and health condition.

The PCA machine (**Figure 27-12**) provides four basic components of a medication order: the medication to be administered (morphine, hydromorphone); the quantity to be delivered per dose; the quantity to be delivered throughout each hour (basal rate); and the total maximum dose allowed in a period of time (from 1 hour up to a 4-hour maximum, depending on the pump guidelines). Safety is maintained in children as long as the safe dose is accurately ordered for the child's weight and needs. Neither the parent nor the nurse should press the button to deliver the medication except under special conditions, such as an impending painful procedure where extra medication is required beyond the

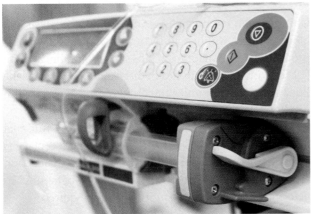

Figure 27-11 *A syringe pump.*

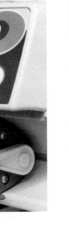

Figure 27-12 *A PCA machine.*

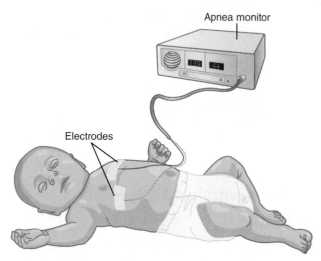

Figure 27-13 *Apnea monitors allow for the continuous measurement of a child's heart rate and respiratory rate.*

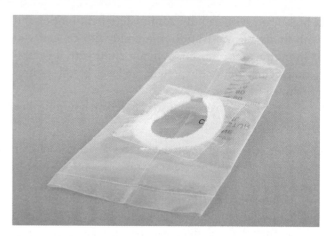

Figure 27-14 *A urine collection bag.*

© Audrius Merfeldas/Shutterstock

provision of the PCA dose order. Only the child should determine when and if a PCA dose in required.

Apnea Monitors

Apnea monitors, also called cardiorespiratory monitors, allow for the continuous measurement of a child's heart rate and respiratory rate (**Figure 27-13**). No electrocardiogram (EKG) strip is produced; rather, the machine allows for a warning alarm to be emitted in case of an abnormally low or high respiratory rate or heart rate, and in the presence of apnea (typically 15 to 20 seconds without a breath). High and low respiratory and heart rate values are programmed into the machine, as well as the criteria for a period of apnea. The pediatric nurse places two electrodes on the child's chest and secures the electrodes with adhesive material; in home apnea monitors, the electrodes may be secured by soft straps. Alcohol should be used to clean the child's skin oils where the electrodes will be placed to ensure better adherence.

Specimen Collection

Urine

Urinalysis specimen collection can be done by the "clean catch" method for older children who can control their stream of urine, cotton ball placement in a child's diaper, or the application of a urinary collection bag. If a urinalysis with culture and sensitivity is required, the child must be able to provide a clean specimen or be catheterized for specimen collection (**Figure 27-14**).

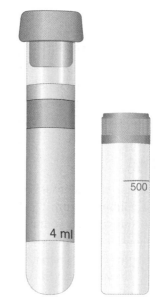

Figure 27-15 *A comparison of full-size lab tubes to pediatric micro-containers.*

Blood Analysis and Blood Culture

Children who require phlebotomy for blood analysis and blood cultures will benefit from pain control during this procedure. Use of pain relief aids such as numbing cream (EMLA) or spray (Pain Ease), distraction, and use of the Buzzy can help minimize the discomfort associated with needle sticks.

Newborns, infants, and toddlers should have minimal blood volumes taken for laboratory analysis. Micro-containers (**Figure 27-15**) are appropriate in most blood collection requirements. Check with the laboratory personnel to determine the smallest quantity of blood required.

Assessment Tips

Due to children's unique anatomy, the pediatric nurse uses skills for assessment that are appropriate for the child's age, size, and developmental ability.

Ear Examination

Given the high incidence of otitis media with and without effusions in pediatric patients, children's ears are frequently inspected. Otoscopes and disposable ear pieces are readily found in pediatric healthcare settings. The pediatric nurse must be skilled at inspecting a child's outer ear and middle ear for the presence of foreign bodies, obstructing cerumen, inflammation, and infection. The nurse gently inserts the otoscope to visualize the ear canal and the tympanic membrane. The tympanic membrane should be intact with a pink color. If it is found to be red, inflamed, perforated, or draining pus or fluids, then infection should be suspected. To best visualize the tympanic membrane of children, the nurse pulls the ear pinna down and back for children age 3 years and younger, and up and back for children older than 3 years of age.

UNIQUE FOR KIDS

Young children can be very resistant and frightened of an otoscope and the inspection of their middle ear. By being playful and asking if the nurse can look for elephants in their ear, young children can be distracted momentarily. If the child is uncooperative, the nurse can place the child in the lap of the parent; the parent then holds the child's head with one hand against his or her chest, while restraining the child's arms with the other arm across the child's chest.

Visual Acuity Screening

A child's vision is assessed according to the child's age. Infants' visual acuity is not assessed beyond their ability to track an object with their eyes. For toddlers, visual acuity is assessed by the HOTV instrument, Snellen E chart, or a picture chart. The HOTV instrument uses only the letters H, O, T and V in a random order, as the toddler may not know the alphabet. A separate card with the HOTV letters can be held close by so that the child can point out what he or she sees on the chart 20 feet away. Older children who have mastered the alphabet will typically use the Snellen chart.

Hearing Acuity Assessment

Every state mandates when and how young children have their hearing assessed via the Early Hearing Detection and Intervention (EHDI) program. The purpose of this nationwide program is to detect significant hearing loss before a child reaches 3 months of age. Many states mandate newborn hearing screening. Hearing acuity is directly related to a child's academic success and language development, so accurate hearing assessment is an imperative. Children of any age can accurately have their hearing screened.

Newborns and Infants

Hearing screening is performed using technology that evokes otoacoustic emissions (OAEs). The OAE machine produces a stimuli sound through the ear canal via a probe that sends and records the sound. The newborn's or infant's ear response (an echo-type response naturally produced in response to sound) is captured. This process is safe and pain free. Many infants sleep right through the screening, and it takes just a few minutes to complete.

Another device used in newborns and infants measures the auditory brain stem response (ABR). This device captures how well sound travels along the hearing nerve to the brain. Electrodes are placed on the infant's head and behind the ear, sound is directed via earphones, and the electrodes record how the brain responds to different sounds. This procedure takes approximately 30 to 60 minutes.

Toddlers

Hearing assessment in the toddler period is done in several ways. For example, in play audiometry (PA), children are taught how to wait, listen, and then perform a play activity whenever they hear a specific sound. Another simpler method relies on visual reinforcement orientation audiometry (VROA), in which a child's hearing is grossly tested by providing sounds in various frequencies during play and the child's response by turning toward the speaker is noted.

Preschoolers

A well-calibrated pure tone audiometry machine is used to assess hearing in cooperative preschool-age children. Earphones are placed on the child and sounds are used to detect hearing. The child must raise the hand in response to hearing the sound provided. Use of this technology requires a quiet environment.

Case Study

A 4-year-old Latino male presents with a month-long history of fever, fatigue, and enlarged lymph nodes. His parents are working-class Central American immigrants who live in a largely Latino neighborhood with their five children (this child is the youngest) plus the mother's parents. The grandparents look after the preschooler while his siblings are at school and the parents are at work. The father speaks fluent English and is a naturalized U.S. citizen; the mother knows English but is more comfortable speaking Spanish; the grandparents speak only Spanish.

During the initial assessment, blood is drawn for a complete blood count (CBC) with differential. The lab results show a white blood cell count of 4300/mm³, with 16% blast cells in the peripheral blood; hemoglobin is 8.8 g/dL and the platelet count is 49,000/mm³. A lumbar puncture and bone marrow aspiration are ordered. The cerebrospinal fluid is found to be negative for blast cells, but the bone marrow is hypercellular, with 64% of the cells being large, low-nucleus blasts; more than 80% of the blast cells are monoblasts, and the rest are promonocytes or monocytes.

The child is diagnosed with acute myelogenous leukemia (AML) and prescribed a chemotherapy regimen (the modified MRC-10 protocol) consisting of daunorubicin 50 mg/m² (days 1, 3, and 5); cytarabine 100 mg/m² in a 1-hour infusion every 12 hours on days 1 to 10; and etoposide 100 mg/m² in a 4-hour infusion every 24 hours on days 1 to 5. Upon being told about the planned treatment, the father looks ill at ease, speaks for a few minutes in Spanish with his wife and in-laws, and then explains that the family members are worried about his son receiving so many injections and punctures during his treatment (Dorantes-Acosta et al., 2009).

Case Study Questions

1. Prior to his diagnosis, this seriously ill preschool-age child experiences three different invasive procedures: a blood draw, a lumbar puncture, and a bone marrow aspiration. What are the key goals of nursing care in this situation?
2. After his diagnosis, the child undergoes a chemotherapy regimen that involves multiple infusions over different time frames. What are the key priorities and challenges of nursing care for this child and his family, given their social history?
3. Which strategies can the nurse employ to effectively address some of the family's concerns around chemotherapy treatments?

As the Case Evolves...

This male child has successfully completed the initial round of chemotherapy. At 27 days after the end of his chemotherapy cycle, he undergoes bone marrow aspiration and is determined by the lack of blast cells to be in remission. Three days later, a second chemotherapy cycle is initiated and proceeds through the full course without complications. A third cycle is halted on day 3 because of a life-threatening episode of pneumonia, which requires that the patient be transferred to the ICU and supported by mechanical ventilation. It is determined that placement of a chest tube would be beneficial.

4. Which of the following accurately describe(s) nursing considerations after placement of the chest tube? (Select all that apply.)
   A. Adhering to strict hand hygiene and infection prevention
   B. Keeping a loose covering over the chest tube insertion site
   C. Monitoring the tubing for debris, clots, or kinks that would prevent proper drainage
   D. Immobilizing the child and tightly clamping the tubing to ensure that nothing moves
   E. Providing adequate pain control measure during the insertion and maintenance of the chest tube drainage system

---

Chapter Summary

- Children of all ages and developmental levels experience the need for nursing skills and procedures. Children, owing to their vast differences in weight, height, and body surface area, need to have equipment available that is appropriate for their variability.
- Pediatric nurses need to demonstrate competence in providing comfort during skills procedures. Protocols for comfort management during painful procedures may include the use of topical anesthetics such as EMLA or Pain Ease, the Buzzy, distraction techniques, and the assistance of Child Life specialists.
- Numerous calculations are unique to the field of pediatric care. The pediatric nurse needs to be able to rapidly calculate fluid maintenance needs, kilocalorie needs, rehydration fluids (oral and IV therapy), safe medication administration, and burn resuscitation

needs, among others. Nurses must also be able to tailor calculations to the specific patient, as situational adjustments may be required in children who are overweight or underweight or who are receiving nephrotoxic chemotherapy.

- Delivery of fluids or medications via IVs, PICCs, pumps, or other devices requires the nurse to become familiar with their use and management of insertion sites as well as the type and nature of various IV fluid solutions.
- Medication safety includes calculating the safe dose range for the child's age and weight and alerting the pharmacist and physician if an ordered dose falls outside that range. Particularly in infants and toddlers, the immaturity of their liver and kidneys alters the pharmacodynamics (absorption), pharmacokinetics (distribution), and drug excretion parameters.
- Due to children's unique anatomy, the pediatric nurse uses skills for hearing and vision assessment that are appropriate for the child's age, size, and developmental ability.

Bibliography

Atkins, D. L., Berger, S., Duff, J. P., Gonzales, J. C., Hunt, E. A., Joyner, B. L., . . . Schexnayder, S. M. (2015). Pediatric basic life support and cardiopulmonary resuscitation quality: 2015 American Heart Association guidelines update for cardiopulmonary resuscitation and emergency cardiovascular care, Part 11. *Circulation, 132*, S519–S525.

Charnock, Y., & Evans, D. (2001). Nursing management of chest drains: A systematic review. *Australian Critical Care, 14*(4), 156–160.

Dabbous, M., Sakr, F. R., & Malaeb, D. N. (2014). Anticoagulant therapy in pediatrics. *Journal of Basic and Clinical Pharmacy, 5*(2), 27–33.

Dorantes-Acosta, E., Arreguin-Gonzalez, F., Rodriguez-Osorio, C. A., Sadowinski, S., Pelayo, R., & Medina-Sanson, A. (2009). Acute myelogenous leukemia switch lineage upon relapse to acute lymphoblastic leukemia: D case report. *Cases Journal, 2*, 154.

GlaxoSmithKline. (2006). Prescribing information: Amoxicillin. Retrieved from http://www.accessdata.fda.gov/drugsatfda_docs/label/2008/050760s11,050761s11,050754s12,050542s25lbl.pdf

Linnard-Palmer, L. (2015). *PedsNotes* (pp. 99–130). Philadelphia, PA: F. A. Davis.

Mayo Clinic. (2016). Drugs and supplements: Amoxicillin (oral route): Proper use. Retrieved from http://www.mayoclinic.org/drugs-supplements/amoxicillin-oral-route/proper-use/drg-20075356

Medscape. (2016). Amoxicillin (Rx). Retrieved from http://reference.medscape.com/drug/amoxil-moxatag-amoxicillin-342473

National Heart, Lung, and Blood Institute. (2013). Parent tips: Calories needed each day. Retrieved from https://www.nhlbi.nih.gov/health/educational/wecan/downloads/calreqtips.pdf

Paes, B. F., Vermeulen, K., Brohet, R. M., van der Ploeg, T., & de Winter, J. P. (2010). Accuracy of tympanic and infrared skin thermometers in children. *Archives of Disease in Childhood, 95*, 974–978.

Pesaturo, K. A., & Matthews, M. (2009). Topical anesthesia use in children. *US Pharmacist, 34*(3), HS-4–HS-7.

Robinson, J. L. (2004). Body temperature measurement in paediatrics: Which gadget should we believe? *Paediatrics and Child Health, 9*(7), 457–459.

Tang, A., Velissaris, T., & Weedon, D. (2002). An evidence based approach to drainage of the pleural cavity: Evaluation of best practice. *Journal of Evaluation in Clinical Practice, 8*(3), 333–340.

United Nations, Food and Agriculture Organization. (n.d.). Infants, children and adolescents; Energy and protein requirements. Retrieved from http://www.fao.org/docrep/003/aa040e/aa040e07.htm

U.S. Department of Agriculture, & U.S. Department of Health and Human Services. (2010). *Dietary guidelines for Americans, 2010* (7th ed.). Washington, DC: U.S. Government Printing Office. Retrieved from https://www.dietaryguidelines.gov

CHAPTER 28

Safe and Legal Aspects of Care

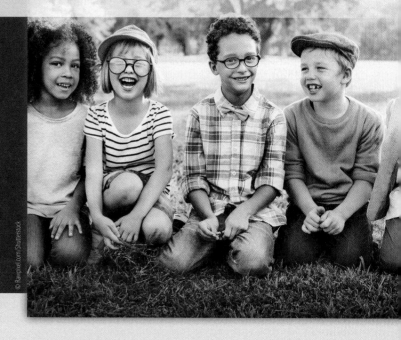

© Rawpixel.com/Shutterstock

LEARNING OBJECTIVES

1. Assess the nurse's responsibilities with respect to legal and ethical parameters regarding pediatric care.
2. Analyze key legal aspects of pediatric nursing care.
3. Differentiate between scope of practice, nurse practice act, and registered nursing licensure requirements.
4. Assess the ability of the child to weigh in on treatment decision making and provide input into care selection based on developmental stage.
5. Analyze the difference between situations involving misconduct and those involving negligence.
6. Discuss legally vulnerable aspects of foster care.

KEY TERMS

Assent
Autonomy
Beneficence
Consent
Delegation
Disciplinary action
Ethics
Incident report
Justice
Licensure
Malpractice
National Council of State Boards of Nursing
Negligence
Nonmaleficence
Nurse practice act
Scope of practice
Tort

Introduction

The professional practice of nursing and the care of those in need have many legal aspects to consider. Nurses need to understand how their professional practice is regulated. The **National Council of State Boards of Nursing** (NCSBN), along with each state's Board of Registered Nursing and its nurse practice act, provides oversight, regulation, and authority over licensure and practice of nursing. Safe practice stems from a solid understanding of hazards, implications, and responsibilities associated with licensed professional practice, scope of practice, and nurse practice acts. Legally safe practice requires knowledge of responsibilities, scope of practice, and legal risks associated with the practice of nursing.

Nurse Practice Acts

The practice of nursing has developed into a highly skilled profession that requires independent decision making, a specialized body of knowledge, and delivery of care that minimizes risks of harm. Because of the complexity surrounding care in multiple settings and with diverse populations, oversight is needed to ensure nursing care is provided by competent, prepared, and responsible people. **Nurse practice acts** (NPAs) provide the nursing profession with guidelines on nursing practice and governance on performance; these acts are set forth by state governments to protect the public. State legislation provides NPAs through both laws and boards of nursing that implement rules and regulations for safety. Each state's Board of Registered Nursing holds the power and authority to license nurses, regulate their education, and provide disciplinary action and remedies for nurses who fail to meet the profession's standards. Practice within the profession of nursing is not a right, but rather a protected professional act that is highly regulated at the state level. Even so, state boards of nursing are in a position to serve as advocates for healthcare consumers as well as advocates for nurses.

Scope of Practice

The **scope of practice** defines the limits of nurses' legal, ethical, and moral practice boundaries. A registered nurse (RN) must first complete an accredited program of study, sit for and pass the NCSBN's National Council Licensure Examinations (NCLEX exams), and meet requirements for continued good standing in practice. One aspect of good standing is that the pediatric nurse provides care within the scope of practice for a licensed RN and maintains the mandates associated with continued **licensure**. According to Brous (2012), maintaining a good standing requires demonstrating a moral character, continuing education,

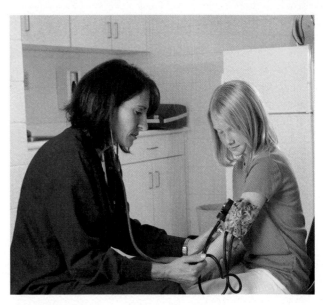

Figure 28-1 *A nurse must practice within the scope of RN licensure within the nurse's state.*

© Brian Eichhorn/Shutterstock

clinical competence, licensure maintenance, English language competency, and a clean criminal record.

Practicing within the scope of licensed RN practice means the nurse understands what is allowed and what is not allowed within the nurse's state (**Figure 28-1**). There are 61 nursing boards in the United States, and they have diverse requirements. Professional guidelines, laws, regulations of practice, practice alerts, and licensure mandates need to be understood for the specific state(s) in which the nurse practices. The nurse provides care for sick and vulnerable populations, groups, and individuals. Each state views these responsibilities as a *social contract* with the public, whose members need protection in the healthcare environment. If the social contract is breached or broken, the state board is legally responsible for enforcing disciplinary action to *protect the public.*

QUALITY AND SAFETY

Is a person's private life and conduct relevant to his or her professional nursing practice and licensure? Yes, it very much is: A nurse's personal life choices can indeed influence licensure.

A common misconception is the belief that only a nurse's clinical practice is regulated by the state board of nursing. Investigations can include a nurse's private conduct, and their results related to moral character, impairment related to substance use, and other illegal activity can lead to disciplinary action. Recreational drug use, driving while

(continues)

To find a summary of the scope of practice for the RN, search for a specific state's Board of Registered Nursing website (e.g., for the state of California, see http://www.rn.ca.gov/).

Professional Practice

The practice of professional registered nursing means the nurse performs care acts that require skills, specialized knowledge, and sound judgment, all based on a foundation gleaned from multiple sciences and disciplines, including mathematics, biology, physiology, pathophysiology, anatomy, **ethics** (the branch of philosophy concerned with decisions about what is right and wrong), communication theory, and social science. Nursing is a complex professional practice that requires application of the nursing process, educational theory, developmental theory, leadership theory, and management theory, as well as the promotion, restoration, and maintenance of health. The nurse must be prepared to care for clients or patients in a variety of clinical settings—hospitals, community settings, business settings, and educational settings. This is no small feat. Not surprisingly, then, the educational preparation of a professional nurse for clinical practice is rigorous, demanding, and complex. The nurse must be prepared to make sound clinical judgments independently but also within complex interdisciplinary teams.

Practicing as a nurse requires accountability, compassion, and highly specialized knowledge, often with a particular population. To best prepare for practice in pediatric nursing, the nurse must understand the needs of patients across the developmental period stretching from prematurity through young adulthood, and be prepared to assist these patients within the context of a family. Maintaining clinical competency, currency in knowledge and theory, application of technological skills, and currency in licensure are all requirements of state boards of nursing.

Licensure

Obtaining an RN license requires that the nurse graduate from an accredited program and pass the NCLEX, a national licensing examination created, validated, and implemented by the National Council of State Boards of Nursing. All states have had a licensure examination since 1923, albeit with wide variations in those examinations. Today, the NCLEX is administered via computerized adaptive technology (CAT), with each examinee being given a different examination and the number of questions ranging from 75 to 260 depending on test performance. The computer adapts to the performance of the licensure candidate during the test procedure until the examinee demonstrates competency equivalent to the performance of a nurse in entry-level practice (**Figure 28-2**).

States have their own particular requirements concerning background checks, felony and criminal disclosures, and fingerprinting as part of the licensure process. Having a history of a felony, fraudulent practice, or violation of certain laws pertaining to crimes may require disciplinary action or investigations prior to being cleared for licensure. Participation in "unprofessional conduct," as defined by a state's Board of Registered Nursing, may be grounds for revoking a professional license. Examples of unprofessional conduct include diverting drugs or narcotics from patients for personal use by the nurse; engaging in the distribution, sale, or possession of illegal substances or controlled substances without legitimate cause; failure to meet minimal standards of nursing practice; inaccurate recording; leaving a nursing assignment; discriminating against or

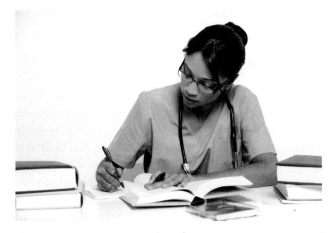

Figure 28-2 *Nurses must graduate from an accredited program and pass the NCLEX in order to obtain RN licensure in the United States.*
© alejandrophotography/E+/Getty Images

bullying others; failing to perform in a way that meets minimal standards; and being deemed unsafe or fabricating information to obtain or maintain a professional license (Becher & Visovsky, 2012; Blair, Kable, Courtney-Pratt, & Doran, 2015; MacLean, Coombs, & Breda, 2016; Olson & Stokes, 2016). See the individual state's nurse practice act for further information.

Organizations of Professional Oversight

The main focus of regulatory bodies is ensuring the safety of healthcare consumers. State, national, and international boards or councils of nursing contribute to that safety by providing licensure oversight, data collection on licensed nurses, data collection on nursing practice, and **disciplinary actions**, including loss of license and support of criminal investigations, as needed. Several bodies provide professional oversight over the attainment and continuation of licensure for registered nursing, including organizations that provide state-based oversight, manage national licensure, and establish international codes of ethics and international practice guidelines.

State Boards of Registered Nursing

State Boards of Registered Nursing (BRNs) provide consumers with protection from harm. By providing licensure oversight via the Department of Consumer Affairs, the BRN implements laws that regulate nursing practice and provide authority to enforce disciplinary actions. State BRNs have an eclectic membership; they include both professional nurses and elected community members with no licensure or healthcare services background. Members serve on the board and have the direct responsibility of protecting consumers of nursing care. Nurses who serve on the BRN must be actively engaged in professional practice.

National Council of State Boards of Nursing

The NCSBN is a regulatory organization that encompasses the various state boards of nursing. The first, overarching aim of the NCSBN is to protect the public's welfare and health by "assuring that safe and competent nursing care is provided by licensed nurses" (NCSBN, 2017). Oversight of the registered nurse's licensure is provided by granting a nurse legal permission to practice safely within a narrow scope of practice. The four areas that the NCSBN manages are standards relating to education, licensure, practice, and discipline. Outlining and communicating standards for safe nursing care is the second major aim of the NCSBN.

International Council of Nurses

The International Council of Nurses (ICN) is a federation consisting of 130 national nurse associations that collectively represent more than 16 million nurses worldwide. This organization's mission is to provide practice standards, global health policies, scientific advancement, and leadership by representing nursing on a worldwide basis. ICN (2015) categorizes its work into three areas: (1) activities that promote the practice of professional nursing, (2) activities that assist in the regulation of the profession, and (3) activities that promote the socioeconomic welfare of the professional nursing global workforce.

In 2000, ICN established an international code of ethics for nurses. This work was organized into four elements:

- Nurses and people: values, rights, confidentiality, and respect
- Nurses and practice: responsibility, education, evidence-based practice, and safety
- Nurses and coworkers: teamwork, cooperation, and interdisciplinary care
- Nurses and the profession: currency in practice, standards of practice, scope of practice, and knowledge

Other Organizations

Other organizations that provide oversight of nurses' professional practice include State Departments of Health and Human Services and The Joint Commission. They provide standards for safe care in healthcare institutions as well as oversight, investigations, and site visits related to the practice of nursing.

Tort Law

A **tort** is a wrongful act that produces harm to a patient, whether that harm was intentional or unintentional. Tort law is the legal aspect of patient care that involves negligence (omitting care) or malpractice (performing a harmful act), with the goal of promoting safer behavior (Zabinski & Black, 2015). Most nurses understand the term **malpractice** as it pertains to an act where specific standards of care were not performed or fully met.

Prevention of Negligence

The term **negligence** is used to describe a breach or failure in behaving in a reasonable and prudent manner. Prevention of negligence in nursing means that the nurse performs his or her duties within the scope of practice using reasonable and prudent judgment and decision making (**Figure 28-3**). A claim of negligence indicates that the nurse failed to practice in such a way that another person, in a similar situation, would identify the actions as neither reasonable nor prudent. Examples of negligence in nursing include failure to provide proper and safe monitoring of recent postoperative patients; failure to provide for the safety of infants by not having suction, oxygen, and resuscitation equipment readily available; and administering an inaccurate dose of insulin to a diabetic child (not double-checking doses with a second RN).

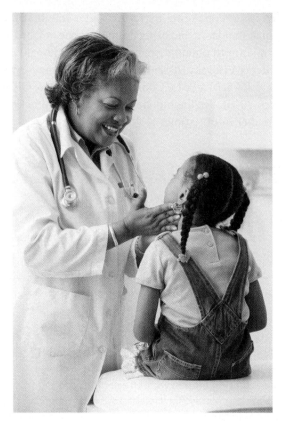

Figure 28-3 *Prevention of negligence in nursing means that the nurse performs his or her duties within the scope of practice using reasonable and prudent judgment and decision making.*
© Blend Images - Jose Luis Pelaez Inc/Brand X Pictures/Getty

Malpractice

To avoid malpractice claims, pediatric nurses must perform their professional duties at the level expected given their responsibilities and licensure. Ensuring that documentation is meticulous, accurate, and thorough is a key consideration in preventing malpractice lawsuits. Thorough assessments, accurate skills, articulate communication, and attention to detail to prevent errors are all part of safe and legal practice. Even if it seems mundane, the pediatric nurse must document daily routine care that represents protection from harm and promotion of health and wellbeing. Written proof of the nurse's care—which should be based on standards, policies, and procedures—via paper or electronic charting consistently offers the best protection against malpractice lawsuits.

Four conditions must be met if a malpractice claim is to succeed:

- A duty between a patient and a nurse was owed.
- The nurse did not perform that duty or violated that duty.
- Injuries were caused by the failure of a nurse to act on his or her duties.

- Actual and measurable injury or harm occurred due to the failure of the nurse to meet the standards of care or duty.

It is far more common for a nurse to become drawn into a civil lawsuit than a criminal lawsuit. Civil lawsuits encompass situations where a patient and family feel their individual rights were infringed upon or violated by a nurse or healthcare team. The family, which is considered the plaintiff, has the responsibility of providing the burden of proof of wrongdoing or violation by the nurse (the defendant).

Unique Issues of Safety in Pediatric Nursing Practice

The care of children entails unique care practices and competencies not found in the care of adults. To be successful in the complex care of children and their families, a pediatric nurse needs to obtain sufficient preparation, to practice role modeling and support, and to secure strong administrative guidance. The presence of vulnerable children in a clinical setting requires a special view of care. Wise pediatric nurses will want to review the following aspects that are unique to providing comprehensive and holistic care to children in any clinical setting.

Hospitalized Children Without Parents or Guardians Present

A child who is hospitalized without having a supportive family member present places the nurse in a situation of needing to provide greater supervision, as such a child is vulnerable to both emotional turmoil and physical risk. When possible, encourage family to stay with a hospitalized child, no matter what the child's age. Provide a sleeping arrangement in close proximity to the child.

Child Maltreatment Reports

The number of child maltreatment cases that are reported to child protection agencies is only the tip of the iceberg—it falls far short of indicating just how prevalent child maltreatment is on a global scale. The most common form of maltreatment in the United States is neglect. Regardless of the type or form of maltreatment, the pediatric nurse is responsible for identifying, reporting, and preventing further child maltreatment.

Parental or Guardian Refusal of Medical Treatments

Given the emotional turmoil that arises when a child is ill or injured, parents may become frustrated, angry, or confused about the care needed by their child. Parental refusal of medical care is a complex phenomenon and can be due to stress, religious beliefs, cultural perspectives, or lack of education. Children are vulnerable to parental influences in treatment refusal. Any suspicion of refusal—whether it involves limiting medical care, refusing medical care, or failing to adhere to a medical or nursing treatment plan—must be reported to the administrative and medical teams.

Floating Outside the Nurse's Usual Unit or Care Setting

Situations in which staffing influences where a pediatric nurse practices can have safety and legal consequences. When pediatric nurses are required to float to care areas other than pediatric settings, their clinical competencies in regard to theory, assessments, care practices, skills, and documentation must be confirmed. For instance, if a pediatric nurse is required to float to an intensive care environment, the nurse must have documented competencies prior to providing care. The same is true when an adult nurse floats to a pediatric care environment. Without documented competencies, nurses should not be asked to provide care to children.

Children on a Police Hold

An uncomfortable but not infrequent situation that occurs in pediatric health care is the need for a child to be placed on a police hold. In this scenario, the child is deemed to need extra protection, even within the hospital setting. Cases of child maltreatment may warrant a police hold, which may ban or limit a parent's visiting rights. The pediatric nurse caring for a child on a police hold must obtain sufficient information to participate in the child's protection.

Children with Developmental or Cognitive Disabilities

Children who are not at the developmental or cognitive level usually associated with their chronological age bring further complexities in care. The nurse must realize that these children may not understand what is occurring to and around them, and they may not be able to participate in their care if they function at a lower level than their same-age peers. For instance, a 10-year-old developmentally delayed child may not be able to comprehend his environment, take medications on cue, or participate in personal hygiene, and may pose greater threats to safety and increased chances of bodily harm.

Informed Consent

Children are not legally able to provide informed **consent** (i.e., permission to initiate a healthcare intervention), but children who are developmentally capable from the age of seven years should be included in assent. **Assent** means that the child is included in the discussions of health care, treatment decisions, and priorities.

Because children cannot provide informed consent, it is imperative that the pediatric nurse participate in meeting the legal and ethical requirements for obtaining informed consent from the parent(s) or legal guardian(s) on the child's behalf. Issues to be discussed during the informed consent process include the procedure, who will be performing the procedure, the nature of the procedure, its risks, its benefits, and any alternatives. The discussion should be expanded to include the potential outcomes or prognosis if the procedure is not performed or is delayed. Three signatures are often required on the informed consent form: the signature of the physician or primary care provider (physician assistant or nurse practitioner) who is responsible for the implementation of the procedure; the signature of the child's parent or legal guardian; and the signature of the witness, who is often the nurse. (For safety and accuracy, check your state regulations on legal consent procedure requirements.)

Tips for Achieving a Successful Career as a Pediatric Nurse

Pediatric nurses should continue to be informed about specific aspects of safe and legally appropriate nursing practice. Among other topics, the pediatric nurse should be well versed in the following issues:

- *Knowing one's scope of practice as it pertains to the registered nurse caring for children from prematurity through adolescence.* Understand that the core of pediatric nursing is the care of not just the child, but the entire family. (See the Society of Pediatric Nurses website at http://www.pedsnurses.org.)
- *Knowing delegation parameters for the role of the pediatric nurse.* Appropriate and safe **delegation** stems from the pediatric nurse understanding how to assign, manage, and supervise other healthcare providers such as nursing assistive personnel. Assuring competence prior to delegation is the responsibility of the healthcare administrative and education team, yet prior to the pediatric nurse delegating any tasks or duties, there must be confidence and assurance that the delegate is able to provide that care, and has sufficient competence and understanding to do so. Delegate tasks only to those persons who have the appropriate legal capacity, educational preparation, and licensure or certification. For instance, do not delegate complex care or advanced assessments to a licensed vocational nurse. Ask nursing assistants to perform only those duties in which they have demonstrated competence. For further guidelines, see the NCSBN (2005) position paper on working with others and delegating.
- *Applying principles of legal and safe charting.* The national movement toward electronic medical records (EMR) is under way, with federal mandates dictating the need for any healthcare institution that accepts federal funds to have an EMR system in place. Regardless of the form of charting required, it is imperative that charting on each child be complete and follow institutional requirements as well as state and federal mandates.
- *Preventing errors in pediatric healthcare treatment settings to save lives and prevent injuries and harm.* The pediatric nurse is safety minded in all clinical settings and in all clinical circumstances. Demonstrating safety mindedness includes conducting safety sweeps using all of one's senses and making the assumption that children are, in general, inherently unsafe and require supervision when receiving care in healthcare settings. Consistently insisting that children wear accurate identification tags with their name, birth date, and medical record identifier allows the nurse to conduct safety checks before initiating nursing care, medication administration, and medical procedures. Parents or legal guardians must also wear identification badges or bracelets.
- *Documenting incident reports to share high-error situations and the need for changes to improve safety.* When an error occurs, or nearly occurs (near miss), the pediatric nurse should communicate what happened via an **incident report** and submit that report to administrative personnel. This allows for an investigation of what occurred prior to, during, and after an error. Without documentation of error or near miss circumstances, changes cannot be made to prevent future errors. Application of the principles of a *just culture* supports a nurse in reporting errors or near misses without fear of reprimand or reprisal.
- *Understanding institutional compliance, including being well versed in institutional policies and procedures.* Because many aspects of caring for children differ from caring for patients at other developmental stages, it is important that the pediatric nurse

is well versed in clinical policies and procedures. Knowing how to rapidly investigate the steps of a skill or the policies associated with care practices is an imperative.

- *Knowing and understanding children's rights.* Children are vulnerable. They may not possess the developmental understanding of what is occurring around them, so they need advocates whose priority is to maintain their dignity, protection, safety, and privacy. The pediatric healthcare team should understand the basic rights of children if they are to be strong and competent child and family advocates. See the websites of the Children's Defense Fund (http://www.childrensdefense.org/) or the United Nations Children's Fund (http://www.unicef.org/) for specific information about child rights.

- *Keeping patient data confidential and consistently applying the provisions of the Health Insurance Portability and Accountability Act (HIPAA).* Regardless of the child's age, the protection of privacy of healthcare information is a legal standard set forth by HIPAA, which was passed in 1996. The pediatric nurse must never discuss or disclose information about a child's health status or medical condition except on a need-to-know basis. Always clarify who is asking for information about a child and why they need to know the information, especially on the phone. Consequences of breaching a child's privacy via a HIPAA violation can include severe penalties such as fines, imprisonment, and loss of licensure. Never share a child's health information, never leave charts or computer screens open when not in use, never search the records of patients who are not your clinical responsibility, never give health information over the phone unless you are certain that the person posing the questions is a legal guardian or a parent, never fax medical information until the fax number is double-checked and a cover sheet is applied, and never leave any healthcare setting with information about a child's clinic visit, home visit, or hospitalization.

- *Maintaining professional malpractice liability insurance.* Nurses have the freedom to purchase individual malpractice liability insurance plans. These plans are generally affordable and will provide coverage for a lawsuit when breach of a standard of care, poor clinical outcome, patient harm, or an act of negligence occurs. The American Nurses Association highly suggests that nurses obtain professional malpractice liability insurance, even if they have coverage as part of their healthcare institution's benefit plan.

Caring for a Foster Child

Legally vulnerable children warrant special consideration from nurses. A foster child, for example, may enter the pediatric healthcare arena requiring nursing care. It is important to provide a holistic and comprehensive assessment of such a child to determine the child's unique needs.

Situations where it is deemed unsafe for a child to live with his or her parents or guardians may be brought to the attention of the legal system. Fostering is a form of socially recognized "family" provided for a child in need of a short-term placement. Typically, there is either no parent to provide for the child, or the child's parents or guardians are considered "unfit" (Blythe, Wilkes, & Halcomb, 2014). As of December 2015, more than 397,000 children were in foster care in the United States, and approximately 32% of these children were waiting for adoption (Congressional Coalition on Adoption Institute, 2015) (**Figure 28-4**).

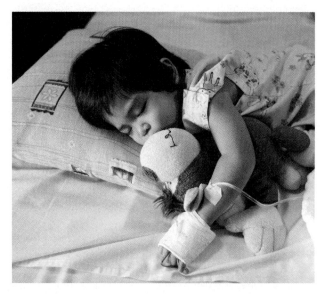

Figure 28-4 *As of December 2015, more than 397,000 children were in foster care in the United States, and approximately 32% of these children were waiting for adoption.*

© Roylee_photosunday/Shutterstock

The most common reasons for placement of children in foster home environments are neglect, abuse, incarcerated parents, or special circumstances preventing the parents or guardians from providing care. The goals of fostering children are to provide a nurturing, safe, and developmentally supportive environment for short-term care, while the parents or guardians receive assistance so that they can resume the child's care. Reuniting the child with his or her siblings and parents is the primary goal of fostering.

Foster children may be adopted by a family, or the child may stay within the foster child infrastructure, sometimes remaining at one home and at other times experiencing a variety of successive foster homes, until he or she reaches the legal age of 18. A foster parent might not have legal decision-making custody for the foster child. Even if the child is not living with an extended family member, it is not uncommon for an aunt, uncle, older sibling, or grandparent to have legal rights over the child while the child remains in a foster home. Emotional and mental health concerns may surface when a foster child is moved from one home setting to another. The period between fostering a child and securing legal adoption is considerable. Some states provide financial support to biological family members who care for a foster child, whereas other states provide financial assistance to only unrelated foster families for the care they provide.

Medical foster parenting is also not uncommon. Children with chronic conditions, with disabilities, or who are technology dependent, and whose parents or guardians are not able to provide sufficient safe care, will be placed into medical foster homes. Foster parents who provide medical care are considered to provide a *protective service* when a child has a special-needs diagnosis. Studies suggest that at least one-third of children in foster care in the United States have disabilities, ranging from minor developmental delays to significant mental and physical disabilities (Blakeslee et al., 2013).

Case Study

Leslie, an experienced pediatric and emergency room nurse, is assisting the pediatric oncology healthcare team in a discussion with the family of a 17-year-old patient who has relapsed from acute lymphocytic leukemia (ALL) for the second time. The mother and stepfather of the teen are describing their desire to consent to further medical treatment including chemotherapy. The teenager, at first very quiet and seemingly depressed, speaks up in the middle of the discussion and states that he is done with further treatments and prefers to go home with palliative care interventions only. The team sits down with the teenager and begins to discuss how he feels, what his interpretation of their discussion for further treatment was, and what his wishes are and why. The teenager, with great clarity, states that he knows he will not respond to further cancer treatment and that he does not wish to endure any further multidrug chemotherapy courses and their severe side effects.

Case Study Questions

1. Which ethical principle is in question in this scenario?
2. Who should be a part of this important conversation?
3. At what age can a minor make healthcare treatment decisions?
4. What does the term *emancipated minor* mean?

As the Case Evolves. . .

In this case study, the care team includes a pediatric oncologist (medical doctor), a licensed social worker (Child Life specialist), a registered nurse, a nurse's aide, and a technician. The bulk of the case's day-to-day workload is handled by the RN and the two unlicensed assistive personnel.

5. Which of the following aspects of patient care can be undertaken only by a licensed provider such as the registered nurse and may not be delegated to unlicensed personnel? (Select all that apply.)
   A. Creation of patient care goals
   B. Evaluation of care goals
   C. Recording intake and output
   D. Assisting with activities of daily living
   E. Reporting changes in a pediatric patient's condition
   F. Providing a nonpharmacologic comfort measure
   G. Assisting with the collection of heart rate, respiratory rate, and temperature measurements

After extensive discussion, the family of the 17-year-old with ALL has decided that they will come to a compromise solution regarding their son's desire to undergo no further treatment: They will initiate palliative care for eight weeks and give the young man a "rest" from therapy before resuming discussion of treatment options. The pediatric oncology team offers

(continues)

Case Study (continued)

appropriate guidance about the potential repercussions of the delay, but recognizing that an uncooperative near-adult is unlikely to comply with the regimen, they agree to the plan, provide a referral to counseling services and a support group for young adults with leukemia, and put a note in the patient's file that he is being discharged against medical advice.

Four days after the young man is released, a middle-aged man arrives at the oncology unit, identifies himself as the youth's biological father, and asks to see his son. The father's name is not listed on the disclosure documents filled out when the youth entered treatment. Told that the young man is not there, he becomes visibly upset and asks why the oncology team is willing to "let his son die." He threatens a malpractice lawsuit. In a later communication with the boy's mother, she confirms that the man is the boy's biological father, but says that although he has a cordial relationship with his son, the father relinquished custodial rights to him many years ago.

6. Which of the following statements best describes the oncology unit's legal liability in this situation?
   A. The oncology unit and its staff are at risk of being held criminally liable for malpractice because they did not require the youth to continue life-sustaining therapy.
   B. The oncology unit and its staff are at risk of being held criminally liable for custodial interference because they did not obtain the biological father's consent to treat his son.
   C. The oncology unit and its staff bear no criminal liability, but they may face a successful civil suit from the father for negligence.
   D. The oncology unit and its staff bear no criminal liability, and any civil suit the father might bring for malpractice or negligence is unlikely to succeed.

The teen has been receiving palliative home care and attending regular support group meetings and therapy sessions with a licensed social worker since his discharge. Five weeks after his decision to refuse further treatment, the family informs the clinic that the teen has changed his mind about therapy; after working with the therapist, he is less depressed and has a more positive outlook on his potential to achieve remission. Two weeks after therapy is reinitiated, the youth's biological father arrives at the clinic and insists, politely, that he be brought up to speed on his son's prognosis.

7. What is the clinic's best course of action in this situation?
   A. The clinic should ascertain whether the father has legal custody of his son and, therefore, should be included in decision making.
   B. The clinic should inform the mother that the boy's father will be given his records unless she obtains a restraining order.
   C. The clinic should inform the father that giving him his son's medical information would be a HIPAA violation and, therefore, is illegal.
   D. The clinic should inform the father that he has no legal rights and will be charged with trespassing if he returns to the clinic.

Chapter Summary

- Nurses must know the laws and regulations that encompass professional nursing practice. Knowledge of and adherence to laws is a nurse's responsibility.
- Nurses must acknowledge the imperative in understanding the oversight, regulation, and authority that is provided by the National Council of State Boards of Nursing and each state's Board of Registered Nursing and subsequent nurse practice act.
- The scope of practice defines the limits of a nurse's legal, ethical, and moral practice boundaries.
- An RN must first complete an accredited program of study, sit for and pass a NCSBN's NCLEX exam, and meet requirements for good standing in practice as part of his or her professional practice.
- The practice of professional registered nursing means the nurse knows and performs acts that require skill, specialized knowledge, and sound judgment, based on a foundation including knowledge from sciences, mathematics, biology, physiology, pathophysiology, anatomy, ethics, physical science, and social science.
- A tort is a wrongful act that produces harm to a patient, whether that harm was intentional or unintentional. Tort law is the legal aspect of patient care that incorporates both negligence (omitting care) or malpractice (performing an act that results in harm).
- Pediatric nurses should review the following aspects of care that are unique to providing comprehensive and holistic care to children in any clinical setting: hospitalized children without parents or guardians present; child maltreatment reporting; parent or guardian refusal of medical treatments; floating outside of the nurse's usual unit or care setting; children on a police hold; and children with developmental or cognitive disabilities.

- Situations where it is considered unsafe for children to live with their parents or guardians may be brought to the attention of the legal system. Fostering is a form of a socially recognized "family" provided for a child in need of a short-term placement.

- Children with chronic conditions, with disabilities, or who are technology dependent, and whose parents or guardians are not able to provide sufficient and safe care, will be placed into medical foster homes. Often referred to as medical homes, foster parents that provide medical care are considered to provide a protective service for children.

Bibliography

Becher, J., & Visovsky, C. (2012). Horizontal violence in nursing. *Medsurg Nursing, 21*, 210–213.

Blair, W., Kable, A., Courtney-Pratt, H., & Doran, E. (2015). Mixed method integrative review exploring nurses' recognition and response to unsafe practice. *Journal of Advanced Nursing, 72*, 488–500.

Blakeslee, J. E., Quest, A. D., Powers, J., Powers, L. E., Geenen, S., Nelson, M., . . . Research Consortium to Increase the Success of Youth in Foster Care. (2013). Reaching everyone: Promoting the inclusion of youth with disabilities in evaluating foster care outcomes. *Children and Youth Services Review, 35*(11), 1801–1808.

Blythe, S. L., Wilkes, L., & Halcomb, E. J. (2014). The foster carer's experience: An integrative review. *Collegian, 21*, 21–32.

Brous, E. (2012). Nursing licensure and regulation. In D. J. Mason, J. K. Leavitt, & M. W. Chaffee (Eds.), *Policy & politics in nursing and health care* (6th ed.). St. Louis, MO: Saunders.

Catalano, J. (2009). *Nursing now: Today's issues, tomorrow's trends* (5th ed., pp. 41-48). Philadelphia, PA: F. A. Davis.

Children's Aid Society. (2017). Overview. Retrieved from http://www.childrensaidsociety.org/adoption-foster-care?gclid=CMnKpdOSndQCFRSGfgodseQEpw

Congressional Coalition on Adoption Institute. (2015). Facts and statistics. Retrieved from http://www.ccainstitute.org/resources/fact-sheets

International Council of Nurses (ICN). (2015). Mission, strategic intent, core values and priorities. Retrieved from http://www.icn.ch/who-we-are/our-mission-strategic-intent-core-values-and-priorities/

Levati, S. (2014). Professional conduct among registered nurses in the use of online social networking sites. *Journal of Advanced Nursing, 70*, 2284-2292.

MacLean, L., Coombs, C., & Breda, K. (2016). Unprofessional workplace conduct: Defining and defusing it. *Nursing Management, 47*, 30–34.

National Council of State Boards of Nursing (NCSBN). (2005). Working with others: A position paper. Executive summary. Retrieved from https://www.ncsbn.org/Working_with_Others.pdf

National Council of State Boards of Nursing (NCSBN). (2017). Nurse practice act and rules. Retrieved from https://www.ncsbn.org/nurses.htm

Olson, L. L., & Stokes, F. (2016). The ANA code of ethics for nurses with interpretive statements: Resource for nursing regulation. *Journal of Nursing Regulation, 7*, 9–20.

Sprung, C. L., Ledoux, D., Bulow, H.-H., Lippert, A., Wennberg, E., Baras, M., . . . Solsona Duran, J., for the ETHICUS Study Group. (2008). Relieving suffering or intentionally hastening death: Where do you draw the line? *Critical Care Medicine, 36*, 8–13.

Zabinski, Z., & Black, B. S. (2015). The deterrent effect of tort law: Evidence of medical malpractice reform. Northwestern Law & Econ Research Paper No. 13-09. Available at https://ssrn.com/abstract=2161362

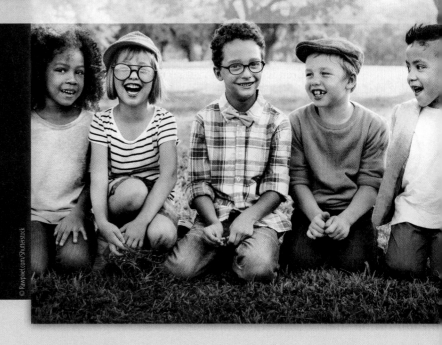

© Rawpixel.com/Shutterstock

CHAPTER 29

Care of the Acutely Ill or Critically Ill Child

LEARNING OBJECTIVES

1. Distinguish the role of the pediatric nurse as a child moves between the emergency department (ED) for initial stabilization, to the pediatric intensive care unit (PICU) for observation, to the pediatric acute care unit for discharge.
2. Discuss the implementation of family-centered care across hospital settings.
3. Critically evaluate safety issues and safety assessments for a child moving from the ED to the PICU to the acute care unit.
4. Evaluate components of a safe nursing handoff for a child transferring care across units.

KEY TERMS

Alarm fatigue
Color-coded alarms
Critically ill
Pediatric acute care
PERRLA
Procedural sedation
Stabilization
Transfer

Introduction

Most children will never have to experience a hospitalization during their developmental period. Nevertheless, many children will need to visit an urgent care center or an emergency department (ED) for an acute condition needing assessment, intervention, or stabilization. When a child suffers a significant injury or illness, he or she may need to be initially triaged in the emergency department, receive assessments and diagnostics to determine the severity of the condition, and then be transferred to a pediatric intensive care unit (PICU) for more observation and stabilization. (**Table 29-1** identifies common reasons for hospitalization across childhood.) As the child heals, he or she will be transferred to the inpatient hospital unit for final treatments and nursing care, followed by a discharge with specific instructions being provided to the family on follow-up care. Each step of this process should focus on the immediate physiological, psychological, emotional, and educational needs of the child and family, keeping in mind the child's developmental stage. Each department involved in this process should have a competent interdisciplinary team prepared to care for children at stages from birth to adolescence.

Both the child and the family will likely experience significant stress and fear surrounding the circumstances of the hospitalization across settings. Three themes affecting the family experience of a hospitalized child have been identified: apprehending the reality, engaging adversity, and advancing forward (Uhl, Fisher, Docherty, &

TABLE 29-1 Childhood Hospitalizations
› Approximately 18% of hospitalizations are for children 17 years or younger, who account for 6.3 million hospitalizations each year.
› Almost two-thirds of hospitalizations are for children in the neonate and infancy stages.
› Children coming through the emergency department (ED) account for 44% of hospitalizations.
› Children who require routine admission with an initial ED visit account for 45% of hospitalizations.

Most Common Reasons for Hospitalization of a Newborn

1. Complications associated with the newborn period (acute life-threatening events)
2. Hemolytic jaundice and perinatal jaundice
3. Complications associated with prematurity, including low birth weight
4. Respiratory compromise or distress
5. Newborn and infant infectious diseases
6. Acute bronchiolitis
7. Complications associated with cardiac and circulatory birth defects
8. Complications associated with gastrointestinal and digestive birth defects
9. Transitory tachypnea of the newborn

Most Common Reasons for Hospitalizations of Children from Infancy Through Adolescence

1. Pneumonia
2. Asthma
3. Acute bronchitis
4. Disorders of fluid and electrolyte status
5. Appendicitis
6. Affective disorders (depression most common)
7. Seizure disorders (e.g., epilepsy)
8. Urinary tract infections
9. Infections of the gastrointestinal system
10. Noninfectious gastroenteritis

Data from American Academy of Pediatrics. (2017). Immunization. Retrieved from https://www.aap.org/en-us/advocacy-and-policy/aap-health-initiatives/immunizations/Pages/Immunizations-home.aspx; The Arc. (2011). Facts about childhood immunizations. Retrieved from www.thearc.org/what-we-do/resources/fact-sheet/facts-about-chidhood-immunizations; Centers for Disease Control and Prevention. (2017). Immunization schedules. Retrieved from https://www.cdc.gov/vaccines/schedules/index.html

Brandon, 2013). Providing support, clear communication and honest explanations of the situation and treatment plan will help the family cope.

Role of the Registered Nurse

The pediatric nurse plays a very important role in the care of a child requiring an ED to PICU to pediatric unit **transfer** across settings. The nurse is responsible for monitoring the patient's condition for changes in clinical status and for the administration of ordered treatments. The pediatric nurse communicates across settings to ensure the most seamless process possible. A commitment to clearly presenting critical information during handoffs across settings will increase the likelihood that the child achieves continued stabilization and receives expeditious care. The nurse should also communicate the nursing and medical treatment plan to the family and, according to the principles of family-centered care, act as the child's and family's advocate and main support system (**Figure 29-1**).

Advocacy

When a family is experiencing a child's hospitalization, it is typically a crisis beset with unknowns and confusing scenarios. Many staff members will interact with the family, and consultants may be called in to provide pediatric-focused specialty care. The nurse assigned to the child must provide clear instructions and explanations for the family, advocating for team members to explain what they are doing and why, and what can be expected to come next. For instance, if a young infant is seen in the emergency department in a critical state from severe dehydration and acidosis related to a prolonged acute viral infection, the child will be stabilized in the ED and transferred to the PICU for further observation and higher level of care. The nurse is the family's advocate and helps them understand all aspects of the child's transfer and subsequent care. The nurse advocates by assessing the family's health literacy level, preferred language, and cultural preferences, while explaining the care plan in an accessible manner.

The registered nurse is often in the position of first recognizing the needs of patients, and is responsible for reporting these needs to the professionals assigned to effect changes. The nurse must frequently assess the patient, perform the functions of the nursing process, initiate and perform complex thinking strategies throughout all phases of the nursing process, and act as an advocate for the patient and family. Advocating for patients is considered a core obligation and core principle of the nurse as he or she commits to protecting the well-being, safety, and health of the patient (American Nurses Association [ANA], 2016). As an advocate, the registered nurse (RN) has a primary ethical responsibility to protect the health, safety, and rights of the patient (ANA, 2016).

Families can have strong reactions to the hospitalization of the child and may feel confused and frightened as the child is transferred between settings. Pediatric patients also have strong reactions based on fear of separation and pain (**Table 29-2**). Research has shown that communication, information, and relationships are the three key areas impacting the experience of pediatric hospitalization, whether that experience is good or bad, from the perspective of providers, parents, and the hospitalized child (Foster, Whitehead, Maybee, & Cullens, 2013).

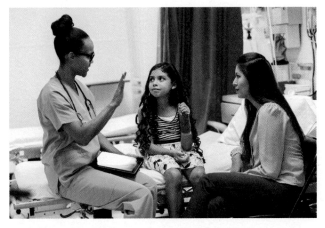

Figure 29-1 *The role of the registered nurse includes communicating the nursing and medical treatment plan to the family.*
© asiseeit/E+/Getty Images

TABLE 29-2   Common Reactions to Hospitalization Across Developmental Stages

Neonate

› Common reactions: Stress reaction, hypoglycemia, hypothermia, sleep deprivation
› Nursing care:
- Provide physical comfort, warmth, a quiet time for uninterrupted sleep, and frequent vital signs checking and temperature monitoring.
- Provide a source of nutrition at regular intervals to stabilize blood glucose.

Infant

› Common reactions: Stress reaction, older infants fear separation
› Nursing care:
- Provide physical comfort.
- Encourage the family to stay with the child around the clock.
- Care for basic needs rapidly to encourage trust.
- Reduce opportunities for overstimulation and allow for uninterrupted sleep time.

Toddler

› Common reactions: Separation anxiety, stranger anxiety, frustration, defiance, regression, fears assessments and procedures
› Nursing care:
- Approach the child with a positive attitude and provide praise for cooperation.
- Encourage the family to stay with the child around the clock.
- Provide play activities, and balance them with rest.
- Minimize stranger interactions.
- Provide developmentally appropriate procedural preparation and involve Child Life specialists for support and assistance.
- Expect the child to be frustrated and defiant and to have tantrums; stay calm and in control.
- Offer choices whenever possible.

Preschooler

› Common reactions: Anxious, fearful, feels punished, magical thinking, fear of body mutilation, aggression, regression
› Nursing care:
- Explain what is coming next in a developmentally appropriate way.
- Engage the family in providing care.
- Provide praise for cooperation.
- Do not use language that provokes fear; use simple explanations and speak in a comforting voice.
- Try to maintain eye contact at the child's level.
- Allow the child to be involved with care and procedures when possible.

School Age

› Common reactions: Stress, emotional withdrawal, fearing procedures, stalling behaviors, fear of "failing"
› Nursing care:
- Explain all procedures and treatment plans at a developmentally appropriate level.
- Include the child (when older than age 7) in treatment decisions and discussions as appropriate.
- Allow a small amount of stalling behavior so the child feels some perception of control, but do not allow the child to interrupt procedures.
- Provide praise for attempts at self-care.
- Give the child duties or small projects to accomplish to increase feelings of industry.

TABLE 29-2	Common Reactions to Hospitalization Across Developmental Stages (*continued*)

Adolescent

› Common reactions: Fears loss of peer interaction, body image fears, rebellion, may withdraw

› Nursing care:

- Provide honesty with medical explanations and explain the treatment plan in detail.

- Encourage the teen to express feelings and ask questions.

- Give choices in timing of procedures and medication administration when able.

- Provide privacy, encourage peer interaction, and give alone time.

QUALITY AND SAFETY

Preventing Accidents or Harm in Emergency Department, PICU, and Acute Care Settings

Security Systems

Because EDs and intensive care environments are often populated with family members in distress, escalation of verbal and physical violence as well as threats of violence are frequently encountered. High levels of anxiety, mixed with the feeling of helplessness and not knowing what will happen next to a vulnerable child, create an environment where outside-the-norm behavior takes place. Access to rapidly responding security services staff members who are skilled in managing escalating behaviors or actual violence is an imperative.

Monitoring Systems

Placing a child on cardiopulmonary monitors that display heart rate, respiratory rate, oxygen saturation, and cyclic blood pressure readings with audible alarms allows the pediatric team to acknowledge and respond to impending critical changes in the child's condition. Accuracy in setting the alarm limits as per the physician's orders or institutional policy provides immediate information if the child's vital signs change.

Hospital Equipment Safety

The primary nurse assigned to the pediatric patient is responsible for rapidly assessing the presence of vital emergency response equipment. Basic emergency response equipment includes a source of oxygen and a variety of delivery systems spanning the array of sizes needed to care for children ranging from small infants to adolescents. A working suction device with all tubing and suction devices is imperative. Airway resuscitation equipment (bag, mask, and valve) in a variety of sizes must be present, as well as a working code button and rapid access to fluid resuscitation equipment. Access to a color-coded crash cart set up according to the variety of weights found across childhood must be within rapid reach and checked daily (per institutional policy) for contents and expiration dates (**Figure 29-2**).

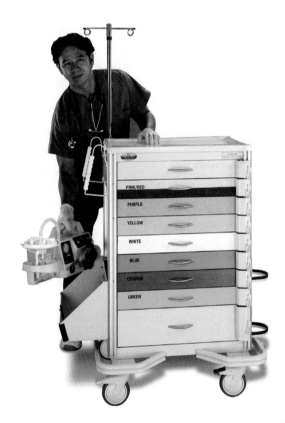

Figure 29-2 *A color-coded pediatric crash cart must be within rapid reach.*
Photo courtesy of Armstrong Medical Industries, Inc.

Entering the Emergency Department

The total number of ED visits made each year across the United States continues to increase. Approximately 25% of all ED visits are for children. Demographic data show that male children outnumber female children in these visits, and families at the lowest economic levels of society account for the majority of visits (32%). The average age for children who are treated in the ED and discharged, as well as those children who are stabilized and admitted to the hospital, is 7 years (AHRQ, 2013).

Pediatric healthcare teams working in emergency room settings must be competent in rapid assessment and **stabilization** (i.e., achievement of homeostasis). Caring for children spanning the developmental periods from newborn through adolescence requires that the emergency team be competent in performing developmentally appropriate assessments. These assessments require recognition of the differences in anatomy and physiology for infants, children, teens, and adults, and use of appropriate assessment tools. Differences in equipment selection and specialized skills are required for transport, assessment of injuries or illnesses in children, and stabilization.

Young children presenting with a critical injury or illness may compensate for that condition for a period of time, then experience rapid deterioration. The pediatric team must be confident in their ability to rapidly assess a child's cardiovascular, respiratory, neurologic, gastrointestinal, metabolic, and genitourinary systems so as to isolate the etiology of the clinical presentation. Once stabilization occurs, the child may need further diagnostics and a transfer into the critical care setting; alternatively, the child may be admitted for further observation and treatment onto the pediatric hospital acute care unit. The determination to transfer should be done with an interdisciplinary focus. **Critically ill** children (i.e., children with a potentially life-altering or life-threatening illness or injury) should not be transferred to a hospital bed where the receiving nurse will be caring for other children as well as the new admission. Knowing which resources, equipment, personnel, and skills are required for stabilization of children means the ED staff must have both specialized training and experience with children across the developmental period (**Table 29-3**).

Priorities of stabilization in the ED start with a visual assessment of the child's status. The Pediatric Assessment Triangle (PAT) is commonly used in emergency medicine and nursing interdisciplinary teams to determine when to

---

TABLE 29-3 Interdisciplinary Priorities When Stabilizing Children in Emergency Care Settings

Initial Assessment

Rapid visual overview of the child, including airway patency, neurologic status, and environmental exposure (heat, fire, toxins, injury), followed by immediate stabilization such as cervical spine immobilization and cardiopulmonary resuscitation (CPR).

Airway

› Position the child supine for maximal visualization of the airway (maintaining cervical spine stabilization and log rolling if required).

› Assess patency and efficacy of the airway.

› Open the airway manually if needed.

› Use the jaw-thrust or chin-lift maneuver as needed to support a patent airway.

› Implement the American Heart Association's guidelines for CPR: Use the acronym CAB—circulation, airway, and breathing.

Breathing

› Assess whether the child is breathing independently.

› Assess respiratory rate adequacy.

› Provide a source of oxygen as required (nasal cannula, mask, nonrebreathing mask).

› Provide artificial breathing with a bag-valve mask.

Circulation

› Assess the child's heart rate; use the brachial artery for infants, and a single-side carotid artery for older children.

› Initiate chest compressions if the child is bradycardic or the pulse is absent.

› Place large-bore intravenous catheters or intraosseous catheters (**Figure 29-3**) if required for administering resuscitative fluid boluses, antiarrhythmic medications, antiseizure medications, bicarbonate for acidosis correction, and other medications as needed.

Neurologic Status (Disability)

› Rapidly assess the child's ability to respond.

› Assess the child's level of consciousness.

› Use the pediatric Glasgow Coma Scale. If the score is 8 or less, intubation is required.

› Assess **PERRLA** (pupil reaction: pupils equal, round, reactive to light, and accommodation).

TABLE 29-3	Interdisciplinary Priorities When Stabilizing Children in Emergency Care Settings (*continued*)

Fluid Status

> › Assess the child's level of dehydration.
> › Assess the child's pulse and blood pressure frequently.
> › Correct fluid status as needed.
> › In case of fluid overload, administer mannitol or albumin infusion as ordered.

Blood Glucose

> › Assess the child's blood glucose level; administer a source of glucose as needed for hypoglycemia.
> › If the child is in diabetic ketoacidosis (DKA), administer insulin as ordered.

Continue assessments and responses to treatments and interventions (e.g., with serial vital signs).

Transfer the child to the level of care required for further stabilization and treatments.

Comfort, support, and educate the family concerning the process of stabilization.

Data from Emergency Nurses Association. (2009). *Core curriculum for pediatric nursing.* (2nd ed.). Retrieved from www.ena.org/publications

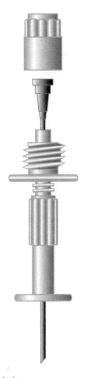

Figure 29-3 *A pediatric intraosseous needle.*

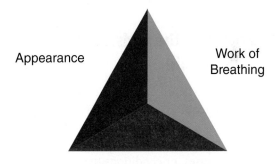

Figure 29-4 *The Pediatric Assessment Triangle.*

Reproduced from Horeczko, T., Enriquez, B., McGrath, N. E., Causche-Hill, M., & Lewis, R. J. (2013). The Pediatric Assessment Triangle: Accuracy of its application by nurses in the triage of children. *Journal of Emergency Nursing, 39*(2), 182—189. Copyright 2013, with permission from Elsevier.

- Circulation to the skin: Considers both bleeding and overall perfusion via the child's skin color (pallor, cyanosis, flushed with fever, mottling)

UNIQUE FOR KIDS

Most Frequent Pediatric Diagnoses in the Emergency Department by Body System

1. Poisoning and injury
2. Disorders of the respiratory tract
3. Central and peripheral nervous tract disorders
4. Infectious processes
5. Gastrointestinal and digestive ailments
6. Integumentary disorders
7. Psychological, behavioral, or mental health issues
8. Disorders and injuries to the musculoskeletal system

Data from Agency for Health Care Research and Quality (AHRQ). (2013). Care of children and adolescents in U.S. hospitals. Retrieved from https://archive.ahrq.gov/data/hcup/factbk4/factbk4.htm

prioritize and triage children who present to an ED (**Figure 29-4**). The PAT focuses on rapid visualization of the child's overall appearance, including color, level of consciousness, respiratory distress, level of shock, and overall failure. The three components of the PAT are as follows (Horeczko, Enriquez, McGrath, Gausche-Hill, & Lewis, 2013):

- Appearance, including mental status changes and patency of the airway
- Work of breathing: Rapidly visualizes a child's respiratory effort, presence of distress including retractions, and pattern of breathing

Transferring Children to the Pediatric Intensive Care Unit

After stabilization in the ED, a child may be either discharged, admitted to the acute care pediatric unit, or transferred to a critical care or pediatric intensive care unit for further monitoring and an advanced level of interdisciplinary care. The objective of the ED personnel is to provide the needed assessment, initial diagnostics, and stabilization in the ED setting, and then, when warranted, transfer the child as soon as possible to the intensive care unit (ICU). Lengthy time periods in the ED are stressful for families, as these environments offer little room for rest, nutrition, and self-care of family members.

Once the child is in the PICU, implementation of family-centered care should include open visitation, family presence during invasive procedures, family-centered rounding, and family conferences (Meert, Clark, & Eggly, 2013).

Supervision at the Bedside of a Critically Ill Child

Children are transferred to intensive care settings when their condition requires an increased level of nursing care and continuous monitoring on cardiac and respiratory monitors. Children with significant injuries, life-threatening infectious processes, or conditions that affect their neurologic status are treated in an ICU setting, where direct nursing care is provided in 1:1 or 1:2 ratios. This high level of monitoring ensures that the interdisciplinary pediatric team receives information on the child's minute-by-minute clinical status and facilitates rapid responses if the child's condition declines. The staff in the pediatric intensive care environment is prepared to respond to hemodynamic instability, airway compromise, cardiopulmonary arrest, or any other status in need of rapid response.

Within the ICU setting, children are typically placed in individual rooms with glass doors facing a central nursing station. This setup provides for visual monitoring of the child's condition and visual access to the cardiopulmonary monitors. The frequency of supervision depends on the acuity level of the child.

Safety Through Handoffs Across Settings

Nursing supervision of children placed in PICU settings requires specialized skills, training, and advanced-level knowledge of critical conditions. One of the most important skills of the PICU nurse is effective professional communication. Such a nurse must be able to participate in bedside rounds and make contributions to the team concerning the outcomes of the higher-level monitoring and supervision.

The PICU nurse must be skilled at taking reports from the ED nurse (or transferring hospital) and giving reports to those receiving the child after PICU discharge. Reports given between nurses are frequently referred to as *handoffs*, as the responsibility for care is being handed to a different care provider in a different setting. Handoffs must be comprehensive enough to provide information on the child's entire care experience, from the time the child came to the ED to the moment of handoff. Most healthcare institutions have established a handoff policy and specific guidelines. Most handoffs include the following components:

- The child's age, weight, height, allergies, primary language, developmental level, and medical diagnosis(es)
- Pertinent past medical history
- Summary of recent care required, including outcomes of laboratory analysis, diagnostics, and interactions with specialists
- Recent vital signs or other monitoring information
- Current medications and timing of critical infusions, such as last antibiotics, and recent peaks and trough values
- Summary of information related to body systems—for example, for the respiratory system: rate, depth, oxygen saturations, need for suctioning, need for oxygen delivery, presence of retractions, and overall respiratory efficacy and status
- Diagnostic results pending
- Status of family dynamics and needs; presence of family at the bedside and their level of involvement
- Known aspects of the medical treatment plan
- Pertinent aspects of the child's temperament, emotional needs, and play needs

Procedural Sedation

The use of conscious sedation during invasive bedside procedures is not uncommon in the PICU setting. Children who require lumbar punctures, bone marrow aspirations or biopsies, and placement of chest tubes or bedside central lines will require a level of **procedural sedation**. This type of sedation involves the child breathing independently but requires constant visual supervision and rapid airway support by a certified team. The PICU nurse may be assigned to obtain the signature for procedural informed consent from the parent or legal guardian and to document the procedure minute by minute at the bedside. The PICU intensivist or other primary caregiver will provide airway management and administration of the sedation medication (e.g., propofol). The team works together seamlessly to provide safety at all times. Alarms require rapid attention to prevent harm.

A full time-out is required for safety before any procedure is begun, and all members of the team who will be involved with the procedure must be present during this meeting. The pediatric nurse makes sure the time-out confirms the patient's full name, birth date, medical record number, diagnosis, procedure to be implemented, and assurance of consent. Due to the risky nature of procedural sedation, it is imperative that the nurse ensures a full time-out is performed and documents that the time-out occurred and who was present.

Transferring Children to the Pediatric Acute Care Hospital Unit

Children who no longer need a higher level of observation and monitoring will be transferred to the pediatric hospital unit in preparation for discharge. Pediatric hospital units, called **pediatric acute care** units, provide continued assessments and, if the technology is available, monitoring, but at a lesser level of intensity, without the need for 1:1 or 1:2 nursing care ratios. Families typically express relief when the transfer occurs, as the transfer of care may signify that the child is now clinically stable and is healing. Other families may become more stressed, however, as they know the child will not be provided the same level of advanced care and frequency of observation that was received in the intensive care environment. Education, support, and anticipatory guidance must be provided to relieve their worries. Eliciting the assistance of a social worker and a Child Life specialist can be helpful if the family expresses concern about the transfer to a lower level of care.

Many pediatric acute care hospitals post the phone number and criteria for calling a rapid response team (akin to the code blue team) if the child's condition worsens while on the pediatric hospital unit (**Table 29-4**). Families may find comfort in knowing that they can call for immediate help by taking steps beyond pressing the call light button at the child's bedside, as this call may not be answered right away. Research has shown that posting the criteria for and phone number of a rapid response team does not lead to an inappropriate use of the service by family members. The pediatric nurse must be very familiar with how to call

TABLE 29-4 Hospital Emergency Codes

Although hospitals vary in their use of **color-coded alarms**, the following codes are often used in ED, PICU, and acute care settings to alert the pediatric healthcare team that support is required. Check with your healthcare institutions for its exact codes used, and become familiar with them to ensure help is provided expeditiously.

› *Code blue:* A cardiopulmonary arrest is taking place. The code team must respond to help provide resuscitation assistance.

› *Code red:* A fire is occurring in the building. Safety procedures for containment, evacuation, and emergency response must be followed to reduce injury or prevent death.

› *Code orange:* A hazardous material has been spilled. A team approach is required for containment, evacuation, rescue, and cleanup. Material Safety Data Sheets (MSDS) are used as guidelines to prevent injury.

› *Code yellow:* A bomb threat is currently happening. A rehearsed approach for safety of the staff and patients is required.

› *Code triage:* A mass-casualty incident has occurred. Institutional policies need to be implemented to prepare for the care of a large number of ill and injured persons, possibly representing ages across the lifespan; the response needs to be rapidly coordinated and resources allocated.

› *Code gray:* A threatening person is currently in the facility. A team approach is needed to provide support to those involved and to provide safety for those near the escalating situation.

› *Code pink:* A newborn or infant abduction has occurred. Procedures need to be activated to secure stairwells, exits, and elevators while a search is conducted to find the baby.

› *Code purple:* An older child has been abducted. Procedures need to be activated to secure stairwells, exits, and elevators while a search is conducted to find the missing child.

› *Code silver:* An active shooter or a person with a gun is threatening an individual or group. Rapid safety and security processes are needed to prevent injury or death.

Code red	Fire
Code black	Bomb threat/ suspicious package
Code purple	Hostage taking
Code white	Actual or potential violent behavior
Code yellow	Missing patient
Code brown	Hazardous material spill/leak
Code grey	Infrastructure loss/air exclusion
Code orange	External disaster
Code green	Evacuation
Code blue	Cardiac arrest/ medical emergency

Figure 29-5 *Hospital emergency codes.*

a code blue team, rapid response team, or any number of possible "codes" that provide rapid assistance (**Figure 29-5**).

The transfer a child from the PICU to the pediatric hospital unit requires a thorough handoff. It is not uncommon for the PICU nurse to accompany the child and family down to the receiving unit to make sure the handoff report is given directly to the nurse who will be providing care. The receiving nurse should then make sure the acute care hospitalist knows about the timing of the transfer, as

new medical orders will need to be written for the care of the child. The family will be anxious to meet the physician assigned to their child's care on the new unit and discuss the revised interdisciplinary care plan.

Preparing the Family for Discharge

When the child's condition improves to the point that discharge is pending, the nurse moves into the role of educator. The family needs to be taught how to safely administer any medication or treatment independently at home. The family also needs to know the indications for and side effects of all medications. Follow-up appointments must be explained. Most importantly, the family needs to know which clinical signs or symptoms arising in the child warrant a call to the physician or a return to the ED.

Discharge should be a celebratory event for families—one that is greatly anticipated and welcomed. Taking the time to explain all discharge instructions will reduce the chance of readmission (also known as recidivism).

QUALITY AND SAFETY

Advanced Emergency Response Certifications

Nurses can become certified in a number of areas where advanced assessments and skills are taught. Four examples include the following certifications:

- Pediatric Advanced Life Support (PALS)
- Neonatal Resuscitation Program (NRP)
- Adult Cardiac Life Support (ACLS)
- Emergency Nursing Pediatric Course (ENPC)

For more information on the PALS, NRP, and ACLS certifications, see the American Heart Association's website (http://www.heart.org/ HEARTORG/). For the ENPC certification, see the Emergency Nursing Association's website (https://www.ena.org).

Case Study

A 4-month-old infant has presented to the emergency department with a history of fevers, poor oral intake, productive cough, and increasing lethargy. The parents have brought the child in at the urgent request of their pediatrician, who saw the infant just prior to the ED visit. The father describes that the infant has been sick for 5 days but just today became more symptomatic with no interest in breastfeeding or bottle feeding and showing increasing "sleepiness." The infant is quiet but demonstrates adventitious

breath sounds, tight persistent coughing spells followed with a short "whooping" sound, fever, and clinical signs of moderate dehydration. The mother states that neither the infant nor the 2½-year-old toddler sibling have had any childhood vaccines.

The ED team begins a process of assessment and stabilization. A length-based resuscitation tape is used to determine the equipment needed for the child's weight and height. Vital signs, oxygenation saturation, arterial blood gases, and

(continues)

Case Study *(continued)*

laboratory analysis specimens are taken for rapid identification of streptococcal infection, respiratory syncytial virus (RSV), and influenza A and B. During the placement of a 23-gauge peripheral angiocatheter, a complete blood cell count with manual differentiation, chemistry panel, and blood culture are all collected. A urinary collection bag is placed over the infant girl's perineum to obtain a specimen for urinalysis and culture. A 0.9% normal saline bolus is given (Y-ed) via the tubing of a $D_{5\frac{1}{2}}NS$ 1× fluid maintenance line and is administered over 30 minutes. The child is placed on droplet and contact precautions and is maintained on NPO (nothing by mouth) status. Oxygen is given to the child via nasal cannula, and the respiratory therapist is paged overhead to stabilize the airway, provide suction, and administer nebulizers. The infection control nurse is paged, as the laboratory specimen for pertussis has come back positive. The child will be transferred to the PICU.

Case Study Questions

1. Which tests are commonly used to rapidly determine if a child is infected with RSV, influenza, and pertussis?

2. What are possible means by which the infant may have been exposed to a person infected with pertussis in the community?

3. Which information needs to be shared with the receiving PICU unit during handoff?

4. Calculate the infant's fluid maintenance needs, 0.9% NS bolus volume, and safe dose for her first dose of an antibiotic for pertussis (azithromycin dose range: 10 mg/kg for the first day, followed by 5 mg/kg for days 2–5, or longer if indicated) if she weighs 13.6 pounds.

As the Case Evolves...

Although it is most likely the infant has pertussis, the child's father is concerned about long-term complications if the infant is infected with RSV.

5. Which of the following are long-term complications of RSV infection?
   A. Respiratory failure
   B. Sepsis
   C. Secondary bacterial infections
   D. Pleural effusion
   E. Carditis

Chapter Summary

- Most children will never have to experience a hospitalization during their developmental period. When they do, pediatric nurses must apply principles of developmentally appropriate assessment, stabilization, education, support, and family-centered care.

- Children may need initial evaluation in the emergency department, where rapid assessments, stabilization, and initial diagnostics are performed. Then, as required, they may need a transfer to the pediatric intensive care unit or be admitted to the pediatric acute care setting.

- The family and the child will likely experience significant stress and fear surrounding the circumstances of hospitalization across all settings. Providing support, clear communication, and honest explanations of the treatment plan will help the family cope.

- Approximately 18% of hospitalizations in the United States involve children 17 years of age or younger, and almost two-thirds of hospitalizations involve neonates and infants. Children who reside in low-income areas (50%) are much more likely to be admitted from the ED to the pediatric hospital unit than children who reside in higher-income areas (25%).

- The pediatric nurse is expected to assist the interdisciplinary team in rapid assessment, stabilization, and transfer of pediatric patients to an appropriate level of care. This process is facilitated by seamless communication via effective handoffs and by supporting, educating, and guiding children and families through the very stressful scenario.

- The pediatric nurse must have the level of skill required to provide advanced assessment, airway management, stabilization, monitoring, and communication of changes in the critically ill or injured child.

Bibliography

Agency for Health Care Research and Quality (AHRQ). (2013). Care of children and adolescents in U.S. hospitals. Retrieved from https://archive.ahrq.gov/data/hcup/factbk4/factbk4.htm

American Association of Critical-Care Nurses. (2013). Strategies for managing alarm fatigue [Newsletter article]. *NTI ActionPak.* American Nurses Association (ANA). (2012). Frequently asked questions: Roles of state boards of nursing: Licensure, regulation and complaint investigation. Retrieved from http://www.nursingworld.org/MainMenuCategories/Tools/State-Boards-of-Nursing-FAQ.pdf

American Nurses Association (ANA). (2016). Code of ethics for nurses with interpretive statements. Retrieved from http://nursingworld.org/DocumentVault/Ethics-1/Code-of-Ethics-for-Nurses.html

Emergency Nurses Association. (2009). *Core curriculum for pediatric nursing* (2nd ed.). Retrieved from https://www.ena.org/publications /ena/Pages/CoreCurriculumPedsNursing.aspx

Foster, M. J., Whitehead, L., Maybee, P., & Cullens, V. (2013). The parents', hospitalized child's, and health care providers' perceptions and experiences of family centered care within a pediatric critical care setting: A metasynthesis of qualitative research. *Journal of Family Nursing, 19*(4), 431–468.

Horeczko, T., Enriquez, B., McGrath, N. E., Gausche-Hill, M., & Lewis, R. J. (2013). The Pediatric Assessment Triangle: Accuracy of its application by nurses in the triage of children. *Journal of Emergency Nursing, 39*(2), 182–189.

Meert, K. L., Clark, J., & Eggly, S. (2013). Family-centered care in the pediatric intensive care unit. *Pediatric Clinics of North America, 60*(3), 761–772.

Uhl, T., Fisher, K., Docherty, S. L., & Brandon, D. H. (2013). Insights into patient and family-centered care through the hospital experiences of parents. *Journal of Obstetric, Gynecologic, & Neonatal Nursing, 42*, 121–131.

Wier, L. M., Yu, H., Owens, P. L., & Washington, R. (2013). Overview of children in the emergency department, 2010. Healthcare Cost and Utilization Project. Statistical Brief. Retrieved from http:// www.hcup-us.ahrq.gov/reports/statbriefs/sb157.pdf

CHAPTER 30

The Dying Child

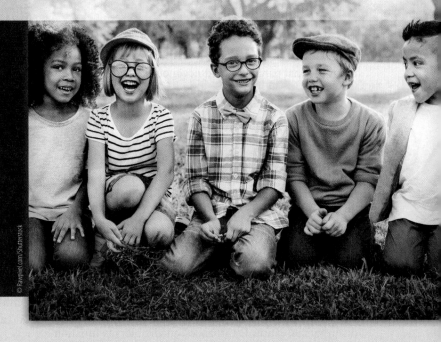

© Rawpixel.com/Shutterstock

LEARNING OBJECTIVES

1. Apply key nursing concepts related to care for the family experiencing the death of a child and the dying process for children.
2. Evaluate the emotional impact of a child going through the dying process on parents, guardians, and siblings.
3. Analyze the physiological dying process of a child versus an adult.
4. Assess the care needs of a dying child.
5. Differentiate the principles of pediatric hospice care from the principles of care provided in the hospital setting.
6. Design nursing care appropriate to a child dying from complications of a chronic disease and to a child dying from a traumatic accident.

KEY TERMS

Dying process
Dysfunctional grief
End-of-life care
Grief
Hospice care
Kübler-Ross, Elisabeth
Palliative care
Palliative measures
Trieste Charter

Introduction

The death of a child can be emotionally traumatic for the immediate family and those within the family's community. Many say that parents should never outlive their child and describe how the death of a child has life-changing effects on those who survive. These life-changing effects can be consequential in daily functioning. **Grief**, or the process of deep sorrow, can last a lifetime, can have impact on the parent's ability to function at work (Fox, Cacciatore, & Lacasse, 2014), and can strain a marriage (Kastenbaum, 2015). Grief can also significantly impact how the parents interact with the surviving siblings.

Because the death of a child is so often unexpected, an unhealthy reaction that can develop is called **dysfunctional grief**. Here, one demonstrates complicated grief over a period of at least a year. Dysfunctional grief entails prolonged emotional reactions, including longing, loneliness, yearnings for the child, depression, low self-esteem, sleep disturbances, eating disturbances, and inability to function in roles such as employment and marriage (Lee, 2015).

For the pediatric healthcare team, the loss of a child can also produce a level of grief that has a significant impact on their ability to function professionally. It is imperative that a pediatric healthcare provider who experiences a child's death be offered opportunities to debrief, talk about the circumstances associated with the death, and receive professional help (**Figure 30-1**).

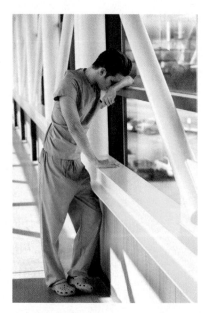

Figure 30-1 *It is imperative that a pediatric healthcare provider who experiences a child's death be offered opportunities to debrief, talk about the circumstances associated with the death, and receive professional help.*

© jonathandowney/iStockphoto.com

BEST PRACTICES

Healthcare professionals who work in environments when there is a potential for the death of a child would benefit greatly from training in how best to communicate with the dying child, the child's siblings, and the child's parents. The pertinent aspects of communication in the dying process include being able to provide support, being honest about death, explaining the process of caring for a dying child or a dead child's body, and describing the care needed for the child's siblings.

Developmental Aspects of Understanding Death

Children's understanding of death is highly dependent on their developmental stage. Most young children do not comprehend what is happening to them and, therefore, might display their emotions by clinging to their primary caregiver and fearing separation. Older children, owing to their concrete thinking abilities, are able to understand the permanence of death and may display their emotions by asking poignant questions, eliciting information about the **dying process** (i.e., the predictable physiological changes and emotional states that occur as the end of life approaches), and sharing their concerns. Each developmental stage has predictable responses to the dying process and predictable levels of understanding of death. Culture, ethnicity, religion, spirituality, and openness of family discussions can all influence how a child comprehends death and dying.

FAMILY EDUCATION

Developmental Factors Associated with Death

Each developmental stage has unique perspectives and levels of understanding concerning death. In general, the nurse can predict the responses and needs of the dying child according to their developmental stage.

Infants
- Have no concept of death
- May show reactions concerning hospitalization, including fears of separation and stranger anxiety
- React to changes in their routine
- Must have their needs cared for immediately to continue the process of building trust

(continues)

Toddlers

- Have little or no concept of the permanence of death
- Will demonstrate egocentric thinking and processing of information
- Often reflect the emotions displayed by the adults— anxiety, sadness, anger
- Continue to show anxiety and powerful reactions to medical procedures, fear of pain and discomfort, and both stranger and separation anxiety
- May be very clingy and emotionally needy

Preschoolers

- Participate in magical thinking—they believe their thoughts have power and can cause events to take place, such as death
- May connect the dying process with punishment
- Often see death as temporary and reversible
- Continue to demonstrate egocentric thinking and processing
- May demonstrate regressive behaviors to an earlier developmental stage (acting in an infant-like or toddler-like manner)

School-Age Children

- By the age of 7 to 8 years, process death as permanent, inevitable, and universal
- May not be able to comprehend their own immortality
- Express fears specific to the dying process
- Respond to factual information and ask many questions related to death; may show fascination with details about death
- May be uncooperative, defiant, and frustrating in their behaviors, which are based in fear of the unknown
- See death as something beyond their control

Adolescents

- See death and the death process as adults do—as universal, inevitable, and irreversible
- May show frustration and anger with dying, as this is the period of time when they are learning their identity and thinking about their future
- Often continue to depend on their peers and their social network for support, though those networks may diminish as peers become frightened or unable to process the teen's death
- May push family away and then feel isolated
- Can be very distressed about changes in their physical appearance associated with the dying process

Data from Webb, N. B. (2010). *Helping bereaved children: A handbook for practitioners* (3rd ed.). London, UK: Guilford Press.

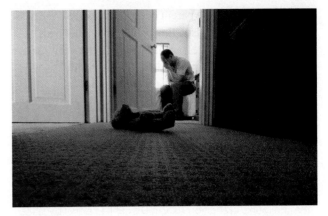

Figure 30-2 *Most parents suffer tremendous feelings of grief and loss.*
© fasphotographic/iStock/Getty Images

Reactions of Parents and Siblings

The reaction to a child's death can be quite individualized for parents and siblings. This reaction may be based on the adult's previous experiences with loss or professional background. Most parents suffer tremendous feelings of grief and loss (**Figure 30-2**). Some parents may have healthy reactions, including being supportive of others, and providing comfort and support to grieving siblings. Other parents who have strained interpersonal relationships, personal stressors, social isolation, and spiritual distress may demonstrate unhealthy responses, including social withdrawal, substance abuse, self-harm, and isolation (Kastenbaum, 2015).

The pediatric nurse must be able to identify the needs of the parents and reach out to them as appropriate. The support provided to a parent of a dying child should be interdisciplinary, family centered, care focused, and non-judgmental. Understanding the widely accepted model of the series of predictable emotional stages experienced by those who are surviving a child's death, as developed by **Elisabeth Kübler-Ross** (1969), can greatly assist the pediatric nurse in understanding the emotional responses of a parent. Kübler-Ross's (1969) stages of grief are usually experienced in the following order and can be applied to a parent's reaction to the impending death of his or her child:

1. Denial: The first reaction experienced by a parent is characterized by shock and disbelief.
2. Anger: The parent realizes that he or she cannot change the situation and the death of the child is imminent and a reality.
3. Bargaining: The parent tries to hold onto hope of avoidance by negotiating for more time, or by negotiating with a spiritual or religious force.

4. Depression: The parent demonstrates great sadness, mournfulness, isolation, grief, and sullenness.
5. Acceptance: The parent embraces the very real or inevitable impending death of the child.

Types of Care for the Dying Child

End-of-life care is a phrase used synonymously with *palliative care*. Nevertheless, one should distinguish the aspects of end-of-life care that are different from palliative care.

The term **palliative care** refers to a multidisciplinary approach to the process of dying that can begin before the physiological aspects of dying start. This kind of care can be offered to the child and the family during the early process of a poor prognosis. Palliative care includes support with last wishes or "bucket lists" that the family wants to experience before the loss of the child, and includes conversations about the wishes of the family concerning the death process and after death plans. Palliative care recognizes that there is no cure for the child's condition, so it focuses on emotional support, resource allocation, symptom management, education, honest and straightforward communication with all family members involved in the child's dying process, and the building and implementation of a therapeutic environment for the dying child. In other words, palliative care is a unique and comprehensive plan to promote quality of life for the time that is left (**Figure 30-3**).

Palliative care can also refer to the types of medical treatments offered to the child. For example, for a child with a terminal oncologic diagnosis, palliative radiation may be administered to shrink tumors that do not respond to chemotherapy or are considered inoperable. Palliative

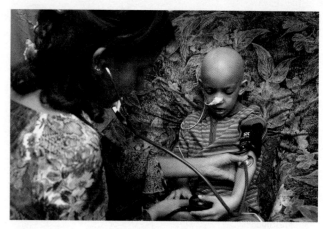

Figure 30-3 *Palliative care focuses on building and implementation of a therapeutic environment for the dying child.*
© LADA/Science Source

chemotherapy may be administered not to seek a cure, but rather to decrease a tumor size or burden and so provide relief from symptoms. These kinds of **palliative measures** may also include surgical debulking of tumor size or removal of a tumor that is causing pain.

The term **end-of-life care** is often used to describe the care aspects of the dying process. It can denote the wishes, cultural practices, and care activities surrounding the imminent death of the child.

Physiological Aspects of the Dying Process

The human body, regardless of the age, goes through predictable physiological changes during the dying process. In general, a child may potentially display 12 signs of impending death (Palliative Care Australia, n.d.):

- Signs of increasing physical weakness, evidence of fatigue, and increased desire to sleep
- Increasing disorientation and confusion; may try to get up to find someone or do something
- Loss of appetite
- Inability to swallow, which poses a choking risk and produces discomfort if attempts are made to drink or eat, or if someone places food or drink in the child's mouth
- Slowed metabolism
- Changes in the gastrointestinal system, including slowed or diminished peristalsis and elimination
- Changes in the genitourinary system, as the kidneys are shutting down and not producing urine
- Buildup of waste products in the blood, which may contribute to an increasing state of lethargy and eventually coma

- Early phases of imminent death: tachypnea and labored breathing
- Later phases of imminent death: a classic breathing pattern called Cheyne-Stokes respiration, marked by gradual hyperpnea or hypoapnea followed by a period of apnea; demonstrates evidence of hypoperfusion of the respiratory center in the brain (**Figure 30-4**)
- Peripheral blood shunting that leaves the hands, fingers, and toes cool to the touch
- Mottling of the skin that leaves a pattern like a jigsaw puzzle of darkened lines

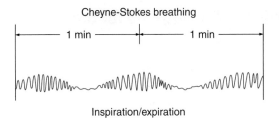

Figure 30-4 *Cheyne-Stokes breathing pattern.*

PHARMACOLOGY

Symptom management for children who are dying is challenging and often the responsibility of the pediatric nurse. Research has shown that only 27% of dying children experience pain relief and that the four most common symptoms experienced during a child's last weeks of life are pain, poor appetite, fatigue, and respiratory distress (Cherny, 2010). Knowledge of palliative care, traditional medications, and adjunctive therapies is a priority in providing holistic care. One must take into consideration the child's previous experiences with narcotics, each medication's half-life, administration guidelines, institutional formulary (approval), tolerance level, potential symptoms, and drug allergy. Medications that may be used in children during the dying process include the following (Gregoire & Frager, 2006; World Health Organization [WHO], 2013):

Pain Control
- Opioids such as morphine, hydrocodone, fentanyl, oxycodone, and hydromorphone

Oral Secretion Control (Antisecretory Agents)
- Transdermal or subcutaneous anticholinergics such as hyoscine hydrobromide, atropine, hyoscine butylbromide, and glycopyrronium/glycopyrrolate
- Antimuscarinic drugs

Antianxiety Agents
- Benzodiazepines such as lorazepam or diazepam

Adjuvant Medications for Breakthrough Pain
- Tricyclic antidepressants such as serotonin–norepinephrine reuptake inhibitors (SNRIs)
- Nonsteroidal anti-inflammatory drugs (NSAIDs)
- Anticonvulsants (for neuropathic pain) such as carbamazepine and gabapentin

Antinausea Medications
- Serotonin 5-hydroxytriptamine antagonist such as ondansetron
- Prokinetic agents such as metoclopramide for delayed gastric emptying

Psychosocial Aspects of the Dying Process

The family of a dying child may be struggling with the cessation of all diagnostic and curative efforts to assist the child's progressing injury, disease, or condition. It is very hard for many parents to accept the process of first participating in aggressive treatment and cure models and then switching to only palliative measures. Often, the application of technology such as monitoring systems, intravenous fluids, and central lines is withheld as the child begins the final dying stages. Parents need tremendous psychological support during this difficult time.

Children who are trying to understand the process they are going through, and trying to understand the emotional reactions of those around them, can struggle with their own psychosocial aspects of dying. Before they experience a decreased level of consciousness or loss of consciousness, they may ask provocative questions about what will happen to them as they die. It is important that the pediatric healthcare team help the dying child both physically with symptom management so comfort can be obtained, and mentally and spiritually. The pediatric nurse should be prepared to be close to the child and answer any questions about spiritual concerns. Open communication is imperative during this difficult time. The nurse should not attempt to proscribe his or her own religious or spiritual beliefs to the child; rather, the nurse should ask questions about the child's beliefs and understandings of death and support whatever the child states or describes. The following open-ended questions may be of value:

- "Tell me about your understanding of your condition. . ."
- "Tell me about your understanding of death. . ."
- "Tell me about your thoughts of what happens after death. . ."
- "Tell me about what is important to you and your family right now. . ."
- "Tell me how I can help you and your family right now. . ."
- "Tell me anything I can get for you for your comfort at this time. . ."
- "Tell me if there is someone you want to talk to right now. . ."

Pediatric Nursing Care for the Dying Child

Caring for the dying child takes specialized skills. Developing a care plan and providing help for the family of a dying child should take the following considerations into account:

- Provide a quiet, warm, nurturing, low-stress environment for the child and family that feels comfortable.
- Continue to provide warm baths, skin care, mouth care, hair brushing, and the basic elements of meticulous nursing care that promote a sense of well-being and comfort.
- Be honest about the expected course of events; explain the diagnosis, prognosis, medications, and resources available.
- Do not isolate the family; frequently check in with them and offer support, even if it is in silence.
- Encourage the family to talk, share, and express their emotions with the team; encourage the child, siblings, and parents to ask questions.
- Secure the assistance of the Child Life team to offer education, support, medical play, and communication with the child's school, teachers, and schoolmates.
- Continue to provide the child with distractions, play opportunities, and moments of joy found only in childhood.
- Promote the disclosure and solicitation of support and assistance from the family's social network, neighbors, and community; encourage others to provide food, comfort, respite care for the siblings, and overall support of the grieving parents.
- Ask the child what his or her wishes are; secure applications for organizations that provide "last wish" fulfillments for terminally ill children.
- Mobilize an interdisciplinary team approach; assemble a team of pediatric professionals who can be comprehensive in their views and diverse in their support. Team members should include physicians, nurses, social workers, chaplains, child psychologists, pharmacists, and case managers.
- Secure involvement with the desired clergy or spiritual support networks.
- Provide comprehensive symptom management for the child and keep the child clean, dry, and in positions of comfort; encourage physical contact and cuddling as tolerated.
- In the last stages of the dying process, assess the child's ability to swallow; provide nutrition and oral fluids only if safe to prevent choking.
- Provide comfort to the child by telling the child that he or she is not alone in the dying process, and offer reassurance that he or she is cared for, cherished, and will be kept comfortable.
- When appropriate, encourage the child to feel permission from loved ones to die; some children may feel fear of hurting their parents and siblings and need encouragement to relax and let go.

Settings for a Dying Child

When able, the pediatric healthcare team should discuss with the family in advance what their wishes are concerning the setting in which the child will die.

Hospital

Children may die in a hospital setting, especially if they experience a traumatic death from an injury or accident. Children who have an expected shorter lifespan from complications associated with a chronic illness or congenital anomaly may not benefit from dying in a hospital setting. Not all urban, suburban, and rural communities in the United States have inpatient hospice units, so the choice may be made to have a child die in the hospital. Not all families desire this outcome, but others may choose the hospital setting over having the child die at home. Because hospital settings focus on diagnostics and treatments, hospital nurses may not feel comfortable or have the competencies required for a peaceful and symptom-controlled death in an acute care setting.

RESEARCH EVIDENCE

According to Dussel et al. (2009), parents who have the opportunity to plan the location of their child's death are more likely to have the child die at home. A significantly greater number who plan for the location of the child's death report feeling prepared for the child's end of life.

Pediatric Hospice Settings

It is important to distinguish between hospice care and palliative care. **Hospice care** is provided to a child nearing the end of the life when the application of medical diagnostics and treatments is no longer considered. Palliative care, which is a part of hospice care, is also a separate area of medical and nursing practice provided while the patient is still receiving treatment for the condition. Hospice care is provided to give the child and the family the best quality of life possible in the last 6 months of the child's life.

Although such facilities are few and far between, children who are dying may be able to have their death experience take place in a hospice setting created especially for children.

When a child is believed to be in the last 6 months of life, the family can be referred to a hospice institution for continued care. The pediatric healthcare hospice team is trained to provide end-of-life care in a setting that mimics a home environment with comfortable furniture, soothing lighting, and minimal stimulation.

UNIQUE FOR KIDS

Hospice care differs for children who are dying versus adults who are dying, as children's developmental needs are incorporated into the hospice care plan. Hospice nurses working with dying children have a foundation of knowledge around developmental stages and developmental theories that enables them to provide comprehensive and supportive care across childhood.

Pediatric Hospice Services at Home

Pediatric home hospice services should be secured whenever possible. Specific conditions must be met for a child to die at home while being assisted with hospice services. An adult must be present who is willing and capable to care for the child both emotionally and via symptom management. Goals of pediatric hospice care provided to families are threefold and should include identifying and reducing stress for all those involved (Baranowski, n.d.; Center for Hospice Care Southeast Connecticut, 2016):

- The provision of hands-on help with the day-to-day care of a child in palliative care or who is actively in the dying phases
- The provision of emotional, spiritual, and bereavement support and the promotion of well-being for both the patient and the family
- The provision of care for the caregivers providing for the child, including education, listening, and backup support

Traumatic Death in the Emergency Department

Although such events are rare, the traumatic and unexpected death of a child is a profound loss. A traumatic loss is a very different experience than the loss of a child who has been battling a chronic or life-threatening condition for a period of time. Both experiences produce great emotional responses, but a traumatic death can also produce tremendous guilt and extreme despair. Etiologies for sudden and unexpected deaths of children in emergency department (ED) settings include sepsis or other severe infections (pneumonia, meningitis, or encephalitis), airway obstruction, aspiration, poisonings or toxic exposures, falls, motor vehicle accidents, seizure disorders, complications of congenital anomalies, and sudden infant death syndrome (SIDS) or sudden unexpected death in childhood (SUDC).

Pediatric healthcare professionals who work in environments where children receive care after traumatic events must have specialized skills in caring for the family during the shock and disbelief phase. The team must immediately mobilize multiple resources such as a social worker, nurse administrator, psychologist, hospital chaplain, and other personnel who are experienced with helping a family during the initial emotional upheaval. Child Life specialists can assist with the collection of hair, footprints, and handprints along with photographs using a preassembled memory box. When possible, the parents should be allowed to witness the resuscitation of the child. Great sensitivity must be displayed to the child's body after prolonged resuscitation efforts, and family members need time with the child to say goodbye before the child is wrapped and taken to the morgue. Ensure that the family has safe transportation home after the loss of a child. Securing follow-up emotional help is also an unwritten responsibility of the team. The child and family should be kept together as long as desired and feasible. When an infant or child dies in the emergency room setting, the medical examiner must also be notified.

Regardless of the setting where a child experiences the dying process, the child should be respected and offered support to ensure an honest, dignified dying process. In 2012, the United Nations General Assembly created the **Trieste Charter**, a list of rights of the dying child within the United Nations' declaration of the rights of the child (Benini, Vecchi, & Orzalesi, 2014):

- To be considered a person until death irrespective of age, location, illness, and care setting
- To receive effective treatment for pain, and physical and psychological symptoms causing suffering, through qualified, comprehensive, and continuous care
- To be listened to and properly informed about his or her illness with consideration for his or her wishes, age, and ability to understand
- To participate, on the basis of his or her abilities, values, and wishes, in care choices about his or her life, illness, and death
- To express and, whenever possible, have his or her feelings, wishes, and expectations taken into account
- To have his or her cultural, spiritual, and religious beliefs respected and receive spiritual care and support in accordance with his or her wishes and choices
- To have a social and relational life suitable to his or her age, illness, and expectations

- To be surrounded by family members and loved ones who are adequately supported and protected from the burden of the child's illness
- To be cared for in a setting appropriate for his or her age, needs, and wishes and that allows the proximity of the family
- To have access to child-specific palliative care programs that avoid futile or excessively burdensome practices and therapeutic abandonment*

The pediatric healthcare team should work collectively to ensure these rights of the dying child are upheld and communicated to the child's family.

Case Study

Kathleen, a 15-year-old girl, has been in the pediatric unit of a large urban hospital receiving end-of-life care. She was diagnosed with acute myeloid leukemia 3 years ago and has experienced a relapse of her leukemia 3 times. She is no longer receiving chemotherapy or any treatment beyond palliative care.

The pediatric oncology team has explained to the family that Kathleen is in and out of a coma-like state and is considered to need total care by the nursing staff. The team further explains to the family that her breathing pattern, decreasing urine production, refusal of food and fluids, and skin mottling are all evidence of Kathleen's impending death. The parents attended a care conference in the morning with the medical staff, pediatric oncologist, pediatric intensive care unit (PICU) director, social worker, nurse manager, charge nurse on duty, child psychologist, and case manager. It was decided that Kathleen's care would be transferred to the pediatric hospice facility as soon as feasible so the family could be together in a setting conducive for the experience of her death.

Kathleen has four male siblings; she is the second youngest in her family. Her eldest brother is overseas, serving in the military. Her youngest sibling is a preschooler.

Case Study Questions

1. What are the common reactions that a pediatric nurse can expect from Kathleen's family members?
2. What are the stages of death and dying according to Kübler-Ross?
3. What are the developmental issues surrounding death for a teenager?
4. Which decisions should be made by the family prior to the final dying process of the child?
5. What are issues and decisions that can be made at the time of the teen's death?

As the Case Evolves. . .

Kathleen's parent asks the nurse to assist in helping their child with the symptoms of dry mouth and lips. When the nurse provides glycerin swabs, the parent breaks down in tears and states, "Why can't I die for her, please?"

6. According to Kübler-Ross's model, which stage of the grief response is the parent in?
   A. Denial and thoughts that the dying process cannot be true
   B. Anger and resentment
   C. Depression
   D. Acceptance of the impending death
   E. Bargaining and guilt

Kathleen's siblings have assembled at her bedside at the hospice. The oldest brother, on leave from military service, is having difficulty accepting his sister's impending death. He tearfully asks if his sister knows that she is dying.

7. What is the most accurate response to this question?
   A. As an adolescent, Kathleen understands fully what death is and that she is dying.
   B. Although children in adolescence understand what death is, Kathleen probably is developmentally unable to recognize that she is in the dying process.
   C. Although children in adolescence lack an understanding of the permanence of death, Kathleen likely understands that she is dying.
   D. It is unlikely that an adolescent fully understands either what death is or accepts that she is dying.
8. The pediatric nurse caring for Kathleen's family should demonstrate which of the following as a priority response?
   A. An empathetic attitude
   B. Disclosure of personal experiences with death and dying
   C. Palliative care model principles
   D. Silence and closeness

---

* Reprinted from Benini, F., Vecchi, R., & Orzalesi, M. (2014). A charter for the rights of the dying child. *The Lancet, 383*(9928),1547–1548, Copyright 2014, with permission from Elsevier.

Chapter Summary

♦ The emotional impact of a dying child on parents, guardians, and siblings is immeasurable. The death of a child can be emotionally traumatic for the child's immediate family and those within the family's community. The death of a child has life-changing effects on survivors. Grief may affect the parents' ability to function at work and in relationships. Grief can also have a significant impact on how the parents interact with the surviving siblings.

♦ The physiological dying process for a child is very similar to that for an adult. The child's body begins to demonstrate evidence of shutting down. The child's hands, fingers, and toes cool to the touch and the skin demonstrates mottling.

♦ Dying children need support, honesty, closeness, comfort, and control of their symptoms to prevent suffering. Family members are highly encouraged to touch, cuddle, and stay with their child.

♦ When the child is in the last 6 months of their life, the family should be referred to hospice care, in which specially trained healthcare professionals assist the family in the final stages of the child's life.

♦ Traumatic deaths are a different experience than the loss of a child from a chronic or life-threatening condition for a period of time. Both experiences produce great emotional responses, but a traumatic death can also produce tremendous guilt and extreme despair.

Bibliography

Baranowski, K. P. (n.d.). Stress in pediatric palliative and hospice care: Causes, effects, and coping strategies. Retrieved from https://www.nhpco.org/mar-06/stress-pediatric-palliative-and-hospice-care-causes-effects-and-coping-strategies

Benini, F., Vecchi, R., & Orzalesi, M. (2014). A charter for the rights of the dying child. *Lancet, 383*(9928), 1547–1548.

Cancer.Net Editorial Board. (2015). Caring for a terminally ill child: A guide for parents. Retrieved from http://www.cancer.net/navigating-cancer-care/advanced-cancer/caring-terminally-ill-child-guide-parents

Center for Hospice Care Southeast Connecticut. (2016). Hospice and palliative care: Pediatric hospice. Retrieved from https://www.hospicesect.org/hospice-and-palliative-care/hospice-requirements

Cherny, N. I. (2010). The problem of suffering and the principles of assessment in palliative medicine. In G. Hanks, N. I. Cherny, N. A. Christakis, M. Fallon, S. Kaasa, & R. K. Portenoy, *Oxford textbook of palliative medicine* (4th ed., Section 2.1). Oxford, UK: Oxford University Press.

Dussel, V., Kreicbergs, U., Hilden, J. M., Watterson, J., Moore, C., Turner, B. G., . . . Wolfe, J. (2009). Looking beyond where children die: Determinants and effects of planning a child's location of death. *Journal of Pain and Symptom Management, 37*(1), 33–43.

Fox, M., Cacciatore, J., & Lacasse, J. R. (2014). Child death in the United States: Productivity and the economic burden of parental grief. *Death Studies, 38*, 597–602.

Gregoire, M.-C., & Frager, G. (2006). Ensuring pain relief for children at the end of life. *Pain Research and Management, 11*(3), 156.

Hospice Foundation of America. (2011). *A caregiver's guide to the dying process.* Washington, DC: Author.

Kastenbaum, R. (2015). *Death, society, and human experience.* New York, NY: Routledge.

Kübler-Ross, E. (1969). *On death and dying.* New York, NY: Routledge.

Kübler-Ross, E. (2005). *On grief and grieving: Finding the meaning of grief through the five stages of loss.* New York, NY: Simon and Schuster.

Lee, S. A. (2015). The Persistent Complex Bereavement Inventory: A measure based on the *DSM-5. Death Studies, 39*, 399–410.

North Central Florida Hospice. (1996). Hospice: Preparing for approaching death. Retrieved from http://www.hospicenet.org/html/preparing_for.html

Palliative Care Australia. (n.d.). The dying process. Retrieved from http://palliativecare.org.au/resources/the-dying-process

Webb, N. B. (2010). *Helping bereaved children: A handbook for practitioners* (3rd ed.). London, UK: Guilford Press.

Wolfe, J., Grier, H. E., Klar, N., Levin, S. B., Ellenbogen, J. M., Salem-Schatz, S., . . . Weeks, J. C. (2000). Symptoms and suffering at the end of life in children with cancer. *New England Journal of Medicine, 342*(5), 326–333.

World Health Organization (WHO). (2013). Essential medicines in palliative care: Executive summary. Prepared by the International Association for Hospice and Palliative Care (IAHPC). Edited by Lillana De Lima. Retrieved from http://www.who.int/selection_medicines/committees/expert/19/applications/PalliativeCare_8_A_R.pdf

Pediatric Nursing Care: Helpful Professional Organizations

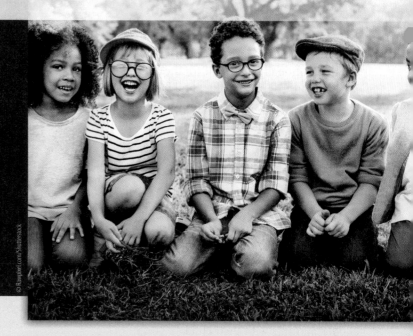

© Rawpixel.com/Shutterstock

Society of Pediatric Nursing (www.pedsnurses.org)

The mission of the Society of Pediatric Nursing (SPN) is to "advance the specialty of pediatric nursing through excellence in education, research and practice." Started in 1990, SPN has grown to have more than 3300 members. Its annual nursing conference provides state-of-the-science information on the care of children and their families, skills, technologies, and research.

American Nurses Association (www.nursingworld.org)

The American Nurses Association (ANA) represents U.S. nurses' interests by providing information and fostering best practices and high practice standards for the profession. This organization focuses on safety, ethics, healthy work environments, and the healthcare needs of the public.

American Association of Nurse Practitioners (www.aanp.org)

The American Association of Nurse Practitioners provides support and education on the advancement of quality in health care. It promotes research, education, advocacy, leadership, and excellence in practice for nurse practitioners.

American Holistic Nurses Association (www.ahna.org)

The American Holistic Nurses Association represents nurses who have devoted their practice to the theories, knowledge, and expertise of care of the human being in totality. It provides practice standards and scope of practice guidelines for the administration of holistic care.

Association of Child Life Professionals (www.childife.org)

The Association of Child Life Professionals provides standards of practice, research, and education for child life professionals involved with patients and families.

American Psychiatric Nurses Association (www.apna.org)

This professional organization advances the science of psychiatric and mental health nursing through research, education, and practice standards.

Association of Camp Nurses (www.acn.org)

The Association of Camp Nurses supports the practice of providing professional nursing care to children and families attending camps. It provides education and support for best practices in the promotion of healthy camp environments and ways to provide care to those with special needs.

International Council of Nurses (www.icn.ch)

Representing more than 130 national nursing associations around the world, the International Council of Nurses (ICN) provides global health policies, advanced nursing knowledge, and education on global health issues.

National Association of Neonatal Nurses (www.nann.org)

The National Association of Neonatal Nurses provides collaboration, education, and research for those who care for high-risk neonates. It promotes best practices for the care of the most vulnerable patients.

Hospice and Palliative Nurses Association (hpna .advancingexpertcare.org)

This professional organization represents nurses who care for patients with serious health issues, complex symptom management needs, and those who are entering end of life.

Association of Pediatric Hematology Oncology Nurses (www.aphon.org)

The Association of Pediatric Hematology Oncology Nurses supports the goals and successful careers of nurses who care for children with hematologic or oncologic disorders or conditions. It provides standards of practice, education, and research for best practices. It also provides a center for advocacy for families who experience a childhood cancer diagnosis or a hematologic disorder; this center offers information on the latest legislation and resources.

Infusion Nurses Society (www.ins1.org)

The Infusion Nurses Society provides state-of-the-science information and care practices for infusion therapy, including standards of practice, evidence-based practice guidelines, and national certification.

National Association of School Nurses (www.nasn .org)

The National Association of School Nurses provides school nurses with continuing education courses, resources, and publications to assist with the administration of nursing care and health in school environments. Its website includes tool kits for best practices and information on pertinent topics such as immunizations, mental health, and children with chronic illnesses and disabilities.

Sigma Theta Tau International Nursing Honor Society (www.nursingsociety.org)

The Sigma Theta Tau International Nursing Honor Society includes nurses from 520 chapters in 90 countries. The society's mission is to advance world health, including the health of children and families.

18 Common Pediatric Medication and Supportive Calculations*

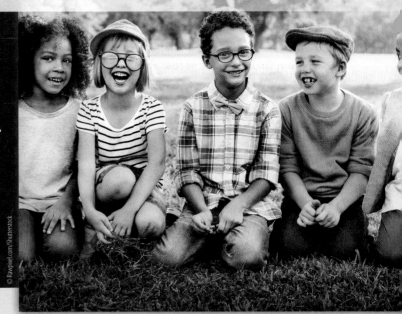

© Rawpixel.com/Shutterstock

1. **Medication Dosing in mg/kg**

   Most medications administered to children are dosed based on their most recent and accurate weight in kilograms (calculated by dividing the child's weight in pounds by 2.2). Dosing may be expressed in terms of mg/kg/dose or mg/kg/day. If a medication is prescribed in mg/kg/day, the pediatric nurse should ask for further clarification to ensure that each dose is accurate.

   Pediatric medications should never be prescribed in milliliters. The actual milligrams per milliliter may be included in the prescription, but clarity of the order should be in mg/kg/dose.

   Example: Give a 40 mg/kg/dose of amoxicillin to a 3-year-old patient with severe and confirmed bacterial otitis media. The medication comes as a suspension with a final concentration of 400 mg/5 mL. The child weighs 42 pounds.

   a. Convert the pounds to kg: 42 divided by 2.2 equals 19.1 kg.
   b. Calculate the dose required in mg: 19.1 kg times 40 mg equals 763 mg.

   c. Convert the dose in mg to dose in mL: 763 mg/dose divided by 400 mg/5 mL equals 9.5 mL of the medication.

2. **Determining Safe Dose Ranges**

   Pediatric medications are given to children across the developmental period. Pediatric patients can run the gamut from the smallest premature infant in the neonatal intensive care unit (NICU) to the adolescent who has the height and weight of an adult. To provide safe dosing, medications for children are administered within a safe dose range according to the child's weight. For instance, the steroid prednisone has a commonly published safe dose range of 0.5 to 1 mg/kg of weight per day for a child 18 months or older, with a maintenance dose of 0.125 mg/kg up to 0.25 mg/kg daily. If a nurse receives an order for a dose that is outside (less than or greater than) this common safe dose range, the nurse should double-check the safety of the dose by clarifying with the prescriber or the pharmacist as to why the medication was ordered outside the safe dose range.

   Example: Give prednisone 11 mg PO BID to a 19-month-old child weighing 23 kg (as a maintenance dose) with an asthma exacerbation. The nurse would check the medication safe dose range for this child and would find that the ordered amount per day (22 mg per day if it was 11 mg BID) is too high for a child weighing 23 kg. The safe dose range for a maintenance dose of prednisone is 0.125 mg/kg to 0.5 mg/kg per day (23 kg weight times the maintenance

---

* The following calculations are based on this author's clinical experience in giving care to children in various clinical settings across the San Francisco Bay Area under the direction of various pediatric multidisciplinary teams. Readers should use caution and follow institutional policy and licensure regulations in their clinical practice settings. Not all providers or healthcare institutions use the following calculations. The prescribing provider's orders must be followed, and all calculations should be double-checked for safety.

safe dose range would be between 4 mg per day up to 8 mg per day or 2 to 4 mg per dose for BID dosing). The nurse would need to clarify why 22 mg per day was ordered and check whether the larger dose was prescribed in error.

3. **Safety in Drawing up the Correct Amount of Medication from a Multidose Container**

   Once the pediatric nurse determines the child's most recent accurate weight and confirms that the prescribed medication was ordered within the safe dose range, the next step in safe medication administration is to determine how much medication to draw up from a multidose vial. Medications can come up prepared for dosing from the pharmacy (such as an oral antibiotic in a prefilled oral syringe ready for double-checking and immediate administration), or they may be found in the unit refrigerator, patient medication cubby, or electronic medication dosing machine (i.e., Pyxis) in multidose vials or containers. In the latter case, the nurse would need to first calculate the amount that should be drawn up from the multidose vial.

   Example: Diphenhydramine (Benadryl) 13 mg slow IV was ordered for a child with a significant rash at 1 mg/kg. The child weighs 13 kg. After double-checking that the medication falls within the safe dose range, the nurse takes the multidose vial of 50 mg/1 mL and calculates how much to safely draw up.

   Diphenhydramine 13 mg IV: Multidose vial is 50 mg/1 mL. Drawing up 0.26 mg from the vial equates to 13 mg per dose: 13 mg desired divided by 50 mg/1 mL on hand equals to 0.26 mg per dose.

4. **Calculating Body Surface Areas**

   Some drugs, such as chemotherapeutic agents, are prescribed according to the child's body surface area (BSA). Body surface area is calculated by multiplying the child's height in centimeters times weight in kilograms, then dividing the number by 3600, then squaring the final number.

   Example: A child who weighs 16.8 kg and is 98 cm tall requires a maintenance dose of vincristine (Oncovin). The safe dose is 2 mg/m². The child's BSA would be 0.68 m²: 16.8 times 97 cm, divided by 3600, then squared. The nurse would then determine that the safe dose of the medication should be 0.68 m² multiplied by 2 mg, for a final dose of 1.35 mg of vincristine.

5. **Fluid Maintenance Calculations**

   Many children who are seen in acute, critical, emergency departments or urgent care centers require intravenous fluids for stabilization and maintenance of fluid stability. IV fluids are often ordered in fluid maintenance calculations.

   0-10 kg: Child will require 100 mL per kg per 24 hours.

   11-20 kg: Child will require 1000 mL plus 50 mL/kg for each 1 kg over the first 10 kg per 24 hours.

   21-70 kg: Child will require 1500 mL plus 20 mL/kg for each 1 kg over the first 20 kg per 24 hours.

   To determine an hourly rate of fluid administration, the nurse would calculate the entire amount needed for the day and divide by 24.

   Examples: A child weighs 8 kg. The fluid maintenance requirement would be 8 kg multiplied by 100 (i.e., 800 mL of fluid) over 24 hours, or 33.3 mL per hour.

   A child weighs 13.5 kg. The fluid maintenance would be 1000 mL plus 3.5 times 50; the total amount per day is 1175 mL per 24 hours, or 48.9 mL per hour.

   Note that fluid maintenance does not provide fluid resuscitation for a child with dehydration.

6. **Minimal Urine Output Calculation**

   To determine the minimal amount of urine required for a pediatric patient, the nurse would calculate the range to be between 0.5 mL/kg/hour and 2 mL/kg/hour for children ranging in age from infants to adolescents. This is not an acceptable amount of urine per day, but rather the minimal amount needed to show kidney perfusion and function.

   Example: An infant weighs 12.8 kg. The minimal urine output (UOP) expected per hour would be 0.5 mL/kg (0.5 multiplied by 12.8 equals 6.4 mL per hour).

7. **Kilocalorie Determinants for Children**

   Kilocalorie determinants include a number of factors, including the child's health status, need for reduced calories for obesity, increased calories for failure to thrive, and the child's amount of daily activity (athletes will need more kilocalories). The following are general guidelines for kilocalorie needs (other guidelines also exist):

   Newborns: 110 kilocalories per kilogram

   Infants: 90-100 kilocalories per kilogram

   Children age 5 months to 5 years: 70 kilocalories per kilogram

   Children older than 5 years: 45-70 kilocalories per kilogram

   Example: A 6-month-old infant weighs 16.4 kg. This child's general kilocalorie requirements per day would be 70 kilocalories multiplied by the child's weight of 16.4 kg, for a total of 1148 kilocalories per 24 hours.

   Pediatric nurses should inquire about the provider's preferences and institutional policies for daily kilocalorie requirements, as they vary widely.

To determine the quantity of breast milk (20 kilocalories per ounce) or standard formula (20 kilocalories per ounce) required per day, divide the daily kilocalorie requirement by 30 (mL per ounce).

Example: A 6-month-old child weighing 16.4 kg requires approximately 1148 kilocalories per day. Dividing 1148 by 30 equals 38: that is, the child needs 38 ounces of formula per day. If the infant feeds 6 times per day, the general guideline would be 6.3 ounces of formula for each feeding.

8. **Equations for Determining Fluid Resuscitation After a Burn**

When a child suffers a significant burn, the wound will weep fluids. The emergency team may request that the nursing team administer a fluid resuscitation intervention. The calculation is based on the child's most accurate or estimated weight and the percentage of body surface burned.

Many burn resuscitation fluid calculations are possible. With the Parkland formula for burn fluid resuscitation, the amount of intravenous fluid (IVF) administered in the first 24 hours is calculated as 4 mL of IVF per kilogram per percentage of body surface burned (4 mL/kg/% burned). The first half of the total IVF calculated is administered in the first 8 hours, with the remainder administered over the next 16 hours. Note that the percentage of body surface burned is entered into the calculation as a whole number.

Example: Based on the "rule of nines," a child weighing 110 pounds (50 kg) has experienced the following burns in terms of body surface area:

Each arm: 9% (both arms burned)

Torso: 18%

One leg: 18%

Therefore the child has experienced a significant burn, determined to be 45% of the child's body surface area.

Using the Parkland formula, 4 mL multiplied by 50 kg multiplied by 45 would equate to 9000 mL (9 L) of fluid needed in the first 24 hours. The team would administer 4500 mL during the first 8 hours (562 mL/hour) and 4500 mL in the next 16 hours (262 mL/hour).

9. **Drip Factors (drops per minute)**

If a pediatric healthcare team is providing health care in a setting without electricity or electronic and computerized intravenous fluid pumps, it is common practice to determine the rate of an IV fluid dose by using the drip factor equation: Amount of fluid ordered multiplied by the drip factor of the tubing (can be found on the product packaging; typically 10 gtt/mL, 15 gtt/mL, or 20 gtt/mL), then that quantity multiplied by the number of minutes ordered, equals the total amount to be administered.

Example: A child who weighs 28 kg was located in the woods after a search and rescue team found the child; the child had been missing for 36 hours. First responders used the drip factor calculation to give the child IVF. The team used a fluid bolus resuscitation calculation of 30 mL per kilogram over 2 hours.

Child's weight multiplied by 30 equals 840 mL.

Drip factor tubing used is 15 gtt/mL.

Time for the infusion is 120 minutes.

840 times 15 divided by 120 equals 105 gtt/min.

The team uses a standard wristwatch to determine the rate of 105 gtt/min and administers the IVF over 2 hours.

10. **One-to-One Body Fluid Replacement**

If a child has a drain located on the body (e.g., a nasogastric tube, jejunostomy tube, or bile tube) and is losing a quantity of body fluids, the surgeon may request the child have the body fluids replaced as a one-to-one quantity. Typically, this amount is determined by looking back at the previous 4 hours of total body fluid loss, and replacing the fluid loss forward over the next 4 hours by dividing the quantity lost per hour.

Example: A child on the second postoperative day has a nasogastric tube set to low continuous suction. The nurse has been asked to replace the fluid with IV lactated Ringer's solution with a 1:1 replacement calculation. At 1100 hours, the nurse looks back at the child's output and sees that the child has lost 112 mL between the hours of 0700 and 1100. For the hours of 1100 to 1500, the nurse would take the quantity lost (112 mL), divide by 4, and run the lactated Ringer's IVF line at 112 mL divided by 4 hours, or 28 mL per hour of IVF.

11. **Blood Transfusion Calculation**

Blood is administered to children based on a dose, not in units as with adults. Children typically need one dose to raise the hemoglobin by 1 g/dL or the hematocrit by 3%. A typical dose is 10 to 15 mL blood per kilogram. This dose may vary if the child is severely anemic and very symptomatic (each dose may be between 3 and 8 mL/kg, and more doses may be ordered to ensure a slower replacement of blood lost and to meet the overall dose required); it may also vary per institutional policy.

Example: A school-age girl presents to the hematology outpatient clinic with anemia; her hemoglobin is 6.2 g/dL and she is very symptomatic, with severe fatigue, tachycardia, and pallor. The hematology team decides to admit her to the hospital's pediatric unit for an observation status (less than 24 hours stay) and to give transfusions to raise her hemoglobin by 4 g/dL. The child's current weight, as measured in the clinic, is 82 pounds (37.3 kg).

Multiplying 37.3 kg times 10 mL of blood per dose up to 15 mL of blood per dose gives a safe range of 370 to 559 mL per dose. Each dose is administered over 4 hours. The patient's final hemoglobin was raised to 10.7 g/dL at discharge.

12. **Fluid Bolus Calculation**
Pediatric teams use a standard calculation when a child with dehydration or fluid loss needs a rapid fluid bolus. The bolus is typically ordered as 30 mL/kg and is administered over 1 hour, with vital signs taken before and after the infusion to check for improved clinical status. The overall time of administration of a fluid bolus can vary depending on the team's decision, the fragile nature of the child, and the child's age and weight.

Example: An infant presents with recent history of high fevers, poor oral intake, and vomiting. The child is lethargic and has a delayed capillary refill time of 2 to 3 seconds. The team orders a STAT IVF bolus of 0.9% normal saline (NS) over 1 hour, repeated as necessary to see clinical improvement and hemodynamic stabilization. The infant weighs 7.2 kg.

To calculate the dose, the nurse multiplies 7.2 kg times 30 mL per bolus, which equals 216 mL of 0.9% NS over 1 hour, followed by reassessment.

13. **High Fevers and Calculation of Body Fluid Loss**
If a child has had several high fever spikes, the team may decide to take into account the fluids lost per degree of fever over the child's normal body temperature. The calculation assumes 7 mL of fluid lost per degree of fever over normal per hour, every 4 hours.

Example: A child with a series of high fevers from acute bacterial gastroenteritis requires a fluid bolus, maintenance fluids, and an extra quantity of IVF based on fever history. The child's temperature has been 39.0°C four times in the last 24 hours. The child weighs 19 kg.

The nurse multiplies 7 mL times 2 degrees of fever over the child's base line temperature. This equates to an additional 14 mL of fluid resuscitation per hour over the next 4 hours, repeated as needed.

A more aggressive fluid replacement for a febrile child is suggested by Cellucci (2014). In this protocol, the care provider is encouraged to increase the maintenance fluids by 12% for every degree of fever over 37.8°C.

14. **Dehydration Calculation**
Although various calculations are used to estimate body fluid loss, pediatric healthcare teams who have access to a recent accurate weight of a child prior to the fluid loss can use the following to guide decision making:

Mild dehydration: approximately 5% of total body fluid loss (lost 5% of previous weight)

Moderate dehydration: approximately 10% of total body fluid loss (lost 10% of previous weight)

Severe dehydration: approximately 15% of total body fluid loss; the child will be in a critical state (lost as much as 15% of previous weight)

Example: If a child with severe cerebral palsy has lost 10% of his previous weight owing to fevers, diarrhea, and severe diaphoresis, the team may determine that the child is moderately dehydrated. They will proceed with fluid boluses and fluid maintenance calculations to provide fluid resuscitation equaling his 10% loss (based on his fluid maintenance requirements).

15. **Rehydrating a Very Sick Child Who Presents with Significant Dehydration**
When a child presents to an emergency room as very sick and needing immediate rehydration, the team will choose to rehydrate the child quickly to prevent complications. The child should receive both the full fluid maintenance quantity calculated over 24 hours plus the percentage of fluid lost (% of deficit) over a 48-hour period of time or less.

Deficit = % dehydration × child's weight in kilograms × 10

Example: A child who weighs 18 kg presents with a 5-day history of diarrhea and vomiting. The child appears toxic and very sick. The team determines the child to be 10% dehydrated.

Based on the weight of 18 kg, the fluid maintenance calculation shows that the child needs 1400 mL over 24 hours. If the child is 10% dehydrated, he needs an additional 1800 mL over 24 hours. This is calculated by multiplying the child's dehydration percent deficit (10%) times the body weight in kilograms (18) times 10. This equals an additional 1800 mL on top of fluid maintenance, for a total fluid resuscitation need of 1400 mL + 1800 mL = 3200 mL over 24 hours.

16. **Albumin Needs in the Premature Infant**
Premature infants are at risk of not receiving adequate daily protein, which they need to achieve safe and expected total growth before discharge. Most term

infants lose between 10% and 20% of their birth weight in fluids soon after birth, but then gain it back by 2 weeks. Premature or small infants can take much longer to regain this weight (Thureen & Heird, 2005).

Most infants who, for instance, require a 12- to 16-week NICU admission do not achieve the 2–3 kg body mass increase desired. Premature infants need adequate protein intake to support protein synthesis, adequate growth patterns, and net protein balance, and to support normal cellular function by way of signaling molecules (Hay & Thureen, 2010).

Protein requirements at 24 to 30 weeks' gestation are as high as 4 g/kg/day, but then decrease to 2 to 3 g/kg/day at term.

17. **Intravenous Immunoglobulin Therapy Infusion Protocols and Calculations**

Intravenous immunoglobulin (IVIG) therapy is administered to help support children who have one of more than 150 medical immunodeficiency diagnoses that are affected by the production and function of immunoglobulins (antibodies). Each dose, which is pooled from donor immunoglobulin G (IgG) antibodies, contains 10,000 to 60,000 units of donated plasma. Due to concerns about reactions to IVIG administration, pediatric nurses use a calculation to determine the small amount of product per kilogram that should be infused over a short time frame to assess for early symptoms of reactions (e.g., fever, headache, myalgia, rash, arthralgia, and hypersensitivity reactions including anaphylaxis) and the need for future premedications (e.g., acetaminophen, diphenhydramine, and steroids).

Example: A child with a primary IgG immunodeficiency requires an IVIG infusion, to be administered over 4 hours, or per a protocol where the product is administered very slowly for the first 5 minutes, with quantities then increasing in small milliliter increments every 5 to 10 minutes. Vital signs should be checked before each increase in volume is delivered.

18. **Body Mass Index (Quetelet Index) Expressed as kg/m²**

Pediatric healthcare team members may need to calculate a child's body mass index (BMI) to determine if the child's overall body size is appropriate for age, growth, and development. BMI is calculated by dividing the child's weight in kilograms by the square of the child's height in meters (weight divided by height^2). The final BMI calculated is then used to determine the percentile in which the child fits on a standardized BMI growth chart. For instance, if a child's BMI is less than the plotted 5th percentile, the child is considered underweight; if it is in the 5th to 85th percentiles, the child is considered in the healthy weight category; and if it is greater than the 95th percentile, the child is considered obese. BMI growth charts are available on the Centers for Disease Control and Prevention (CDC, 2015) website.

Example: An 11-year-old boy presents to the clinic with a weight of 108 pounds (49.1 kg) and a height of 52 inches (130 cm).

The calculation would be:
1 foot equals 12 inches or 3.3048 meters
1 inch equals 0.025 meter
Child's height: 52 inches or 1.3 meters (0.025 × 52)
Child's weight: 49.1 kg
Divide 49.1 kg by the height in meters squared (1.69)
Child's BMI: 49.1 kg/1.69 m² = 29

The BMI of 29 places this 11-year-old boy in the 96th percentile on a CDC BMI growth chart. The child would be considered obese.

Bibliography

Cellucci, M. F. (2014). Dehydration in children. Retrieved from https://www.merckmanuals.com/professional/pediatrics/dehydration-and-fluid-therapy-in-children/dehydration-in-children

Centers for Disease Control and Prevention (CDC). (2015). Healthy weight: About child and teen BMI. Retrieved from https://www.cdc.gov/healthyweight/assessing/bmi/childrens_bmi/about_childrens_bmi.html

Hay, W. W., & Thureen, P. (2010). Protein for preterm infants: How much is needed? How much is enough? How much is too much? *Pediatric Neonatology, 51*(4), 198–207. doi.10.1016.S1875-9572

Hockenberry, M. J., & Wilson, D. (2010). *Wong's essentials of pediatric nursing* (9th ed.). St. Louis, MO: Elsevier.

Linnard-Palmer, L. (2015, revised). *PedsNotes* (p. 71). Philadelphia, PA: F. A. Davis.

Thureen, P., & Heird, W. C. (2005). Protein and energy requirements of the preterm/low birth weight (LBW) infant. *Pediatric Research, 57*(95R–98R). doi:10.1203./01.PDR.0000160434.69916.34

Younger, E. M. (Ed.). (2012). *IDF guide for nurses: Immunoglobulin therapy for primary immunodeficiency diseases* (3rd ed., pp. 1–31). Towson, MD: Immune Deficiency Foundation.

Pediatric-Focused Laboratory Values

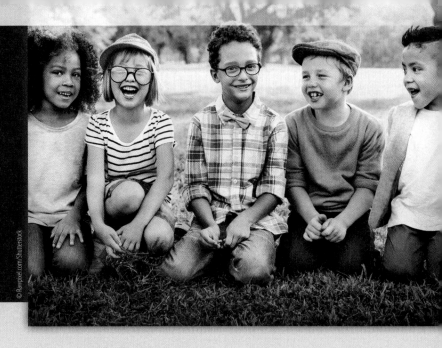

© Rawpixel.com/Shutterstock

The pediatric laboratory values listed here are for children older than 1 year of age. Please consult your hospital or service regarding the standard pediatric lab values that it prefers you to use.

Complete Blood Cell Count (CBC)

Hemoglobin	10.2–14.8 g/dL
Hematocrit	31.5–43.9%
WBC	3000–10,000 cells/μL
Platelets	170,000–380,000 mm^3
MCV	70–85 femtoliters
MCHC	32–36 g/dL RBC
Neutrophils	1500–7500 mm^3
Monocytes	275–825 mm^3
Eosinophils	40–390 mm^3
Basophils	7–140 mm^3

Comprehensive Metabolic Panel

Sodium	135–144 mEq/L
Potassium	3.5–5.2 mEq/L
Chloride	98–110 mEq/L
CO_2	17–30 mEq/L
Glucose	60–100 mg/dL
BUN	5–8 mg/dL
Creatinine	0.2–0.8 mg/dL
Calcium	8.4–10.4 mg/dL
Magnesium	1.5–2.4 mg/dL
Phosphorus	3.2–6.1 mg/dL

Thyroid Panels

T_4	0.90–1.72 μg/dL
Thyroxine	6.1–12.6 μg/dL
TSH	0.55–7.10 mU/L

Liver Function Tests

ALT	0–55 U/L
AST	0–50 U/L
Total bilirubin	0–1.4 mg/dL
Conjugated bilirubin	<10 μmol/L

Arterial Blood Gases

pH	7.35–7.45
P_{CO_2}	32–48 mm Hg
P_{O_2}	50–83 mm Hg
Bicarbonate	24–34 mEq/L
Base excess	-4 to +2 mmol/L

Urinalysis

pH	4.6–8.0
Specific gravity	1.010–1.030

Clotting Factors

PT	11–15 seconds
PTT	20–30 seconds

Nationally Normed Growth Charts

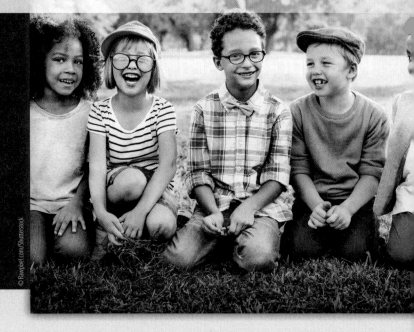

© Rawpixel.com/Shutterstock

One of the most effective ways to determine a child's healthy growth pattern is to document the child's anthropometric measurements on nationally normed growth charts. Provided by many national organizations, such as the Centers for Disease Control and Prevention (CDC; www.cdc.gov/growthcharts), the National Institutes of Health (NIH), and the U.S. Department of Agriculture's WIC Resource System (https://wicworks.fns.usda.gov/assessment-tools/growth-charts/wic-growth-charts), growth charts provide a visual depiction of a child's growth trends and a documented pattern over time. The information provides a visual diagram of percentile curves that show a distribution of a child's body measurements. First created in 1977, these charts help a pediatric healthcare team determine whether an infant's, child's, or adolescent's growth is adequate. Plots on a nationally standardized growth chart are not diagnostic in value, but rather provide trends to assist a team in decision making.

There are now a total of 16 charts (8 charts for each sex), including the latest addition of body mass index-for-age charts. Charts are provided in English, Spanish, and French.

Infants: Birth to 36 Months

Boy: length for age
Boy: weight for age
Boy: head circumference for age
Boy: weight for length
Girl: length for age

Girl: weight for age
Girl: head circumference for age
Girl: weight for length

Children and Adolescents: 2 Years to 20 Years

Boy: stature for age
Boy: weight for age
Boy: BMI for age
Girl: stature for age
Girl: weight for age
Girl: BMI for age

Preschoolers: 2 Years to 5 Years

Boy: weight for stature
Girl: weight for stature

Sites such as www.infantchart.com/child provide children's growth chart calculators that enable pediatric healthcare professionals to rapidly enter a child's measurements and trend them over time. In addition, with the adoption of electronic medical charts, most institutions have internal means to plot and trend a child's growth patterns. In addition, paper or downloadable growth charts are available from the CDC and the NIH for general use.

Parents often appreciate being able to see how their child's growth patterns are trending. It is common practice to share a child's growth chart with the family.

Examples

1. Infant girls to second birthday: weight to height ratio

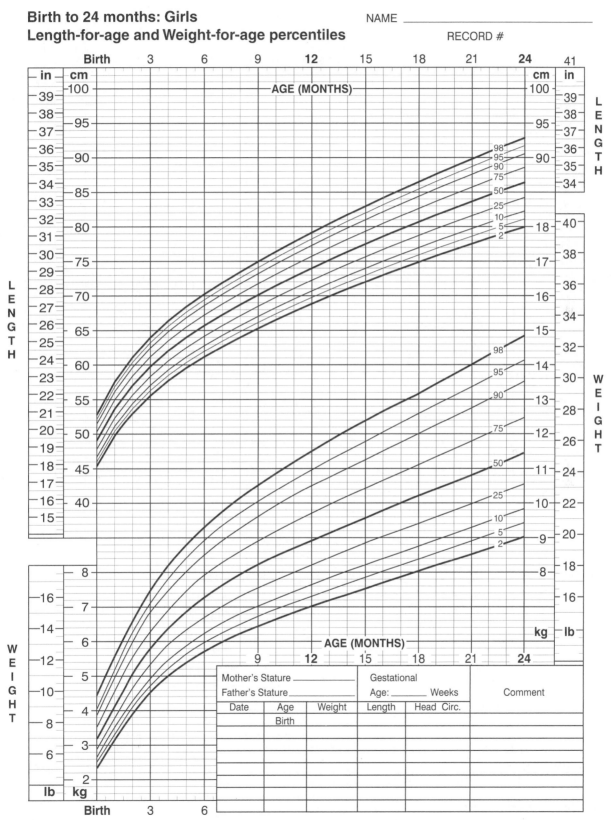

Birth to 24 months: Girls
Length-for-age and Weight-for-age percentiles

NAME _____

RECORD # _____

Published by the Centers for Disease Control and Prevention, November 1, 2009
SOURCE: WHO Child Growth Standards (http://www.who.int/childgrowth/en)

2. Infant boys to second birthday: weight to height ratio

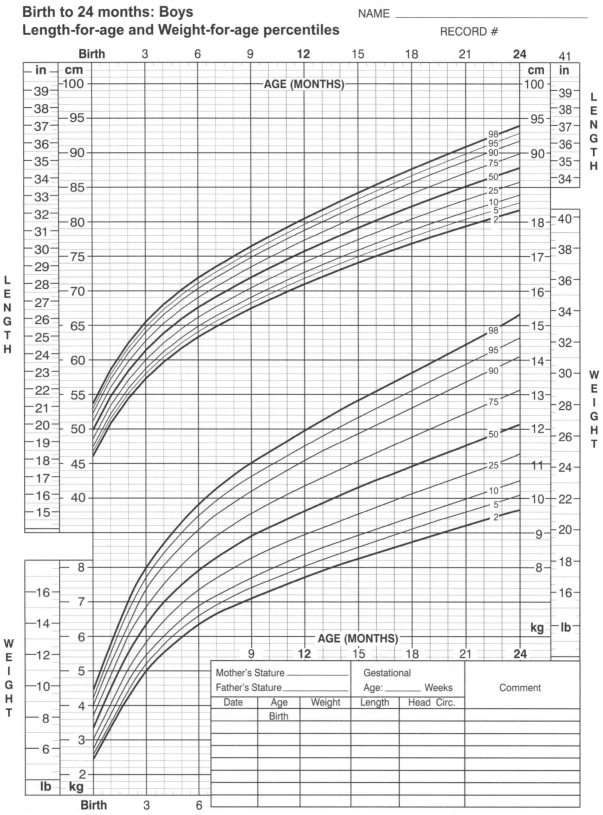

Birth to 24 months: Boys
Length-for-age and Weight-for-age percentiles

NAME _____

RECORD # _____

Published by the Centers for Disease Control and Prevention, November 1, 2009
SOURCE: WHO Child Growth Standards (http://www.who.int/childgrowth/en)

3. Girls 2 to 20 years of age: weight to height ratio

2 to 20 years: Girls
Stature-for-age and Weight-for-age percentiles

Mother's Stature _____ Father's Stature _____

Date	Age	Weight	Stature	BMI*

*To Calculate BMI: Weight (kg) ÷ Stature (cm) ÷ Stature (cm) x 10,000
or Weight (lb) ÷ Stature (in) ÷ Stature (in) x 703

AGE (YEARS)

4. Boys 2 to 20 years of age: weight to height ratio

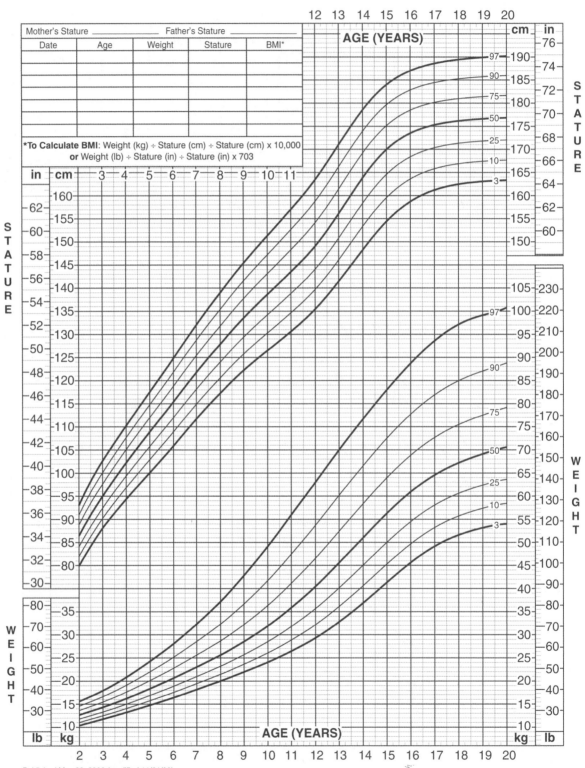

2 to 20 years: Boys
Stature-for-age and Weight-for-age percentiles

NAME _____

RECORD # _____

Mother's Stature _____ Father's Stature _____

Date	Age	Weight	Stature	BMI*

*To Calculate BMI: Weight (kg) ÷ Stature (cm) ÷ Stature (cm) x 10,000
or Weight (lb) ÷ Stature (in) ÷ Stature (in) x 703

AGE (YEARS)

STATURE

WEIGHT

Published May 30, 2000 (modified 11/21/00).
SOURCE: Developed by the National Center for Health Statistics in collaboration with
the National Center for Chronic Disease Prevention and Health Promotion (2000).
http://www.cdc.gov/growthcharts

Best Practices in Pediatric Nursing Care: Handoff Sheets and Huddle Tips

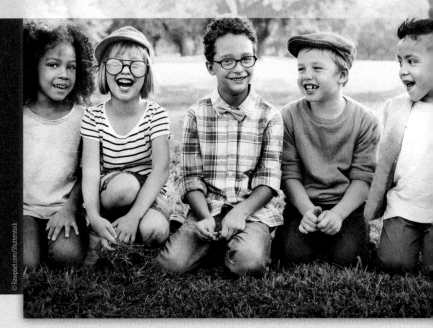

© Rawpixel.com/Shutterstock

What Should Be Required in a Safe and Thorough Pediatric Handoff?

At the end of care, one nurse provides the oncoming nurse with a report of information that is considered essential to give safe and comprehensive care to patients. The terms *report*, *handoff*, and *end-of-shift report* are all used to describe this process of sharing information. Some handoffs are done in small groups, others are done individually; some are done in writing with a brief period of questions and answers. Other institutional-wide handoffs occur when transporting the pediatric patient from one department to another (i.e., emergency department [ED] to pediatric intensive care unit [PICU], PICU to the pediatric unit, pediatric acute care unit [PACU] to the pediatric unit, pediatric unit to magnetic resonance imaging [MRI]).

No matter how a healthcare institution selects its preferred best practices, the responsibility of giving and getting patient information is considered an essential aspect of quality care. Legally, nurses are responsible for providing information to the oncoming nurse that allows the next nurse to effectively provide care *with continuity*.

Excellence in pediatric handoffs takes planning, thoughtfulness, critical thinking, respect, and practice. A formal handoff is a collaborative effort; without it, the nurse and the healthcare institution can be liable for *care failures* (Logsdon, 2014). Some institutions, such as

Boston Children's Hospital, have reported significant reductions in medical errors (from 32% of admissions to 19%) by formalizing handoffs (Logsdon, 2014). The Joint Commission has made standardized handoffs one of its annual National Patient Safety Goals (Arora & Johnson, 2006).

Example of a Pediatric Care Handoff Sheet

Patient Name: Age: Weight: Height: Known Allergies: Code Status: Developmental Stage:	IV in Place: Date of Insertion: Gauge: Location: Last Flush: Next Tubing Change:	Pertinent Medical History:
Presence of Family/ Support Systems:	Developmental Pain Scale Used: Last Pain Score: Last Pain Med Administered:	Pertinent Lab Values: Date Drawn: Reported?
Play Needs:	Other Symptoms:	Pending Labs to Draw:
Medical Diagnosis:	Pulse Oximetry:	Pertinent Diagnostic Exams:
Isolation Precautions:	Oxygen Therapy in Use:	Findings Reported?:
Diet:	Type of Oxygen Delivery Device:	Pending Diagnostics?
Activity Orders:	Wounds or Drains:	Output:
Previous Nurse:		Toileting Needs:

(continues)

Example of a Pediatric Care Handoff Sheet (*continued*)

Body System Assessment:	Medications Due:	Vital Signs:
Respiratory:	0800:	_____
Cardiac:	0900:	_____
Neuro:	1000:	
Endocrine:	1100:	
Skin:	1200:	
GI:	1300:	
GU:	1400:	
MS:	1500:	
Sensory:		
Nutrition:	PRNS Ordered:	
Cognition:		
Emotional State:		

Who Should Attend a Huddle?

During a huddle, the pediatric healthcare team gathers together for a quick interdisciplinary check-in about the children currently on the unit. Important information on clinical status, clinical stability, impending transfers, impending surgeries or diagnostic exams, and possible discharges is shared during this gathering. In some settings, the team may ask the nurse to provide a child's pediatric early warning score (PEWS) system, which shows the severity of the child's clinical status and may guide the hospitalist and his or her team to see that child first during the shift.

How Should a Handoff or Huddle Be Implemented?

The process of sharing patient information between caregivers or between departments should be formalized and protected. The following tips are from The Joint Commission:

- Always allow for clarifications and questioning between caregivers and care receivers.
- Commit yourself to update information right before sharing it.
- Encourage the use of read-backs, repeat-backs, and other forms of verification.
- A review of the patient's relevant past medical history should be shared.
- Allow for minimal disruptions or interruptions so information is both conveyed and heard.

Bibliography

Arora, V., & Johnson, J. (2006). National Patient Safety Goals: A model of building a standardized hand-off protocol. *Joint Commission Journal on Quality and Patient Safety, 32*(11), 646–655.

Gephart, S. M. (2012). The art of effective handoffs: What is the evidence? *Advances in Neonatal Care, 21*(1), 37–39.

Joint Commission on Accreditation of Healthcare Organizations. (2007). 2007 National Patient Safety Goals: Hospital version manual chapter, including implementation expectations. Retrieved from http://www.jointcommission.org/PatientSafety/National PatientSafetyGoals/07_hap_cah_npsgs.htm

Logsdon, T. (2014). Improving handoffs, communication and patient safety. Retrieved from https://www.childrenshospitals .org/newsroom/childrens-hospitals-today/issue-archive/issues/ summer-2014/articles/improving-handoffs-and-safety

Pediatric-Focused Checklists and Helpful Mnemonics

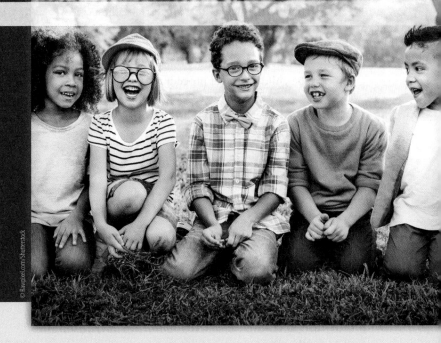

© Rawpixel.com/Shutterstock

Preoperative Teaching Checklist for Children Going to Surgery: 22 Tips and Concerns

Used to ensure adequate preparation and safety prior to transferring a child from a pediatric unit to the operating room.

1. Has the consent form been signed by the parent or primary care provider/legal representative?
2. Does the child or the parent have any questions? Do the parents feel they have provided informed consent?
3. Has a member of the Child Life team visited the child and helped educate him or her with anatomically correct dolls?
4. Have recent vital signs, oxygenation saturation, and pain scale scores been taken and documented? Are there any current symptoms that need to be reported to the operating room team (nausea, discomfort)?
5. Any pertinent recent or past medical history that should be shared with the surgical team?
6. Any experiences with previous surgeries that would influence the child's current experience?
7. Are recent laboratory data complete, including complete blood cell count (CBC), clotting factors, and glucose?
8. Are the child's allergies clearly communicated to the surgical team? Is there a safety allergy wristband on the child?
9. Current medications clearly communicated? Last dose taken of each medication?
10. Latest height, weight, and head circumference (for children younger than 2 years) documented?
11. Any loose teeth that could cause complications with intubation prior to surgery?
12. Any metal in the child's body (implanted central line ports, metal nails, screws or plates from previous orthopedic surgeries, implanted pumps, infusing pumps, hearing aids)?
13. Last urination and stool documented, including date, time, and quantity?
14. Last food or fluid taken, including date, time, and quantity? (Describe exactly what was consumed and when.)
15. Is a name badge including the child's full name, date of birth, and medical record number securely placed on the child's wrist or ankle?
16. Any premedications ordered to be administered before surgery such as antibiotics?
17. Has the child's peripheral or central line been flushed and saline locked (or heparin locked per institutional protocol)?
18. Will the child return with a new device such as a patient-controlled anesthesia (PCA) machine, and has the child/family been taught the protocols on how to operate the machine?
19. Any safety issues concerning transporting the child to the operating room (special devices for transfer from bed to gurney)?
20. Are the child's bed or crib side rails up for safety? Is the bed locked?

21. Where will the child return to (post-anesthesia recovery room to pediatric intensive care unit [PICU] or the pediatric unit)? Where should the parents wait? How will the parents be notified of the conclusion of the child's surgical procedure?

22. Has the pediatric nurse given an adequate handoff to the operating room nurse prior to sending the child to surgery?

CIAMPEDS: Emergency Nursing Association Mnemonic for Triage and Physical Assessment

Used to organize a health history from the parents or caregivers of a child brought into an emergency setting, urgent care setting, or clinic.

C = Chief complaint
I = Immunizations and need for isolation precautions
A = Allergies
M = Medications currently on and most recently taken
P = Past medical history and parents' impression of the child's current condition
E = Events surrounding the injury, illness or condition of concern
D = Diet and diapers; recent bowel and bladder output
S = Symptoms associated with injury, illness or child's current condition

Data from Emergency Nurses Association. (2003). *Core curriculum for pediatric emergency nursing*. Sudbury, MA: Jones and Bartlett Publishers.

Standardized Approach to Pediatric Triage Assessment (Emergency Room Prioritization)

Step 1:   Appearance/work of breathing/circulation
Step 2:   Airway/breathing/circulation/disability/ exposure–environmental control (ABCDE)
Step 3:   Pertinent history
Step 4:   Vital signs
Step 5:   Fever?
Step 6:   Pain?

Reproduced from Agency for Healthcare Research and Quality. (2014). Emergency Severity Index (ESI): A triage tool for emergency department. Retrieved from https://www.ahrq.gov/professionals/systems/hospital/esi/esi6.html

SIGNOUT? Mnemonic

Can be used as a rapid communication tool to update interdisciplinary team members or to update the charge nurse for decisions concerning patient assignments.

S = Sick? Do not resuscitate? Unstable?
I = Identifying data, gender, weight, age and diagnosis(es)
G = General course of hospitalization
N = New events of the day, including vital signs, diagnostics, lab results, and medications
O = Overall health status/clinical condition
U = Upcoming possibilities, with the plan and rationale
T = Tasks to complete, plan, timing, rationale
? = Any questions or concerns?

Data from Horwitz, L. I., Moin, T., & Green, M. L. (2007). Development and implementation of an oral sign-out skills curriculum. *Journal of General Internal Medicine, 22*(10), 1470-1474.

SBAR(R)

Used for safety when communicating with other healthcare team members. Especially useful when asking a primary provider to give a new medical order or clarify an existing order.

Situation
Background
Assessment
Recommendation/request
Read-back

Chemotherapy Administration Safety in Children

Used as a safety check when preparing for the administration of chemotherapy to children. Provides a three-part safety check: (1) prior to administration of chemotherapy drugs, (2) during the administration of chemotherapy drugs, and (3) after the drugs have been administered to check for longer-term safety and symptom management.

Before Chemotherapy Starts

C   Consent signed by the family? Do they feel informed? Has the pediatric oncologist signed the consent?

H   Health assessment: vital signs, developmental status of the child and pertinent laboratory analysis

E   Evaluation of family education and knowledge of treatment plan; need for an interpreter

M	Mother or father? (securing of the presence of a supportive family member before treatment)
O	Overview of the chemotherapy treatment plan and review of the treatment roadmap; review of any required pretreatment requirements such as minimal required platelet count or absolute neutrophil count, urine specific gravity, or urine pH

During Chemotherapy Administration

S	Safe administration with double-blind verification by two chemotherapy-certified nurses of the orders, roadmap, child's body surface area (BSA) calculation, chemotherapy dosing per recent weight, timing, and route
A	Assessments of the central venous catheter's patency and confirmation of a strong blood return to prevent extravasation of a vesicant drug
F	Intravenous fluids to maintain hydration and adequate urine output (UOP)
E	Electrolyte assessments; if roadmap requires specimens between chemotherapy drugs to check for electrolyte wasting

After Chemotherapy Is Administered

S	Symptoms that may need assistance, such as anxiety, fear, fatigue, and nausea
O	Observations for chemotherapy side effects; drug allergy reactions
U	Urine output must be adequate for appropriate excretion of the drugs
N	Nursing care and education needed during the post-chemotherapy period, such as home supplies, home care, follow-up plans, and nadir and symptoms of anemia, thrombocytopenia, and neutropenia
D	Drugs needed for home treatment of symptoms management; mouth care or chemoprotective medications

Pediatric Code Blue Skills Mnemonic

A = Assess the child's level of alertness and airway patency

B = Is the child breathing on his or her own, and is the breathing effective?

C = Check the child's circulation for 8 to 10 seconds. Can you feel a pulse?

CAB = Initiate cardiopulmonary resuscitation (CPR) via compressions, airway support, and breathing.

C = Crash cart; bring the cart to the child, open the cart, place the child on cardiac leads and turn on the cardiac monitor, use the vital signs equipment.

O = Place the child on a source of oxygen (tank on the side of the crash cart) and attach the oxygen line to the Ambu bag/mask/valve tubing being used.

P = Place the child on the backboard for stabilization and effectiveness of cardiac compressions.

I = Start IV lines, draw blood tubes (green, red, purple, and gold), draw arterial blood gases (ABGs), and begin fluid resuscitation with 0.9% normal saline (NS) boluses.

M = Move all of the extra equipment, furniture, other patients in the room, and the family to a safe area (encourage family presence with a supportive team member).

E = Explain to the code team information about the child, including age, weight, height, medical diagnosis, condition prior to code, and events surrounding the code.

Data from Linnard-Palmer, L., Phillips, W., Fink, M., Catolico, O., & Sweeny, N. (2013). Testing a mnemonic on response skills during simulated codes. *Clinical Simulation in Nursing, 9*(6), e191–e197. doi: 10.1016/j.ecns.2011.12.004

Steps to Prevent Pediatric Medication Errors: Safety Tips

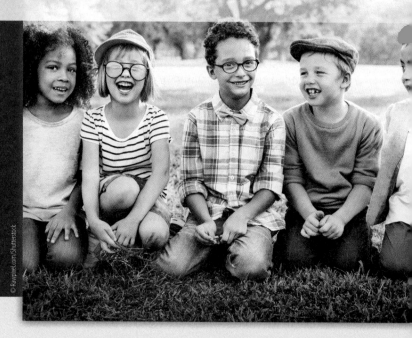

Administering medications to children is very different from administering medications to adults. Children are more prone to medication errors, and administering doses accurately takes skill and requires double-checking each step. Safeguards are needed to safely administer medications to infants and young children, beyond those safeguards applied to adult patients (American Academy of Pediatrics, 2003). The medications most prone to dosing errors are those that are intravenously administered (Crowley, Williams, & Cousins, 2001).

Keep vulnerable infants and children safe! The nurse is the final step in safety and accuracy!

Before Administration

1. Wash your hands to prevent any contamination of the medication; wear gloves when required and when administering IV medications.
2. Know the child's most recent weight, height, and body surface area (BSA), as needed.
3. Understand the indication for the medication.
4. Know the pharmacologic properties of the medication, and be aware of the toxicities, adverse effects, delayed clearance, and potential allergic reactions for all medications.
5. Clarify the order with the prescriber if there is any doubt about it.
6. Never hesitate to call a pharmacist for clarification, support, or education about a drug or its dosing,

safe duration of administration, or compatibility with other drugs or infusing IV fluids.
7. Do not accept verbal or handwritten orders unless it is an emergency; ask that all orders be placed into the electronic medical chart so the pharmacy has access and time to confirm the safety of the order.
8. Do not accept orders that have a terminal zero (require 5 mg rather than 5.0 mg), and do not accept orders without a zero on the left side of a dose less than 1 (require 0.75 mg rather than .75 mg).
9. Do not accept orders that include "do not use abbreviations" such as MSO4 for morphine or U for units or milligrams. Milligrams and micrograms should be written out.
10. Determine whether any laboratory analyses are required before administration of the agent (i.e., serum potassium level for potassium supplementation, last aminoglycoside serum trough level before vancomycin administration, blood cultures required before first-dose antibiotics).
11. Calculate the child's safe dose range by using an approved pediatric formulary.
12. Determine the accurate means and correct quantity when drawing the medication up from a multidose vial.
13. Double-check the medication drug, dose, time, route, and patient identification with a second nurse as needed or required.

14. Confirm your accuracy by completing three safety checks: right drug, right dose in milligrams and quantity in milliliters, right patient.
15. Before leaving the medication room, label the medication with the date, time, patient, medication name, and dose.
16. Bring the original packaging in for parental confirmation and scanning for the electronic medical record.
17. Conduct premedication assessments as warranted, including heart rate and blood pressure for cardiac medications, allergies, and tolerance of previous doses.
18. Do not administer an oral medication to a crying child due to the choking risk.
19. Place the child in an upright position when administering oral medications.
20. Ensure a patent IV for parenteral medications; conduct a visual tracing from the bag hanging to the tubing; check the date on the tubing down and the IV catheter size, location, and patency. Assess the site for infiltration or signs of infection. Wear gloves to prevent contamination. Scrub the IV site hub per institutional policy with sterile alcohol pad, and allow it to dry before instilling medication into the line.
21. Check the patient's identification with two sources (full name, date of birth, medical record number).
22. Prevent vomiting, spilling, or loss of any amount of the medication to ensure the full dose is received.

After Administration

23. Never leave medications at the bedside or leave medications for a parent or other caregiver to administer; return the medication to the medication room if the child does not take the dose.
24. Document carefully, accurately, and thoroughly.
25. Address any medication success tips for a child during rounds, huddles, or handoff reports.

Bibliography

American Academy of Pediatrics, Committee on Drugs and Committee on Hospital Care. (2003). Prevention of medication errors in the pediatric inpatient setting. *Pediatrics, 112(2)*, 431–436.

Crowley, E., Williams, R., & Cousins, D. (2001). Medication errors in children: A descriptive summary of medication errors reports submitted to the United States Pharmacopeia. *Current Therapy Research, 26*, 627–640.

Rapid Response, Code Blue Skills, and PEWS Tool

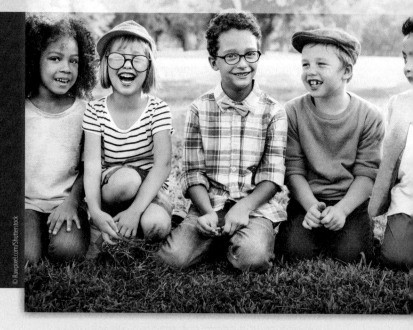

© Rawpixel.com/Shutterstock

Rapid Response

A rapid response team is a coordinated effort that enables a staff member or a family member to receive immediate assistance in evaluating the clinical status of a child. Typically those who respond are either the full code team, a partial code team, or specific team members such as the pediatric intensive care unit (PICU) charge nurse, PICU hospitalist, and the emergency department (ED) primary provider. The goals are to rapidly respond to any concern about the safety and status of a child, to escalate the concern to those who have the advanced skills needed to assess and respond to the child's condition, and to prevent a code blue. The rapid response phone number may be unique, or it may be the same as the code blue number.

Evidence-Based Practice

Research has shown that the use of rapid response teams with members who have specialized skills significantly reduces the rate of in-hospital code blue events and the number of unplanned intensive care transfers (Dacey et al., 2007). The current rate of pediatric survival to discharge after an in-hospital code blue event is 16% (Ray et al., 2009). Rapid response teams, including early activation of these teams by families, have been shown to decrease full pediatric codes, to decrease mortality, and to decrease the duration of pediatric clinical instability (Ray et al., 2009).

Code Blue Skills

The activation of a code blue button or a call to the code blue phone line should initiate a rapid response by a designated team of advanced responders. This team comes as quickly as possible, often avoiding elevators, and provides lifesaving assistance when a child is experiencing a respiratory arrest, severe respiratory distress, shock, cardiovascular arrest, or a combination of these conditions. Responders can include the PICU hospitalist, PICU nurse, respiratory therapist, pharmacist, anesthesiologist, nursing supervisor, surgery representative, emergency room charge nurse, and a central supply representative who can coordinate bringing a new stocked crash cart if the primary one is opened and supplies exhausted. A laboratory assistant may also be a part of the team to run specimens to the lab for rapid evaluation.

Code blue response skills include the following (not in order of priority):

- Rapid assessment, determination of need, and initiation of cardiopulmonary resuscitation
- Care of the family present
- Application of cardiac leads and cardiac monitoring
- Placement of a firm backboard to increase the effectiveness of chest compressions
- Frequent vital signs assessment
- Initiation of IV access, fluid boluses, and laboratory analysis
- Ability and skill to use a length-based color-coded pediatric resuscitation tape
- Accurate confirmation of the child's cardiac dysrhythmia
- Use of code blue algorithms to determine research-based interventions
- Advanced skills in medication preparation and safe administration

- Team work and leadership
- Accurate documentation
- Code blue response team debriefing

Evidence-Based Practice

Predetermined team member roles, team organization, uninterrupted and timely high-quality CPR, rapid defibrillation, and the correction of identified reversible causes of the need for resuscitation efforts lead to an effective code blue team (Prince, Hines, Chyou, & Heegeman, 2014). Regular practice of code blue response skills via simulations and mock code blue scenarios has been shown to increase staff confidence, improve patient outcomes, and reduce child morbidity and mortality (Corey, 2016).

Bedside PEWS Tool

The pediatric early warning score (PEWS) system was developed to provide an objective evaluation of a child who may require a team response due to a deteriorating clinical status (Parshuram, Hutchison, & Middaugh, 2009). The goal when applying the bedside PEWS tool is to use information that is collected in what is considered a routine clinical assessment by various team members, with the outcome being a decision to intervene or transfer the child to a higher level of care. There are many renditions of a bedside pediatric early warning system of communication via a scoring system, all centered around a theme of safe early warning to prevent a child from experiencing poor clinical outcomes or death.

The PEWS tool consists of three categories: behavior, cardiovascular, and respiratory status. Each of these three categories is assessed according to the child's severity on seven specific objective measures: heart rate, systemic blood pressure, capillary refill time (CRT), respiratory rate, respiratory effort, transcutaneous oxygen saturation, and oxygen therapy. The final score ranges from 0 to 9. Reporting of scoring varies per healthcare institution. *Always follow your institution's policies carefully, and never hesitate to call for an assessment or call for help.*

Scoring Guidelines

0-2 = Child is stable

3 = Reassess; report findings to hospitalist and charge nurse; document and reassess frequently

4 = Notify hospitalist and charge nurse; consider respiratory therapist evaluation; reassess frequently

5 = Notify hospitalist, charge nurse, and call respiratory therapist immediately; consider a rapid response

6 = Consider transfer to a higher level of care; call for a rapid response team

7 = Call for a rapid response team; transfer to a higher level of care

	0	1	2	3
Behavior	• Playing • Alert • Appropriate • At baseline	• Sleep • Fussy but consolable	• Irritable • Inconsolable	• Lethargic • Confused • Reduced response to pain
Cardiovascular	• Pink • Capillary refill: 1–2 seconds	• Pale • Capillary refill: 3 seconds	• Gray • Capillary refill: 4 seconds • Tachycardia at 20 beats/min above normal rate	• Gray • Mottled • Capillary refill: 5 seconds or longer • Tachycardia of 30 beats/min above normal rate or bradycardia
Respiratory	• Within normal parameters • No retraction	• Greater than 10 breaths above normal parameters • Use of accessory muscles • $\geq 30\%$ FiO_2	• Greater than 20 breaths above normal parameters • Retractions • $\geq 40\%$ FiO_2 • Oxygen ≥ 6 L/min • Tracheostomy or ventilator dependent	• Below normal parameters with retractions • Grunting • $\geq 50\%$ FiO_2 • Oxygen ≥ 8 L/min

Modified from Gold, D. L., Mihalov, L. K., & Cohen, D. M. (2014). Evaluating the Pediatric Early Warning Score (PEWS) System for admitted patients in the pediatric emergency department. *Academy of Emergency Medicine, 21*(11), 1249–1256. © 2014 by the Society for Academic Emergency Medicine. With permission of the publisher, Wiley.

Evidence-Based Practice

Research has demonstrated that with adequate training for healthcare team members and with consistent use, the bedside PEWS scoring system can often prevent adverse outcomes (Parshuram, Hutchison, & Middaugh, 2009). With a PEWS system implemented in an ED, and with early identification of pediatric patients at risk for deterioration, elevated scores on the tool are associated with appropriate direct intensive care unit (ICU) admissions (Gold, Mihalov, & Cohen, 2014).

Bibliography

Corey, P. J. (2016). *The effectiveness of adult and pediatric code blue simulation-based team trainings*. Doctoral dissertation, Walden University. Retrieved from http://scholarworks.waldenu.edu/dissertations/2804

Dacey, M. J., Mirza, E. R., Wilcox, V., Doherty, M., Mello, J., Boyer, A., . . . Baute, R. (2007). The effect of a rapid response team on major clinical outcome measures in a community hospital. *Critical Care Medicine, 359*(9), 2076-2082.

Gold, D. L., Mihalov, L. K., & Cohen, D. M. (2014). Evaluating the pediatric early warning score (PEWS) system for admitted patients in the pediatric emergency department. *Academy of Emergency Medicine, 21*(11), 1249-1256.

Parshuram, C. S., Hutchison, J., & Middaugh, K. (2009). Development and initial validation of the bedside paediatric early warning system score. *Critical Care, 13*(4), R135.

Prince, C. R., Hines, E. J. Chyou, P.-H., & Heegeman, D. J. (2014). Finding the key to a better code: Code team restructure to improve performance and outcomes. *Clinical Medicine and Research, 12*(1-2), 47-57.

Ray, E. M., Smith, R., Massie, S., Erickson, J., Hanson, C., Harris, B., & Wills, T. S. (2009). Family alert: Implementing direct family activation of a pediatric rapid response team. *Joint Commission Journal on Quality and Patient Safety, 35*(11), 575-587.

Tips for Maintaining Professional Boundaries in Pediatric/Family Nursing Care

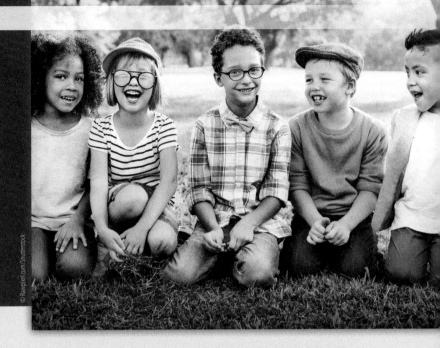

© Rawpixel.com/Shutterstock.

As health care professionals, nurses strive to inspire confidence in their patients and their families, treat all patients and other health care providers professionally, and promote patients' independence. Patients can expect a nurse to act in their best interests and to respect their dignity. This means that a nurse abstains from obtaining personal gain at the patient's expense and refrains from inappropriate involvement with a patient or the patient's family members.

—National Council of State Boards of Nursing (2017)

Caring for Families with Healthy Boundaries

A very special relationship can develop between a pediatric nurse and his or her patients. During the course of providing intimate assessments, symptom management, education, and support, it is possible for a professional relationship to become transformed into a true friendship. Nevertheless, it is the best interest of the nurse and the family to maintain professional boundaries so that the therapeutic nurse–patient relationship is not jeopardized and trust continues to grow. This is not always easy to do when families are cared for over a long period of time and deep relationships develop. To be therapeutic and effective, the professional nurse must set goals for the patient and family that are upheld while maintaining their privacy and dignity. Sensitive information about a child's health history or family dynamics must be kept in confidence and remain in the professional workplace.

According to the National Council of State Boards of Nursing (2014), nurses may describe their care as being "under-involved, therapeutic, or over-involved." Obviously, the "therapeutic" level of care is the goal. To ensure the nurse meets this standard, it is important to be able to identify when boundaries are blurred.

Offering Support Outside of Work

The therapeutic relationship should not extend beyond the workplace. According to the National Council of State Boards of Nursing (2014), red flags include the following:

- Sharing personal information or intimate details of one's life and relationships between the patient, the patient's family, and the nurse
- Spending more time with the patient than is required for professional nursing care
- Meeting patients and families outside of work
- Any display of favoritism or asking to care for a family when it is not an appropriate assignment
- Continuing a relationship with the child and family after the patient is discharged

Not Taking Photos or Filming Children

The use of cell phones to take photographs of a child or family is a direct violation of the child's and family's right to privacy and should be avoided—no matter how cute the child is. This practice violates institutional policies and can lead to loss of employment and legal ramifications. The best practice is to not take any photographs while caring for patients in any healthcare setting. Even taking a picture of a fellow staff member in which a child appears in the background can be a direct violation of privacy laws.

Social Media and Families

Making comments on social media sites about a pediatric patient or the patient's family is a breach of privacy and confidentiality. This sort of behavior is a relatively new violation of boundaries, and it can prove very tempting when the family encourages the nurse to post the comments. Whether the posting of pictures or information about a child or their family takes place during work hours or at home, it is a direct violation of privacy and confidentiality and can lead to the loss of employment.

Attending Funerals

Many healthcare professionals are invited to attend the funeral services of patients for whom they have cared over a period of time. Attending funeral services is a show of respect, but is also a very personal decision that must be made by the individual healthcare professional. For some, attending the service provides a sense of closure and peace. For others, it may be seen as crossing over boundaries. Nurses who find themselves in this position should first check with their institutional policies. If none exists, attending the funeral will be a personal decision to be made by each care provider.

Bibliography

Benbow, D. (2013). Professional boundaries: When does the nurse-patient relationship end? *Journal of Nursing Regulation, 4*(2), 30-33. doi.org/10/1016/S2155-8256(15)30154-X

Cronquist, R., & Spector, N. (2011). Nurses and social media: Regulatory concerns and guidelines. *Journal of Nursing Regulation, 2*(3), 37-40. doi.org/10.1016/S2155-8256(15)30265-9

National Council of State Boards of Nursing. (2014). A nurse's guide to professional boundaries. Retrieved from https://www.ncsbn.org/ProfessionalBoundaries_Complete.pdf

National Council of State Boards of Nursing. (2017). Professional boundaries, p. 1. Retrieved from https://www.ncsbn.org/professional-boundaries.htm

Formula Feeding Guidelines for Infants

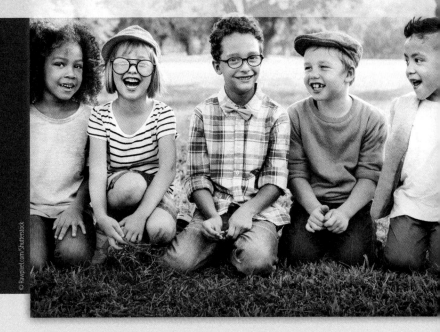

© Rawpixel.com/Shutterstock

Breast milk is the perfect and ideal food for newborns and infants. Breast milk is sterile, is abundant, and provides antibodies to help protect the child from pneumonia, otitis media, and diarrhea. The World Health Organization (WHO) encourages exclusive breastfeeding until the child is 6 months of age, with breastfeeding then continuing, with appropriate complementary foods, until the child's second birthday. Breastfeeding should begin within 1 hour of birth, pacifiers and bottles should be avoided, and breastfeeding should occur on demand throughout the night and day.

Breast milk provides components not found in commercially prepared infant formulas. Specifically, it contains lactoferrin, secretory immunoglobulins (IgA), white blood cells, healthy fats, vitamins, minerals, and carbohydrates—all of which collectively represent the perfect nutrition for infants, provide protective components against infection (e.g., respiratory infections, gastrointestinal infections, and necrotizing enterocolitis), and promote brain development. Breast milk has been shown to improve visual acuity and lead to larger amounts of brain white matter and gray matter (important for memory, speech, learning, decision making, and self-control), larger head circumference, higher neurocognitive test scores, improved motor development, and overall better health and wellness (Belfort et al., 2016; Grace, Oddy, Bulsara, & Hands, 2017; Tawia, 2013).

Breastfeeding has both health and social benefits for the mother. It helps protect women against ovarian cancer, breast cancer, diabetes type 1, and postpartum depression, In addition, it provides up to 98% natural (although not guaranteed) birth control for the first 6 months after delivery.

The skill of breastfeeding must be learned, and a woman should be provided support to initiate and continue breastfeeding her infant. Workplaces should give nursing mothers a place and time for expressing breast milk, as well as a storage area for the breast milk (WHO, 2017).

When a child cannot breastfeed, or when a mother cannot or chooses not to breastfeed, infant formula must be provided. No other substance should be given to an infant younger than 6 months.

Infant Formula Overview

- Infant formulas should be commercially produced, not made at home from other substances (e.g., cow's or goat's milk and sugar or honey).
- Three types of formulas are currently available: premixed liquids, liquid concentrations that require dilution, and powders.
- Infant formulas are provided in the following general types:
  - Cow's milk protein-based formulas
  - Soy-based formulas
  - Protein hydrolysate (broken down into component amino acids for infants with protein allergies to cow's milk or soy-based formulas)
- Infants need iron; an iron-fortified formula should be used for feeding an infant unless instructed otherwise by the primary care provider.
- Cow's milk formulas contain lactose, milk proteins (whey and casein), and minerals, along with vegetable oils and vitamins.

- Compared to human breast milk, commercially prepared formulas have far less lactoferrin (a multifunctional protein with antimicrobial properties) and lysozyme (an antimicrobial wall enzyme that fights infection).
- If an infant is showing signs of colic, switching formulas will not improve the symptoms.
- True allergies or inability to tolerate cow's milk-based formula warrants switching to a different formula per the direction of the primary care provider.
- Soy formulas are available; they do not contain lactose.
- If a child has galactosemia (an inborn error of metabolism), he or she will require a lactose-free formula.
- Formulas to assist an infant with reflux who is not gaining weight are prethickened with rice starch.
- Premature infants will require a formula that has more calories than the 20 kilocalories per ounce provided in standard formulas.
- Toddler formulas should not be used as a replacement for complete nutrition or for picky/fussy eaters.
- Infants should not be weaned off formula until their 1-year birthday.
- Although breastfed infants feed more often than formula-fed infants, formula feeding should take place 6 to 8 times per day
- General guidelines for formula feeds are as follows:
  - Newborns take 2 to 3 ounces of formula per feed, every 3 hours, for a total of 16 to 24 ounces per day.
  - Sterile water should be used when preparing formulas for newborns and young infants.
  - Bottles should be sterilized during the newborn and young infant period, and cleaned well with hot water for the older infant.
  - Hands and counter surfaces should be thoroughly washed before preparing formulas.
  - The exact mixing and storing requirements should be followed to ensure the safety of the child, as over-dilution or under-dilution of formulas can cause health risks.
- The total number of formula feeds will decrease as the child grows older, and the quantity of each feed will increase to 6 to 8 ounces.
- At 6 months, the infant may be ready to start solid foods (i.e., baby cereals), but the amount of formula should not decrease until the infant shows mastery of oral solid foods.
- If the geographical area where the family lives does not have tap water with fluoride, prescribed fluoride will need to be administered.

The pediatric nurse should be a breastfeeding advocate. In fact, the pediatric nurse can have a positive impact on breastfeeding initiation and continuation (Robinson, 2016).

Bibliography

Belfort, M. B., Anderson, P. J., Nowak, V. A., Lee, K. J., Molesworth, C., Thompson, D. K., & Inder, T. E. (2016). Breast milk feeding, brain development, and neurocognitive outcomes: A 7-year longitudinal study in infants born at less than 30 weeks' gestation. *The Journal of Pediatrics, 177,* 133–139.e1. doi: 10.1016/j.jpeds.2016.06.045

Binns, C., Lee, M., & Low, W. Y. (2016). The long-term public health benefits of breastfeeding. *Asia Pacific Journal of Public Health, 28*(1), 7–14.

Grace, T., Oddy, W., Bulsara, M., & Hands, B. (2017). Breastfeeding and motor development: A longitudinal cohort study. *Human Movement Science, 51,* 9–16. doi: 10.1016/j.humov.2016.10.001

Robinson, K. M. (2016). Perinatal nurses: Key to increasing African American breastfeeding rates. *Journal of Perinatal & Neonatal Nursing, 30*(1), 3–5.

Salone, L. R., Vann, W. F., Jr., & Dee, D. L. (2013). Breastfeeding: An overview of oral and general health benefits. *Journal of the American Dental Association, 144*(2), 143–151.

Tawia, S. (2013). Breastfeeding, brain structure and function, cognitive development and educational attainment. *Breastfeeding Review, 21*(3), 15–20.

World Health Organization (WHO). (2003). Global strategies for infant and young child feeding. Retrieved from http://whqlibdoc.who.int/publications/2003/9241562218.pdf

World Health Organization (WHO). (2017). Ten breast feeding facts. Retrieved from http://www.who.int/features/factfiles/breastfeeding/facts/en

How to Effectively Talk to Children

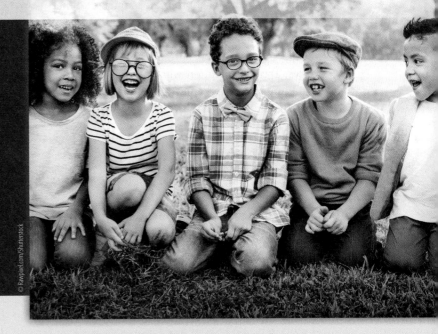

© Rawpixel.com/Shutterstock

Children are not little adults. How we communicate with children, therefore, should be based on a foundation of understanding of growth and development for each of the five developmental stages: infancy, toddler, preschool, school age, and adolescence.

Pediatric nurses might find themselves challenged regarding how to start a relationship with a child in a clinical setting, and then further challenged about how to maintain that relationship. Children are often frightened of nurse-related procedures involving injections and needles (Karlsson, Rydström, Enskär, & Englund, 2014). Consequently, it is important for the nurse to see each individual child as a unique person and understand his or her specific perspective. The uniqueness of the patient–nurse relationship in pediatrics should be based on trust, respect, and kindness. A child should be honored during communication exchanges, he or she should never be belittled or judged, and the interaction should not be full of power struggles. With study, foresight, and experience, the pediatric nurse will develop his or her own ways of engaging with children from infancy to adolescence, while maintaining a playful but professional role in the healthcare team.

The following subsections provide tips for successful communication with children across the developmental stages.

Young Infancy

1. Show trust. Approach the young infant slowly and gently.
2. Use a quiet, kind voice; sing to the infant; smile and hold the infant close to your face so the infant's immature eyes can focus on you.

3. Provide a quiet and consistent environment; take care of the young infant's basic needs.
4. By 4 months of age, young infants will know that when they make a noise, people look and respond. This interaction gives infants pleasure.

Older Infancy

1. Start slowly, but show the growing infant that you and the parents have a positive and trusting relationship.
2. When approaching an older infant, talk to and smile to the parents first.
3. Babble to the infant and encourage return of vocal sounds. Give positive reinforcement when the infant relates to you.
4. Remember that stranger anxiety and separation anxiety start in this developmental period. Be sensitive to older infants' dismay.

Toddler

1. Know that tantrumming and saying "NO!" is expected and normal for this developmental period.
2. Offer just a few (limited) choices when possible. Do not allow the child to "run the show." Say, "Do you want your medication with orange juice or cherry syrup?"
3. Give simple consequences for unwanted behaviors (taking a break from a movie until medications are taken).
4. Talk to children at their level; crouch down if possible and look the child in the eye.

5. Use developmentally appropriate language so that the toddler can have a basic understanding of the purpose of your conversation.
6. Toddlers speak in one- and then two-word sentences. Try to expand on what a toddler is saying by adding nouns and adjectives back to the child. Keep it simple.

Preschooler

1. Preschoolers understand and use longer sentences than toddlers.
2. Cause and effect understanding is intact and can be used to explain reasons behind actions (e.g., getting out of bed and walking will help you go home faster).
3. Preschoolers love to ask why.
4. Preschoolers may talk incessantly, especially when you have developed a trusting relationship. They like to tell and hear the same story over and over. They enjoy talking about their past (but recent) experiences.
5. Preschoolers like to be read to and enjoy picture books to explain concepts.
6. Communicate via play, fantasy, dress up, and pretend.

School Age

1. School-age children like to be talked to and listened to. They want to be a part of decisions, and they want situations explained to them. Most school-age children enjoy conversations with adults. Do not talk down to them.
2. School-age children do well with medical books that explain procedures and interventions.
3. School-age children like to talk about their lives, schoolwork, and peers.
4. To solicit a relationship, school-age children can be engaged when they are offered an important task (feelings of industry).

Adolescence

1. Teenagers enjoy talking about their lives, activities, and friendships.
2. Not all teens will want to establish a friendly relationship with their pediatric nurse.
3. Good conversational openers start with conveying a genuine interest in the teen's life, health, relationships, and accomplishments.
4. When shy, teens may respond to an offer to play a game or do a craft.
5. Teens may want more concrete information about their diagnosis.
6. Silence should be respected and honored.
7. Time alone and privacy should be offered.

Overall

- Smile infectiously.
- Include all family members.
- Never break a promise.
- Never say, "Don't cry" or "You are too big to cry."
- Never compare children to each other.
- Use silence; it is okay.

Bibliography

Fastaff Travel Nursing. (2015). Pediatric nurse: A crash course in talking to kids. Retrieved from http://www.fastaff.com/blog/pediatric-nurse-crash-course-talking-kids

Karlsson, K., Rydström, I., Enskär, K., & Englund, A.-C. D. (2014). Nurses' perspectives on supporting children during needle-related medical procedures. *International Journal of Qualitative Studies on Health and Well-being, 9,* 10.3402/qhw.v9.23063. doi:10.3402/qhw.v9.23063

Ranmal, R., Prictor, M., & Scott, J. T. (2008). Interventions for improving communication with children and adolescents about their cancer. *Cochrane Database of Systematic Reviews, 4,* CD002969. doi:10.1002/14651858.CD002969.pub2

Traub, S. (2016). *Communicating effectively with children.* University of Missouri Extension. Retrieved from http://extension.missouri.edu/p/GH6123

Quick Guide to Selected Developmental Theorists

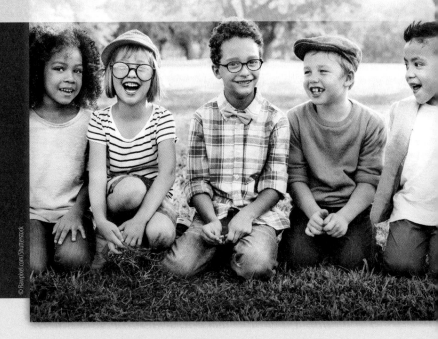

Theoretical foundations provide a platform that bridges between concepts and clinical practice. The application of theory guides the pediatric nurse to not only predict the behaviors and developmental progression of a child, but also understand why children behave the way they do. Theories are intended to help make sense of individual human behavior and the world in which individuals live. In particular, developmental theories provide a structure on which to plan care for children and predict behavioral outcomes.

Erik Erikson (1902–1994): German Scholar

Created the psychosocial developmental theory.

- Childhood's social interactions have the greatest influence over full development.
- Humans pass through eight stages of development, from infancy to geriatrics.
- Mastery of the positive nature of each stage of conflict must occur for the child to function well during further growth and development, the stages finally ending with death.
  - Stage 1: Infancy—trust versus mistrust. An infant needs continuity, consistency, and reassurance that the world is a safe place. Mistrust develops when the child feels rejected, is harmed, or has few needs met.
  - Stage 2: Toddler—autonomy versus shame and doubt. A young child needs encouragement to try skills and tasks without feeling shamed. Otherwise, children may develop the feelings that they cannot act on their own and doubt their abilities.
  - Stage 3: Preschool age—initiative versus guilt. The child needs to have positive reinforcement of new skills and new responsibilities through encouragement. The child needs to feel purposeful through play.
  - Stage 4: School age—industry versus inferiority. Growing children need to learn how to act and perform in school, feeling that they have the skills and abilities to accomplish what is expected of them. Feelings of inferiority develop when they do not feel accepted or able.
  - Stage 5: Adolescence—self-identity versus role confusion. Teens need to develop a sense of who they are and what their purpose in life is. Their self-image is based on what they have learned and how they see themselves able to be successful. Role confusion occurs when there are poor role models, poor communication, and uncertainty about the teen's place in society.
  - Stage 6: Young adult—intimacy versus isolation. The young adult needs to have a sense of value in intimate relationships (siblings, friends, lovers, and partners) versus a feeling of isolation without commitment.
  - Stage 7: Middle age—generativity versus stagnation. The middle adulthood period is the time of less selfishness and more concern for children, family, society, and the future.

- Stage 8: Elder years—self-actualization versus despair. The older adult will experience a sense of coming to terms with his or her life and not fearing death, versus feelings of uselessness and personal despair.

Sigmund Freud (1856–1939): Austrian Neurologist

Authored the grand theory of psychosexual development.

- The grand theory of psychosexual development is based on a series of stages representing the conflicts the child must satisfy as part of libidinal desire. The various stages play a significant role in the child's development. If children do not complete a psychosexual stage, they will become fixated, which later influences their adult behaviors.
- The pleasure-seeking energy (id) focuses on specific erogenous areas of the body, whereas the ego attempts to mediate and control the id's demands.
- Successful mastery and completion of each stage leads to a healthy personality in adulthood.
  - Stage 1: Infancy—erogenous zone is the mouth (oral). The infant experiences the oral passive stage during the first 6 months after birth, and the oral aggressive stage during the second 6 months. The infant obtains stimulation through sucking and tasting and obtaining comfort from oral sensations.
  - Stage 2: Toddler—erogenous zone is the bowel and bladder control (anal). The primary focus of the libido during this phase in on controlling elimination. Parental leniency can lead to an anal-expulsive personality, which then develops into a destructive personality. Parental control or strictness can lead to an anal-retentive personality, which is characterized by an obsessive, orderly, and rigid nature. Penis envy is the outcome of desire to be the opposite gender for girls.
  - Stage 3: Preschooler—erogenous zone is the genitals. The child discovers differences in gender. The Oedipus complex is the desire to possess the mother figure while replacing the father figure. Castration anxiety is considered an outcome of fear of the father figure's punishment.
  - Stage 4: School age—erogenous zone is considered inactive (latency). In this stage, sexual energy is directed toward learning and creative pursuits.
  - Stage 5: Adolescent—erogenous zone is a powerful maturing sexual interest, starting in adolescence but persisting throughout life (genital).

Jean Piaget (1896–1990): Swiss Scholar

Created the cognitive developmental theory.

- The cognitive developmental theory explains the development of children's thought processes, mental status, and knowledge (epistemology),
- How a child's thought processes develop influences how the child interacts with the world.
- The theory assumes that children do not think the way adults do, but rather think differently.
- The theory provides a sequence of steps to cognitive development:
  - Step 1: sensory motor. The infant uses the senses and motor exploration to learn about the environment.
  - Step 2: preoperational. The toddler and the preschooler learn about symbols, creative play, and manipulation while tending to be egotistical in their thinking; that is, they lack the ability to see the world from another's point of view or understand other people's feelings.
  - Step 3: concrete operational. The school-age child focuses on logical operations and specific principles to solve problems and learn about the academic world.
  - Step 4: Formal operational. The older school-age child and teen become more adult-like in their thinking; they start to use hypothetical thinking and early abstract thinking.

Lawrence Kohlberg (1927–1987): American Scholar

- Kohlberg proposed a theory on how children grow into moral beings.
- He based his theory on three levels of moral development spanning childhood:
  - Level 1: Preconventional. During the young childhood years, the child has little to no sense of what is considered right or wrong behavior. Motivation comes from wanting to avoid punishment and securing rewards.
  - Level 2: Conventional. During the school age years, the child knows what is wrong or right and tends to want to follow rules through respecting authority. Children of this age have a strong sense of what others around them want of their behaviors.
  - Level 3: Postconventional. During the teenage years, children develop individual principles to guide their moral behavior. Motivation comes entirely from within but is influenced by the significant adults in their lives.

John Bowlby (1907–1990): British Scholar

- Proposed an early childhood theory on social development called the attachment theory.
- Attachment theory assumes that a child's early relationship with specific caregivers plays a significant role in the growing child's social relationships throughout life.
- Each child is assumed to be born with a programmed (biologic) tendency to seek out and then maintain close relationships; this is considered a survival tactic. Separation can lead to unsatisfactory personal relationships later in life.

Abraham Maslow (1908–1970): American Scholar

- Proposed a needs pyramid based on five stacking concepts. The first four levels are deficiency needs; the top level comprises being and growth needs.
- Maslow believed that everyone has the potential to progress to the top-level need, but often this progression is disrupted by an inability to meet the lower-level needs.
  - Physiological needs: Feelings of fulfillment and one's needs being met in relation to sleep, rest, warmth, comfort, food, and water
  - Safety needs: Feelings of security and safety in one's various environments
  - Belonging needs: Feelings of satisfaction in intimate relationships, partnerships, and friendships
  - Esteem needs: Feelings of accomplishment, prestige, and being needed
  - Self-actualization needs: Feeling of living to one's highest and full potential

Bibliography

Harmon Hanson, S. M. (2001). *Family health care nursing* (2nd ed., pp. 45–46). Philadelphia, PA: F. A. Davis.

Hockenberry, M., & Wilson, D. (2017). *Essentials of pediatric nursing* (10th ed., pp. 45-50). St. Louis, MO: Elsevier.

Kaakinen, J. R., Gedlay-Duff, V., Coehlo, D. P., & Harmon Hanson, S. M. (2010). *Family health care nursing* (4th ed., pp. 64-65). Philadelphia, PA: F. A. Davis.

Linnard-Palmer, L. (2015). *PedsNotes* (rev. ed., pp. 7-8). Philadelphia, PA: F. A. Davis.

McLeod, S. (2016), Maslow's hierarchy of needs. *Simply Psychology*. Retrieved from https://simplypsychology.org/maslow.html

Ollendick, T. H., & Vasey, M. W. (1999). Developmental theory and the practice of clinical child psychology. *Journal of Clinical Child Psychology, 28*(4), 457-466.

Peterson, L., & Tremblay, G. (1999). Importance of developmental theory and investigation to research in clinical child psychology. *Journal of Clinical Child Psychology, 28*(4), 448-456.

Glossary

Absence seizure A seizure in which the child "checks out" and is nonresponsive for a brief period.

Abstract thinking Thinking in terms of concepts and general principles.

Abuse Child maltreatment that consists of acts of commission (physical abuse, sexual abuse, and psychological abuse).

Abusive head trauma A severe form of nonaccidental cerebral trauma leading to encephalopathy.

Acidosis Increased acidity of the blood.

Acne An accumulation of pimples—comedones, papules, pustules, nodules, and or cysts—that is caused by blocked pilosebaceous glands.

Acquired heart disease Cardiovascular disease that occurs sometime after birth.

Acquired immunity Immunity that is not inherited.

Active immunity Immunity developed through contact with a disease-causing agent.

Acute care pediatric nursing Team-oriented care for children who have complex healthcare needs that require expanded medical treatments and nursing care beyond what can be offered in clinic or ambulatory settings.

Acute diarrhea A gastrointestinal condition characterized by increased intestinal motility and rapid emptying, leading to frequent loose or liquid stools that may be foul smelling.

Acyanotic Left-to-right cardiac blood flow.

Adaptive immunity Components of the lymph system (lymphocytes) that are responsible for identifying self versus non-self, and therefore that do not react until activated by a foreign invader.

Addison syndrome A metabolic disorder caused by reduced production and secretion of cortisol and aldosterone, the hormones of the adrenal gland.

Adolescence The time period from the beginning of secondary sex characteristics through the end of the period of rapid growth in height and complete reproductive maturity called primary sex characteristics.

Adventitious breath sounds Abnormal breath sounds that include rales, rhonchi, wheezing, and stridor.

Alarm fatigue Sensory desensitization caused by exposure to excessive monitor alarms, which cause the nurse to become immune to the sound of the alarm and not hear it.

Alkalosis Abnormally low hydrogen ion concentration in the blood.

Allodynia A pain experience due to a type of stimulus that normally does not induce or provoke pain.

Anemia A condition in which the blood lacks adequate numbers of red blood cells or hemoglobin.

Anorectal malformations Congenital absence of a patent anorectal canal, a severe narrowing of the anal canal, or the presence of only a fistula (external to the peritoneum).

Anthropometric measurements Height, weight, head circumference, and body mass index.

Anticipatory guidance The process of preparing parents, guardians, or caregivers for what to expect as the child grows, develops, and matures.

Anxiety A mental disorder characterized by restlessness, difficulty concentrating, being irritable or fatigued, and feeling insecure or powerless.

Apgar scores A system for scoring the stability of the newborn's first few hours.

Ascites Edema concentrated in the abdomen.

Asphyxiation Choking.

Aspiration Inhalation of a substance or foreign body so that it enters the larynx or lower respiratory tract.

Assent Inclusion of a child in the discussions of the child's health care, treatment decisions, and priorities.

Associative play Play characterized by loose rules, creativity, and pretend or dramatic play; it typically starts as spontaneous with little preparation, thought, organization, or role delineation.

Asthma A chronic inflammatory disease of the lungs that affects the small and large airways; it stems from the airways' hyper-responsiveness to specific triggers.

Atelectasis Collapse of the lung owing to blockage of the small airways; a complication of bronchiolitis.

Autism spectrum disorders A group of disorders that affects brain development.

Autoimmune response Reaction of the immune system against a "self" antigen on normal body tissues that it is supposed to ignore.

Autonomy The ability to act without another person's control or influence; independence.

Bacteria Single-cell organisms capable of causing infection.

Barlow's sign A method of assessing for congenital hip dysplasia; it is positive if, when adducting the child's hip joint, the femoral head slips back out of the socket to a state of dislocation.

Beneficence The provision of ethically correct intention acts of good (without errors).

Binuclear family A family in which a child's living time is divided between two or more households.

Body image A person's perception of the attractiveness of his or her own body.

Breakthrough pain The experience of continued and increasing pain above the child's baseline pain experience; pain that emerges during a period of symptom management and may be associated with new activity or increased movement.

Bronchiolitis A viral respiratory infection of the lower airway structures.

Brudzinski's sign A sign associated with meningitis, in which severe neck stiffness causes the child's hips and knees to flex when the neck is flexed.

Burn Damage to the skin and other tissues caused by heat, chemicals, electricity, sunlight, or radiation.

Camp nursing Health support for children who attend day or overnight camps.

Carriage The presence of microbes that do not cause illness.

Carrier A person in whom microbes are present, but who is asymptomatic and well, though capable of spreading the pathogen to others.

Cephalocaudal growth pattern The growth pattern for an infant, in which growth proceeds from the head downward.

Cerebrospinal fluid A fluid found in the brain and spinal cord, which is produced and reabsorbed by the choroid plexus lining the four ventricles of the brain.

Child maltreatment According to the CDC, "any act or series of acts of commission or omission by a parent or other caregiver (e.g., clergy, coach, teacher) that results in harm, potential for harm, or threat of harm to a child."

Child Protective Services A government agency that protects children from abuse or maltreatment.

Chronic diarrhea Ongoing loose and watery stools, typically associated with malabsorption syndrome, lactose intolerance, inflammatory bowel disease, and food allergens.

Clinical judgment The analysis of, interpretation of, and conclusions made about a patient's condition, including that individual's holistic needs, concerns, health problems, and areas of needed action or intervention.

Club foot A congenital condition in which the foot is twisted into an unusual position.

Cognition Mental capacity and awareness.

Cognitive development Development of the ability to think and reason.

Cognitive impairment Overall mental deficiency or mental difficulty.

Colic A nonpathologic condition in which an infant cries for more than 3 hours per day for more than 3 days per week.

Color-coded alarms Codes used in emergency department, pediatric intensive care unit, and acute care settings to alert the pediatric healthcare team that support is required.

Communication The sharing of information and meaning.

Competencies Skills and knowledge needed to provide care appropriately and effectively.

Concept-based learning A dynamic approach to the ever-growing body of scientific nursing knowledge that focuses on learning key concepts that can be applied to various situations and settings.

Concrete operations In Piaget's theory, the phase of development in which logical thinking and basic inductive reasoning about the world and life's events guide the school-age child in processing information and developing thinking strategies.

Concussion A mild traumatic brain injury, in which the impact of a direct hit to the head causes the brain to develop neuropathy such as micro-bleeds and axonal injury.

Congenital heart defect A malformation of the physical structures in the heart that is present at birth.

Congenital heart disease Heart disease that is present at birth and predominantly involves structural issues that affect blood flow and, therefore, perfusion.

Congestive heart failure A chronic or acute decrease in the ability of the heart to pump adequate amounts of blood to the body, which causes congestion or backup of fluid into the systemic vascular and/or pulmonary vasculature, negatively impacting perfusion; directly related to a malfunctioning ventricular muscle.

Congenital hip dysplasia Developmental dysplasia of the hip, in which either the hip joint is shallow enough to allow the head of femur to slip slightly (preluxation) from the acetabulum, or it is so shallow that the femoral head can move around the hip socket (subluxation).

Consent Permission to initiate a healthcare intervention.

Constipation Infrequent and difficult passage of stool.

Contact dermatitis A skin rash that can be caused by a variety of irritants.

Contagious Readily spread through direct and indirect contact.

Coping Skills for handling stressful events, stressful circumstances, and other stressors.

Cortisol A stress hormone released from the adrenal cortex (i.e., the outer segment of the adrenal gland).

Critical thinking A problem-solving means of thinking through a complex situation and drawing the conclusions that will best help a child and family; it is used to separate what is known from what is unknown while helping a team of concerned healthcare providers devise a plan to assist a child in need.

Critically ill Having a potentially life-altering or life-threatening illness or injury.

Crohn disease Inflammation of all layers of the gastrointestinal mucosa, affecting any portion of the gastrointestinal tract.

Croup Acute inflammation, edema, and mucus production within the larynx, trachea, and bronchi caused by a virus such as parainfluenza, influenza, enteroviruses, and respiratory syncytial virus; also called laryngotracheobronchitis.

Cryotherapy Use of liquid nitrogen to kill cells.

Cultural assessment tools Tools that can provide a structure for nurses to provide culturally driven care for pediatric patients and their families.

Cultural awareness An ability to stand back and view other cultural groups as unique, distinct, important and influential while demonstrating respect.

Cultural beliefs Patterns of behavior, communication, and human encounters that are based on a shared and learned framework.

Cultural competence Skills in cultural assessment and culturally driven care.

Cultural diversity The presence of multiple groups within a population, including groups other than those considered traditional cultural or ethnic groups.

Cultural humility An ability to see the perspectives of another outside of one's own cultural group, especially those aspects that are most important to the other.

Cultural intelligence The ability to differentiate whether a behavior is driven by an individual's cultural background or is characteristic of a specific person.

Cultural sensitivity A set of skills that enable an individual to study and learn about diverse cultures and come to an understanding of cultural practices and needs.

Culture A set of learned behaviors or beliefs that are shared among members of a group.

CUS protocol A means of encoding a level of concern by selecting key phrases that staff must be trained to recognize as indicating that a red-flag issue exists.

Cushing syndrome A metabolic disorder caused by hypersecretion of the adrenal hormone cortisol.

Cyanosis Bluish discoloration of the skin due to low oxygen saturation.

Cyanotic Right-to-left cardiac blood flow.

Cycle of abuse A pattern of behavior in which children who experience child maltreatment grow up and abuse their own children.

Cystic fibrosis (CF) An autosomal recessive genetic disorder caused by a mutation in the protein cystic fibrosis transmembrane conductance regulator (*CFTR*) gene on chromosome 7, which regulates digestive secretions, sweat, and mucus production.

Decibel dB; a unit of measurement of the intensity of sound.

Deciduous teeth The first set of teeth; also known as baby teeth.

Dehydration A condition in which fluid loss exceeds fluid intake.

Delegation Assignment of tasks to those persons who have the appropriate legal capacity, educational preparation, and licensure or certification.

Depression A persistent mood disorder characterized by a state of sadness and loss of interest in life activities.

Developmental theory Theory related to the developmental stages of childhood.

Differentiation How closely a tumor cell resembles its mother cell.

Disciplinary action Punishment for violation of a regulation or standard, which may include loss of license and support of criminal investigations, as needed.

Discomfort Lack of comfort or ease.

Dislocation Displacement of a bone from a joint, such as the femoral head from the hip socket.

Disparities of health outcomes Poorer clinical or health outcomes associated with particular races, ethnicities, and cultural groups due to, among other things, the intersection of cultural factors with acceptance of therapy.

Distress Stress that is not managed or becomes chronic, such that the individual feels the effects of stress beyond emotional reactions and the body begins to respond to the stressful stimuli.

Diurnal enuresis Daytime urinary incontinence.

Duchenne muscular dystrophy A recessive disorder linked to a mutation on the X chromosome, which leads to progressive skeletal muscle abnormalities in children.

Dying process The predictable physiological changes and emotional states that occur as the end of life approaches.

Dysfunctional grief Complicated grief over a period of at least a year, which includes prolonged emotional reactions such as longing, loneliness, yearnings for the deceased person, depression, low self-esteem, sleep disturbances, eating disturbances, and inability to function in roles such as employment and marriage.

Early intervention Support for children and families that begins soon after birth, so as to minimize the extent of the problem experienced by the young child.

Eczema Atopic dermatitis; an allergic reaction to an agent, which causes a dry rash from a disruption of the skin barrier.

Egocentric Related to the perspective that the world revolves around "me."

Emetogenic The property of inducing vomiting.

Empowerment The process through which a family comes to feel competent to provide care for their child due to the support, education, and trust built through interacting with the healthcare team.

Enabling Providing situations and opportunities for a family to gain and show mastery of the care required by their child.

Endemic A more widely spread occurrence of an infectious disease within a larger geographical area or beyond a particular community.

End-of-life care The care aspects of the dying process; the wishes, cultural practices, and care activities surrounding the imminent death of the child.

Enucleation Removal of the eye.

Enuresis A voiding dysfunction that occurs after a child has mastered urinary toilet training.

Enzyme A substance that catalyzes a chemical reaction, but is itself unchanged by the reaction.

Epidemic A widespread occurrence of an infectious disease within a community found at a particular time.

Epidural hematoma A rapid arterial bleed where a clot forms above the dura mater.

Epiglottitis A severe, life-threatening infection of the epiglottis caused mainly by *Haemophilus influenzae* type B bacteria.

Epinephrine A stress hormone released from the adrenal medulla (i.e., the inner segment of the adrenal gland).

Epiphyseal plate The growth plate found in bones.

Epispadias Abnormal positioning of the urinary meatus on the upper side (dorsum) of the penis.

Ethics The branch of philosophy concerned with decisions about what is right and wrong.

Ethnicity The beliefs and practices of a group whose members identify with one another based on common language, ancestry, nationality, or other factors.

Evidence-based practice Best practice based on the integration of clinical expertise, scientific evidence, and the patient's and family's perspectives.

Extended family Family members beyond the parents and siblings.

Extensor surfaces Surfaces of muscles that move a body part, such as the elbows, knees, shins, and forehead.

Family-centered care A model of care based on the premise that the family is the constant in the child's life; it compels healthcare providers to recognize that all family members are affected by the injury, illness, hospitalization, or healthcare need that the child is experiencing.

Family strengths Assets of a family that develop as a family grows, interacts, and has experiences; they include affection and appreciation, commitment, ability to cope with stress and crisis, positive communication, time spent together as a unit, and spiritual well-being.

Fatigue A state of being tired, exhausted, wearied, or unmotivated, with poor energy and poor concentration.

Febrile seizure A seizure that occurs in children ranging from 3 months to 6 years of age, and which is not classified as an epileptic seizure disorder.

Fetal circulation The blood flow in the fetus; the right ventricle and atrium circulate deoxygenated blood to the lungs, and then the oxygenated blood returns to the left atrium and ventricle to be pumped to the rest of the body.

Fluid maintenance Fluid needs as determined in milliliters per kilogram of body weight, which is then converted to identify the appropriate dose rate to provide the needed amount per unit of time, usually 1 hour.

Fungi Yeasts and molds capable of causing infection.

Galactosemia An inborn error of metabolism that occurs when a child is unable to convert galactose, a simple carbohydrate found in dairy products and milk, to glucose-1-phosphate.

Gas exchange The movement of oxygen from the lungs into the bloodstream, and the corresponding movement of carbon dioxide from the bloodstream into the lungs.

Glomerulonephritis A kidney condition that develops following an infectious process—typically 1 week to 10 days after a streptococcal infection.

Good faith In regard to reporting child abuse/neglect, acting out of genuine belief that maltreatment is present, rather than for some other rationale.

Grand mal seizure A generalized seizure that affects the entire body; it involves a combination of abnormal muscular activity including tonic (sustained contraction) and clonic (jerking movements) features.

Graves's disease An immune-mediated disorder associated with hyperthyroidism and caused by stimulated B-lymphocyte immunoglobulins that bind to the thyroid hormone-releasing receptors, mimicking the action of thyroid-stimulating hormone.

Grief The process of deep sorrow.

Handoff The passing or transfer of information and responsibility between healthcare providers.

Health literacy The ability of an individual or group to obtain, process, and understand basic health information and services needed to make appropriate health decisions.

Healthcare disparities Differences in access to health care among different groups.

Hearing loss Loss of auditory abilities; characterized as conductive (problems with the ear canal, eardrum, or middle ear structures), sensorineural (damage to the auditory nerve or the inner ear structures), or mixed.

Hematopoiesis The process by which normal stem cell proliferation and differentiation takes place.

Hemolytic uremic syndrome (HUS) a rare and potentially lethal form of kidney failure in children who develop an infection caused by either *Escherichia coli* 0157.H7 or *Escherichia coli* 0111.

Hernia Protrusion of an organ through the cavity in which it resides. For example, a *diaphragmatic hernia* is a protrusion of abdominal contents (intestines) through an opening in the diaphragm muscle.

Hirschsprung disease A structural anomaly of the lower segment of the large intestine and rectum.

Histology The types of cells found in tumor tissue.

Holistic Care for the whole person, including not only his or her medical condition, but also any mental, social, and environment concerns.

Hormones Substances released by the glands in minute quantities into the bloodstream, which serve as chemical messengers in the body.

Hospice care Care provided to a child nearing the end of life when the application of medical diagnostics and treatments is no longer considered.

Hospice nursing The comprehensive emotional, spiritual, psychosocial, and physical care of the terminally ill child and the family members.

Hyperbilirubinemia Jaundice; a yellow discoloration of the skin caused by the deposition of unconjugated bilirubin in the skin.

Hyper-responsiveness Overreaction of the immune system against a genuine foreign body.

Hypertonic A type of dehydration in which the child's body water loss is greater than the electrolyte loss.

Hypertrophic pyloric stenosis Excess growth of the circular areas of muscle that surround the pyloric valve, which then blocks gastric emptying.

Hypospadias An abnormally positioned opening of the urinary meatus, which may be located in various areas of the penis or base of the penis—most commonly on the underside of the penis.

Hypotonic A type of dehydration in which the child's electrolyte loss exceeds the water loss.

Hypoxemia An abnormally low level of oxygen in the blood.

Idiopathic pain Pain described or experienced by a child even in the presence of no identifiable pathological condition that would contribute to the source of the discomfort.

Immunization schedule The recommended doses and agents for routine vaccinations.

Immunotherapy In the context of childhood cancer, immune cells such as cytotoxic T lymphocytes that are treated with Epstein-Barr virus to stimulate cancer-fighting properties.

Impaired immunocompetence Reduced ability to fight off infections, such that even minor microbial encounters can become extremely serious.

Inborn error of metabolism A congenital genetic defect that affects one of the metabolic pathways.

Incident report Documentation of an error or near miss, which is submitted to administrative personnel.

Increased intracranial pressure Increased pressure inside the skull.

Industry A feeling of competence and mastery of skills.

Infection Invasion of the body by microorganisms, which then reproduce in the body.

Informatics The application of information and computer science to health care.

Initiative versus guilt In Erikson's theory, the preschool stage, in which the child attempts to try out new skills, try out new relationships, and participate in new activities, but may develop a sense of self-doubt and guilt if unsuccessful or discouraged.

Innate immunity Cells and proteins—such as macrophages, neutrophils, and natural killer cells—that are programmed to quickly identify and react to the invasion of microorganisms.

Interdisciplinary team A group of healthcare professionals from diverse fields who work in a coordinated fashion toward a common goal for the patient.

Intravenous immunoglobulins Pooled antibodies that are administered to provide artificial passive immunity.

Intuitive thinking A practice in which the child centers his or her thinking on one characteristic of something and then forms a judgment or decision based on that single characteristic.

Intussusception An invagination or telescoping of a segment of bowel into a section just distal, which usually occurs at the junction of the ileum with the lower colon.

I-PASS A mnemonic for the elements to be included in handoff communication; illness severity, patient summary, action list, situation awareness and contingency planning, and synthesis by the receiver.

Isotonic A type of dehydration in which equal loss of water and sodium occurs.

Justice Demonstration of fairness, justness, and impartiality in all care and patient interactions.

Kernicterus A condition in which the neonate's bilirubin levels are high enough to become absorbed by the brain tissue, potentially causing severe brain damage.

Kernig's sign A sign associated with meningitis, in which severe hamstring stiffness leaves the child unable to straighten the leg when the hip is flexed to 90 degrees.

Kübler-Ross, Elisabeth The developer of a widely accepted model of the series of predictable emotional stages experienced by those who are surviving a child's death.

Latch-key child A child who returns home after school, but is not supervised by an adult until the parent returns home from work.

Legg-Calvé-Perthes disease A muscular disorder characterized by avascular necrosis of the femoral head.

Leukemia Cancer in tissues where blood cell production occurs.

Leukocoria An abnormal whitish glow on the child's retina when light falls on the eye in a particular angle, which is indicative of the presence of a retinoblastoma.

Licensure Possession of a state license to work as a professional nurse.

Limb-length discrepancies Differences in the lengths of the arms or the legs.

Lund-Browder chart A tool used to determine total body surface area damaged by burns in pediatric patients.

Lymphoma Cancer that develops from lymphocytes.

Macroparasites Organisms visible to the naked eye, such as nematodes (worms) or arthropods (insects), that live in and feed on other organisms' tissues.

Macule Color change to the skin that is flat, not palpable, and less than 1 cm in diameter.

Magical thinking The idea that merely thinking about or wishing an interaction, person, or event will cause it to occur.

Malignant Cancerous.

Malpractice An act where specific standards of care were not performed or fully met.

Mandatory reporter A person who is legally obligated to report to authorities the actual or suspected abuse of a child (or other vulnerable person).

Maple syrup urine disease An autosomal recessive metabolic disorder that results in accumulation of three amino acids and their keto acids, which cause the urine to have a sweet odor.

Meningitis Inflammation or infection of the meninges, which can be viral, bacterial or aseptic in nature.

Metabolic pathway Any of the complex mechanisms of carbohydrate, lipid, and protein synthesis or catabolism, as well as the production, secretion, and mechanism of action of various hormones.

Metabolism The chemical reactions that occur via metabolic pathways; these biochemical processes sustain life.

Metastasis Distant growth of tumor cells.

Mitotic index The percentage of tumor cells currently in the process of division.

Mnemonics Memory tools used to rapidly recall complex information, sets of steps for skills, or components of treatment plans.

Moral development Development of a sense of right and wrong, and the ability to perform moral reasoning.

Morning huddle A meeting of healthcare personnel at a predetermined time each morning to discuss the day's schedule and clarify patient needs.

Mummy wrap A type of soft restraint used with pediatric patients that gives them a sense of security, while enabling the healthcare provider to access the extremity that is the target of the skill procedure.

Munchausen syndrome by proxy A rare, sometimes fatal form of child maltreatment in which a caregiver with some healthcare education or experience—often the mother—fabricates, exaggerates, or induces the symptoms of a medical condition in a child as a way of getting attention.

Nadir In the context of childhood cancer, the point at which antineoplastic drugs have suppressed the production of red blood cells, neutrophils, and thrombocytes to their lowest level.

Narcotic An opioid pain reliever.

National Council of State Boards of Nursing (NCSBN) A national organization that provides oversight, regulation, and authority over licensure and practice of nursing.

National Standards for Culturally and Linguistically Appropriate Services in Health Care (CLAS) A set of mandates, guidelines, and recommendations, developed by the Office of Minority Health within the Department of Health and Human Services, to inform, guide, and facilitate recommended and required practices related to culturally and linguistically appropriate health services.

Natural immunity Immunity developed through contact with an agent in the environment.

Nausea Upset stomach, which may be followed by vomiting.

Neglect Child maltreatment that consists of acts of omission (physical neglect, emotional neglect, medical/dental neglect, educational neglect, and failure to supervise).

Negligence A breach or failure in behaving in a reasonable and prudent manner.

Neonatal intensive care unit (NICU) A specialty unit for neonatal patients whose care requires advanced training and experience.

Nephrotic syndrome Minimal change nephrotic syndrome; the development of large pores on the final filtration membrane of the kidney, which leads to a significant loss of serum protein into the urine.

Neuroblastoma A cancer of the central nervous system that arises from the branches of nerves that run out of or exit from the spinal cord.

Neurochemicals Hormones and other substances released by the nervous system that cause a number of physiological symptoms.

Neuropathic pain A sensory dysfunction that occurs in the presence of structural damage, lesions or disease, or nerve cell dysfunction or injury within the central or peripheral nervous system.

Neutropenia A low number of neutrophils in the blood.

New morbidity A term coined in the 1980s by pediatrician Robert Haggerty to denote concerns associated with current environmental and social issues that decrease quality of life, as distinguished from issues of concern during earlier centuries, such as infectious disease.

Night terrors A sleep disorder characterized by screaming, intense fear, and flailing.

Nightmares Bad dreams.

Nonmaleficence Doing no harm, reducing risk, and reducing pain or discomfort.

Norepinephrine A stress hormone released from the adrenal medulla (i.e., the inner segment of the adrenal gland).

Normal inhabitants The normal flora; the billions of bacteria found on the skin of a child.

Nurse practice act (NPA) State legislation and regulations established through state nursing boards that provide the nursing profession with guidelines on nursing practice and governance on performance.

Obesity Extremely excessive weight that, in children, occurs when dietary intake exceeds the child's energy expenditure on a daily basis.

Oral rehydration therapy Replacement of dehydration or fluid losses.

Ortolani's sign A method of assessing for congenital hip dysplasia; it is positive if a clicking sound is heard while the femoral head is slipping back into the acetabulum.

Osmolality The number of dissolved particles in 1 liter of fluid.

Ossification Replacement of cartilage (embryonic connective tissue) with osteoblasts during the maturation process.

Otitis media Ear infection.

Overweight Weighing more than is normal for the child's age group.

Oxygenation The addition of oxygen to the body's systems.

Pain Physical and emotional suffering or discomfort caused by illness or injury.

Pain assessment tools Biophysical assessments of pain through vital signs measurement and oxygen saturation findings, objective pain assessment tools that utilize the clinical judgment of the nurse to determine the level of pain the child is experiencing, and subjective pain assessment tools that allow the child to express his or her experience of pain.

Pain threshold The minimal sensory stimuli needed to be perceived as a source of discomfort or pain.

Palliative care An area of specialization that provides assistance to give the child the best possible quality of life by reducing suffering, improving discomfort, controlling symptoms, and, when possible, restoring functional capacity; it focuses on emotional support, resource allocation, symptom management, education, honest and straightforward communication with all family members involved in the child's dying process, and the building and implementation of a therapeutic environment for the dying child.

Palliative measures The types of medical treatments offered to the dying child, which are intended to reduce symptoms and increase comfort, rather than to provide a cure.

Pandemic The presence of an infectious disease breakout within a large or wide geographical area such as across a country, a continent, or the world.

Papule A solid raised lesion with distinct borders that is 1 cm or less in diameter.

Parallel play A type of play in which toddlers move toward and play near each other, but typically end up back to back, or alongside each other, not sharing toys or craft supplies.

Passive immunity Immunity developed through exposure to antibodies, such as through breast milk.

Pathogen A microbe that has the potential to cause infection.

Pediatric acute care Pediatric hospital units that provide continued assessments and, if the technology is available, monitoring, but at a lesser level of intensity, without the need for 1:1 or 1:2 nursing care ratios.

Pediatric intensive care unit (PICU) A specialty unit for pediatric patients whose care requires advanced training and experience.

Perfusion Delivery of blood to the body's cells.

PERRLA Pupil reaction: pupils equal, round, reactive to light, and accommodation.

Phallic–locomotion In Freud's theory, the preschool stage, in which the child recognizes that there are differences in the genders and shows an interest in discovery and understanding of the genital area.

Phenylketonuria (PKU) An inborn error of metabolism in which children lack the enzyme phenylalanine hydroxylase and therefore are unable to convert phenylalanine—an essential amino acid consumed in the diet that is typically used for protein synthesis—to tyrosine in the liver.

Pica The consumption of material not associated with food substances.

Power distance The feelings and perceptions of inequality that exist between people and teams.

Precocious puberty A rare condition in which prepubescence and subsequent puberty occur earlier than expected—before the age of 9 for boys and before the age of 8 for girls.

Preconceptual thought In Piaget's theory, the type of thinking that occurs in preschoolers, who are unable to distinguish members of the same class.

Preconventional In Kohlberg's theory, the preschool stage, in which the child's moral thinking and behavior are based on notions of obedience and punishment.

Prepubescence The stage of development in which the school-age child develops secondary sex characteristics.

Primary sex characteristics Maturation of testes, ovaries, and external genitalia.

Primary skin lesion The initial change of skin integrity.

Prions The smallest known disease-causing agents; they are made of infectious protein, but lack DNA and RNA.

Procedural sedation Conscious sedation during invasive bedside procedures; the child breathes independently but requires constant visual supervision and rapid airway support by a certified team.

Proximal–distal growth pattern The growth pattern for an infant, in which growth proceeds from the center point outward.

Psychosexual development In Freud's theory, the development of libido fixed on specific areas of the body, which proceeds through five stages (oral, anal, phallic, latent, genital).

Psychosocial development In Erikson's theory, the development of personality over the life span based on social influences and environmental factors.

Puberty The time period of completed sexual maturation when a teen is able to reproduce.

Pustule A raised lesion filled with a fluid exudate, giving it a white or yellow appearance.

Quality and Safety Education for Nurses (QSEN) A program created to address some of the challenges encountered when trying to prepare nurses for professional practice, which focuses on the knowledge, skills, and attitudes needed to consistently and continuously improve the practice of professional nursing.

Race A group identified on the basis of supposedly shared genetic or physical traits.

Radiation High-energy X-rays that take the form of either external radiation beams directed at a tumor or internal radiation via implantation of radioactive seeds, wires, catheters, or injection.

Rales Crackles; popping, bubbling, or high-pitched crackling sounds that occur from air passing through pockets of pulmonary fluids and alveoli.

Reasonable suspicion Suspicion of child abuse based on visual evidence or "gut feelings," "bells going off," or "being uncomfortable" by the child's emotional and physical presentation.

Reflux Regurgitation of gastric contents into the esophagus due to the incompetence or relaxation of the lower esophageal sphincter.

Religion The practice of one's spiritual beliefs.

Respiratory distress Difficulty in breathing.

Respiratory syncytial virus (RSV) A pathogen that causes mild, flu-like symptoms in most people.

Retinoblastoma A rare tumor of the retina.

Retinopathy of prematurity A disorder in which the blood vessels in the retina develop abnormally, potentially leading to blindness.

Retractions Pulling of the muscles between the ribs inward during breathing.

Rhonchi Rattling breath sounds that resemble snoring.

SBAR protocol A mnemonic that represents a series of steps to organize one's thinking prior to communicating; it stands for Situation, Background, Assessment, and Recommendation.

Scalp veins An option for peripheral intravenous access that may be used infants.

School nursing Consultation and hands-on care for children in academic settings.

Scoliosis A lateral curvature of the spine with no known etiology that is typically identified during the rapid growth period of adolescence, but in some instances manifests earlier and may be present from birth.

Scope of practice The limits of nurses' legal, ethical, and moral practice boundaries.

Secondary sex characteristics Pubertal changes triggered by the secretion of estrogen and testosterone: pubic hair, underarm hair, breast development, facial hair and voice changes in males, increased production of skin oils, and distribution of fat.

Secondary skin lesion A change in skin integrity that evolves from poor healing due to picking, scratching, or infection of a primary lesion.

Seizure disorder A disorder in which a wave of abnormal and excessive electrical activity in the brain causes changes in motor movements, levels of awareness, and behavior.

Sensory integration The process of managing and translating sensory inputs obtained through vestibular, proprioception, tactile, auditory, and visual senses.

Sensory perception The use and experience of the sensory organs across the developmental period.

Sensory processing The process of translating all incoming sensory stimulation in a meaningful way.

Sexual latency In Freud's theory, the school-age child's minimal attention to bodily details and greater attention on activities, hobbies, socialization, and schoolwork.

Shame and doubt In Erikson's psychosocial development theory, self-questioning about one's ability to handle problems.

Sleep disturbances Conditions that impair the ability to sleep well on a regular basis.

Slipped capital femoral epiphysis An injury in which the upper section of the femoral epiphysis slips from its normal position, leading to an acute and painful slip of the femoral head at the site of the femoral head's epiphyseal growth plate.

Special needs Disabilities in medical, psychological, or mental functioning that affect a child's development, such as developmentally disabled or medically fragile children.

Specialists Healthcare professionals with extensive knowledge in a particular area.

Spina bifida A weakened area or gap in the bony spinal column, which allows for protrusion of the meninges and cerebral spinal fluid sac (meningocele) or protrusion of the meninges, cerebrospinal fluid, and a portion of the spinal cord nerve roots (myelomeningocele).

Spirituality A broad concept encompassing how an individual views situations and experiences a sense of well-being and internal peace.

Stabilization Achievement of homeostasis.

Stem cell A cell that may proliferate to form the various types of new cells that are needed by the body: either the myeloid cell line or the lymphoid cell line.

Stress A physiological reaction that occurs when the challenges experienced exceed one's ability to control and manage the environment.

Stressors Stimuli that create stress, such as factors related to daily life, marital relationships, childrearing and disciplinary issues, health issues, elder care, and finances.

Stridor High-pitched, grating breath sounds.

Subdural hematoma A slower venous bleed leading to a clot below the dura mater but outside of brain tissue.

Suicidal ideation Preoccupation with suicide.

Suicide attempt An unsuccessful attempt to commit suicide, in which the person survives.

Suicide gesture An attempt at self-harm that is suggestive of suicide, but in which the person does not intend to die.

Surfactant A phospholipid that keeps the alveoli open and able to provide adequate gas exchange through a membrane.

Symbolic functioning A type of play engaged in by preschoolers, in which the child takes an item and turns it into an object of the child's reality.

Syringe pump A type of small infusion pump system that holds syringes rather than intravenous fluid bags.

Tanner stages An illustration of the maturity phases of adolescents, which include pubic hair growth and distribution, breast changes during puberty, and penile enlargement.

Temperament The dominant disposition of an individual; an aspect of personality.

Therapeutic relationship A positive alliance between healthcare providers and patients/families that is based on trust, respect, sensitivity, helpfulness, and emotional/spiritual support, which improve motivation and promote empowerment.

Tonsillitis Inflammation of the tonsils, which can be bacterial or viral in origin.

Tooth caries Breakdown of the teeth because of bacterial actions.

Tort A wrongful act that produces harm to a patient, whether that harm was intentional or unintentional.

Transfer Movement of a pediatric patient from one unit to another—for example, from the emergency department to the pediatric intensive care unit to the pediatric unit.

Trieste Charter A list of rights of the dying child within the United Nations' declaration of the rights of the child.

Tumor burden The number of cancer cells, the tumor size, or the amount of cancer in the body.

Ulcerative colitis Inflammation of the colonic mucosa.

Uremia Buildup of urea and other waste products in the body.

Urticaria Hives.

Vaccination Administration of weakened or dead pathogens; the vaccine is intended to provoke the production of antibodies that confer immunity against the full-blown disease.

Vaso-occlusive episode An event caused by the presence of abnormal sickle S hemoglobin in sickle cell disease; in the resulting vaso-occlusive state, the child experiences both chronic pain and acute peaks of pain, significant hemolytic anemia, and buildup of cellular waste products in the spleen.

Venous access Insertion of a needle into a vein.

Ventilation The process of breathing air into and out of the lungs.

Vesicle A raised lesion filled with clear fluid that is less than 1 cm in diameter.

Viruses Noncellular organisms composed of a protein capsule surrounding genetic material that can cause illness by taking over a human cell and reproducing themselves.

Vomiting The forceful expulsion of gastric contents through the mouth.

Well-child visits Routine healthcare visits that include a recent health history, complete physical examination, plotting of measurements on a standardized growth chart, immunizations as indicated, and a discussion of wellness topics and anticipatory guidance.

Index

Note: Page numbers followed by *b*, *f*, or *t* indicate entries in boxes, figures, or tables, respectively.